CANADIAN NURSING
ISSUES AND PERSPECTIVES

THIRD EDITION

CANADIAN NURSING
ISSUES AND PERSPECTIVES

JANET ROSS KERR, RN, PhD
Professor, Faculty of Nursing
University of Alberta
Edmonton, Alberta

JANNETTA MacPHAIL, MSN, PHD, FAAN, LLD (Hon)
Professor Emeritus, Faculty of Nursing
University of Alberta
Edmonton, Alberta

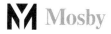 Mosby

St. Louis Baltimore Boston Carlsbad Chicago Naples New York Philadelphia Portland
London Madrid Mexico City Singapore Sydney Tokyo Toronto Wiesbaden

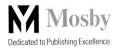

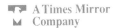

Vice President and Publisher: Nancy L. Coon
Executive Editor: N. Darlene Como
Project Manager: Mark Spann
Production Editor: Holly Roseman
Electronic Production Coordinator: Terri Bovay
Designer: David Zielinski

THIRD EDITION
Copyright © 1996 by Mosby–Year Book, Inc.

Previous editions copyrighted 1988, 1991

Printed in the United States of America
Composition by Mosby Electronic Production
Printing/binding by R.R. Donnelley

Mosby–Year Book, Inc.
11830 Westline Industrial Drive
St. Louis, Missouri 63146

♲ Printed on recycled paper.

International Standard Book Number 0-8151-5225-6

96 97 98 99 00 / 9 8 7 6 5 4 3 2 1

To the University of Alberta nursing students whose enthusiasm and desire for knowledge about professional issues and trends in nursing inspired us to write this book. Also, to nursing educators who value the histroy and philosophy of the profession and who have helped make opportunities available for students to study nursing issues and trends at the undergraduate and graduate levels.

Preface

I t is sometimes difficult to see progress and feel a sense of pride or satisfaction with the events in a profession when you are in the middle of the action. Every nurse is a part of that action because each one of us contributes in a unique way to the development of the profession. There are matters of critical and fundamental importance to the provision of nusing that require careful attention in the health-care reform movement now sweeping the country. Although things may not always appear to be positive to individual nurses and to the profession, and although progress often seems to be slow and uneven, the pursuit of our goals is important to us, and in working for them individually and collectively, we can and do make a difference in the course of events over time. Nurses have been known both for their altruism and high standards of practice. The integrity of the individuals and the profession itself has been seen in the quality of the service provided and in the vigilance of the profession in ensuring that the recognized standards are upheld.

The publication of three editions of our book within the relatively brief span of 7 years has allowed us to identify and evaluate developments in the profession and has given us the opportunity to measure the extent of progress over this period. Despite the fact that we would want things to move faster in some areas, it is evident that there has been steady and measurable progress in a relatively short period. Movement toward the entry to practice goal of the profession has been considerable in some areas of the country, and the realization of five doctoral programs in nursing since January 1991 has been a remarkable achievement within this period of time. Nurses are asserting their needs and are using political skills and labour relations processes to their advantage. Our issues are being taken more seriously by politicians, employers, and institutions. In some cases, governments have literally been brought to their knees by the voices of nurses.

Disruptions to the nursing workforce in the face of health-care reform have had negative repercussions for individuals and groups of nurses. Some have been able to turn adversity into advantage while others have had more difficulty in doing so when demand for certain types of services has changed. It is clear that the health system of the future will look substantially different from that of the past and that nursing roles are in transition. It is clear to the authors that, despite the complexity of the issues and the difficult problems presented by the changing nature of practice, the profession of nursing will survive and will grow stronger in the process. These and other developments have been explored in the third edition.

The addition of a new chapter on nursing research utilization is complementary to the other chapters in the section on the development of nursing knowledge. As in previous editions, the historical basis of developments in nursing is a strong thrust thoughout and forms an integral part of each chapter. It is our belief that it is important to know and recognize the evolution of patterns of practice as well as the contributions of nurses over time. The attention to the way in which nursing has evolved throughout the book is complementary to the four chapters that are devoted to the history of nursing and nursing education.

The primary health-care movement in Canada is being nurtured and led by nurses, and there have been positive steps forward in this area. It is also evident that nursing research has been enhanced by the quality of work done by an increasing number of nurses with research preparation. The success of the two previous editions confirmed our view that there was a tangible need for a resource book on issues and trends in contemporary Canadian nursing. The intent has been to provide a resource for nursing students as well as all pracitising nurses, including those involved in direct care, educating nurses, doing research, and administering nursing systems. It is our hope that this book will inspire our colleagues to consider issues that will positively influence the health care of Canadians. The opportunity to step back and identify and evaluate what has happened has given us satisfaction and pleasure. It is our hope that readers will be able to share with us a renewed appreciation of the accomplishments of nurses and the rewards of being involved in professional developments.

Janet Ross Kerr
Jannetta MacPhail

Acknowledgments

We are indebted to the following authors who contributed chapters to this book:

Marion N. Allen, RN, BN, MScN, MN, PhD
Professor
Faculty of Nursing, The University of Alberta
Edmonton, Alberta

Heather F. Clarke, RN, BNSc, MN, PhD
Nursing Research Consultant
Registered Nurses Association of British Columbia
Vancouver, British Columbia

Louise A. Jenson, RN, BScN, MN,PhD
Associate Professor
Faculty of Nursing, The University of Alberta
Edmonton, Alberta

Doreen Reid, RN, MEd
Research Assistant
Faculty of Nursing, The University of Alberta
Edmonton, Alberta

Eleanor Ross, RN, BScN, MScN
Chief of Nursing Practice, Women's College Hospital
Doctoral Candidate, University of Toronto, and
President, Canadian Nurses Association
Toronto, Ontario

Richard Splane, MA, MSW, PhD, LLD (hon)
Professor Emeritus, School of Social Work, University of
British Columbia, and Consultant in Social Policy, Splane Associates
Vancouver, British Columbia

Verna Huffman Splane, RN, MPH, LLD (hon)
Associate Professor (Associate Faculty), Faculty of Nursing, University of
Alberta, and Nursing Consultant (International Health Policy), Splane Associates
Vancouver, British Columbia

Contents

PART I   THE PROFESSION IN CANADA

 1   Early Nursing in Canada, 1600 to 1760: A Legacy for the Future, 3
 JANET ROSS KERR

 2   Nursing in Canada from 1760 to the Present: The Transition to Modern Nursing, 11
 JANET ROSS KERR

 3   Professionalization in Canadian Nursing, 23
 JANET ROSS KERR

 4   The Role of the Canadian Nurses Association in the Development of Nursing in Canada, 31
 JANNETTA MacPHAIL

 5   The Professional Image: Impact and Strategies for Change, 54
 JANNETTA MacPHAIL

 6   Nursing and Feminism, 67
 JANET ROSS KERR

 7   Men in Nursing, 74
 JANNETTA MacPHAIL

PART II   NURSING KNOWLEDGE

 8   Knowledge Development in Nursing, 85
 MARION N. ALLEN AND LOUISE A. JENSEN

 9   Theory Testing and Theory Building: Research in Nursing, 105
 HEATHER F. CLARKE

10   Research-Mindedness in the Profession, 118
 JANNETTA MacPHAIL

11   The Financing of Nursing Research in Canada, 135
 JANET ROSS KERR

12   Scope of Research in Nursing Practice, 146
 JANNETTA MacPHAIL

13   Utilizing Research Findings in Practice: Issues and Strategies, 162
 HEATHER F. CLARKE

PART III   NURSING CARE DELIVERY

14   Quality of Care: Where Have We Come From—Where Are We Going?, 182
 JANET ROSS KERR AND DOREEN REID

15   From Shortage to Oversupply: The Nursing Work Force Pendulum, 196
 ELEANOR ROSS

16   Political Awareness in Nursing, 208
 JANET ROSS KERR

17 The Organization and Financing of Health Care: Issues for Nursing, 216
JANET ROSS KERR

18 Organizing for Nursing Care: Primary Nursing, Traditional Approaches, or Both?, 228
JANNETTA MacPHAIL

19 The Practising Nurse and the Law, 241
JANET ROSS KERR

20 Ethical Issues and Dilemmas in Nursing Practice, 251
JANNETTA MacPHAIL

21 Emergence of Nursing Unions as a Social Force in Canada, 268
JANET ROSS KERR

22 Unionism and Professionalism: Conflicting or Compatible Processes, 282
JANET ROSS KERR

PART IV   EDUCATING NURSES FOR THE FUTURE

23 The Origins of Nursing Education in Canada: An Overview of the Emergence and Growth of Diploma Programs: 1874 to 1974, 291
JANET ROSS KERR

24 A Historical Approach to the Evolution of University Nursing Education in Canada: 1919 to 1974, 306
JANET ROSS KERR

25 Entry to Practice: Striving for the Baccalaureate Standard, 321
JANET ROSS KERR

26 Collaboration Between Nursing Education and Nursing Practice for Quality Nursing Care, Education, and Research, 334
JANNETTA MacPHAIL

27 Monitoring Standards in Nursing Education, 350
JANNETTA MacPHAIL

28 Credentialing in Nursing, 363
JANET ROSS KERR

29 Developing Specialty Certificate Programs with Credit toward the Baccalaureate Degree in Nursing, 373
JANET ROSS KERR

30 Distance Education in Nursing: Increasing Accessibility of Degree Programs, 381
JANET ROSS KERR

31 Primary Health Care: The Means for Reaching Nursing's Potential in Achieving Health for All, 390
JANNETTA MacPHAIL

32 The Growth of Graduate Education in Nursing in Canada, 407
JANET ROSS KERR

PART V   THE VIEW BEYOND

33 International Nursing: Looking Beyond Our Borders, 427
RICHARD SPLANE AND VERNA HUFFMAN SPLANE

34 Looking Ahead, 441
JANNETTA MacPHAIL AND JANET ROSS KERR

PART I

The Profession
in Canada

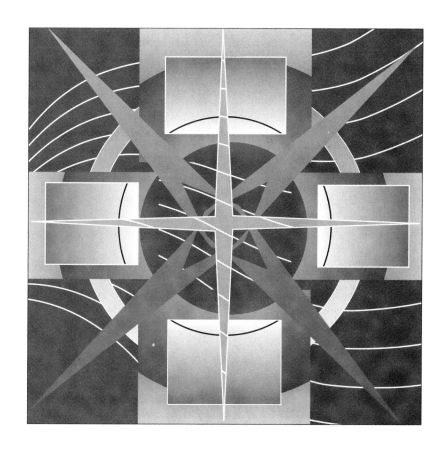

Early Nursing in Canada, 1600 to 1760: A Legacy for the Future

JANET ROSS KERR

As a result of Jacques Cartier's numerous voyages across the Atlantic, including his 1535 landing on Newfoundland, France laid claim to the vast area along the St. Lawrence River that was later to become Canada. Exploration and establishment of the first French settlement in the new land occurred over the next century. Samuel de Champlain, who made his first voyage to the new territory in 1603, was well qualified for his prominent role as explorer and leader, for he had already attained the rank of royal geographer in France before setting off for New France (Repplier, 1931). In 1608 he selected Quebec as the site for a colony of settlers because this sheltered and beautiful spot would serve as an ideal trading centre for the growing fur trade.

The story of the early colonization of New France parallels the development of nursing because the establishment of hospitals and a health-care system preceded the general settlement of the colony. The development of health care in the new land was considered to be of prime importance in the civilization of the colony. At the outset, and for many years thereafter, human services, including health care, education, and social welfare, focused on the indigenous peoples—the numerous Indian tribes populating the region. Spurred by religious fervour and zeal, nuns and priests made great efforts to befriend and subsequently convert natives to Christianity. These and other early settlers endured considerable hardship and were subject to hazardous living conditions in the early years. These first colonists in the new land had to provide their own health care, as had the native peoples before them. The first physician-surgeons in this part of New France were:

> Jehan de Brouet, who sailed up the St. Lawrence to Tadoussac in A.D. 1600 as surgeon of Chauvin's fleet; one Bonnerme, who, in 1608 accompanied Champlain to Quebec and thus became its first surgeon, but who died the following year from either scurvy or dysentery (Abbott, 1931, p. 15).

■ ■ ■ ■

THE FIRST NURSES IN NEW FRANCE

The legacy of the first nurses in New France has received considerable attention as a result of their courage, sacrifice, altruism, and skill. It should be noted, though, that the several thousand Indians living in the region before the immigration of French colonists, had developed a system of health care characterized by numerous herbal remedies for particular ailments. The concept of nurse in the new and struggling colony was somewhat different from that of today. The first nurses to tend the sick were male attendants at a "sick bay" established at the French garrison in Port Royal in Acadia in 1629 (Gibbon and Mathewson, 1947). In addition, the Jesuit priests who were missionary immigrants to New France, found themselves caring for the sick in the course of their primary mission, the conversion of the natives to Christianity. "The Jesuits singly or in pairs travelled in the depth of winter from village to village, ministering to the sick and seeking to commend their religious teachings by their efforts to relieve bodily distress" (Parkman, 1897, p. 176).

Marie Rollet Hébert

The first lay woman who regularly cared for the sick, both in her home and in other homes in the community, was Marie Rollet, married to the surgeon-apothecary, Louis Hébert. The Hébert family emigrated to Quebec in 1617 at the request of Champlain. Louis Hébert had previous experience in the New World, having made journeys to île St. Croix in 1604 to 1605 and to Port Royal in 1606 to 1607 and 1610 to 1613. On his fourth journey, he embarked from Honfleur in 1617 accompanied by Mme Hébert and their three children. Mme Marie Hébert thus became the first woman to emigrate from France to the new colony in what was to become Canada (Brown, 1966). In Quebec Louis Hébert's "apothecary skill and his small store of grain were a godsend to the sick and starving winterers. In spite of the company's demands on his and his servant's time, he succeeded in clearing and planting some land" (Brown, 1966, p. 368).

"Marie Rollet aided her husband in caring for the sick and shared his interest in the savages" (Brown, 1966, p. 578). This was quite natural, as it was common practice for French wives of the early seventeenth century to collaborate with their husbands in their work. Of special attention was Mme Hébert's genuine concern for the indigenous people as intelligent human beings. The efforts of Mme Hébert and her husband, to care for the natives and share health knowledge with them, appear to have been welcomed and appreciated (Thwaites, 1959).

A Call for Nurses

The people of France learned about the new colony through the *Jesuit Relations,* informative reports written regularly by the Jesuit missionary priests to spread word about colonial life and to stimulate needed support. These were written over a 72-year period and provide a marvellous account of life in early Canada. "It was clear to the fathers that their ministrations were valued solely because their religion was supposed by many to be a 'medicine' or charm, efficacious against disease and death" (Parkman, 1897, p. 179). Thus they sent urgent requests for nurses to come to the colony to assist with their work. In 1634 Father LeJeune wrote in his *Relation*:

> If we had a hospital here, all the sick people of the country, and all the old people, would be there. As to the men, we will take care of them according to our means; but, in regard to the women, it is not becoming for us to receive them into our houses (Kenton, 1925, p. 49).

Evidently questions of propriety, an important part of the culture of the times, made it a problem for the Jesuit priests on missionary premises to treat native women who were ill. This presented another pressing reason for female members of a nursing order to come to Canada to assist with the work. It is somewhat curious to reflect on the fact that "Quebec, as we have seen, had a seminary, a hospital, and a convent, before it had a population" (Parkman, 1897, p. 259).

Hospitalières De La Miséricorde De Jésus

The Duchesse d'Aiguillon, a niece of Cardinal Richelieu, read and was moved by the *Relations* and developed a plan to build the Hôtel Dieu at Québec. She used her influence to obtain a grant of land and arranged for the careful selection of three nuns of the Hospitalières de la Miséricorde de Jésus to go to Canada to establish the hospital. The three nuns, who all came from good families, were Marie Guenet de St. Ignace (later Mère de St. Ignace), Anne Lecointre de St. Bernard, and Marie Forestier de St. Bonaventure de Jésus. Aboard ship at Dieppe the "hospital nuns" encountered three Ursuline nuns, whose mission was to teach the natives, and Madame de la Peltrie, who intended to help establish a convent school for the native children. The voyage was perilous, lasting from May to August 1639 (Juchereau & Duplessis, 1939), and upon their arrival the women began work immediately.

> The Hospital Nuns arrived at Kebec on the first day of August of last year. Scarcely had they disembarked before they found themselves overwhelmed with patients. The hall of the hospital being too small, it was necessary to erect some cabins, fashioned like those of the savages, in their garden. Not having furniture for so many people, they had to cut in two or three pieces part of the blankets and sheets they had brought for these poor sick people (Kenton, 1925, p. 157).

As there was no time to make any preparations, the nuns had to throw themselves into their work from the first day.

> . . . instead of taking a little rest and refreshing themselves after the great discomforts they had suffered upon the sea, they found themselves so burdened and occupied that we had fear of losing them and their hospital at its very birth. The sick came from all directions in such numbers, their stench was so insupportable, the heat so great, the fresh food so scarce and so poor, in a country so new and strange, that I do not know how these good sisters, who almost had not even leisure in which to take a little sleep, endured all these hardships (Kenton, 1925, p. 157).

The smallpox epidemic, which was raging on the sisters' arrival and for a considerable length of time thereafter, also required the labours of the Ursuline nuns, whose school convent became a hospital, "and they found themselves nursing instead of teaching" (Millman, 1965, p. 424). Jamieson commented on the fact that the Ursulines used native Indian women for assistance in their hospitals, and that "their teacher training was instrumental in providing the earliest instruction and supervision of nurses in America" (Jamieson, Sewall, and Gjertson, 1959, p. 196).

New recruits from Dieppe were sought, and the first two arrived the following summer. The nuns also moved their base of operations to Sillery, a settlement outside Quebec, in a more convenient location for the Indians. The structure in which they had spent the first winter had proved woefully inadequate to withstand the winter elements, and a new building was constructed in Sillery. Soon the hospital was inundated with Indian patients, and many had to be cared for in adjacent cabins. With considerable regret, the nuns had to abandon their white habits for a more serviceable brown. The sisters also applied themselves to learning the language of the Hurons and Algonquins, for whom they cared (Gibbon and Mathewson, 1947).

In 1644 Governor De Montmagny implored the sisters to return to the safety of Quebec, because the Iroquois were reported to be on the warpath, and the sisters would be in danger by staying in Sillery. They returned and were lodged in temporary quarters while a new hospital was constructed. The latter was not completed until 2 years later, and during the smallpox epidemic of 1650, the number of patients received was so great that they could not all be accommodated in the hospital. The sisters also considered it their duty to assist new settling families in Quebec as much as they could. The archives of the Hôtel Dieu of Quebec contain a letter from Vincent de Paul written in April, 1652. "I consider this enterprise as one of the greatest accomplished within fifteen hundred years" (Gibbon and Mathewson, 1947, p. 15).

Another addition to their hospital, begun in 1654, was completed 4 years later. A series of epidemics started in the year after the addition's completion, beginning with typhus and followed by smallpox. This was to be a series of epidemics that had started with the sisters' arrival in 1639 and would continue over the years. Danger from the Iroquois Indians was a serious concern at some periods. Because of this danger, for 3 weeks in 1660, the Governor ordered that only three or four sisters should stay overnight in their hospital convent and the rest would stay in the safer Jesuit monastery. By 1671 the nuns were obtaining sufficient local recruits to the order and no longer depended on assistance from France.

In 1690 hostilities broke out once more between the British and the French, and the sisters of the Hôtel Dieu de Québec found themselves in the middle of the conflict. It is reported that 26 cannonballs hit the hospital on one day of heavy fighting. The siege was over in 4 days, and the British withdrew. Epidemics followed from time to time, but the worst appears to have been a smallpox epidemic in 1703, when more than a quarter of the nuns died.

> Our sisters fell ill in such numbers from the very first that there were not enough of those who were well to look after the infected cases in our rooms and wards. We accepted the offer of service from several good widows (Gibbon and Mathewson, 1947, p. 35).

Jeanne Mance

La Société de Notre Dame de Jésus was composed of a group of philan-thropists who wanted to establish a colony of a religious character to work with the Indians on the Island of Montreal. This was no easy matter because they had to secure the charter for the land and raise sufficient funds to send a carefully selected group of people to create the society they had in mind. They thought, however, the hospital might be begun at once. Jeanne Mance had read the *Jesuit Relations* regularly and believed she had been called to serve in the New World. Through the wealth of Mme de Bullion, Jeanne Mance was asked to take charge of building a hospital in the settlement that was to be established at Montreal. Thus she sailed from La Rochelle, along with 3 women and 40 men, under the leadership of Paul de Chomédy, Sieur de Maisonneuve (Canadian Nurses Association [CNA], 1968). Their two ships arrived in Quebec, but their reception was not a welcoming one. They

> . . . arrived too late in the season to ascend to Montreal before winter. They encoun-tered distrust, jealousy, and opposition. The agents of the Company of the Hundred Associates looked on them askance; and the Governor of Quebec, Montmagny, saw a rival governor in Maisonneuve. Every means was used to persuade the adventurers to abandon their project, and settle at Quebec (Parkman, 1897, p. 296).

Steadfast in his resolve to accomplish the mission to establish a settlement at Montreal, Maisonneuve "expressed his surprise that they should assume to direct his affairs. 'I have not come here,' he said, 'to deliberate, but to act. It is my duty and my honour to found a colony at Montreal; and I would go, if every tree were an Iroquois!'" (Parkman, 1897, pp. 296-297). The group had difficulty find-ing housing for the winter, but through the generosity of one colonist, they were housed at St. Michel. Jeanne Mance found that her neighbours were the hospital nuns who lived in their mission at Sillery, not far from Quebec. Here Jeanne Mance spent a good deal of her time assisting in the work of the hospital, and this undoubtedly served her well as she ventured to Montreal as the only person with health-care knowledge.

When on May 17, 1642, Maisonneuve and his followers landed at Montreal, the Associates of Montreal took possession of the land that "Champlain, thirty-one years before, had chosen as the fit site of a settlement" (Parkman, 1897, p. 302). They gave thanks, then proceeded to establish their settlement. The hospi-tal was one of the first buildings constructed in the colony, although there were apparently some misgivings.

> It is true that the hospital was not wanted as no one was sick at Ville Marie and one or two chambers would have sufficed for every prospective necessity; but it will be remembered that the colony had been established in order that a hospital might be built . . . Instead then of tilling the land to supply their own pressing needs, all labour-ers of the settlement were set at this pious though superfluous task (Parkman, 1897, p. 362).

The hospital was 46 m × 18.5 m and contained a kitchen, living quarters for Jeanne Mance and for the servants, and two large areas for the patients. "It was amply provided with furniture, linen, medicine and all necessaries and had two oxen, three cows and 20 sheep. A small oratory of stone was built adjoining it" (Parkman, 1897, pp. 362-363). A palisade was constructed around it because of considerable danger of Iroquois attacks. " . . . here Mlle Mance took up her abode and waited the day when wounds or disease should bring patients to her empty wards" (Parkman, 1897, p. 363). All of the new settlers were committed to the objective of converting the Indians to Christianity and sought to gain their favour in whatever way they could. "If they could persuade them to be nursed, they were consigned to the tender care of Mlle Mance" (Parkman, 1897, p. 364). A year after its founding, Montreal became the target of the Iroquois, and Jeanne Mance had

> . . . her hands full attending to men wounded by their arrows. She dressed wounds of all kinds. Chilblains and frost-bite frequently required her attention. According to the Clerk of the Court, she had mortar, scales, a syringe with ivory tube, razors and lances. She had sufficient skill to compound her own medicines, and also had experience in blood letting (Gibbon and Mathewson, 1947, pp. 25-26).

As she was soon in need of more help than the one young girl who had come with her, she enlisted the assistance of two others to cope with the patient load. Jeanne Mance made three trips back to France, one 4 years after her arrival, one in 1657, and one in 1663. All of these trips were made primarily for the purpose of meeting with members of the Associates of Notre Dame of Montreal and other benefactors to generate resources for her hospital. She managed to arrange for assistance from a nursing order in France in 1659. Thus three nuns of St. Joseph de la Flèche arrived to assist in nursing the sick in her hospital, of which she remained the administrator. By 1663 the Associates were bankrupt and could no longer continue their assistance to the colony and the hospital. They transferred their interests to the Gentlemen of Saint Sulpice, and Jeanne Mance witnessed the transfer of ownership to this group. When she died in 1673, she was "universally respected and beloved by the Colony which she had helped to found" (Gibbon and Mathewson, 1947, p. 30).

The Grey Nuns of Montreal

The Grey Nuns of Montreal were considered the first visiting nurses in Canada. This uniquely Canadian order of nuns was formed in 1738 by Marguerite d'Youville, a widow who was a niece of the explorer, La Vérendrye. Les Soeurs Grises were also the first noncloistered order to be established in Canada, patterned after the model initiated by St. Vincent de Paul. Madame d'Youville organized this group of women with charitable intentions, and they "agreed to combine their possessions in a house of refuge chiefly for the poor, taking the names of Soeurs Grises or Grey Nuns" (Gibbon and Mathewson, 1947, p. 45).

Life was by no means easy for them because they had to raise funds to subsist and carry on their work with the sick and the poor. For the purpose of raising money, wealthy paying guests were taken in, and the sisters did handiwork that they sold. Because the order was not cloistered, and because it took up the nursing of patients in their homes, something not previously done in Canada, there was originally some mistrust of its work and intentions. "Though they usually did their visiting in pairs for self-protection, the Grey Nuns were innovators and subject to misunderstanding" (Gibbon and Mathewson, 1947, p. 46). It is important to recognize that the other orders of nuns working in Canada, the Augustinians in Quebec and the St. Joseph's Hospitallers of Montreal, were cloistered and were not permitted to venture into the community except in an emergency by special permission of the Bishop.

A fire in 1745 destroyed their house, and the Grey Nuns were forced to move from one place to another for the next 2 years to carry on their work. Then the Gentlemen of Saint Sulpice gave permission for Madame d'Youville and the Grey Nuns to take over the General Hospital under a charter as the Soeurs de la Charité de l'Hôspital Général de Montréal. Their debts were so great that they had to resort to all sorts of new fund-raising activities, including making military garments and tents, establishing a brewery and a tobacco plant, and operating a freight and cartage business. Patients who regained health as a result of the nuns' charitable efforts were put to work to aid in the fund-raising effort (Gibbon and Mathewson, 1947, p. 47).

When war broke out between the British and the French in 1756, a section of the hospital called the Ward of the English was opened to care for the wounded English soldiers. The sisters were sufficiently generous of spirit to provide refuge to escaped English soldiers fleeing from the Indians. " . . . one of these English showed his gratitude, in 1760, by saving the hospital from the artillery fire of the army of invasion" (Gibbon and Mathewson, 1947, p. 48). In 1760 the transfer of authority over Montreal to the British brought with it statements testifying to the respect in which the sisters were held. General Amherst stated:

> Of the goodwill I have to a Society so worthy of respect as that of the Monastery of St. Joseph de l'Hôtel Dieu de Montréal, which can count so far as the British Nation is concerned on the same protection that it has enjoyed under French rule (Gibbon and Mathewson, 1947, p. 48).

Although French nursing orders extended invitations of welcome to the Canadian sisters after the war, and a Canadian philanthropist offered to pay all expenses of the voyage, only two sisters accepted the offer. Most were thoroughly Canadian by now and did not wish to leave. However, abject poverty ensued after the war when communication became difficult with the wealthy citizens in France who had provided donations during the war. The sisters remaining in Canada became dependent on charity for some time.

■■ ■■ ■■ ■■

THE STATUS OF NURSING IN CANADA IN THE SEVENTEENTH AND EIGHTEENTH CENTURIES

There was a marked contrast between Canada and Britain in the status of nursing and the quality of care provided in the seventeenth and eighteenth centuries. Nursing in Britain had fallen into disrepute after Henry VIII's renunciation of the Catholic Church. The nursing orders of nuns, which had previously provided the nursing service in the large London hospitals, were expelled and replaced by those of Charles Dickens' "Sairey Gamp" ilk. Gibbon and Mathewson (1947) recount a number of descriptions of such nurses in England, noting the negative effects on hospitals of incompetent staff more concerned about personal pleasure than the welfare of patients.

These conditions did not occur to any great extent in early Canada because of the historical fact that the first settlement at Quebec developed as a colony of France. In France, nursing did not undergo the regressive period that occurred in England. Young women of good character, who came from reputable families, were recruited to nursing in France—primarily under the auspices of the Catholic Church—throughout this period of time.

> If the settlements along the St. Lawrence River had been colonized in the seventeenth century by the English instead of by the French, the history of nursing in Canada might have been very different. Fate, however, decided in favour of the French, and that was fortunate both for the Huron and Algonquin Indians and for the white pioneers, since in the wake of the fur traders and coureurs de bois, came the Augustinian Hospitallers or Nursing Sisters of Dieppe to Quebec and the St. Joseph Hospitallers of La Flèche to Montreal on their missions of healing and of mercy—missions which had no counterpart in the colonizing efforts of the Protestant English in North America (Gibbon & Mathewson, 1947, p. 1).

The health-care system was firmly established and in operation when the English defeated the French in the battle of the Plains of Abraham in 1759. Undoubtedly, geographic separation from England ensured the continuation of the French traditions of good nursing in Canada.

Voluntarism, philanthropy, and a concern for others figured prominently in the values of both lay and religious French citizens who came to New France to provide health and social services. As such, the new society that developed over the next three and a half centuries was inherently Christian in its character, based on Roman Catholicism, and outwardly focused on the health, well-being, and religious life of the inhabitants of the new land. Such a heritage would prove to be an enduring strength that would persist through clashes with the aboriginal peoples and war with Britain and, later, with the Americans to the development of a new and independent Canada in the nineteenth and twentieth centuries.

REFERENCES

Abbott, M.E. (1931). *History of medicine in the province of Quebec.* Montreal: McGill University.

Brown, G. (Ed.). (1966). *Dictionary of Canadian biography: 1000 to 1700* (Vol. 1). Toronto: University of Toronto Press.

Canadian Nurses Association. (1968). *The leaf and the lamp.* Ottawa: Author.

Gibbon, J.M., and Mathewson M.S. (1947). *Three centuries of Canadian nursing.* Toronto: The Macmillan Co.

Jamieson, E., Sewall, M., and Gjertson, L. (1959). *Trends in nursing history.* Philadelphia: W.B. Saunders.

Juchereau, J-F., and Duplessis, M-A. (1939). *Les annales de l'Hôtel Dieu de Québec: 1636 - 1716.* Québec: l'Hôtel Dieu de Québec.

Kenton, E. (1925). *The Jesuit relations and allied documents.* New York: The Vanguard Press.

Millman, M.B. (1965). In G. Griffin and J. Griffin (Eds.), *Jensen's history and trends of professional nursing* (pp. 423-439). St. Louis: The C.V. Mosby Co.

Parkman, F. (1897). *The Jesuits in North America in the seventeenth century.* Boston: Little, Brown & Co.

Repplier, A. (1931). *Mère Marie of the Ursulines.* New York: Sheed & Ward.

Thwaites, R.G. (1959). *The Jesuit relations and allied documents: Travels and explorations of the Jesuit missionaries in New France* (Vols. I to XII). New York: Pageant Book Co.

CHAPTER TWO

Nursing in Canada from 1760 to the Present: The Transition to Modern Nursing

JANET ROSS KERR

After the war of 1756-1763, the transition to British rule was difficult for the nursing orders, which were now firmly established in Quebec. The nuns received little or no financial support because their wealthy benefactors had returned to France, and donations from previous supporters of health services in the New World were cut off. Without a regular income the nuns were impoverished at the outset of the new regime. However, in correspondence with the Duchesse d'Aiguillon, William Pitt, Prime Minister of Great Britain, stated that the commanding general of the British troops had "the satisfaction to be able to state that our officers, who are very strong in their praises of the charitable care of our sick and wounded by these nuns, have paid them every attention required by piety and misfortune" (Gibbon and Mathewson, 1947, p. 52). In addition, there is a record of some financial assistance from the British for the sisters. "By instruction of Pitt, General Murray relieved the Hôtel Dieu of a debt of taxes to the extent of 3,389 livres, which had reverted to the British at the change of the regime, and also paid £808 for rent of lodgings to the troops, and £3,085 for the use of furniture, laundry and utensils of the hospital" (Gibbon and Mathewson, 1947, pp. 52-53). Nevertheless, all of the hospital systems remained in place at the transfer of power; the nuns were thoroughly Canadian by this time and most had no desire to return to France.

From 1775 to 1776, during the American War of Independence, the American attack on the Canadian border brought patients from each side of the battle to the Hôtel Dieu, where all were cared for with warmth and humanity. An American lieutenant recorded the following in his diary on March 10, 1776:

> Was removed to the Hotel Dieu, sick of the scarlet fever, and placed under the care of the Mother Abbess, where I had fresh provisions and good attendance. For several nights the nuns sat up with me, four at a time, every two hours. Here I feigned myself sick after I had recovered, for fear of being sent back to the Seminary to join

my fellow-officers, and was not discharged until I acknowledged that I was well. When I think of my captivity, I shall never forget the time spent among the nuns who treated me with so much humanity (Gibbon and Mathewson, 1947, p. 55).

Among other hospitals that also cared for the sick and wounded were the Hôtel Dieu at Trois Rivières, which had been established in 1697. In 1778 another hospital, L'Hôtel des Invalides, was built at Sorel, and in 1781 La Samaritaine was opened across the Richelieu River. The tradition of caring for all, regardless of race, nationality, or creed, stayed with these nursing sisters from the beginning of their tenure in Canada in the seventeenth century. Preservation of human life and nourishment of the spirit through religious beliefs and practices remained central characteristics of their work.

■■ ■■ ■■ ■■

EFFECTS OF IMMIGRATION ON NURSING

After the defeat of the French forces at the Plains of Abraham, the Treaty of Paris of 1763 established certain rules for the government of the colony of Quebec. Its thrust was anglicisation in order to attract English-speaking settlers to help rebuild the shattered economy after the war. Although the British had imagined a flood of settlement would soon help anglicise Quebec, "in fact few people came" (Morton, 1983, p. 23). Soon the people of Quebec were recognized as Canadians, and the Quebec Act of 1774 restored many of their former freedoms and rights. The Act was also designed to win the support of these Canadians in the upcoming conflict with the Americans. With some difficulty, the British were able to hold Quebec in that conflict.

After the war, United Empire Loyalists, who wanted to remain loyal to Britain, immigrated to Canadian territory. Their numbers eventually totalled 50,000. These settlers were joined by large numbers of immigrants from Britain and Ireland. "Late Loyalists" followed during the early nineteenth century. There was also a sizeable increase in the French Canadian population, from 60,000 in 1760, to 110,000 by 1784, and 330,000 by 1860. The Act of 1791 divided Quebec into Upper and Lower Canada, each with its own system of government, and confirmed the rights for French colonists as laid down earlier in the Quebec Act.

The devastating effects of the Napoleonic wars on trade in England led many from the British Isles to emigrate to new areas where there might be some hope of overcoming poverty. "Factory folk, miners, and farmers became equally distressed, and the British Government could do little more than divert the resulting emigration to countries where the British flag still flew" (Gibbon and Mathewson, 1947, p. 71). This meant that a majority of these immigrants were poorly nourished and travelled in "vessels which were overcrowded and unsanitary," so disease found easy prey among the new settlers.

The United Empire Loyalists did not have to travel in disease-infested vehicles or under unsanitary conditions, and thus escaped the devastation that followed the voyages of the Europeans. Nevertheless, diseases brought by new arrivals spread rapidly among residents of the new colony. Dramatic increases in the population gave epidemic diseases more scope, and these epidemics seriously affected the colony. Immigrants and travellers brought with them cholera, typhus, smallpox, and trachoma. In 1832 an epidemic of cholera wiped out one seventh of the population of Montreal, or 4000 people (Gibbon and Mathewson, 1947). To protect the Canadian population, the necessity of health examinations for new immigrants was recognized, and a quarantine station and hospital were established at Grosse Isle in the St. Lawrence river.

The rapid increase in population in English-speaking Canada of the late eighteenth and early nineteenth centuries made it difficult to keep up with the need for health-care facilities. The persistent waves of epidemics, however, made them a necessity. The dismal state of nursing in Britain was parallelled in new areas of the country opened up by the English and not served by the French nursing orders. It is noted that "nursing in English-speaking Canada remained primitive for many years" (Canadian Nurses Association [CNA], 1968, p. 30). Lay women attempted to do nursing in the hospitals that were established, but they were largely without the proper training and skill to do what was needed. The established French-speaking sisterhoods expanded, and new English-speaking orders were formed to try to fill the need.

Because so many of the arriving settlers were destitute and ill, they needed a great deal of assistance. The Female Benevolent Society was organized in Montreal in 1816 and was responsible for the establishment of what would be called the Montreal General Hospital. In Kingston the Kingston Compassionate Society secured a grant of land from the government and constructed the first version of what would become the Kingston General Hospital. Likewise, in York the Toronto General Hospital was founded by a philanthropic group with funds designated to buy medals for the War of 1812 (Gibbon and Mathewson, 1947). The introduction of lay nurses in areas previously served by nursing sisterhoods met with some opposition at first, but the needs of the sick and the poor had to be met. Meanwhile, the Grey Nuns continued to visit the sick in their homes and "had accommodation for incurables and the insane" (Gibbon and Mathewson, 1947, p. 74).

■ ■ ■ ■

THE INFLUENCE OF FLORENCE NIGHTINGALE ON NURSING IN CANADA

In 1854 Florence Nightingale set off with her small band of 38 carefully selected nurses to tend the British soldiers in the Crimea. Up to that time, British military hospitals had been staffed exclusively by male attendants. It had not been easy to secure permission to nurse the sick and wounded military personnel during the Crimean War. However, Florence Nightingale came from a prominent and wealthy family and had many connections with powerful people. She managed not only to obtain permission to go to the Crimea but also to stir the British consciousness about the need for good nursing for the sick. "Her onslaught on the appalling lack of sanitation in the wards of the General and the Barrack hospitals at Scutari contributed greatly to the reduction in the deaths of cases treated from 315 per thousand to 22 per thousand" (Gibbon & Mathewson, 1947, pp. 109-110).

The outpouring of public support for Florence Nightingale's cause was overwhelming, and a fund was established, even before she returned from the Crimea, to allow her to organize a training school for nurses (Nutting & Dock, 1937). At last nursing was to become a suitable occupation for women.

> Mark what by breaking through customs and prejudices Miss Nightingale has effected for her sex. She has opened to them a new profession, a new sphere of usefulness . . . a claim for more extended freedom of action, based on proved public usefulness in the highest sense of the word (Gibbon and Mathewson, 1947, p. 110).

Florence Nightingale's influence was worldwide and reached Canada by way of both Britain and the United States when, during the American Civil War, there was an attempt to establish Nightingale's standard of nursing to minimize suffering. In 1873 training schools based on the Nightingale model were opened in three American hospitals: Bellevue in New York, Massachusetts General, and New Haven (Gibbon and Mathewson, 1947). Canadian hospitals, particularly the secular hospitals in English-speaking settlements, considered educating nurses to raise the standards of care, a direct result of Nightingale's influence. The establishment of schools of nursing is discussed in some detail in Chapter 23. However, it is important to recognize the profound influence that Florence Nightingale had on the initiation of an organized system of nursing education for lay nurses throughout the world.

■ ■ ■ ■

OPENING UP OF THE WEST AND THE GREY NUNS

On April 24, 1844, four nuns set out in long canoes bound for St. Boniface, Manitoba. The measure of courage required for the strenuous journey is difficult to appreciate in an age in which superhighways are commonplace. A description of the 2-month trip by one of these nursing pioneers, who had twisted her ankle en route, draws attention to the rigours involved.

> Most of the portages are frightful, above all those which are after the Great Lakes. One has to climb mountains, clamber over rocks, descend precipitous slopes, do four or five miles in the Savannas and by unblazed trails—you understand what I must suffer, being obliged to be carried over difficult roads (Gibbon and Mathewson, 1947, p. 86).

Beginning in 1846, the onslaught of a series of epidemics was the first big challenge facing the nuns after their arrival. These epidemics were extremely serious, and the death toll was high. Sister Laurent has described how they coped with the patient load:

> Each of us was appointed to do that which she was best fitted for. Some of us went into the houses where sick people were. They used to have measles and dysentery and inflammatory rheumatism, and smallpox sometimes. We had medicines from Montreal, but we also learned the uses of herbs that grew in this country, and how to help the sick people so as to ease their pain and aid them to get better (Gibbon and Mathewson, 1947, p. 89).

In Saskatchewan and Alberta the Grey Nuns were again the pioneers who trekked west to establish health-care facilities and systems for the populace. In

1860 three nuns of this order from St. Boniface arrived at île à la Crosse, an Indian settlement 200 miles north of Prince Albert. In 1881 the Grey Nuns established the first hospital in Alberta, located at the St. Albert Mission near Edmonton. Arriving before most of the settlers, the sisters established systems of quality health care that were available to people who needed assistance. The Grey Nuns performed a great deal of visiting nursing, regularly visiting the sick in their homes as they had since the founding of their order.

■ ■ ■ ■

ESTABLISHMENT OF NATIONAL PROFESSIONAL NURSING ORGANIZATIONS

A leading figure in British nursing was Mrs. Bedford Fenwick. Bedford Fenwick was influential in the formation of nursing organizations, and editor of the forerunner of the *British Journal of Nursing*. Attending the 1893 Congress of Charities, Corrections, and Philanthropy in Chicago, Mrs. Fenwick met the leaders in American nursing at the time: Isabel Hampton, Adelaide Nutting, and Lavinia Dock. It is of interest to note that, of these three American leaders, two were Canadians living and working in the United States—Isabel Hampton and Adelaide Nutting. They discussed the need for a concerted effort to secure legislation for the registration of nurses in order to raise the standard of professional nursing and to ensure that those practising were qualified and able.

Mrs. Fenwick had been struggling to achieve such legislation in Britain at the time and became convinced that, to have any hope of achieving their goals, nurses had to band together and form professional organizations. The three American leaders were so impressed with the case Mrs. Fenwick made for establishing organizations that they immediately organized the American Society of Superintendents of Training Schools for Nurses of the United States and Canada, of which Isabel Hampton became the first president. Although in 1912 this was to become the National League for Nursing, the major thrust of the organization never strayed from its original goal "to work for higher standards of nurse preparation" (CNA, 1968, p. 35).

Soon after the formation of the society, alumnae associations began at the large schools of nursing in the United States. In 1896, under the leadership of its first president, Isabel Hampton Robb, The Nurses' Associated Alumnae of the United States and Canada was formed. The criteria for membership for alumnae was that they must have graduated from a school associated with a hospital more than 100 beds in size, and the training program must have been at least 2 years long. The organization first directed its efforts at improving the quality of educational programs, but this proved to be too difficult for a voluntary organization. Instead, they directed their efforts toward working for legislation to ensure the registration of nurses. This organization was the forerunner of the American Nurses Association that began in 1911. The *American Journal of Nursing* began to publish in 1900 and provided a vehicle for information to assist with the development of the organization (CNA).

One of Mrs. Bedford Fenwick's major goals was the formation of an international organization of nurses. She had initiated discussions about such an organization with American nursing leaders in 1893 in Chicago. Because it was decided that the first step was the formation of national groups, these became a matter of priority. Although the North American organization had initially included both Canada and the United States, it was necessary to separate the organizations because of the concept of membership by country in an international organization. In addition, the responsibility for health was vested at provincial and state levels; thus the fight for registration of nurses was decentralized. A structure involving separate national organizations seemed more useful to pursue the goal of registering nurses. Accordingly, the International Council of Nurses (ICN) was formed in 1899 with Britain, the United States, and Germany as charter members. Canada was represented at this meeting by five nurses, and Mary Agnes Snively of Canada became the first honorary treasurer of the fledgling organization.

In Canada the Canadian Society of Superintendents of Training Schools for Nurses was the first completely Canadian national organization of nurses; it was formed in 1907 with Mary Agnes Snively as President. The next year the society invited representatives from all nursing organizations in Canada to meet and establish a national association of nurses. The result of the meeting was the inception of the Provisional Society of the Canadian National Association of Trained Nurses (CNATN), and Mary Agnes Snively was inducted as founding president. Initially, membership took place through member societies composed primarily of graduate nurse and alumnae associations. The first alumnae association in Canada had been founded in 1894 at the Toronto General Hospital (Gibbon and Mathewson, 1947). Nearly every school formed such an organization shortly thereafter, and many of these amalgamated with other groups regionally, and eventually provincially. The CNATN applied for membership in the ICN in 1908, and formal admission took place the next year at the international meeting in London.

Because the CNATN had been organized somewhat hastily for the purpose of joining the ICN, a structure that would be suitable for the national organization and would recognize the historical division of powers between the provincial and federal governments had yet to be considered. According to Mrs. E.G. Fournier, who studied the question for the CNATN:

> It should be the object of the national Association to organize the unorganized provinces, to strengthen the weak ones, to encourage the disheartened, bind all together, inform all of the nursing achievements, and suggest work to be taken up (CNA, 1968, p. 37).

A full-time executive secretary, Miss Jean Wilson, was appointed in 1923, and the first national office was opened in Winnipeg; later it was moved to Montreal and then to Ottawa. In the meantime, *The Canadian Nurse* had begun publication in 1905. Membership of affiliated organizations in the CNATN went from 28 in 1911 to 52 in 1924 when the association changed its name to the Canadian Nurses Association (CNA). In 1930 the organization became a federation of the provincial nurses associations that "made the provincial association the official representative of registered nurses in each province and automatically ensured that all members of the CNA were registered nurses" (CNA, 1968, p. 39).

The Provisional Council of the Canadian Association of University Schools and Departments of Nursing held its first meeting in 1942. Representatives from eight university schools and departments of nursing met to consider how university schools might respond to a proposed program of federal financial assistance for university schools of nursing (J. Bouchard, personal communication, 1987). The organization was a small one for a considerable period of time after its founding because of the small nursing population within its purview. The work of the organization was accomplished entirely on a volunteer basis until 1970, when a part-time executive secretary was hired for the first time. Also at that time the name of the organization became the Canadian Association of University Schools of Nursing (CAUSN). It was not until 1984 that the position of executive secretary became full-time.

An ongoing discrepancy in the way the organization collects fees to finance its operations has continued to be a problem. At the national level, fees are paid by member schools. At the regional level, Ontario and Quebec collect fees from institutions. But in the Atlantic provinces and in the West, individual faculty members of university schools of nursing pay fees on an individual and voluntary basis. The total fees collected tend to be rather small, and it is difficult to finance committee travel, projects, and other programs the organization might desire to undertake. However, the organization has provided a vehicle for communication between faculty members in university schools of nursing, and has addressed some important questions about university education for nursing.

In 1962 the Canadian Nurses Foundation (CNF) was incorporated as an organization separate from the CNA in order to provide scholarships, bursaries, and fellowships for graduate study in nursing. Because the CNF was a charitable organization, donations could be accepted on a tax-exempt basis, thus facilitating the collection of funds for scholarship. A grant of $150,000 from the W.K. Kellogg Foundation in 1962 helped build the fund at its inception; memberships, collected on a voluntary basis, provided the financial base for operations. However, the Foundation has had some difficulty in soliciting the number of memberships needed to maintain a solid financial base for the organization. It continues to seek memberships from affiliates of provincial nurses associations to support a national program of scholarships and fellowships for university-level study in nursing, and for research.

At the outset the CNA and the CNF operated quite autonomously. However, when it became clear that the financial structure of the CNF was not strong, closer links were developed between the two organizations. The executive director of the CNA is the secretary-treasurer of the CNF, the CNF is housed in CNA House in Ottawa, and in the years of CNA biennial conventions, annual meetings of the CNF are held in association with the CNA meeting. In recent years the CNF has broadened its activities to work closely with the CNA on matters of importance to both organizations. "Operation Bootstrap" involved seeking funds for a doctoral program in nursing, doctoral fellowships for nurses pursuing a doctoral degree in nursing, and other supportive activities. Although the effort was not successful in achieving external fuding for these projects, CNA, CNF, and CAUSN participated in the effort as equal partners.

Although it is reported that provision was made in 1966 to include assistance for study at the baccalaureate level (CNA, 1968, p. 11), in practice, fellowships were awarded almost exclusively for master's and doctoral study. However, a resolution, passed at the 1982 annual meeting in St. John's, Newfoundland, provided a mandate for the awarding of one scholarship for study at the baccalaureate level in each province or territory each year.

■■ ■■ ■■ ■■

NURSING DURING THE WORLD WARS

Nurses have played pivotal roles during military conflicts throughout Canadian history. Reference has already been made to the important, bipartisan role played by the nursing sisters of the Hôtel Dieu hospitals in Quebec and Montreal during the hostilities between the French and English. During the Northwest Rebellion of 1885 a military request for nursing services shows the influence of Florence Nightingale and the experience gained during the American Civil War. "No volunteer nurses. If you can send an organized body under a trained head, they will be welcome" (CNA, 1968, p. 63). Two groups of nurses responded to the call, one headed by Mother Hannah Grier from the Anglican order of St. John the Divine in Toronto, the other by Miss Miller, a head nurse at the Winnipeg General Hospital (CNA, 1968). In 1898 nurses with the Victorian Order of Nurses (VON) were attached to the Yukon Military Force and accorded considerable praise for their efforts (Gibbon and Mathewson, 1947).

In 1899 an offer of a Canadian contingent of nurses for the Boer War was made by the Canadian government to Mr. Joseph Chamberlain. The first group of four nurses was sent to assist in South Africa under the leadership of Georgina Fane Pope, a Bellevue Hospital-educated nurse from Prince Edward Island. She described the conditions under which nursing took place.

> We nursed in huts and found the work at times very heavy, often times having our dinner between nine and ten p.m. We received our first convoy of wounded a few days after the Battle of Maggersfontein and Modder River when the beds were filled with men of the Highland Brigade. We remained at Wynberg for nearly a month, when No. 3 General Hospital of 600 beds was pitched under canvas at Rondesbosch, a few miles away—Here we arrived on Christmas Day and remained almost six months, having at times very active service; sometimes covered with sand during a "Cape South-Easter;" at others delayed with a fore-runner of the coming rainy season, and at all times in terror of scorpions and snakes as bed-fellows (Gibbon and Mathewson, 1947, pp. 290-291).

The South African nursing experience was sufficient to persuade the Canadian Army Medical Corps that an army nursing service ought to be an integral part of the permanent corps. Georgina Pope and Margaret Macdonald thus were appointed to the staff on a permanent basis in 1906. When World War I broke out, the Army Nursing Corps consisted of five nurses. However, within three weeks of the declaration of war, thousands of nurses had volunteered for service overseas. Margaret Macdonald, who was appointed Matron-in-Chief of the Army Nursing Corps, described the first group of volunteers:

The selection, from coast to coast, of over one hundred nurses from thousands of applicants, the vast majority of whom were entirely unacquainted with Army Life and regulations, constituted somewhat of a problem. However, when all the formalities incident to the appointment of these as Nursing Sisters were concluded, it was astonishing how quickly and naturally in becoming military minded they fell into place. Their example and esprit de corps became the pattern for the many hundreds that followed (Gibbon and Mathewson, 1947, p. 296).

There are many accounts of the nature of service rendered by Canadian nurses during the war, all of which make note of the flexibility and devotion to duty that was required. Matron Macdonald described the introduction of the first group of nursing sisters to field nursing.

Their first introduction to Field Nursing began at Salisbury Plain in 1914; patients, many seriously ill, poured into huts that were ill-equipped to receive them. Cold, damp weather with continuous rain prevailed, adding much to the general discomfort. The sisters literally ploughed their way through mud and water from hut to hut; their living quarters left much to be desired. In the matter of rations, assuredly, vitamins were not the order of the day (Gibbon and Mathewson, 1947, p. 297).

Margaret Macdonald, who was given the rank of major, was succeeded by Edith Rayside as Matron-in-Chief of the nursing service. In all, approximately 1800 nurses saw service during World War I, 47 losing their lives as a result of the conflict. Fourteen nurses perished in the sinking of the Canadian hospital ship, Llandovery Castle (CNA, 1968).

The significant service provided by nursing sisters during World War I led to the establishment of a permanent corps of nursing sisters by the Royal Canadian Army Medical Corps (RCAMC), as well as a registry of nurses who could be available for active service in the event of war.

Matron-in-Chief of the nursing service of the Army Medical Corps from 1940 to 1944 was Elizabeth Smellie. In civilian life, Miss Smellie had been chief superintendent of the VON; she became the first Canadian woman to achieve the rank of colonel. The number of nurses who served during World War II was approximately double the 4000 that served in World War I. Twenty-four Canadian general hospitals were established to care for the wounded during World War II, compared with 16 during World War I. In addition, there was a convalescent hospital in France, a neurologic and plastic surgery hospital in England, and casualty clearing stations transferring the wounded from many locations on the continent to Britain, totalling 34 overseas hospitals. Sixty hospitals were maintained in Canada, as well as two hospital ships, all staffed with nurses (Gibbon and Mathewson, 1947). In response to a request from South Africa, nurses under the leadership of Matron-in-Chief Gladys Sharpe were sent to care for wounded British soldiers.

For the major part of the war, Canadian nurses staffed the military hospitals in England and Canada and did not serve under battle conditions in Europe until 1943, when they were sent to assist after the invasion of Italy.

Canadian nurses were the first to reach Sicily after the invasion . . . The unit was recruited largely from Winnipeg, and other Western cities, but the first girl ashore was

Lieutenant Elizabeth Lawson of St. John, New Brunswick . . . Lieutenant Trennie Hunter, of Winnipeg, was a close second. The Matron of this hospital is Miss Agnes J. MacLeod, of Edmonton. They were described as a 'group of grimy, tin-hatted girls, perspiring in the terrific heat and burdened with cumbersome equipment' (Gibbon and Mathewson, 1947, p. 465).

"Comfort was a rarity to them that first winter. Often casualties were heavy, and they were on duty in the wards night and day," said one Red Cross officer (Gibbon and Mathewson, 1947, p. 467). Gladys Sharpe described conditions in South Africa and the response to the arrival of Canadian nurses.

> Our beds filled rapidly, the first convoy via hospital train brought casualties from Burma, Madagascar, the Middle East and Singapore, at the rate of 257 admitted in just two hours—the highlight was the official opening ceremony at which Field Marshall Smuts took the opportunity of publicly thanking 'Canada' for sending nurses (Gibbon and Mathewson, 1947, p. 462).

It is reported that, up to this point, nurses in military service held the relative rank of officers, but did not actually have the official status of officers or the authority that accompanied the rank. This was changed about half-way through the war by order of the privy council, who granted nurses commissions equivalent to those of other commissioned officers. By contrast, nurses in Britain and the United States did not achieve this until the end of the war (CNA, 1968, p. 65).

■ ■ ■ ■

THE EMERGENCE OF PUBLIC HEALTH NURSING

The development of public health nursing as both an area of specialization in nursing and an integral part of nursing in all settings is largely a process that occurred in the twentieth century. The idea of preventing illness and the spread of disease by educating people about beneficial health practices and life-style modifications was not recognized until the twentieth century. Further, it was realized that good nutritional practices were important for all, but essential for the health of young children and pregnant women. Some of the first public health nursing was performed by visiting patients with tuberculosis, and teaching preventive measures in the home.

The first school nurses were appointed in Hamilton, Ontario, in 1909, and then in Toronto in 1910. Lina Rogers, a Canadian nurse who was graduated from the Hospital for Sick Children, had achieved international fame for her work that correlated the absence of children from school with lack of medical care. Her appointment to the School Nursing Service of the Toronto Board of Education led to the recruitment of a staff of nurses and dentists, and emphasis on teaching children and their families hygienic practices to prevent disease. The Nursing Service was transferred to the Health Department several years later. Its work provided a model for the rest of the country to gradually initiate a system of public health nursing in each province (Gibbon and Mathewson, 1947).

After World War I the Canadian Red Cross Society facilitated the development of public health nursing by providing grants for the establishment of certificate courses in public health nursing at six universities across the country

(Canadian Red Cross Society, 1962). The VON also encouraged nurses to study public health nursing at the universities by initiating a program of bursaries for advanced study in 1921. These programs continue to the present day and have been very important in encouraging the study of public health nursing.

The development of public health nursing throughout the twentieth century has been a gradual process. The entrenchment of a hospital-based system of health care, encouraged by Canadian federal health legislation since 1948, has undoubtedly retarded recognition of the need for preventive services, home-based services, and consumer involvement in health care. The Lalonde Report (1975) provided the first evidence of concern about disease prevention and health maintenance at the federal level. However, skyrocketing costs of care in hospitals have at last focused attention on the need to care for people in different ways. Day surgery services, ambulatory care, outpatient services, and home care are now being used as substitutes for hospital-based care, and the nurse is play-ing a prominent role in all of these areas. Even though many of these services can be described as "illness care," the need to teach health practices for disease prevention and health maintenance is an important facet of nursing care in all of these areas. The Epp Report's (1986) continued emphasis upon prevention, poverty reduction, and enhancement of people's ability to cope with their lives, indicated that federal health officials had moved to an approach to health pro-motion that took account of the determinants of health and the problems that people faced in their lives.

Public health nursing was also the driving force behind the establishment of nursing courses at universities in Canada, as noted above. Gradually these cer-tificate programs were phased into baccalaureate degree programs, and prepa-ration in public health nursing became an essential component of the basic cur-riculum. Notwithstanding its essential role in the development of university education for nursing in Canada, the fact remains that public health services are only just beginning to be recognized as critical to the health of Canadians. Acute care has for years usurped much of the attention and most of the funds desig-nated for health. However, there is now renewed public interest in community health services, and their development is an important step in maximizing the investment of Canadians in health.

The history of nursing in Canada is long and distinguished. Nurses have been caring for people from the time of the earliest French settlements on the shores of the St. Lawrence. Over time they have adapted to the changing health-care needs of society. In the beginning the primary health-care needs centred around care of those with infectious diseases, which often became epidemics. Nurses also distinguished themselves in caring for the wounded in various con-flicts. As time went on, cures were found for many of the most troublesome infectious diseases, leading to a dramatic extension of life span and adding a new dimension to health care. Nurses have been at the heart of new develop-ments in high technology acute care, and they have pressed for more emphasis on encouraging the populace to adopt behaviour that is beneficial to health. Altruism has characterized nursing and nurses from the outset, and a review of the deliberations of organized nursing over time reveals that commitment to the public good has been a firmly entrenched principle guiding professional activities. The future is likely to hold many new and difficult challenges for the nursing profession. With such a historical record, nurses will likely continue to distinguish themselves in meeting the challenges ahead.

REFERENCES

Canadian Nurses Association. (1968). *The leaf and the lamp*. Ottawa: Author.

Canadian Red Cross Society. (1962). *The role of one voluntary organization in Canada's health services: A brief presented to the Royal Commission on Health Services on behalf of the Central Council of the Canadian Red Cross Society*. Toronto: Author.

Epp, J. (1986). *Achieving health for all: A framework for health promotion*. Ottawa: Health and Welfare Canada.

Gibbon, J.M., and Mathewson, M.S. (1947). *Three centuries of Canadian nursing*. Toronto: The Macmillan Co.

Lalonde, M. (1975). *A new perspective on the health of Canadians*. Ottawa: Health and Welfare Canada.

Morton, D. (1983). *A short history of Canada*. Edmonton: Hurtig Publishers Ltd.

Nutting, M.A., and Dock, L. (1937). *A history of nursing* (Vols. 1-4). New York: Putnam's.

CHAPTER THREE

Professionalization in Canadian Nursing

JANET ROSS KERR

T he *raison d'être* of any profession is to be found in the contribution it makes to society. Nurses and nursing have made an enormous contribution to the delivery of care. Founded on an acute-care and physician-centred model, the first piece of federal health legislation that was enacted provided funding for the construction of hospitals through the National Health Grants Act of 1948. The establishment of a system of national health insurance emerged from passage of the Hospital Insurance and Diagnostic Services and Medical Care Acts of 1957 and 1968, respectively. Nurses have been making the case for health care reform eloquently and articulately for the better part of 2 decades.

Although there has been some openness to the need for a fundamental rethinking of the existing system, as in the provision in the Canada Health Act of 1984 to extend provisions for remuneration from physicians and dental surgeons to include "health practitioners," provincial and federal governments have done little to change a system that is still focused almost entirely upon diagnosis and treatment of disease, with little attention to health promotion, prevention of illness, and identifying and addressing the determinants of health.

The restructuring that is currently taking place in Canada has meant major downsizing of tertiary care, with widespread losses of nursing positions. Despite this negative effect upon the traditional role of nurses in the system, the move to a more community-oriented and consumer-driven model makes it likely that nurses will be the linchpin in the health system of the future. They are uniquely situated to function effectively in new roles based on the primary health care, community-based model.

The advancement of nursing as a profession has occurred gradually over the 350 years of nursing history in Canada, which began when three Augustinian nuns from France arrived to provide nursing care to the small population at Quebec. From this humble beginning nursing evolved as an essential service in the New World at a time when knowledge of disease was in a primitive state, technology was virtually nonexistent, and a few herbal remedies were the only drug therapies available. Over the centuries the practice of nursing was refined and perceived as important to the health and well-being of the community. In the twentieth century a concerted effort was made to develop educational standards and programs to prepare nurses for practice. Efforts were also made to gain control over the practice of nursing through registration of nurses, and development of professional standards.

The process of professionalization, or the evolution of nursing from an occupation to a profession, can be clearly seen and identified. However, there is considerable diversity of opinion about the characteristics of a profession and the extent to which particular occupational groups may possess these characteristics.

■ ■ ■ ■

DEVELOPMENT OF PROFESSIONS

Categorizing an occupation as a profession has traditionally been based on fairly standard criteria, developed by people with expertise in the study of professions. The nursing profession has generated controversy and conflict, and much time has been spent debating whether nursing is a profession; some have termed it a semiprofession. With the passage of time and the phenomenal changes in the nature and scope of nursing over the past 2 decades, this debate has seemed less relevant. "The significant question to ask about occupations, however, is not whether or not they are professions but to what extent they exhibit characteristics of professions" (Moloney, 1986, p. 9).

The debate began shortly after the turn of the century when Abraham Flexner (1915, pp. 578-581) identified six characteristics of a profession based on his observations of the traditional professions of law, medicine, and theology.

1. It is basically intellectual, carrying with it high responsibility.
2. It is learned in nature, because it is based on a body of knowledge.
3. It is practical rather than theoretical.
4. Its technique can be taught through educational discipline.
5. It is well organized internally.
6. It is motivated by altruism.

These characteristics were presented to address the question of whether social work was a profession. Flexner (1915) observed that nursing did not appear to be a profession because ". . . the responsibility of the trained nurse is neither original nor final"(p. 581). It should be noted that his assessment of how nursing met the stated criteria was made before the passage of laws regulating the practice of nursing in most provinces and before nursing education first appeared in a university prospectus in Canada.

"Although the term 'profession' is sometimes used in a purely descriptive way, a careful analysis of the nature of a profession will show that the idea of a profession carries with it some important ethical implications"(Quinn and Smith, 1987, p. 3). The ethical dimension may be the critical one in determining the esteem in which members of a profession are held by the public.

. . . the idea of a profession can be examined sociologically, which results in a descriptive account of the professions. The sociologist would first identify those occupations usually called professions and then determine what characteristics they have that nonprofessional occupations do not have. That list of characteristics is sometimes used as a way of classifying other occupations as either professions or nonprofessions. This is a descriptive approach and does not entitle us to draw any conclusions about what one's own occupation ought to be (Quinn and Smith, 1987, p. 3).

In arriving at a definition of a profession, Quinn and Smith (1987) have melded the descriptive and ethical models of professionalism.

The professions are those forms of employment that require an uncommonly complex knowledge base, used by persons committed to the direct benefit of human beings, with minimal societal control placed on their practice, and organized among themselves to ensure that they continue to provide those benefits (Quinn and Smith, 1987, p. 4).

Moloney (1986) has referred to the "natural history of professionalization" as a description of the milestones in the development of professions. Some of these milestones include the date the profession first became a full-time occupation, the date of the first educational program to prepare practitioners of the profession, and the date the first university school for the profession was established. Also included as significant events are the date the first national professional association was formed, the date of the enactment of the first provincial registration act, and the date of the development and adoption of a formal code of ethics. Although these events are static and finite, they allow for comparisons between professions and assessment of where a particular group is in terms of the process of professionalization.

Flexner (1915) saw the development of a formal base of knowledge, the first criterion, as the most central for professions. It appears that others concur, as an articulated knowledge base is common to the vast majority of categorizations of professions. The knowledge needed to practise a profession is complex and cannot be mastered by the ordinary person. Practitioners require a lengthy period of preparation and supervised practice before they can function competently on an independent basis. The educational process is considered important and complex enough that programs are offered within universities, and the first professional degree often follows a 4-year university arts or science degree. The knowledge base of a profession is continually upgraded through research performed by members to expand and update knowledge for practice. Members of the profession also maintain control over educational standards for the admission of new practitioners into the profession. The "direct benefit" idea referred to by Quinn and Smith (1987), is a key element in the definition of a profession that places emphasis on the ethical dimension. The knowledge of the professional practitioner must be used for the direct benefit of the public.

Because the professions are inherently important to the public, some form of licensing or registration of those qualified to practise is necessary. Control of this process, while vested in legislation, is normally left to the profession. Professions are organized for the purpose of regulating practice; their associations seek to improve standards of practice and education, register members, monitor professional conduct, and judge practice of professionals where disputes have arisen. Thus professions retain the authority to remove from practice those who are incompetent.

Professional commitment to the public is demonstrated by the development of a code of ethics, or statement of moral or ethical duty. A code of ethics has been described as "a set of principles to guide the individual practitioner" and as addressing "some of the most common temptations that professionals might experience in the course of their practice, temptations to take advantage of the special power that their expertise gives them over clients" (Quinn and Smith, 1987, pp. 9-10). "Codes are an essential characteristic of a profession, and are a statement of the acceptance of the trust and responsibility the public has placed in a profession" (Storch, 1982, p. 20). Although codes of ethics are important for the health professions, they are limited by their purpose to guide professional practice and they may not "include all issues of importance to the patient" (Storch, 1982, p. 20).

■■ ■■ ■■ ■■

EVOLUTION OF NURSING AS A PROFESSION

In Canada the nursing profession has been prominent in the life of society since the first nurses were encouraged to emigrate to the shores of New France. Later, in the nineteenth century, members of the Order of the Sisters of Charity of Montreal (Grey Nuns) bravely set out, without benefit of reliable transportation, to provide needed health care to remote parts of the country where small settlements were opening.

Around the turn of the twentieth century, there was a movement to secure legislation to regulate nursing practice to differentiate qualified from unqualified practitioners. The first provincial statute governing the practice of nursing was passed in Nova Scotia in 1910. By 1922, with the passage of legislation in Ontario, there were statutes governing nursing in all provinces. The development of stronger legislation, which would differentiate the actual practice of nursing with the title of Registered Nurse (RN), occurred later, with the initial passage of legislation in Newfoundland in 1953. Eight provinces today have mandatory acts, leaving only two, Manitoba and Ontario, to achieve this goal. Achieving exclusive right to practise, embodied in law, is an important step in professionalizing nursing. The profession in Canada is well on its way to uniform acceptance of the need for this legislation.

Nursing education in Canada began in 1874 in St. Catharines, Ontario, after worldwide recognition of Florence Nightingale's efforts in nursing education. Nightingale believed that nurses needed to be educated to care for patients properly. She demonstrated her point by dramatically lowering mortality and morbidity rates of soldiers in the Crimea in 1856, when she and a small group of nurses provided care for wounded soldiers. Nursing education moved into the universities in 1919 with the inception of a degree program in nursing at the University of British Columbia under the direction of Ethel Johns. In 1959, master's degree education in nursing was initiated at the University of Western Ontario, and nursing research development began in earnest. Although initial preparation is still largely based in community colleges and hospitals across the country, the adoption and active promotion of the entry to practice position by the Canadian Nurses Association (CNA) and various professional associations is significant. The position seeks to ensure that those entering the practice of nursing in the year 2000 and thereafter qualify at the baccalaureate level. Master's level preparation has been available since 1959; the first doctoral program, at the University of Alberta, admitted students on January 1, 1991.

The development of a code of ethics for a profession normally occurs relatively late in the process of professionalization. "Toward the end, legal protection appears; at the end, a formal code of ethics is adopted" (Wilensky, 1964, pp. 143-144). A historical review indicates that this was the case for the nursing profession in Canada. The first North American Code of Ethics for nursing was published by the American Nurses Association in 1950; in 1953 the International Council of Nurses (ICN) approved a code of ethics. The latter was generally accepted and used by professional associations until 1980, when the first CNA code of ethics was developed. Disagreement about the wording of the initial code resulted in the development of a new code, adopted in 1985. Recently the CNA has taken the position that the code of ethics should be reviewed every 5 years. An ad hoc committee of four members and an ethics consultant reviewed the code in 1990, and a new code was published in 1991 (CNA, 1991). Committee members were being sought for the next review in late 1994.

■ ■ ■ ■

EMERGENCE OF A SCIENTIFIC KNOWLEDGE BASE FOR NURSING

Research to create and extend the knowledge base in nursing has been enhanced by the establishment of graduate programs in nursing at the master's level since 1959. There are now 13 master's programs in nursing in Canada. Many of these programs have a strong research thrust, and graduates of such programs are engaged in advancing the scientific basis of nursing. The movement to prepare nursing scholars who have the skills to undertake research was inhibited by the delay in establishing a doctoral-level nursing program in Canada, a development that has been discussed publicly since the 1978 Kellogg National Seminar on Doctoral Education in Nursing (Zilm, LaRose, and Stinson, 1979). The initiation of a doctoral program by the Faculty of Nursing at the University of Alberta on January 1, 1991, was followed by the approval of a second program at the University of British Columbia in May, 1991, which got underway in the fall of that year. Three other universities have subsequently initiated programs including: McGill University/the University of Montreal joint program (1993), the University of Toronto (1993), and McMaster University (1994).

The importance of studying nursing questions has been emphasized by leaders in the profession, who have stressed scientific testing of traditional nursing care practices.

For members of the professions, being expert is more than a matter of personal pride; it becomes a matter of professional ethics. Clients come to a professional expecting and trusting that the professional has knowledge and expertise that the client needs but does not have. The implicit promise that the professional makes in accepting a client or patient involves their mutual understanding that the professional has a special knowledge and will use it for the benefit of the client (Quinn and Smith, 1987, p. 103).

There is a scientific knowledge base for nursing, and a review of the chapters in Part 2 will help the reader gain an appreciation of this basis of the professional nursing practice.

■■ ■■ ■■ ■■

PROFESSIONAL EDUCATION FOR NURSING: ISSUES OF STATUS AND CONTROL

Nursing education has been the subject of considerable controversy. However, the entry to practice proposal has possibly engendered more heated debate than other issues in recent decades. Initially proposed by a government-appointed committee in Alberta, the proposal, stating that all nurses entering the profession be qualified at the baccalaureate level by the turn of the century, has been ratified by the CNA and provincial associations. Implementation of the position is a much more difficult matter, requiring public consent because nursing education is funded under federal-provincial programs for post-secondary education. Although universities, colleges, and hospital schools of nursing operate under boards of governors, independent of governments, difficulties may arise if special funding or funding increases are required to support baccalaureate-level education in a period of retrenchment of higher education. The CNA has advised that it is unwise to assume the entry to practice proposal will result in higher costs.

> Contrary to the popular assumption we suggest that the institutional costs of educating nurses through universities are very likely to be overstated relative to those of other post-secondary institutions . . . costs . . . may well be lower in universities than in other institutions and that in any case, the assumption that a baccalaureate program is necessarily costlier is unwarranted. (1986, p. 1)

It is becoming increasingly evident in parts of the country that arrangements are being made to facilitate the baccalaureate entry to practice standard. The School of Nursing of the Vancouver General Hospital and the School of Nursing of the University of British Columbia initiated a collaborative degree program in 1989. This was followed by a program arranged collaboratively between the University of Alberta and Red Deer College in 1990. The program was extended to include the other four diploma schools of nursing in Edmonton in 1991. Other collaborative programs are being initiated or planned in other parts of the country (please see Chapter 25 for a complete discussion).

The professional association monitors standards in initial programs of nursing education in all provinces except Alberta, Ontario and Quebec; this is discussed in Chapter 27. Nursing remains different from most other professions in terms of this process. The difference is that the majority of nurses graduating from educational programs are prepared in non-university programs, whereas in law, medicine, theology, pharmacy, engineering, architecture, and other professions, all educational preparation is centred in the universities. When all practitioners enter the field of nursing as graduates from university programs in nursing, the monitoring function will no longer be necessary.

The nursing profession is bound to be preoccupied for some time with establishing educational programs within universities. This process is likely to extend over several decades because the majority of new graduates are still prepared in diploma programs. The establishment of five doctoral programs since 1991 is providing for the preparation of nurse researchers with the expertise to undertake theory-building and theory-testing research. The placement of the professional program is an issue likely to arise after the establishment of initial programs of nursing education. Within the university it remains to be seen whether some university-level study in the liberal arts and sciences will be required before admission to the program.

▬ ▬ ▬ ▬

CONTROL OF PROFESSIONAL NURSING PRACTICE

The first phase of the drive by nurses to gain control of the professional nursing practice extended from the enactment of the first provincial legislation regulating nursing, in Nova Scotia in 1910, to the conclusion of the process, in Ontario in 1922. Prowse (1983) drew attention to the importance of "aspects of nursing legislation which (a) expedite effective utilization of nursing knowledge and expertise, (b) influence the supply of qualified competent nurses, and (c) ensure regulation and monitoring of both practice and practitioners"(p. 33).

The second phase of this process was the development of mandatory acts regulating nursing in each province. This ensured that the practice and practitioners would be more strictly regulated. Legislation incorporating mandatory registration requires a definition of nursing, and a description of the scope of nursing practice. The first mandatory nursing legislation in Canada was enacted in 1953 in Newfoundland. Other provinces did not follow suit until Prince Edward Island passed such legislation in 1972, followed by Quebec in 1973 (with significant amendments in 1974). Although the Manitoba statute passed in 1980 is permissive and protects only the title of registered nurse, it requires employers to demonstrate that those employed as registered nurses are actually registered. Alberta passed a mandatory Nursing Profession Act in 1983, and New Brunswick, Nova Scotia, and Saskatchewan and British Columbia followed suit in 1984, 1985, and 1988 respectively. Thus only two provinces, Manitoba and Ontario, have not developed mandatory legislation to regulate nursing practice. These issues are discussed in more detail in Chapter 28.

The tremendous change in nursing roles over the past 25 years has altered the nature and scope of practice extensively. Specialization is almost a requirement because of changes in the knowledge required to practise in a specific area. Certification of practitioners in specialty areas is a concern; the way in which the CNA has addressed this issue is described in Chapter 29. The trend toward increased specialization can be expected to continue as health-care knowledge and technology continue to develop.

■■■ ■■■ ■■■ ■■■

FACILITATING PROFESSIONALIZATION

It is likely that changes in the way in which nursing is practised will continue as society becomes more aware of the benefits of health promotion and the need to develop healthier lifestyles to prevent disease. Alternatives to hospitalization for tertiary and long-term care, in the form of home care and ambulatory care, appear attractive at both the personal and societal levels. Nurses have been preparing for their new roles in community and long-term care settings and have the knowledge and the communication and interactional skills to assist consumers in meeting health goals. They are thus well-poised to serve society in a health system that is centred in the community and based on the primary health-care model.

The initiation of doctoral education is an important milestone for the nursing profession because preparing nurses to contribute to the discovery of nursing knowledge through theory and research will lead to improved care. Increased availability of baccalaureate programs in nursing will provide a stronger basis for the practice of nursing. The profession will need a great deal of political expertise to surmount the obstacles that will arise while implementing the entry to practice proposal. Dynamic leadership will be required to provide direction to new generations of skilled practitioners and to ensure that their talents are used to the fullest extent for the benefit of the public.

REFERENCES

Canadian Nurses Association. (1986). *Entry to Practice Newsletter*, 2(1).

Canadian Nurses Association. (1991). *Code of ethics for nursing*. Ottawa: Author.

Flexner, A. (1915). Is social work a profession? In *Proceedings of the National Conference of Charities and Corrections* (pp. 578-581). Chicago: Heldermann Printing Co.

Moloney, M.M. (1986). *Professionalization of nursing: Current issues and trends*. Philadelphia: J.B. Lippincott Co.

Prowse, A.J. (1983). *Nursing legislation in Canada: An overview for health services administrators*. Edmonton: Department of Health Services

Administration and Community Medicine, The University of Alberta.

Quinn, C.A., and Smith, M.D. (1987). *The professional commitment: Issues and ethics in nursing*. Philadelphia: W.B. Saunders.

Storch, J. (1982). *Patients' rights: Ethical and legal issues in health care and nursing*. Toronto: McGraw-Hill Ryerson Ltd.

Wilensky, H.L. (1964). The professionalization of everyone? *American Journal of Sociology, 70*(2), 143-144.

Zilm, G., LaRose, O., and Stinson, S. (1979). *Proceedings of the Kellogg National Seminar on Doctoral Education for Canadian Nurses*. Ottawa: Canadian Nurses Association.

CHAPTER FOUR

The Role of the Canadian Nurses Association in the Development of Nursing in Canada

JANNETTA MacPHAIL

T he Canadian Nurses Association (CNA) has played a key role in the development of nursing in Canada since its establishment in 1924, as did its forerunner, the Canadian National Association of Trained Nurses (CNATN), which was initiated in 1908. The CNATN comprised affiliated member societies, including alumni associations of hospital schools of nursing and local and regional groups of nurses, with a total of 28 such groups by 1911 (CNA, 1968). By 1924 each of the nine provinces "had a provincial nurses' organization with membership in the CNATN, and in that year the national group changed its name to the Canadian Nurses' Association" (CNA, 1968, p. 38). Fifty-two nursing organizations were affiliated with the CNA in 1924; some nurses had multiple memberships and some organizations had members who were nonregistered nurses, so it was decided in 1930 that the CNA would become a federation of the nine provincial nurses' associations. This change established the current policy that the provincial/territorial nurses' association is the official representative of registered nurses in each province/territory and that all members of the Canadian Nurses Association are registered nurses (CNA, 1968).

Membership in the CNA has increased dramatically, from about 8000 in 1930 to 111,470 members of nine provincial and two territorial nurses' associations in 1992. This excludes 57,330 potential members from Quebec because of the decision made by the Order of Nurses of Quebec in 1985 to disaffiliate from the CNA. Some Quebec nurses who were thus excluded from the CNA, have joined as individual members through other provinces/territories. In addition, the 111,470 membership figure takes into account for the decrease in members from Ontario in 1987 as a result of the decision made by the nurses' union, the Ontario Nurses Association (ONA), to terminate the arrangement for block memberships of 40,000 in the Registered Nurses Association of Ontario (RNAO). Current membership of RNAO in the CNA is 12,024 (1992), which represents 14% of 86,413 registered nurses employed in nursing in Ontario in 1992.

The CNA Board of Directors consists of a President; a President-Elect; a Vice-President; five members-at-large representing nursing administration, nursing education, nursing practice, nursing research, and socio-economic welfare; one representative of the CNA Advisory Council; three public members, appointed by the Board from nominees from the provinces; and the presidents of the provincial/territorial nurses' associations.

The CNA Advisory Council was established in 1985 and held its first meeting on June 21, 1986. It includes representatives from recognized CNA Interest Groups and the Executive Committee of the CNA Board of Directors. The Council's function is to provide information and advice to the Board of Directors on selected nursing and health care issues; the first issue identified was certification. The number of national nursing interest groups holding membership on the CNA Advisory Council increased to 20 by 1992 (CNA Connection, 1993b). As the number of groups has grown and the Advisory Council has become more focused and productive, criteria for membership has been an ongoing concern. Although some groups have asked for a decrease in the 70% CNA membership criterion required to have a representative on the Advisory Council, the Board of Directors has maintained that basic policy.

From its inception the CNA has focused on the needs of the profession and the needs of Canadians served by professional nurses. Priorities, established by the Board of Directors at the beginning of each biennium, are responsive to changes in society, the health care system, and the educational system for the preparation of nurses. In her last official address as CNA President in 1990, Judith Ritchie identified the two major issues of the past biennium as "the need to articulate the nature of nursing practice and nurses' working environments, and the escalating need for major change in the philosophy, structure and approach of the health care system" (CNA Connection, 1990d, p. 15).

Reform of the health care system evolved as the major priority for the CNA in the 1990-92 biennium. Attention focused on identifying threats to the principles of medicare, designing approaches to continue having care accessible to all, addressing the problems of over-reliance on acute care, and failure to increase funding for community-based care. President Alice Baumgart urged CNA members to take action to effect needed changes despite decreases in funding (CNA Connection, 1991i). She emphasized the need for nurses to develop new working skills, including "learning to work within a multi-disciplinary team in which traditional career boundaries are increasingly blurred, and developing greater flexibility and resourcefulness to make the most of new health care opportunities" (CNA Connection, 1992e, p. 9).

In June 1991 the CNA Board of Directors identified the following six goals as the foci of CNA activities over the next 5 years:

raising the visibility of nursing's contributions to the health of individuals, families and communities; examining and shaping the impact of the health care system on the health status of the individual, the family, the community, the provider of services and the use of resources; investing in primary health care; developing and refining new models of nursing practice; enhancing quality of work-life issues; [and] advancing specialization and certification initiatives (CNA Connection, 1991j, p. 10).

The role of the CNA in the development of nursing in Canada will be presented in relation to CNA's corporate objectives and the priorities established for recent bienniums, along with some historical perspective in relation to each priority.

■ ■ ■ ■

THE IMAGE OF NURSES AND NURSING

Improving the image of nurses and nursing was deemed by the CNA Board of Directors as the top priority for the 1986-88 biennium and is still a priority. The image has become a cause for increasing concern among nurses in provincial/territorial nurses' associations, as well as at the national level. Nurses and the professional associations are concerned about how nurses and nursing are perceived by the public because this influences who is attracted to and retained in nursing. The outcomes of the recruiting process have a great effect on the growth of the profession and the quality of care that can be delivered. Public perceptions of nurses and nursing also affect resource allocation for education and service, the influence that nurses have in shaping health policy, and the structure and functioning of the health care system.

A description of the way in which nurses and nursing are perceived by the public and by nurses themselves is included in Chapter 5. It is sufficient at this point to state that the efforts of the CNA are directed at communicating with the public to produce a more positive image. CNA's President Ritchie stated:

> We must find better ways of describing [our] practice so that the complexity of our assessments and judgments are understood. With such understanding, others will value the visible and the invisible aspects of our work. Such value will lead to adequate remuneration and working conditions, and the assumption that such complex work requires solid educational preparation and continuing education (Ritchie, 1988, p. 3).

In her closing address in 1990 Ritchie stated: "Many of the difficulties we face in having adequate resources and feeling undervalued are related to the basic lack of awareness of nursing's work. . . . We must mount a campaign to portray what nursing really is" (CNA Connection, 1990d, p. 15).

■ ■ ■ ■

NURSING PRACTICE

The involvement of the CNA in nursing practice centres on efforts to develop standards for nursing care, the issue of the expanded role of the nurse, statements pertaining to primary health care and health promotion, statements addressing major issues in health and illness care, the issue of specialization in nursing, certification for specialty nursing practice, and development of a code of ethics. Because of the emphasis on functional aspects of nursing [education and administration] one finds limited reference to practice issues in the early development of the CNA. In 1967 the CNA endorsed a statement by the Canadian Public Health Association (CPHA) listing functions and qualifications for the practice of public health nursing in Canada. In 1970 the CNA issued position statements on the delivery of health services, delivery of nursing care, the transfer of functions, and health services for the poor. This was followed by a CNA "Statement on the Expanded Role of the Nurse—the Physician Assistant," which reinforced the strong belief that the professional nurse was best qualified to assume the functions and responsibilities that have been suggested for the proposed category of physician's assistant. At a subsequent conference about the physician's assistant, held jointly by the CNA and the Canadian Medical Association (CMA) in 1971, it was agreed that the role of physician's assistant would not be introduced in Canada (CNA, 1981).

In 1971 the CNA issued statements on family planning programs and nurses' rights relative to nursing care of patients having therapeutic abortions. To assist in developing standards for nursing care, in 1972 the CNA published *Guidelines for Developing Standards of Nursing Care*. In 1973 the organization also issued a statement, "The Expanded Role of the Nurse—Part 3: The Nurse in Primary Care, supporting the CNA's emphasis on health promotion and maintenance. This was followed by statements in 1975 concerning nurses in health promotion, and a 1976 survey of nurses regarding their expanded role (CNA, 1981).

In 1986 the CNA Board of Directors appointed a Special Committee on Health Issues to include nurses representing all areas of practice and each member jurisdiction. The committee's charge was to meet twice yearly to identify and discuss nursing and health care issues needing a national perspective. In 1990 the committee's name was changed to the Special Committee on Clinical Practice Issues, and it was given the following mandate:

> to assist in identifying emerging clinical practice issues and recommend priorities, positions and strategic actions to the Board; recommend specific clinical practice issues for discussion at regular meetings with the Canadian Medical Association and with other relevant national associations; and receive from the Board selected clinical practice issues for identified action (CNA Connection, 1990e, p. 16).

To date, the issues addressed include: "biomedical technology and its impact on home care, quality of life, nursing care and financial demands on the health care system" (CNA Connection, 1989a, p. 7); the use of tobacco as a hazard to health; the habits and attitudes of nurses and nursing students about smoking; acquired immune deficiency syndrome (AIDS) as a major health problem and its implications for nursing practice; and the pervasive and complex problems of family violence and sexual abuse of children. Position statements have been developed, on these issues, some by the CNA alone and others collaboratively with other health disciplines and members of the community. For example, the CNA developed a position statement on mandatory drug screening in which "CNA goes on record as opposing mandatory pre-employment or random drug screening in the workplace" (CNA Connection, 1989a, p. 7). The CNA "supports the development and maintenance of prevention programs and Employee Assistance Programs in the workplace . . . which are designed to identify problems early and provide a confidential method for employees to seek assistance" (CNA Connection, 1989d, p. 10). Similarly, the CNA has developed position statements on human rights; mental health care reform; "a healthy environment as fundamental to life, free of violence and discrimination, with the right to autonomy and self-determination" (CNA Connection, 1990c, p. 4); protection of the environment from health hazards; reproductive technologies to prevent infertility; fetal alcohol syndrome; opposition to companies distributing free breast milk substitutes, which tends to discourage breast feeding; and a strategic plan on the safety and social implications of the use of health care technologies in health care. On the other hand, the CNA has employed an interdisciplinary approach to the complex problems of family violence, in conjunction with physicians, psychologists, teachers, social workers, lawyers and the police. In addition, the CNA developed a position statement on family violence, as well as clinical guidelines for nurses caring for its victims. The CNA also presented a brief to the Canadian Panel on Violence Against Women, which "travelled across the country listening to women and groups with the hope of heightening public awareness of the problem and enabling participants to seek solutions related to the root causes of violence against women" (CNA Connection, 1991l, p. 10).

In 1990 the CNA received from the Federal Centre for AIDS of Health and Welfare Canada a 3-year grant of $200,000 for developing educational modules for nurses working with persons living with AIDS, and for schools of nursing (CNA Connection, 1991d). Representatives of the Canadian Association of University Schools of Nursing (CAUSN), the Canadian University Nursing Students' Association (CUNSA) and the Canadian Hemophilia Society assisted in identifying the subject areas to be addressed, namely, "social support; sexuality and homophobia; counselling; death, dying and grief; and ethics" (CNA Connection, 1991k, p. 4). Additional CNA goals are "facilitating access by nurses to current relevant information on HIV/AIDS and the nurse's role; promoting individual and collaborative research on aspects of HIV/AIDS related to nursing; and advocating for the development of socio-economic policy with respect to HIV/AIDS and seeking involvement in such policy formulation" (CNA Connection, 1992c, p. 8).

The CNA has made many health promotion efforts, including a strategic plan to reduce tobacco use and promote a smoke-free society over the years. The CNA banned smoking at meetings of the Board of Directors in 1973, issued a statement on smoking in 1975 and another on smoking and health in 1989, and made its headquarters in Ottawa, CNA House, a smoke-free environment in 1987 (CNA Connection, 1986b, 1986c, 1986e). Smoking was banned at all CNA functions, including social gatherings, and another Statement on Tobacco and Health, published in 1987, communicates clearly that the CNA "actively supports efforts to reduce, discourage and eradicate the use of tobacco . . . and actions leading to a smoke-free society" (CNA Connection, 1988b, p. 10). Although some health care agencies have taken steps to ensure a smoke-free environment, the CNA recommended to the Canadian Council on Accreditation in 1987 "that consideration for hospital accreditation include the availability of smoking cessation resources for staff and establishment of a goal to move toward a smoke-free environment" (CNA Board of Directors' Minutes, February 18-20, 1987). In 1989, with the aid of a $72,000 grant from Health and Welfare Canada's Health Promotion Directorate, the CNA conducted a study to assess the smoking prevention and cessation needs of Canadian nurses and nursing students. The final report received by the Board in 1990 revealed that "17 percent of the RN respondents and 30 percent of the nursing student respondents were current smokers; and that nearly half the RN's, but only 10 percent of the students started smoking in nursing school" (CNA Connection, 1991b, p. 6). The data collected are to be used to design a strategic plan to reduce tobacco use among nurses by 50%, to measure future trends in tobacco use, and to enhance the position of nurses as non-smoking role models and health educators (CNA Connection, 1991b).

A code of ethics is very much a part of nursing practice. Although the CNA adopted the International Council of Nurses (ICN) Code of Ethics as its official code of ethics in 1966 (CNA, 1968), a code of ethics project was undertaken in 1979. This resulted in the publication of a paper, *CNA Code of Ethics: Ethical Basis for Nursing in Canada*, in 1980. This was followed by the appointment of another ad hoc committee on ethics, which culminated in the approval and publication of the *CNA Code of Ethics* in 1985. However, it soon became apparent that this code needed further study and assessment based on nurses' experience in using it in practice. The outcome was a revised *Code of Ethics for Nursing* published in 1991 and distributed to all CNA members through *The Canadian Nurse* journal. More information about it is in Chapter 20. Most provincial/territorial nursing associations have adopted it as the standard for professional conduct in their jurisdictions.

■ ■ ■ ■

WORK-LIFE AFFAIRS

Closely related to nursing practice are the environments in which nurses practise and issues pertaining to the working lives of nurses. In 1985 severe budgetary constraints caused a number of CNA staff positions to become part-time, including Manager of Work-Life Affairs. However, this position was restored to full-time in 1988 because of the importance of work-life affairs, the need to systematically collect information on the working environment of nurses, and the need for much more attention to occupational health and safety (CNA Connection, 1989c). Funds were allocated to collect background information on the subject of nursing personnel involved in the direct delivery of care, in response to the increasing attention given by government to the study of the nursing care system and assessment of productivity (CNA Connection, 1989j).

The issues of attracting and retaining nurses have presented major problems, particularly in hospitals. Much is spent on advertising and other recruitment strategies; however, much less attention has been given to the even more perplexing problem of retention. The CNA and the Canadian Hospital Association (CHA) undertook an extensive review of the literature on nurse retention as a first step in preparing a project proposal to further investigate factors that help to retain nurses in places of employment. The CNA matched CHA's contribution of $5000 by providing in-kind services of the CNA Research Manager (CNA Connection, 1989b). Twenty-three Canadian nursing workforce studies were analyzed, 21 of which had been conducted between 1987 and 1988. The findings showed common threads regarding "lack of adequate staffing, too many non-nursing tasks, lack of involvement in organizational decision-making, lack of educational opportunities, inflexible work schedules, inadequate compensation, limited autonomy in professional practice, and lack of respect from other health care colleagues for nursing's contribution to the care of patients" (CNA Connection, 1991a, p. 6).

Another approach used by the CNA to obtain information from practising nurses about work-life issues was organizing conferences to involve them in "identifying work-life issues in the nursing environment; examining strategies to increase recognition of nurses' contributions; exploring avenues to provide nurses with a more meaningful voice in work-life issues; and addressing the impact of work-life issues on caring" (CNA Connection, 1989h, p. 8). Two such conferences were held in late 1989 and early 1991, one in the west and one in the east. In 1993 the CNA again sponsored four conferences using the theme, "Work-life Issues: Value, Vision and Visibility," to be held in Victoria, Regina, Ottawa, and Charlottetown. They were designed to focus on issues in the changing environment of health care, the difficulties those issues present for nurses, and strategies to overcome them (CNA Connection, 1992f).

As a consequence of the findings of the literature review and input from practising nurses gained through the conferences, the CNA developed a position statement on the quality of work-life, recognizing that it has "a direct correlation with job satisfaction, work production, recruitment and retention, and ultimately, the quality of patient care" (CNA Connection, 1991c, p. 4). The statement emphasizes an environment that "promotes collegiality, . . . recognizes and respects nurses' contributions; involves nurses in decision-making; fosters a spirit of inquiry; protects and promotes nurses' health; supports quality nursing care; fosters professional growth; and facilitates continued learning" (CNA Connection, 1991c, p. 4). A CNA position statement on safe work environments, also published in 1990, points out the responsibility of employers to protect and promote the health and safety of employees.

During the 1990-92 biennium the CNA employed another strategy to obtain input from practising nurses about work-life affairs. A group of staff nurses working in hospitals, long-term care, and the community met regularly with the Executive Director of the CNA to share the realities of nursing practice. Beginning in February 1991 they reported problems of lay-offs with some units being closed or altered drastically; concerns about increased workload with lay-offs in other departments, such as pharmacy; concerns about safety and stress among nurses with decreased staffing and increased level of patient acuity; administration of medications by registered nursing assistants; need for technically-skilled nursing care in the community with earlier discharge from hospitals; elimination of visits to "healthy families"; and under-utilization of respite beds (CNA Connection, 1992b).

CNA's Work-life Affairs Department analyzed reports from across Canada pertaining to human resources in nursing and the recruitment and retention of nurses. The findings and recommendations are strikingly similar with a recurring theme about the quality of nurses' working lives. Nurses are concerned about the feasibility of providing quality care under existing staffing; the need for more support staff; the need for more input in decision-making; and the need to foster staffing innovations such as job sharing, flexible scheduling, and self-scheduling. They emphasize the importance of strong and supportive leadership in nursing administration, including the head nurse level. Concern is also expressed about compensation issues, such as appropriate salaries and benefits, broader salary scales, opportunities for advancement, and recognition of clinical expertise by such means as the clinical ladder (CNA Connection, 1989i). These issues are not new; they have been addressed in the literature and by some health care agencies. However, they need to be addressed in individual hospitals and other health care agencies where changes can be made, and by the governments who fund the health care system. Now with severe cutbacks in health care funding, resulting in lay-offs of nurses, increased workloads, and concerns about safety and quality of care, new problems and challenges have arisen in work-life affairs. Nurses need to work together through the CNA and the provincial/territorial associations to address the problems systematically and help to shape health policy during difficult times.

On January 1, 1988, the CNA established a vitally important service to fill the gap that resulted from changes in the liability protective insurance available to nurses in Canada. The Canadian Nurses Protective Fund (CNPF) is managed by nurses for nurses and "is designed to protect nurses from professional liability claims and to address inequities in the present insurance system." It "will provide protection for any nurse who is, or was, a member in good standing or a permit holder of a subscribing provincial association" (CNA Connection, 1988a, p. 7). At the outset the subscribing associations were Alberta, Manitoba, Newfoundland, Nova Scotia, and Saskatchewan. Policymaking and fund administration is the responsibility of the CNPF Committee, which reports directly to the CNA Board of Directors. Requests for assistance are considered by the Adjudicating Committee, which has available the expert services of the largest independent claims adjusting company in Canada as well as legal counsel retained by the CNA to investigate occurrences and advise on settlement and defense of claims. The CNA has also engaged a nurse lawyer as Coordinator of the Professional Liability Project to provide support, advice, and help with documentation to eligible nurses who report a claim or occurrence that might give rise to a claim (CNA Connection, 1988a).

■ ■ ■ ■

CERTIFICATION

Certification is also closely linked to nursing practice in that the program is designed to recognize the clinical expertise of nurses in specialty practice. The question of specialization in nursing has been discussed for a number of years. In 1973 the CNA published a discussion paper on specialization in nursing, written by Dr. Alice Baumgart, which is "a summary of collected views on specialization in hospital and community nursing practice in Canada" (CNA, 1981, p. 21). In the 1970s and 1980s increasing specialization in nursing led to the creation of specialty practice groups interested in gaining recognition and eager to have a certification program in Canada. Many nurses wishing to obtain recognition of their competence level in a specialty area of practice were seeking certification through certification programs in the United States offered by the American Nurses Association and a variety of specialty nursing organizations. In an effort to avoid multiple certification bodies in Canada the CNA has focused on establishing a certification program under the auspices of the CNA to serve nurses practising in a variety of specialty areas.

The first ad hoc Committee on Certification, established in 1980, developed basic principles and guidelines for establishing a certification system. This was followed by the appointment of two other committees, and finally a third committee that proposed a system for certification that was approved by the CNA Board of Directors in 1986. A mechanism for establishing certification in a given nursing specialty is now available through the CNA. "The three-part certification program involves designation of a specialty area of certification, development of a certification examination and certification of individuals" (CNA Connection, 1987, p. 7). To become involved in the certification process, a group of nurses must demonstrate that their specific area of nursing should be recognized as a specialty. Once specialty designation is achieved the group may continue to the development of an examination, and finally to certification. Criteria for designation of a nursing specialty, as well as the other steps in the process, are described in the CNA publication *Certification Program: An Information Booklet*. A Special Committee on Certification was established in 1986 to review requests for specialty designation and to make recommendations to the CNA Board of Directors.

Since the certification program was approved by the CNA Board of Directors in 1986, the following four areas of specialty practice have qualified for specialty designation: neuroscience nursing, occupational health nursing, nephrology nursing, and emergency nursing. A Department of Certification also has been established within the CNA organizational structure with a designated manager. After three years of negotiation with the Canadian Council of Occupational Health Nurses (CCOHN), which had developed its own certification examination, an agreement was signed to integrate it into the CNA certification program (CNA Connection, 1992a). Following field testing that simulated examination conditions, the first-ever CNA certification examination offered was the CNA Neuroscience Nursing Examination in January 1991, (CNA Connection, 1990d). The examinations are developed, tested, administered, and scored through the CNA Testing Service, which has had many years of experience in developing and administering the registration/licensure examinations for both nurses and nursing assistants. With a development cost for each examination of $280,000 over a 2-year period, it was decided that the CNA collaborate with specialty groups in seeking certification funding and "that this be considered in the context of the development of long-term planning, priority setting and the evolution of the certification program" (CNA Connection, 1991e, p. 10).

It is important to understand that the process of certification differs from group to group in Canadian nursing. To date, 20 specialty practice groups that are organized outside the CNA have met the criteria to become a CNA Interest Group (CNA Connection, 1993b) and a member of the CNA Advisory Council, established in 1986 "to provide a formal liaison structure to strengthen CNA's relationship with the national nursing groups and to promote unity and enhance interorganizational communication in a spirit of cooperation and collaberation" (CNA Advisory Council Minutes, June 21, 1986). In addition to having a representative of each of the national nursing groups who have met CNA's criteria serve on the Advisory Council, CNA welcomes representatives from other groups as observers at Advisory Council meetings. Five groups that do not meet the basic criterion of 70% membership in the CNA have chosen to send a representative and are classified as affiliate members. Thus the Advisory Council is representative of interest groups and not of specialty practice. Further, "certification does not require the establishment of a specialty organization prior to designation as a specialty practice" (CNA Connection, 1989m, p. 10). Based on recommendations of the ad hoc Long-Range Planning Committee on Certification, the CNA Board of Directors decided to work toward:

> "modifying the existing process and criteria to ease and expedite the designation of specialty areas and exam development; shortening the test development process from 20 months to 10 months; and giving priority in the next few years to the designation and development of certification exams for specialties in which there are large numbers of nurses (over 10,000); and placing smaller, designated specialty areas on a waiting list and proceeding with the development of exams for these specialties as soon as possible once the certification program is financially self-sufficient" (CNA Connection, 1993a, p. 8).

■ ■ ■ ■

NURSING EDUCATION

In the past few bienniums, high priority has been given to the goal of requiring a baccalaureate degree in nursing for entry to practice by the year 2000. Nonetheless, the CNA has supported and promoted the enhancement and expansion of graduate education in nursing, and more recently, increasing opportunities for continuing education for all nurses. Although nursing education is a provincial matter, the CNA has prepared background materials on the issue and goal of entry to practice to be used by the provincial nursing associations and by individuals to communicate this goal and educate a variety of audiences. Background material prepared by the CNA, entitled *Entry to the Practice of Nursing: A Background Paper* (1982), provides an excellent historical perspective that clearly describes the rationale for the position taken for entry to practice. For several years the CNA published an Entry to Practice Newsletter on a bi-monthly basis for use by the provincial nurses' associations so they would not have to expend funds for this purpose. The contents were very useful in educating and lobbying. In August 1991 the CNA launched a new education newsletter, *Edufacts*, and its French counterpart, *Eduneuf*, published quarterly and distributed to the provincial/territorial nurses' associations and to libraries of nursing schools. It is designed to keep educators and other nurses up-to-date on new developments, including collaborative programs between universities and former diploma programs in nursing, the development of new graduate programs, and educational innovations (CNA Connection, 1991m).

The position on entry to practice originated with the Weir Report, *Survey of Nursing Education in Canada*, published by the CNA in 1932. "Among the major recommendations was one suggesting that schools of nursing should be incorporated into the general education system of the country and be subsidized by government funds" (CNA, 1968, p. 86). The first professional nursing organization to endorse the goal of requiring a baccalaureate degree for entry to practice by new graduates by the year 2000 was the Alberta Association of Registered Nurses (AARN, 1976). The position was adopted by the Board of the CNA in 1982 and affirmed by delegates to the biennial convention in 1982. At this time the background paper cited above was published to make known the rationale for the CNA Board's policy stance on entry to practice.

Throughout the course of the CNA's history there are references to efforts to upgrade the preparation of nurses. In 1957 a statement was made that preparation for nursing should be an educational experience. In 1960

> . . . the Director of Special Studies for the CNA was appointed as the CNA liaison member to the Canadian Conference of University Schools of Nursing, which marked one of the first major moves to link the CNA with progress in higher education for nurses and to establish close working relationships with the university schools of nursing (CNA, 1968, pp. 92-93).

The establishment of the Canadian Nurses Foundation (CNF) in 1962 was further evidence of support for nursing education. The CNF provided "scholarships, bursaries and fellowships for post-graduate study in nursing. Provision was made in 1966 to include assistance for study at the baccalaureate level" (CNA, 1968, p. 93). In 1978 the CNA published *Standards for Nursing Education*— a first in education in Canada—and urged universities with baccalaureate programs to include preparation for primary-care nursing as an integral part of basic nursing education as soon as possible (CNA, 1981). In the same year the CNA sponsored a national forum on nursing education that was attended by 350 nurses. The focus was to identify concerns and priorities in relation to nursing education. The forum was financed in part by the W.K. Kellogg Foundation.

Entry to practice continues to be a high priority for the CNA and the provinces. Remarkable progress has been made over the past 4 years in the design and implementation of collaborative efforts between university and diploma programs to attain the goal. All provincial nursing associations accepted the goal by 1988 with New Brunswick being the last to make the decision. Just 3 years later in 1991 Premier McKenna of New Brunswick became the first premier to commit his government to support the baccalaureate as entry point into nursing by the year 2000 (CNA Staff, September 1991a). Reference is made in Chapter 25 to the decisions taken in Prince Edward Island, British Columbia,

Alberta, Manitoba, Saskatchewan, New Brunswick, Nova Scotia, and Newfoundland to phase out one or more diploma programs and either replace or integrate them into baccalaureate degree programs (CNA Connection, 1989e; CNA News, 1989b; CNA Connection, 1991m; CNA Staff, June 1991b; CNA Staff, September 1991a; CNA Staff, September 1991b; CNA Staff, September 1991c; CNA Staff, March 1992a; CNA Staff, March 1992b; CNA Staff, June 1992; CNA Staff, September 1992; CNA Staff, Winter '92-93c; CNA Staff, Summer 1993a). Prince Edward Island became the first province to offer only baccalaureate as entry to nursing when their one diploma program was phased out and replaced by a Bachelor of Science in Nursing (BSN) program in 1991.

In Alberta in early 1990 the University of Alberta Faculty of Nursing and Red Deer College Department of Nursing announced their plan to provide an option for the college's diploma students to earn a baccalaureate degree while remaining on the Red Deer campus. The first two years of the university's baccalaureate degree program are offered by Red Deer College as a university transfer program, and students who choose take third year university courses taught by college faculty. In the fourth year courses are taught by university faculty using teleconferencing, self-learning modules, and on-site lectures. Clinical practice takes place in Red Deer clinical agencies, supervised by university faculty. For students who choose not to take the baccalaureate option at the end of 2 years, Red Deer College will also offer a diploma program of 23 weeks. The collaborative endeavour was designed over a 5-year period and is being implemented as a 5-year pilot project approved and funded by Alberta Advanced Education with a joint evaluation incorporated (University of Alberta, January 18, 1990). Also reported in Chapter 26 is the comprehensive collaboration between the University of Alberta Faculty of Nursing and four diploma programs in Edmonton (University of Alberta Hospitals, Royal Alexandra Hospital, Misericordia Hospital, and Grant McEwan Community College), launched in 1992. It provides opportunity for all students enrolled in the diploma programs to take the first 2 years of the baccalaureate program within their own schools and then proceed to the third and fourth years at the University of Alberta, or to not choose the baccalaureate option and complete a diploma program of 32 weeks. This model demonstrates the positive outcomes that can be achieved when each institution involved is able to "let go of the territorial boundaries associated with the existing programs and work toward the development of a new program" (Anderson et al, 1993, p. 30).

The most recent Alberta collaborative model between the University of Calgary and the diploma programs at Foothills Hospital and Mount Royal College, was implemented in September 1993. It has the potential of increasing the supply of baccalaureate graduates by 3.5 times and also offers the option of a diploma exit (CNA Staff, Summer 1993a). Most of the other collaborative programs offer the option of a diploma exit, namely the University of Saskatchewan and the Saskatchewan Institute of Applied Science and Technology (CNA Staff, June 1992), the University of Victoria and six colleges (CNA Staff, Summer 1993b), and the University of Manitoba and six diploma programs (CNA Staff, September 1991b). Four exceptions to date are the merger of the University of British Columbia and the Vancouver General Hospital Schools of Nursing (CNA Staff, Summer 1993a), Dalhousie University and two diploma programs in Nova Scotia (CNA Staff, September 1992), the Universities of New Brunswick and Moncton with five diploma programs in that province (CNA Staff, September 1991a), and Memorial University of Newfoundland with four diploma programs (CNA Staff, Winter '92-93b). All plan to offer only the baccalaureate degree exit. In Ontario with nine university programs and 23 diploma programs in colleges, the groupings for collaboration are more complex to design. However, two restructuring initiatives have been funded by the Ontario government and will help to move forward toward the goal of baccalaureate for entry to practice (CNA Staff, 1992-93a).

The CNA has been a strong proponent of graduate education in nursing also and urged the development of master's and doctoral programs so nurses would not have to go to the United States to undertake graduate study in nursing. As described in Chapter 32, the first master's program in nursing was established at the University of Western Ontario in 1959. There are now 13 master's programs in nursing with three established in the 1960s (McGill University, 1961, University of Montreal, 1965, University of British Columbia, 1968), four in the 1970s (University of Toronto, 1970, University of Alberta, 1975, Dalhousie University, 1975, University of Manitoba, 1979), three in the 1980s (University of Calgary, 1981, Memorial University of Newfoundland, 1982, University of Saskatchewan, 1986), and two in the 1990s (Laval University, 1991; and University of Ottawa, 1993). The University of Ottawa's program is the first master's program in nursing to be offered in both English and French (Edufacts, Winter '92-93b).

Efforts to establish a doctoral program in nursing in Canada began in 1978. In that year the CNA sponsored a national Seminar on Doctoral Preparation for Canadian Nurses, and published the *Proceedings* (Zilm, Larose and Stinson, 1979). An outgrowth of this seminar was the development by the CNA, CNF, and CAUSN of a proposal, "Operation Bootstrap," seeking $5.2 million from the W.K. Kellogg Foundation. Its purpose was to obtain establishment grants for PhD in Nursing programs, two nursing research consortia, emergency fellowships for doctoral preparation, as well as funding for communicating nursing research and maintaining an inventory of nurses with doctoral preparation. Unfortunately, funding was not granted.

Since 1978 several universities have initiated efforts to establish a PhD in Nursing program. In 1980 the nursing faculties at McGill University and l'Université de Montréal proposed a joint, bilingual program, but it was not approved. In the same year the University of Toronto approved in principle the development of a PhD in Nursing program, but their proposal was not approved. Consequently the faculty of nursing at that university obtained input into the PhD program offered by the Institute of Medicine there, so selected nurses could study in a program more closely related to their own discipline than doctoral programs in such disciplines as sociology, anthropology, and education. Nonetheless, the University of Toronto nursing faculty did not desist in their efforts to establish a PhD in Nursing program, nor did the nursing faculties at McGill University or l'Université de Montréal.

In 1986 the proposal for a PhD in Nursing program developed by the University of Alberta (UA) Faculty of Nursing, with input from the University of Calgary's Faculty of Nursing, was approved by the UA Board of Governors and the Alberta Universities Coordinating Council. When the Alberta government had still not provided funding by 1988, the Faculty of Nursing obtained approval to admit three predoctoral students on a "special case" basis, an option available on a very limited basis, in the absence of program funding. After 2 years of skilled lobbying by the nurses of Alberta, the PhD in Nursing program was funded by the Alberta government, effective January 1991. Thus the first doctoral program in nursing in Canada began with four students, including the three "special case" students and one new admission. To date, 17 predoctoral students have been admitted and three have graduated.

While efforts to obtain approval of the conjoint PhD in Nursing program continued at McGill University and l'Université de Montréal, McGill admitted three "special case" students and graduated their first one in October 1990 (CNA Staff, June 1991a). The second PhD in Nursing program in Canada was approved and funded at the University of British Columbia with the first two admissions in September 1991 (CNA Staff, September 1991c). The University of Toronto established the third such program in September 1993 with the admission of six predoctoral students (CNA Staff, Winter '92-93b). In May 1993 the conjoint program developed by McGill University and l'Université de Montréal was funded by the Quebec government. It became the fourth nursing doctoral program and the first bilingual program of its kind in Canada with predoctoral students admitted through both universities in September 1993 (CAUSN Staff, December 1993). The CNA has continued to promote doctoral education and provide a strong lobbying force for this important goal for nursing in Canada.

■■ ■■ ■■ ■■

NURSING RESEARCH

In addition to promoting graduate education in nursing, the CNA has been a very strong proponent of nursing research. Up until 1969 its only involvement in relation to research was emphasis on making the CNA Library the most outstanding collection of nursing literature in Canada. In 1969 the CNA submitted a brief to the Special Senate Committee on Science Policy, which included a statement "that research in nursing practice and more prepared nurse researchers are vital to the provision of health care for Canadians" (CNA, 1981, p. 18).

Further evidence of support for research and education was the allocation of $10,000 by the CNA to support the CNF, which was established in 1962 to provide financial support for nurses enrolled in baccalaureate and graduate programs, and finally in 1984 for small nursing research project grants up to $2500. The CNA's Board of Directors then appointed a special committee on nursing research in 1971. In 1978 this committee became a standing committee of the Association, one of only two standing committees in the organization. The other is the Committee on Testing, which is advisory to the CNA Testing Service. In 1976 the CNA's bylaws were amended to include a member-at-large for nursing research on the Board of Directors.

The CNA has strongly supported the series of 10 national nursing research conferences held between 1971 and 1985, as described in Chapter 12. CNA sponsored the 1977 conference on Research Methodology in Nursing Care in cooperation with the University of Ottawa with the aid of a grant from Health and Welfare Canada (CNA, 1981). The CNA has published research abstracts and a few research articles in *The Canadian Nurse*. Reference has been made to the "Operation Bootstrap" proposal, which sought funding for both nursing research and doctoral education.

In 1980 the CNA published the first inventory of Canadian nursing doctoral statistics, reporting 81 nurses with an earned doctorate and 72 nurses enrolled in doctoral study (Larsen and Stinson, 1980). An update in 1982 reported 124 with an earned doctorate and 121 enrolled in doctoral study (Stinson, Larsen, & MacPhail, 1984). A second update in 1986 reported 193 nurses with an earned doctorate and 224 enrolled in doctoral study (Stinson, MacPhail, & Larsen, 1988). A third update in 1989 reported 257 nurses holding an earned doctorate and 265 nurses enrolled in doctoral study (Stinson and Lamb, 1990). The data reflect notable increases in the number of nurses prepared at the doctoral level and the number of nurses engaged in doctoral study; however, the proportion of those with a focus principally in nursing remains small, at 23 percent (CNA Connection, 1991f). The findings also emphasize the need for more nurses prepared at this educational level, particularly with a major in nursing. It is hoped that this will be facilitated by the development of the four PhD in Nursing programs established to date, although the constraints imposed by decreases in educational funding will serve as deterrents unless priority is given to doctoral education.

One of the major accomplishments of the CNA's Committee on Nursing Research in the 1980s was the publication in 1984 of *The Research Imperative*, a 10-year plan for nursing research in Canada. It included recommendations for the establishment of at least one, and preferably several, PhD in Nursing programs, as well as increased funding for nursing research. A major problem has been and continues to be a dearth of funding for nursing research. Although Medical Research Council (MRC) funds are supposed to be available to nurses, very few nurses have been able to obtain funding from this source because preference is given to medical research and to investigators with a track record. Although a nurse was appointed to the MRC in 1971, this was a 1-year term only and did not result in increased funding for nursing research. A special nursing committee, appointed by the MRC, presented a proposal to the Council in 1985 recommending separate funding for nursing research and the establishment of a doctoral program in nursing. However, the MRC failed to produce a response after the report was tabled. Active lobbying efforts were finally effective in obtaining the appointment of another nurse, the Executive Director of the CNA, to the MRC in 1986 for a 3-year term. It was hoped that having nursing representation on the MRC would prove to be effective in accomplishing the goals for funding of nursing research and doctoral education in nursing; however, this has not happened.

In 1987 the MRC, in collaboration with the National Health Research and Development Program (NHRDP) of the Health Promotion Directorate, Health and Welfare Canada, announced a new competitive research funding program to support programmatic research in nursing. Universities were invited to submit letters of intent to develop a research program around a central theme. Seventeen letters of intent were submitted from the 27 university nursing faculties/schools; six were invited to submit full proposals (Alberta, McGill, McMaster, Montreal, Ottawa, and Toronto). All took advantage of the opportunity and expended a great deal of time and effort in the process; however, the outcome was very disappointing with no proposals approved. Instead, three career awards were made to individuals in different universities to support research that was part of the total research program proposals. Once again efforts by nurses to gain access to MRC research funds failed. Nursing still has less than 1 percent of the health sciences research funding in Canada. Moreover, when the term of the nurse appointee to the MRC expired in 1989, she was replaced by a physiotherapist. Another nurse was appointed to the MRC in 1991. Although she was not nominated by the CNA or CAUSN, there is communication between her and both organizations (CAUSN Staff, September 1992).

CNA's Nursing Research Committee has continued to work on new approaches to increase nursing research endeavours and research funding. During the 1986-88 biennium the committee presented to the CNA Board of Directors a proposal to develop a Canadian Centre for Nursing Research. The intent was to design this centre to stimulate and coordinate research in nursing across Canada through programmatic and multi-site research of national relevance. The board of the proposed centre was to include representation from the CNA and the CNF, CAUSN, the Canadian Nursing Research Interest Group, major funding bodies, and the public (CNA Connection, 1988c). Although the boards of the CNA, CNF, and the Canadian Nursing Research Interest Group supported the proposal, CAUSN's Board did not. Because their support was considered essential for the project to succeed, no further action was taken on the proposal (CNA Connection, 1989n).

In 1990 the CNA Board "approved a revised Research Imperative as the strategic plan for nursing research for 1990-93, as well as a new mandate for the Research Committee for 1990-92" (CNA Connection, 1990a, p. 11). In addition to providing consultation and advice related to research matters and initiating actions specified in the Research Imperative, the committee is to strengthen relations with CAUSN, CNF and the Canadian Nursing Research Group (CNRG) to facilitate the advancement of nursing research in Canada (CNA Connection, 1990a). One of their recommendations accepted by the Board in 1992 was to seek funding from the CNF "for a nurse historian to write a history of nursing research in Canada that reflects the role of CNA in its development" (CNA Connection, 1992d, p. 8).

During the 1990-92 and subsequent bienniums the CNA continued to lobby vigorously for both recognition and funding of nursing research, including the submission of a brief to the Royal Society of Canada's University Research Committee. The presentation included infrastructure models to support nursing research in Canada (CNA Connection, 1991i). Two new nursing research grants were established and administered through the CNF, namely the $15,000 Dorothy J. Kergin Research Grant in primary health care and the $10,000

Pharmaceutical Manufacturers Association of Canada Health Research Foundation/CNF Research Grant (CNA Connection, 1991g).

▬ ▬ ▬ ▬

NURSING ADMINISTRATION

Because of the general focus on functional nursing in the early years of the development of nursing, it is logical that the CNA attended to issues and needs pertaining to nursing administration. This is reflected in the historical record of CNA actions in this domain. The first reference found was a "Report on Nursing Service," submitted by the CNA in 1926 at the request of the federal Department of Health. The report "contained statistical data; statement of issues and trends in nursing; the increasing difficulties of recruitment and the large number of drop-outs; the need to reduce wastage and conserve nurse power" (CNA, 1968, p. 85). In 1943 the CNA cooperated with the National Selective Service and the Canadian Medical Procurement and Assignment Board in conducting a survey of nursing service in Canada. The study disclosed a shortage of general duty nurses and recommended improved salaries and working conditions, comparable to other occupations requiring equivalent preparation, to alleviate the shortage and attract the quality of student desired (CNA, 1968).

Concern about the role of the nurse administrator and the lack of preparation for administrative positions was reflected at mid-century. In 1953 the CNA conducted a study of the functions and activities of head nurses in a general hospital, which led to publication of a manual for head nurses in 1960. In the early 1960s nurses could obtain 1-year certificate preparation in nursing administration, designed to provide them with better preparation for assuming administrative responsibilities. With elimination of these certificate programs and increased emphasis on post-RN baccalaureate preparation, there was continued concern about the preparation of nurses for administrative roles. The problem centred on the fact that few courses in management were included in baccalaureate programs, which emphasized clinical preparation. As a result other alternatives were developed. An example is the collaboration of the CNA and the CHA in 1961 to develop an extension course in nursing unit administration, which resulted in the Nursing Unit Administration Program, a home-study, distance-education program that still exists.

Because of continued concern about problems in nursing service and the preparation of nurses for administrative roles, in 1963 the CNA became a member of the Canadian Joint Committee on Nursing, as did the Canadian Medical Association (CMA) and the CHA. Each organization had equal representation, a pattern that continues today. In the same year a brief presented to the Royal Commission on Health Services by the CNA made 25 recommendations for the improvement of nursing service within the health services of Canada (CNA, 1968).

In 1966 the CNA published three major studies that had been initiated in 1960. One was an evaluation of the quality of nursing service. As a means of promoting improvement the CNA sought opportunities for involvement in the Canadian Council on Hospital Accreditation. Thus a CNA representative was appointed to the Canadian Council on Hospital Accreditation Standards

Committee in 1969, and the CNA obtained a seat on the Canadian Council on Hospital Accreditation in 1973 and a second seat in 1976. Such involvement in policy making and decision making about accreditation allowed nurses' views to be heard. Nurse surveyors have been included on the hospital accreditation teams since 1974. In 1969 the CNA published *Standards for Nursing Service in Health Care Facilities, A Self-evaluation Guide* to help nursing personnel evaluate their service in the light of established philosophy and objectives (CNA, 1981, p. 18).

In 1980 at the CNA Biennial Convention the membership asked that the CNA study the education of nurses for nursing administration (CNA, 1981). The CNA commissioned a paper by Leatt (1981) to delineate issues and make recommendations on the education of nurses for nursing administration. The publication *Education for Nursing Administration in Canada: A Discussion Paper* "described the state of the art of education for nursing administration in Canada, identified some of the critical issues related to preparation for nursing administrative positions in nursing, and outlined some possible strategies for the future" (CNA, 1985, p. 1).

After this paper was published the CNA Board established an ad hoc committee to clarify the role of the nurse administrator at various levels in health care organizations, to develop standards for nursing administration, and to critically review the quality and availability of existing educational programs in nursing administration. At a time when the entire Canadian health-care system was undergoing review, the committee produced a publication (CNA, 1982), *Position Paper on the Role of the Nurse Administrator and Standards for Nursing Administration*, that was widely circulated because of the urgent need for change and the significance of the area. The CNA Board of Directors decided to give priority to nursing administration in the 1984-86 biennium; another ad hoc Committee on Nursing Administration was established and charged with responsibility for developing a national plan for nursing administration. Lorine Besel, then president of the CNA, stated, "Our profession urgently needs politically and economically astute leaders who have a solid background in management, a broad philosophical perspective on health services and a clear vision of the type of health care system we ultimately want to see in place" (CNA, 1985, p. 1).

A National Plan for Nursing Administration in Canada, recommended by the committee and approved by the Board of Directors in 1985, included objectives, strategies for attaining them, and target dates, and designated groups to be involved. One of the objectives was to enhance educational opportunities for nursing administrators, a continuing major inadequacy in the nursing education system and a concern for nursing administrators (CNA Connection, 1986a). The ad hoc committee also recommended to the CNA Board regular monitoring of the National Plan at the beginning of each biennium to ensure continued attention to its implementation. The National Plan is still monitored and some progress has been made in its implementation. In December 1987 a joint meeting was held for representatives from the CNA, CAUSN, CHA, CPHA and the Canadian Council of Health Service Executives (CCHSE). The main topic of discussion was continuing education for nurse administrators. Priorities established were to promote support for universities to develop continuing education programs and to increase access to educational opportunities for nursing administrators who do not have access to university programs (CNA Board of Directors Minutes, February 18-19, 1988). In 1989 representatives from the same five organizations collaborated again to develop a strategic plan for the education of nursing administrators. "It includes objectives of increasing the number of graduate degree programs to prepare nurse administrators, providing additional continuing education opportunities and working to increase the understanding of issues faced by nurse administrators" (CNA Connection, 1989g, p. 5).

Subsequently staff from the five organizations met to develop a plan to implement the 1989 Joint Strategies for Nursing Administration. The two major thrusts endorsed by the CNA Board were access to educational programs in nursing administration and advocacy initiatives (CNA Connection, 1990b).

During the 1986-88 biennium nursing groups that discussed the National Plan for Nursing Administration, and other national association groups identified the need to update the position paper on the Role of the Nurse Administrator and Standards for Nursing Administration that had been published in l983. The new document (CNA, 1988) "attempted to balance the professional and corporate aspects of current nursing administration and to address the complex issues faced by nursing administrators today" (CNA, 1988, p. v). It should serve as an excellent resource to practising and potential nursing administrators, to teachers in nursing administration, and to other admistrators in all types of health-care agencies whose support is so vital to attaining the goals of nursing administrators and the nursing staff to whom they provide leadership.

■■ ■■ ■■ ■■

HEALTH-CARE REFORM

One of the CNA's long-term objectives has been to promote changes in the health-care system to use nurses' abilities more fully. Another objective is to place more emphasis on health promotion and maintenance and less emphasis on illness care in use of funds and priorities in programming. In 1984 the CNA had a major influence on the development of the Canada Health Act. CNA members lobbied vigorously against extra billing and user fees, and were successful in obtaining an amendment to the Canada Health Act to include "other health professionals" as potentially qualifying for reimbursement for services by the federal government. This meant that health-care providers other than physicians and dentists could be named as entry points to the health-care system in provincial health-care plans. This was a notable achievement because it was the only amendment made in the Canada Health Act and it provided an example of the potential power of lobbying efforts when nurses remain unified. As a result of this change the CNA is promoting reform of the health-care system to enable nurses to assume greater responsibility, and function more effectively in the system. Such a change has implications for health-care costs because nurses can deliver quality care at decreased cost, particularly in health promotion and health maintenance.

In the 1988-90 biennium, the CNA published a major paper on health-care reform that calls for the creation of a primary health-care infrastructure in

Canada by restructuring and reforming the present health-care system. This comprehensive document mandates a health-care system that is accessible, provides equal emphasis on promotion and prevention with curative care, encompasses lay participation, promotes cooperation with other disciplines and government departments, and uses appropriate technology. The CNA confirms a strong commitment to "continue to work within nursing and with other disciplines, consumers and politicians to ensure that a primary health-care system is implemented" (CNA, 1988, p. 30; CNA Connection, 1989f).

In keeping with the CNA's firm belief in the need for health-care reform, the CNA published *Health Care Reform for Seniors* in 1990. The major assumption in this document is that "the current organization of the health-care system presents barriers for seniors in Canada and therefore requires reform. Other assumptions are: (l) seniors wish to maintain their independence for as long as possible, and (2) the present health-care system is bureaucratic and crisis-oriented and it is, therefore, difficult for seniors to access appropriate services" (CNA 1990, p. 1). The strategies set forth are based on the five principles of primary health care. The role of the nurse in the proposed reformed system is described as "direct care provider, teacher/educator of health personnel and the public, the supervisor and manager of primary health-care services, and researcher and evaluator of health care" (CNA, March, 1989).

Beginning in October 1987 the CNA's work in relation to health-care reform focused on mental health, the elderly and children. In 1991 a discussion paper, *Mental Health Care Reform*, was published that identified five key areas in need of reform: "accessibility; public participation; health promotion and prevention; cooperation; and appropriate technology" (CNA Connection, 1991h, p. 4). The CNA advocated a cost-effective system based in the community with nurses coordinating care in community health centres, linking consumers to a full range of treatment and support services, and emphasizing mental health promotion and prevention of illness, and in time reducing costs (CNA Connection, 1991h).

With reform of the health-care system and influencing national health policy as top priorities, the CNA joined a lobby group, the Health Action Lobby (HEAL), in 1991. It is a coalition of seven national health care organizations (CNA, CMA, CHA, CPHA, Canadian Long Term Care Association, Canadian Psychological Association, Consumers' Association of Canada) dedicated to saving the principles of medicare and thrusting health into the federal spotlight (CNA Connection, 1991j). By 1993 HEAL had expanded to include 26 national health and consumer groups working together to make health care a key issue in the federal election. Their election messages emphasized Canada's health care system as one of the best in the world; the need to reform but not replace the system to control costs and thereby help to reduce the deficit; and the importance of collaboration by governments, consumers, and HEAL to find solutions (CNA Today, August 1993).

■ ■ ■ ▀

CONCLUSION

The CNA clearly recognizes the importance of collaboration with other health professionals and their professional organizations in addressing problems and in endeavouring to reform the health-care system. The CNA has endorsed the formation of a Canada Health Council that has had input from 11 national professional associations. The proposed Canada Health Council would have a primary purpose of providing a national and independent perspective on health and health-related issues. It would identify important issues in maintenance and enhancement of health and health-care delivery in Canada, and through research and analysis, would seek ways to improve the health of Canadians. It would also provide objective information on the costs and benefits of existing services and new technologies (CNA Connection, 1986d). Involvement in the development of this council and in other joint endeavours reflects the CNA's goals of collaborating with others, being an integral part of future-oriented projects that have important implications for the health care system of the future in Canada, and the meaningful involvement of nurses in that system.

REFERENCES

Alberta Association of Registered Nurses. (1976). *Response to the Alberta Task Force on Nursing Education.* Edmonton, Alberta: Author.

Anderson, H.M., Day, R.A., Gibson, B.A., Profetts-McGrath, J., Shantz, S.J. & Young, N.J. (1993). Innovation through collaboration. *The Canadian Nurse, 89*(4), 29-30.

Canadian Association of University Schools of Nursing. (September 1992). *CAUSN Newsletter/ACEUN—Bulletin d'Information,* p. 1.

Canadian Association of University Schools of Nursing. (December 1993). *CAUSN Newsletter/ACEUN—Bulletin d'Information,* p. 3.

Canadian Nurses Association. (1968). *The leaf and the lamp.* Ottawa: Author.

Canadian Nurses Association. (1981). *The seventh decade 1969-1980.* Ottawa: Author.

Canadian Nurses Association. (1982). *Entry to the practice of nursing: A background paper.* Ottawa: Author.

Canadian Nurses Association. (1982). *Position paper on the role of the nurse administrator and standards for nursing administration.* Ottawa: Author.

Canadian Nurses Association. (1984). *The research imperative.* Ottawa: Author.

Canadian Nurses Association. (1985). *A national plan for nursing administration in Canada.* Ottawa: Author.

Canadian Nurses Association. (1988). *Health for all Canadians: A call for health care reform.* Ottawa: Author.

Canadian Nurses Association. (1988). *The role of the nurse administrator and standards for nursing administration.* Ottawa: Author.

Canadian Nurses Association. (March 1989). *Position statement on the nurse's role in primary health care.* Ottawa: Author

Canadian Nurses Association. (1990). *Health care reform for seniors.* Ottawa: Author.

Canadian Nurses Association Advisory Council Minutes, June 21, 1986.

Canadian Nurses Association Board of Directors' Minutes, February 18-20, 1987.

Canadian Nurses Association Board of Directors' Minutes, February 18-19, 1988.

CAUSN Staff. (September 1992). *CAUSN Newsletter/CAUSN ACUEN-Bulletin d'Informacion,* p. 2

CAUSN Staff. (December 1993). *CAUSN Newsletter/CAUSN ACEUN-Bulletin d'Informacion,* p. 3.

CNA Connection. (1986a). New national plan unveiled for nursing administration. *The Canadian Nurse, 82*(1), 11.

CNA Connection. (1986b). Smoking and health. *The Canadian Nurse, 82*(3), 12.

CNA Connection. (1986c). Committee on health issues: smoking. *The Canadian Nurse, 82*(4), 9-10.

CNA Connection. (1986d). 1986 Biennial convention report. *The Canadian Nurse, 82*(9), 16-20.

CNA Connection. (1986e). CNA position on smoking and health. *The Canadian Nurse, 82*(10), 8.

CNA Connection. (1987). Certification project now complete. *The Canadian Nurse, 83*(1), 7.

CNA Connection. (1988a). CNA initiates protective liability plan. *The Canadian Nurse, 84*(2), 7.

CNA Connection. (1988b). CNA statement on tobacco and health. *The Canadian Nurse, 84*(4), 10.

CNA Connection. (1988c). Nursing research. *The Canadian Nurse, 84*(8), 18.

CNA Connection. (1989a). Despite deficit, practice issues prevail. *The Canadian Nurse, 85*(1), 7.

CNA Connection. (1989b). Nurse retention study. *The Canadian Nurse, 85*(1), 8.

CNA Connection. (1989c). Work-life affairs position reaffirmed. *The Canadian Nurse, 85*(1), 8.

CNA Connection. (1989d). Mandatory drug screening. *The Canadian Nurse, 85*(2), 10.

CNA Connection. (1989e). Baccalaureate comes to PEI. *The Canadian Nurse, 85*(3), 10.

CNA Connection. (1989f). CNA endorses primary health care. *The Canadian Nurse, 85*(5), 8.

CNA Connection. (1989g). Strategic plan for administrators. *The Canadian Nurse, 85*(5), 5.

CNA Connection. (1989h). Work-life focus of conference. *The Canadian Nurse, 85*(5), 8.

CNA Connection. (1989i). Work-life issues. *The Canadian Nurse, 85*(6), 10.

CNA Connection. (1989j). Focus: Nursing practice. *The Canadian Nurse, 85*(8), 10.

CNA Connection. (1989k). Nursing research. *The Canadian Nurse, 85*(8), 10.

CNA Connection. (1989l). Smoking cessation project funded. *The Canadian Nurse, 85*(9), 10.

CNA Connection. (1989m). Specialization stimulates debate. *The Canadian Nurse, 85*(9), 10.

CNA Connection. (1989n). September 15 meeting with the Minister of Health and Welfare re: MRC. *The Canadian Nurse, 85*(10), 8.

CNA Connection. (1990a). Nursing research. *The Canadian Nurse, 86*(5), 11.

CNA Connection. (1990b). Joint strategies for nursing administration. *The Canadian Nurse, 86*(5), 11.

CNA Connection. (1990c). CNA's position statement on nurses and the environment. *The Canadian Nurse, 86*(6), 4

CNA Connection. (1990d). Ritchie's parting words. *The Canadian Nurse, 86*(8), 15

CNA Connection. (1990e). A focus on clinical practice issues. *The Canadian Nurse, 86*(8), 16.

CNA Connection. (1990f). Field testing of neuroscience exam. *The Canadian Nurse, 86*(9), 8.

CNA Connection. (1991a). Work environment must change. *The Canadian Nurse, 87*(2), 6.

CNA Connection. (1991b). Nurses and smoking. *The Canadian Nurse, 87*(2), 6.

CNA Connection. (1991c). Quality of worklife and safe workplaces subjects of CNA statements. *The Canadian Nurse, 87*(3), 4.

CNA Connection. (1991d). AIDS education for nurses receives financial boost. *The Canadian Nurse, 87*(3), 4.

CNA Connection. (1991e). Certification update. *The Canadian Nurse, 87*(5), 10.

CNA Connection. (1991f). Canadian Nursing Doctoral statistics. *The Canadian Nurse, 87*(6), 4.

CNA Connection. (1991g). Research grants. *The Canadian Nurse, 87*(6), 4.

CNA Connection. (1991h). A new direction for mental health reform. *The Canadian Nurse, 87*(6), 4.

CNA Connection. (1991i). Act now or miss opportunity, warns Baumgart. *The Canadian Nurse, 87*(8), 9.

CNA Connection. (1991j). Future of health care consumes board agenda. *The Canadian Nurse, 87*(8), 10.

CNA Connection. (1991k). AIDS consultations a success. *The Canadian Nurse, 87*(9), 4.

CNA Connection. (1991l). Violence against women. *The Canadian Nurse, 87*(10), 10.

CNA Connection. (1991m). Education newsletter launched. *The Canadian Nurse 87*(10), 10.

CNA Connection. (1992a). Certification. *The Canadian Nurse, 88*(1), 6-7.

CNA Connection. (1992b). Lay-offs, rumors and anxiety. *The Canadian Nurse, 88*(4), 4.

CNA Connection. (1992c). Technology, HIV/AIDS & health promotion on agenda. *The Canadian Nurse, 88*(5), 8.

CNA Connection. (1992d). Research activities. *The Canadian Nurse, 88*(5), 8.

CNA Connection. (1992e). Baumgart steps down. *The Canadian Nurse, 88*(8), 9-10.

CNA Connection. (1992f). Nursing practice conferences. *The Canadian Nurse, 88*(10), 4.

CNA Connection. (1993a). CNA committed to certification. *The Canadian Nurse, 89*(1), 8.

CNA Connection. (1993b). Interest group status. *The Canadian Nurse, 89*(5), 10.

CNA News. (1989). VGH school joins UBC. *The Canadian Nurse, 85*(2), 12.

CNA Staff. (June 1991a). The PhD comes to Canada. *Edufacts, 1*(1), 1.

CNA Staff. (June 1991b). VGH/UBC prepare for third year of collaboration: Universities and diploma school match minds. *Edufacts, 1*(1), 3.

CNA Staff. (September 1991a). NB for BN: Province joins nurses' call for degree. *Edufacts, 1*(2), 1.

CNA Staff. (September 1991b). Manitoba phasing out two programs: Joint program begins. *Edufacts, 1*(2), 1 and 4.

CNA Staff. (September 1991c). UBC gets PhD. *Edufacts, 1*(2), 2.

CNA Staff. (September 1991d). Towards an all-baccalaureate system: The Edmonton collaboration nursing program. *Edufacts, 1*(2), 4.

CNA Staff. (March 1992a). Building a degree nursing program in PEI. *Edufacts, 2*(1), 1 and 4.

CNA Staff. (March 1992b). University-college collaboration in B.C.: A new program incorporates participatory learning, praxis and humanism. *Edufacts*, 2(1), 3.

CNA Staff. (June 1992). Collaboration among all Saskatchewan nursing schools. *Edufacts*, 2(2), 4.

CNA Staff. (September 1992). New BN education - Nova Scotia style: Three nursing schools collaborate to offer a baccalaureate program. *Edufacts*, 2(3), 1.

CNA Staff. (Winter '92-93a). Ontario edging closer to entry to practice? *Edufacts*, 2(4), 1 and 3.

CNA Staff. (Winter '92-93b). New PhD and master's programs in Ontario. *Edufacts*, 2(4), 1 and 3.

CNA Staff. (Winter '92-93c). Joint funding for Newfoundland collaboration. *Edufacts*, 2(4), 4.

CNA Staff. (Summer 1993a). Calgary conjoint nursing program: A dream realized. *Edufacts*, 3(2), 1.

CNA Staff. (Summer 1993b). B.C. on target for B.N.: Collaboration leaps ahead with new partnerships. *Edufacts*, 3(2), 1 and 4.

CNA Staff. (August 1993). Working together to heal Canada's health care system. *CNA Today*, 3(3), 3.

Larsen, J., and Stinson, S.M. (1980). *Canadian nursing doctoral statistics 1980*. Ottawa: Canadian Nurses Association.

Leatt, P. (1981). *Education for nursing administration in Canada: A discussion paper*. Ottawa: Canadian Nurses Association.

Remkes, T. (December 1991). Life in the lobby lane. *CNA Today*, 1(3), 6.

Ritchie, Judith A. (1988). Editorial. On becoming president. *The Canadian Nurse*, 84(8), 3.

Stinson, S.M., Larsen, J., and MacPhail, J: (1984). *Canadian nursing doctoral statistics: 1982 update*. Ottawa: Canadian Nurses Association.

Stinson, S.M., MacPhail, J., and Larsen, J. (1986). *Canadian nursing doctoral statistics: 1986 update*. Ottawa: Canadian Nurses Association.

Stinson, S.M., and Lamb, M. (1990). *Canadian nursing doctoral statistics: 1989 update*. Ottawa: Canadian Nurses Association.

University of Alberta. Collaborative nursing program with Red Deer College approved. *Folio*. January 18, 1990, p.3.

Zilm, G., Larose, O., and Stinson, S. (1979). *Proceedings of the Kellogg National Seminar on Doctoral Education for Canadian Nurses*. Ottawa: Canadian Nurses Association.

CHAPTER FIVE

The Professional Image: Impact and Strategies for Change

JANNETTA MacPHAIL

I n the 1980s the image of nursing became the centre of much attention in nursing literature and in deliberations of professional associations. It is also of concern to nurse educators seeking to attract the best students into nursing, to nurse administrators endeavouring to staff health-care agencies, to nurse researchers who encounter difficulty in explaining nursing research to others, and to all nurses who encounter negative or indifferent responses when identifying themselves as nurses in social situations. The Canadian Nurses Association's (CNA) Board of Directors made the nursing image a top priority for the 1986-88 and 1988-90 bienniums. Their goal was "to develop a plan of strategic actions to enhance the image of nurses and nursing" (CNA Connection, 1987, p. 7). In addressing the issue of the image of nursing it is important to reflect on historical and current factors that influence the image of nurses and nursing. Such a perspective is needed to determine what can be done to enhance the image and who might or should be involved in addressing this important issue.

■ ■ ■ ■

EXTERNAL AND INTERNAL IMAGES

One often hears or reads about the image of nursing as if there were only one image. Nursing actually has many images, because nurses relate to a variety of audiences. For example, the image presented to attract students or to recruit nurses in health-care agencies is different from the image presented to legislators whose main concern is cost-effectiveness. These are external images; internal images are the views that nurses have of themselves as individuals and of the profession. In examining studies of nursing images conducted through 1964, Simmons and Henderson (1964, p. 222) found:

> . . . two popular and competing images of the nurse . . . At one pole is the image of
> the humanitarian and altruistic person, more or less competent and endowed with

54

sympathy, compassion, and exceptional capacities for establishing rapport—one who gives of herself. At the other pole is the image of the professional, well-trained, technically efficient and cool-headed individual who can be relied upon for able performance within her specialty, and relatively independent of feeling components—one who may seem to keep herself out of her work.

Probably few nurses can be classified at the two extremes; most fit at various points between the two poles.

Emanating from the time of the Romans, the first persons identified with the nurse role were wealthy Roman matrons who gave nurturance, self-sacrifice, and mothering. Nursing continues to be sex stereotyped even though those who cared for the injured during the Crusades were men. Today some men are entering nursing. The proportion of male nurses in Canada and the United States continues to be very limited, at 3.5% (Statistics Canada, 1994) and 4.0% (USPHS, 1994), respectively. The proportion in the United Kingdom is considerably higher at approximately 10% (Gaze, 1987; Skevington and Dawkes, 1988).

Images of any profession or work group are influenced by the values and orientations learned from family and friends, and by individuals' experiences with particular members of a profession. Images are also influenced by the mass media, particularly with today's variety of media. Two recent studies of the public's perception of nurses and nursing found that respondents' views were strongly influenced by personal contact with nurses or the experiences of others (Lippman and Ponton, 1989; Payne, Cook, and Associates, 1990; Giovannetti, 1990). Hence observational learning is an important means of developing images of various professions, including nursing. Such learning promotes a concept of a particular profession and has great impact on how a profession is regarded by members of society and how attractive the profession is to individuals.

■ ■ ■ ■

THE MASS MEDIA AND THE IMAGE OF NURSES AND NURSING

Kalisch and Kalisch (1982) surveyed mass media products, pertaining to nursing, from the past century and a half. These included: "the print media (200 novels, 143 magazine short stories, poems and articles and 20,000 newspaper clippings), as well as the newer non-print media (204 motion pictures, 122 radio programs, and 320 television episodes)" (p. 5). From these products they classified the image into five dominant types characterizing five successive time periods.

The "Angel of Mercy" image of the nurse was portrayed "as noble, moral, religious, virginal, ritualistic and self-sacrificing" (Kalisch and Kalisch, 1982, p. 7). Although it has been said that Florence Nightingale epitomized this image, she was a scholar and has been termed the first nurse researcher. Nightingale's achievements were astounding. She saved the lives of many wounded soldiers during the Crimean War; she restored order from chaos by assuming responsibility for the soldiers' environment as well as nursing care, despite strong resistance from the physicians in charge; and she brought innovation and advancement to the fields of nursing, health, and hospital planning. Nightingale was of high social class, well educated, and a true scholar. If her model for nursing had been followed, the nursing profession would be in a much more advantageous position today. The "Angel of Mercy" image, as identified by Kalisch and Kalisch, existed from 1854 to 1919. It continued through World War I, when nurses were presented by the media as noble and heroic. A typical film from that time period portrayed the nurse enlisting in the service to be near her sweetheart, finding him wounded, and restoring him to health (Kalisch and Kalisch, 1982).

The next image, "Girl Friday," existed from 1920 to 1929; it was very different and reflected considerable deterioration. The nurse was portrayed as "subservient, cooperative, methodical, dedicated, modest, and loyal" (Kalisch and Kalisch, 1982, p. 11). In essence she served as a handmaiden, an image that grew out of the deprofessionalization of nursing that occurred in the 1920s with declining standards of nursing education. The decline was the result of a proliferation of hospitals accompanied by schools of nursing to staff them, as well as poor working conditions and the ruthless exploitation of students. Some of these conditions continued into the 1940s, although the image of the nurse as portrayed by the media changed.

The third image, "The Heroine," existed from 1930 to 1945, when the media portrayed the nurse as "brave, rational, dedicated, decisive, humanistic, and autonomous" (Kalisch and Kalisch, 1982, p. 11). Motion pictures in the 1930s and 1940s depicted this image. Biographies were written about heroines such as Florence Nightingale; Edith Cavell, who was shot by a German firing squad during World War I for helping wounded soldiers escape; and Sister Kenney, whose treatment of poliomyelitis victims enabled many to recover muscle function at a time when the victims were being kept immobilized by the medical profession. Adventure dramas about air or sea travel involved nurse heroines. Airlines required flight attendants to be graduate nurses. Delivering babies, assisting in emergency surgery, and even landing the plane safely when pilots were disabled were among the heroic acts of flight attendants portrayed in movies and other media (Kalisch and Kalisch, 1982). World War II intensified the "Heroine" image; nurses were portrayed very positively on recruitment posters. Many volunteered for military service and were highly regarded by society. When television became available in the mid-1950s, the "Heroine" image was portrayed to a larger audience.

The fourth image, "the Mother Image," existed from 1945 to 1965. It seems almost incredible that women went home to function as wives and mothers after enduring the hardships of war, but they did. At that time the place for married women was perceived to be in the home, and society frowned on working mothers. Although nursing remained a high status occupation for women, nurse characters were portrayed by the media as "maternal, nurturing, sympathetic, passive, expressive, and domestic" (Kalisch and Kalisch, 1982, p. 15).

As this image faded in the mid-1960s, the most negative media image of the nurse since Dickens' imbibing Sairey Gamp developed—the nurse as a "Sex Object." This negative image that portrayed the nurse as "a sensual, romantic, hedonistic, frivolous, irresponsible, promiscuous individual" (Kalisch and Kalisch, 1982, p. 17) continues today on television and particularly in movies. This image is readily identified in such television programs as "M*A*S*H" and "Trapper John, M.D." The nurse is depicted as a sex object with no evidence of being intellectual or professional. The nurse is also depicted as a sex object on greeting cards and in advertisements.

The ideal image, proposed by Kalisch and Kalisch (1982), is "The Careerist," "an intelligent, logical, progressive, sophisticated, empathic, and assertive woman or man who is committed to attaining higher and higher standards of health care" (p. 21). To what extent has such an image been achieved? Do nurses perceive themselves in this image? What can be done to promote such an image?

■ ■ ■ ■

PUBLIC'S PERCEPTION OF NURSES AND NURSING

During the past decade nurses have become increasingly concerned about their image and its effect on recruitment into nursing programs and the retention of nurses in the workforce. One way to address these concerns is to conduct studies to ascertain the public's perceptions of nurses and nursing as a career to obtain data for formulating plans of action.

Lippman and Ponton (1989) conducted a survey of faculty in all disciplines in 19 northeastern United States universities with accredited baccalaureate degree programs in nursing. They obtained perceptions of nurses and nursing from a random sample of 535 faculty members, 11% of whom were nursing faculty. The 42-item questionnaire, developed by the investigators from literature and their experience, focused on three categories: images of nursing practice, attitudes about nursing education, and the nurse as a sex symbol. Most of the respondents, as indicated by the demographic data collected, had nurse friends or colleagues or had been cared for by a nurse. The findings reflected a different and more positive view of nursing than that presented by the media. Nurses were perceived as "educated, autonomous and compassionate individuals whose role is vital to health care" (Lippman and Ponton, 1989, p. 27). They were viewed as knowledgeable about good health, and as good sources of information about health and its promotion. The majority did not perceive nurses as handmaidens to physicians and believed nurses should be treated as equals to physicians. Most were not averse to their daughters entering nursing, although 18% stated that "bright young women should study medicine rather than nursing." The investigators indicated that the responses may have been influenced by the personal contact the respondents had had with nurses. It is also possible that nursing faculty had communicated effectively about nursing and nursing education within the 19 universities from which the sample was drawn.

Because of past concerns about the nursing shortage and how to attract more people to nursing, a survey was conducted in Indiana to ascertain the public's attitudes, values and beliefs about nursing as a career. Subjects included college freshmen (27.1%), students in grades 6 through 12 (29.6%), and "enablers" (those who had potential to influence career selection). The "enablers" included parents (29.2%), teachers and counsellors (7.3%), and school nurses (6.8%). The subjects were selected at random from these categories. Questionnaire items were designed to determine attitudes about the "ideal career" compared with nursing as a career, and were derived from literature on careers and nursing. The findings indicated that, for these respondents, nursing and the ideal career were similar in "opportunities for employment, use of intellectual abilities, caring for people as a career attribute, need for academic achievement, and scholastic achievement as a prerequisite for career development" (May, Austin, and Champion, 1988, p. 7).

However, an ideal career was viewed as "more financially rewarding, more respected, more appreciated, and more powerful," providing "more opportunities for leadership, more safety in the workplace, more opportunities for making decisions, and more opportunities for obtaining and applying knowledge," and involving "less emphasis on manual skills, less utilization of high technology, lighter workload, and easier work" (May et al., 1988, p. 7). Differences were noted in the respondent subgroups. "School-age students had more positive attitudes toward nursing as a career than other groups, and parents and school-age students valued nursing more than other groups" (May et al., 1988, p. 26). Based on the findings, a number of recommendations were made to enhance the positive attitudes and improve the negative perceptions, including ways to increase respect and appreciation for nurses, reduce workloads, promote more autonomy in practice and more safety in the workplace, achieve more competitive salaries, increase leadership opportunities and empowerment of nurses, and place less emphasis on manual skills and high technology in publicity materials. Many of the recommendations reiterate strategies that nurses have advocated for years, both as individuals and as members of study commissions established to address the problems of recruitment and retention in nursing.

Another study was part of a "Public Image of Nursing Campaign" undertaken by nurses in the United Kingdom in 1984. A company skilled in survey techniques was engaged to conduct a survey to determine what the public thinks of nurses and nursing, interviewing a representative sample of 1963 persons aged 15 and over in 172 sampling points (Rayner, 1984). A split sample technique was used; approximately one half of the respondents were asked to state their ideas and impressions of what nurses are like and the other half to delineate what ideal nurses would be like. Although the survey indicated that the public's image of nurses closely matched their ideal, some of the findings need to be examined to create the ideal image of nursing. For example, nurses were perceived as hard working by 82% of the respondents, whereas 70% said they should be (Rayner, 1984). It is doubtful that this image would attract young people into nursing, as reflected in the previous study. Another cause for concern was that only 27% of the respondents believed that nurses are given the opportunity to use initiative in their work, but 39% perceived this opportunity as ideal. This perception needs to be examined in relation to another response: 42% of the respondents indicated that nurses obey physicians' orders without question, and 34% believed they should (Rayner, 1984). Another interesting finding was that younger persons had more positive views than older persons about nurses using their initiative and the extent to which they should obey. Eighty-one percent of the respondents believed that nurses are caring and understanding, and 86% thought they should be. Only 42% thought nurses are well educated and only 47% believed they should be (Rayner, 1984). This result indicates a lack of understanding of what nursing involves and should be a cause of concern to all nurses.

A study conducted in Canada in 1988 was commissioned by the Alberta Association of Registered Nurses (AARN) to assess public attitudes about nursing in Alberta. A telephone survey using a structured interview guide and trained interviewers was conducted by a company skilled in survey techniques

(Payne, Cook and Associates, Inc., 1990). A computerized random digit dialing procedure was used, accessing unlisted and listed numbers and ensuring confidentiality. The instrument was reviewed by a committee of representatives of AARN with background knowledge and experience in nursing and some expertise in questionnaire design (Payne et al.). The instrument was also pretested using a small sample of South Edmonton residents. The study sample included 1087 adults, randomly selected from all regions of Alberta. Respondents were asked to describe in their own words their perception of the nursing profession. More than 87% of the responses were positive, using descriptors such as caring, compassionate, knowledgeable, intelligent, helpful, devoted, dedicated, professional, responsible, and hard-working. The few negative images pertained to nursing being a hard, tough, and demanding job, and nurses being overworked and underpaid. Although the media influenced about 60% of the respondents' images of nursing, more than 80% formed their opinions through personal contact with nurses or experiences of others with nurses. Response to items rated on a 5-point Likert scale indicated that respondents viewed nursing as mentally and physically demanding and as requiring special people. Most also viewed it as challenging and interesting, and for the most part, nursing was highly respected. "Despite the fact that 91% of the respondents believed nursing is a highly respected profession, only 76% would recommend nursing as a career" (Giovannetti, 1990, p. 7). Support for nursing as a career was found to be lowest among persons under age 25 and persons with some postsecondary education, two groups from which potential nursing students could be recruited and who are likely to have strong peer influence. As level of income of respondents increased, positive views of nursing as challenging and interesting decreased, and strong support for nursing as a career decreased. Also disconcerting was that 79% of the respondents believed nurses should always consult a physician before administering patient care, and 72% perceived physicians as having total authority over patient care. These attitudes were less prevalent among the younger persons, the more highly educated, and those with higher incomes. On a more positive note, most respondents perceived nurses as accountable for their own practice and conduct, and as having a role in patient education. Moreover, the majority supported nurses' involvement in research to improve practice and believed that nurses should be required to upgrade their education continually. On the controversial issue of nurses being allowed to strike, 47% were firmly opposed, although almost 70% conceded that strike action might be necessary to keep nurses' salaries on a par with those of other professions (Payne, Cook, and Associates, 1990). This is interesting because the province of Alberta has experienced four nurses' strikes since 1977. Because of these study findings the AARN undertook a province-wide public education campaign to enhance the image of nurses and nursing (Giovannetti, 1990).

Some of the findings of the AARN public opinion survey are corroborated by another study; Reichelt (1988) conducted a telephone survey of a stratified sample of 1686 American adults to determine their perceptions of nursing. Reichelt (1988) found that the public perceived nurses "more as demonstrating care and concern than as providing unique services or utilizing cognitive skills" (p. 475).

As in Alberta, the youngest age group held a more negative view of nursing than other age groups, and respondents in higher income brackets held more positive views than others. The youngest age group (18 to 24 years) was the least likely to perceive nurses as thinking for themselves and as having their own distinctive practice domain. On the other hand, respondents with high incomes were most likely to view nurses as providing unique services and making independent decisions in providing patient care.

Not all members of the public perceive the need for nurses to continue their education, as found in two of the studies. Nurses prepared at the diploma level who earn a baccalaureate degree in nursing have reported that they are asked by family, friends, or patients why they wish to continue their formal education. These reports reflect the misconception that a registered nurse has all the education needed. They also indicate that the individuals responding in this manner have no concept of the pattern of nursing education or why nurses need to be knowledgeable and continue to learn. Describing nursing and nursing education to the public is not easy, but it is the responsibility of the profession and individual nurses to use the findings of research to clarify misunderstandings and communicate clearly and concisely the role and potential of nursing in providing health care and improving the health-care system. The communication must be adapted for a variety of publics—patients, students, prospective applicants to nursing programs, colleagues in medicine and other health professions and disciplines, legislators, and the public in general.

■ ■ ■ ■

SELF-IMAGE OF NURSING

Nurses' view of themselves may be referred to as self-image or internal image. Self-image is vitally important because the public's perception of nurses and nursing is influenced by their interactions and experiences with nurses. The studies cited indicated that these interactions were considerably more influential in shaping images of nursing than were the media.

Nurses have been criticized in the literature for having low self-esteem. This may be reflected in appearance, approach to patients, relationships with other health-care professionals, and behaviour in the community. Many factors contribute to the development of self-image, including the values and attitudes one brings to a profession. These values and attitudes are influenced by life experiences before entering the educational system to prepare for the profession. The educational system then influences the learner's concept of nursing practice, the role of the nurse, relationships with other health professionals, and professional responsibilities as a member of the profession and the community.

Nurse educators can help change the self-image of nursing through their teaching and role-modelling. They may also contribute unknowingly to some negative aspects of image development. The importance that they attach to the individual nurse and to the work of nursing can have a major effect on how the students view themselves for many years. Students are also strongly influenced by the nurses—practitioners, administrators, researchers—with whom they interact in clinical practice settings, and by the relationships they observe between nurses and other health professionals.

Nurses have the opportunity to effect changes now and assume responsibility for the future of nursing. Individuals can affect the image of nursing through their daily performance in nursing practice and their reactions to various publics—patients, family members, friends, students, potential recruits, other professionals, legislators, policy makers, or colleagues. As indicated by the studies cited, these interactions contribute to other people's views of nursing. Moreover, one's personal experiences as a nurse and one's own perception of nursing have a great impact on daily encounters with the public. Styles (1982) points out that we must view nursing with a sense of collegiality and collectivity, thus sharing responsibility and authority for nursing and working together to preserve the wholeness of the profession. Achieving unified action is difficult, however, because of the disparity in nursing over issues such as educational preparation for nursing; preparation for specialty practice; unionism; research to improve practice; and allocation of funds among practice, education, and research. It is well known that others can use such disparities to deter or defeat efforts to make constructive and desirable changes that will help achieve unity.

Nursing is more complex than most people think. Developing the knowledge, skills, attitudes, and values needed to practise nursing is a very complicated undertaking. The list of the knowledge and skills needed is endless. Differentiating nursing from medicine, nurses often cite the focus of nursing as "care," where as "cure" is viewed as the focus and end goal of medicine. Perhaps the essence of nursing practice is caring, and caring is not easy Diers (1984) points out that:

> . . . it is not easy to care for people—any people—anytime, anywhere. It is especially difficult when there are no ties of blood or common interest that bind the nurse and the patient. In nursing, caring requires authentic altruism that must be titrated precisely so as not to overwhelm on the one hand, nor be lost on the other. Caring takes enormous energy, even when genuine liking is present, for it is impossible to care equally for and about everyone. Yet that is precisely nursing's assignment (p. 24-25).

The self-image of nursing affects how nurses think students should be educated; whether they encourage others to enter nursing, particularly daughters or sons; the importance they attach to nursing research; how they think nursing services should be organized; how they view nurses strikes; the importance they attach to helping people take responsibility for their own health; and how much influence they think people should have in decisions about their own care. Although nurses do not have to agree on everything, they should agree on basic goals and have sound rationale to support their positions. Too much internal disparity weakens the profession and undermines the power of nurses, which is potentially great because the number of persons in the nursing profession far exceeds that of any other health profession.

■ ■ ■ ■

STRATEGIES FOR CHANGING THE IMAGE

Because of the negative image of nurses and nursing that continues to exist, it is important to identify strategies that may be undertaken by individuals and the profession, through professional associations, to help enhance the image. A basic requirement is to change the self-image held by a nurse if it is a deterrent to developing the positive image nurses wish to portray. A change in the self-image would logically begin with nursing education promoting the "careerist" image projected by Kalisch and Kalisch (1982). While this is presumably the objective of all nursing programs, particularly those in universities, in view of the entry to practice goal, nurse educators need to examine their teaching strategies to ensure that they promote the "careerist" image of nursing.

In discussing nursing education's responsibility for developing nursing's self-image, Hammer and Toughs (1985) state that any sustained change will emanate from educational programs in nursing that develop a positive self-concept encompassing both self-image and self-esteem. They further point out that:

> . . . self-concept is learned. It is derived from all life experiences, from successes, failures and humiliations. It is also derived from feedback from others, particularly those in authority or those most respected . . . Individuals with a positive self-concept are more likely to reach their aspirations and are generally healthier and more productive than those with a more negative concept (p. 280).

Hammer and Toughs (1985) perceive nurse educators as having the opportunity to help change the image of nursing in a very positive way by providing a supportive and challenging learning environment that engenders a positive self-concept. They emphasize the importance of providing constructive feedback on a consistent basis, particularly in the clinical setting. They believe that faculty convey the importance they attach to nursing practice through their own actions and underscore the need for mutual respect between faculty and staff nurses.

Other methods of changing the image of nursing during the process of education pertain to the attributes or characteristics of a profession that students learn during their basic education. Probably the characteristic of a profession that is least often conveyed to students is that it has its own body of knowledge, defined through research. Research is not emphasized in diploma programs because it is not a component of the programs, but it is important that students know about research development and recognize its importance in advancing nursing knowledge and improving nursing practice. Educators can help students develop research awareness and understand the importance of applying valid and reliable research findings in practice. This inadequacy will be eliminated when all nurses are required to earn a baccalaureate degree to enter practice.

Since mass media influence the public's image of nursing, it is important that nurses be alert and educated to assess the media for the type of images portrayed. Kalisch and Kalisch (1987) advocate a deliberate process of intervention that "involves four key steps: (1) getting organized; (2) monitoring the media; (3) reacting to the media; and (4) fostering an improved image" (p. 187). The "media watch" has been promoted and implemented by professional nursing associations in Canada and the United States. Nurses are encouraged to assess the media for the portrayal of undesirable images and take action by identifying the inadequacies to the producers (Evans, Fitzpatrick, and Howard-Ruben, 1983; Kalisch and Kalisch, 1983; Kalisch and Kalisch, 1987). An example of a positive result from media watch is the organized protest by many nurses and the professional organizations in 1989 to the National Broadcasting Corporation's television series "Nightingales." The series portrayed an extremely demeaning and grossly outdated image of nurses and nursing students. The result of a mass letter-writing campaign, organized by professional nursing associations, and meetings with the producers, was a victory for nursing: the series was cancelled and the producers and the public became keenly aware of the reasons for nursing's protest. They also became aware of the image that nursing wishes to convey and its importance in attracting and retaining nurses to provide quality health care.

Porter, Porter, and Lower (1989) describe a comprehensive strategy, developed by a task force in a teaching hospital, that is designed to enhance the image of nursing in the hospital and the community. The task force started with a review of literature and developed specific recommendations and strategies, giving first priority to internal enhancement of the image, then addressing the community. The internal changes recommended included: increasing staff participation within the nursing department, empowering nurses, developing a system of reward and recognition, and improving communications. An administrative position was established to implement and coordinate the task force's suggestions, and a survey was conducted to determine nurses' perceptions of nursing in this hospital. A follow-up survey in 1 year was planned to determine the extent of change in self-image among the nursing staff at that hospital. The administration's financial investment in this endeavour, and their strong support, reflect the priority level of enhancing the image of nursing in this institution. Many of these ideas could be implemented by other health-care agencies.

Another approach that has been used with considerable success by professional organizations is presenting awards for media presentations that portray the most positive images of nursing. This strategy was implemented by the CNA in 1988, when three awards and five Certificates of Merit, in the areas of television, radio, and journalism, were presented by the Minister of Health and Welfare at a dinner organized by the CNA (CNA Connection, 1988). In 1989 five award recipients and five certificate-of-merit recipients were selected from 29 entries, including national newspapers and magazines, private and public radio and television, and individual publications (CNA Connection, 1989). CNA's media awards have become an annual event, initially during Nurses' Week in May but changed to March to help increase visibility and impact when parliament is likely to be in session. The importance of the awards to the media is reflected in an increase in entries from 29 in 1989 to 69 in 1992 when six Awards of Excellence and six Certificates of Merit were awarded. That year CNA President Baumgart "noted that many entries looked at the support system consumers have developed to help them face the difficulties of disease and handicaps. A number also dealt with the funding crisis in the health care system" (CNA Connection, 1992, p. 14). In 1993 the number and quality of entries increased even more and 10 Awards of Excellence and 11 Certificates of Merit were awarded (CNA Connection, 1993). In addition to helping to foster greater public understanding of health-care issues, the media awards are having a positive effect on the image of nurses and nursing.

Nurses themselves have designed and presented radio and television programs to educate the public and also portray the desired image of nurses as intelligent, knowledgeable, articulate and caring health professionals. For example, in January 1993 a television news series, *Nursing Approach*, made its debut on American cable television. Hosted by a nurse executive and media executive, it is an informative half-hour monthly program designed to improve nursing care and increase nursing knowledge. "Research information on this series shows the cutting edge of nursing research and presents a positive image of the nurse as a key professional in a changing health care system" (CNA News, 1993, p. 11). Although designed to educate nurses and nursing students, the program is available to the public and can help to enhance their image of nursing.

Public opinion surveys are important to enhancing the image of nursing. The samples used must be random and of sufficient size to allow generalization, and instruments must be tested for validity and reliability. The results of such surveys should be used in marketing the nursing profession to the public as the AARN has done. The younger age groups should be targeted, not only to increase recruitment into nursing, but also to ensure favourable public opinion in the future. Reichelt (1988) emphasizes the importance of regular assessment of public opinion of nursing, both to formulate marketing strategies and to assess the results of the strategies that are implemented.

Recruitment materials, both to attract persons into nursing and to attract nurses into positions in health-care agencies, must be scrutinized carefully for the image presented. They should apply to both men and women. To attract staff in times of scarce resources, health-care agencies often use gimmicks that promote a negative and sexually oriented image by emphasizing nonprofessional aspects of the place of employment. An example is advertisements emphasizing the advantages of social life in a particular setting rather than the challenges of professional practice. Another means of promoting the positive and careerist image of nursing is to eliminate some of the traditions and rituals of graduation ceremonies. The graduation ceremony for nursing students in university and college programs should be the same as for other students, not set apart for long-standing rituals. Similarly the language used in educational programs and among nurses themselves must be changed to eliminate sexist and paternalistic phrases, such as "the girls."

The practice of nursing should be envisioned and interpreted by students as primarily independent and interdependent, with some dependent aspects pertaining to the prescription of therapies. The focus of practice should be on the promotion and maintenance of health, not illness care, with the goal of helping people attain, maintain, and regain their optimal levels of health and function. Nurses should be portrayed as in interdependent practice, where they have an important role in collaborative decision making and in making independent decisions related to nursing care. They should also be depicted as playing an active role in making policies that pertain to health care and financing of health care, not merely serving in a reactive manner. In an effort to portray the desired image of nurses as intelligent, capable and equal partners in health-care delivery, Grant and Dow (1992) developed a series of 10 interactive television programs about issues in nursing, to be used in teaching nursing students.

The nurses selected to serve on the panels presenting each topic "showed themselves to be intelligent, articulate and caring and demonstrated respect and appreciation for the opposing opinion. Thus positive images of nurses were displayed (p. 33)."

Nurses can play a key role in explaining the image of nurses and nursing to society in general and to the other health professionals with whom they work on a daily basis. The image of nursing held by practitioners themselves is of vital importance, as is their skill at communicating that image to others. Unless nurses have a concept of the careerist image, as proposed by Kalisch and Kalisch (1982), nursing will not succeed in changing the image and developing a cadre of intelligent, sophisticated, assertive, competent, empathic, and supportive individuals whose major goal is to assist persons in assuming increased responsibility for their own health. The concept of nurses marketing their services in an increasingly competitive health-care system, as proposed by Krampitz and Coleman (1985), is a strategy that would help change the image. This approach is needed in the United States, where physicians organize to protect their practices and work to limit nursing practice and competition from nonphysician providers, and because nursing services are eligible for third-party reimbursement in some states. Some physicians in Canada have voiced similar fears as nurses continue toward their goal of a baccalaureate degree for entry to nursing practice and as some nurses venture into independent practice. Krampitz and Coleman (1985) believe that nurses must identify services unique to their profession and market them to succeed in a competitive marketplace.

■ ■ ■ ■

CONCLUSION

Although the image of nurses and nursing may be changing to overcome the sex object image that still exists in mass media, the challenge for nurses is to change both the internal and external images of nursing to promote the careerist image. Only nurses can change the image, and change will be effected only by commitment on the part of individuals and the profession as a whole. The priority given to enhancing the image of nurses and nursing by professional associations needs to be continued. In addition, individual nurses need to accept the challenge of promoting the ideal careerist image of nurses, which will help attract the kind of person needed to develop the potential of nurses to advance knowledge and improve practice, and to be known as persons committed to knowing and especially to doing. This will require changes in the nursing educational system, in keeping with the profession's goal for entry to nursing practice. Kelly (1989) states:

> If enough nurses practice professionally with competence and caring, if they create, direct and/or practice in innovative settings that provide needed care to patients, if they are risk-takers not afraid to develop or assume "different" roles in health care, if with research they find answers to better patient care, if they look beyond the crisis-centred here and now to anticipate and search out ways to meet the public's health care needs, if they simply demonstrate the existing diversity in nursing, there will be like-minded men and women who will see nursing as a worthwhile career opportunity (p. 17).

REFERENCES

Anatomy of a profession. (1986). *Nursing Times, 82*(13), 24-26.

CNA Connection. (1987). Staggering agenda set by directors for 1987. *The Canadian Nurse, 83*(1), 7.

CNA Connection. (1988). CNA media awards a hit. *The Canadian Nurse, 84*(7), 6.

CNA Connection. (1989). Media excellence. *The Canadian Nurse, 85*(7), 9.

CNA Connection. (1992). Media awards. *The Canadian Nurse, 88*(7), 14.

CNA Connection. (1993). 1993 Media award winners. *The Canadian Nurse, 89*(3), 8.

CNA News. (1993). Prime time nursing. *The Canadian Nurse, 89*(6), 11.

Diers, D. (1984). To profess—to be a professional. *Journal of the New York State Nurses' Association, 15*(4), 22-29.

Evans, D., Fitzpatrick, T., and Howard-Ruben, J. (1983). A district takes action. *American Journal of Nursing, 83*(1), 52-59.

Gaze, H. (1987). Men in nursing: Man appeal. *Nursing Times, 83*(20), 24-27.

Giovannetti, P. (1990). News release. *AARN Newsletter, 46*(1), 7.

Grant, N.K. and Dow, M. (1992). The promotion of the image of nurses. *AARN Newsletter, 48*(6), 32-33.

Hammer, R.M., and Toughs, M.A. (1985). Nursing's self-image—nursing education's responsibility. *Journal of Nursing Education, 24*(7), 280-283.

Kalisch, B., and Kalisch, P. (1982). Anatomy of the image of the nurse: Dissonant and ideal models. In C. Williams (Ed.), *Image-making in nursing* (pp. 3-23). Kansas City: American Academy of Nursing.

Kalisch, B., and Kalisch, P. (1983). Improving the image of nursing. *American Journal of Nursing, 83*(1), 48-52.

Kalisch, P., and Kalisch, B. (1987). *The changing image of the nurse.* Don Mills, Ontario: Addison-Wesley Publishing Company.

Kelly, L.S. (1989). Editorial: Updating nursing's image. *Nursing Outlook, 37*(1), 17.

Krampitz, S.D., and Coleman, J.R. (1985). Marketing, a must in a competitive health care system. *Nursing Economics, 3*(4), 286-289.

Lippman, D.T., and Ponton, K.S. (1989). Nursing's image on the university campus. *Nursing Outlook, 37*(1), 24-27.

May, F., Austin, J.K., and Champion, V. (1988). *Attitudes, values and beliefs of the public in Indiana toward nursing as a career: A study to enhance recruitment into nursing.* Indianapolis: Sigma Theta Tau International Honor Society of Nursing, Inc.

Payne, Cook, and Associates, Inc. (1990). *Insight: The 1989 provincial public opinion study of nursing in Alberta.* (Available from the Alberta Association of Registered Nurses, 11620-168th Street, Edmonton, Alberta, T5M 4A6.)

Porter, R.T., Porter, M.J., and Lower, M.S. (1989). Enhancing the image of nursing. *Journal of Nursing Administration, 19*(2), 36-40.

Rayner, C. (1984). Images of nursing: What do the public think of nurses? *Nursing Times, 80*(35), 28-31.

Reichelt, P.A. (1988). Public perceptions of nursing and strategy formulation. *Western Journal of Nursing Research, 10*(4), 472-476.

Simmons, L.W., and Henderson, V. (1964). *Nursing research: A survey and assessment.* New York: Appleton-Century-Crofts.

Skevington, S. and Dawkes, D. (1988). Fred Nightingale. *Nursing Times, 84*(21), 49-51.

Statistics Canada. (1994). Registered nurses employed in Canada by sex and province, *1992. Registered Nurses Management Data, Canadian Centre for Health Information,* Ottawa: Author.

Styles, M.M. (1982). *On nursing: Toward a new endowment.* Toronto: The C.V. Mosby Company.

U.S. Public Health Service, Department of Health and Human Services, Division of Nursing. (1994). *Registered nurse population: Findings from 1992 national survey of registered nurses.* Washington, DC: Author.

CHAPTER SIX

Nursing and Feminism

JANET ROSS KERR

Feminism is an outgrowth of reactions against forms of social organization in which women are not valued as highly as men; the norms of such a system condone systematic bias toward women. Although feminism is commonly thought of as a movement that grew out of the 1960s, feminist ideas are reflected in writing by women in the seventeenth century (Spender, 1982). In more recent history the suffragette movement of the late nineteenth and early twentieth centuries had a powerful impact on society and resulted in important changes in the treatment of women. Nightingale's work in this era is "recognized by feminist scholars as reflecting remarkable feminist insight" (Chinn and Wheeler, 1985, p. 74).

Nurses were profoundly influenced by the thinking of the suffragettes and were in an important position to demonstrate women's capabilities. Politically active nursing leaders had recently become a respected profession and was one of few careers open to women. Politically active nursing leaders were able to accomplish critical professional goals that would allow the profession remarkable development throughout the twentieth century. The entrenchment of nursing registration in legislation in Canada and other countries during this time period was a victory that was an important step forward for the status of women.

Chinn and Wheeler (1985) have documented four philosophic views of feminism. The liberal feminist stance derives its tenets from the belief that women are an oppressed group, and it suggests that the solution is to equalize opportunities for women. According to Marxist feminist thinking, capitalism and the acquisition of property has created a class system that favours men; resolution of the inequality is seen as an important consequence in a society in which materialism and capitalism are rejected for a system of collective organization and ownership. Socialist feminist ideas derive from analyses of sociocultural phenomena and institutions where "the oppression of women and socioeconomic class oppression are equally fundamental and mutually reinforcing" (Chinn and Wheeler, 1985, p. 75). In contrast, radical feminist theory emphasizes the importance of defining issues from a female approach to the world. In this stance attention is not focused on the relation of women to men, as in some other perspectives, but on "discovering, analyzing, and valuing women's experience without the imposed standards of male ideology or systems" (Chinn and Wheeler, 1985, p. 75).

Kleffel (1991) has suggested that the ecofeminist framework as described by Warren (1990) has much to offer beyond the more limiting psychosocial paradigm and has the potential to "revolutionize our profession by liberating us from patriarchal oppression, changing our relationships with our clients and with each other, allowing us to develop new tools and approaches to knowledge development, moving us into areas where we have had no voice, and opening up our profession to limitless possibilities." (Kleffel, 1991, p. 16).

The ideology of feminism is threatening to some, undoubtedly because its framework is one that is a radical departure from traditional thinking. Although feminism may be seen as a movement which is in opposition to both men and traditional institutions such as the family, its fundamental ideas espouse valuing both women and men. Systems and institutions favouring one sex over the other are targets of feminist criticism. Feminists also model behaviour that may not be thought of as feminine, undoubtedly unsettling to some. In this respect, modern feminists are like the suffragettes in the way their ideas are presented. Independent thought and action, straightforward and hard-hitting commentary on issues of concern, and generally assertive behaviour characterize the feminist modus operandi. McHale (quoted in Eisler, 1988) suggested that it will be necessary to

> leave behind the hard, conquest-oriented values traditionally associated with "masculinity." For is not the need for a "spirit of truly global cooperation, shaped in free partnership," "a balancing of individualism with love," and the normative goal of "harmony with rather than conquest of nature," the reassertion of a more "feminine ethos"? And to what end could "drastic changes in the norm stratum" or a "metamorphosis in basic cultural premises and all aspects of social institutions" relate if not to the replacement of a dominator with a partnership society (p. 106)?

■ ■ ■ ■

THE RELATIONSHIP BETWEEN FEMINISM AND NURSING

The relationship between feminism and nursing has been described as uneasy, but this was not always the case. Although nursing was at the forefront of the women's movement early in the century, predominantly male professions have been the focus of recent feminist concern. This has largely been a successful thrust because women are now entering nontraditional professions in greater proportions than ever. Sex stereotyped views of nursing emphasize subservience, lack of assertiveness, and domination of nurses, who are primarily female, by physicians, who are primarily male. The real status of modern nursing may be difficult to appreciate from a view outside the profession. Technologic advances and increases in health-care knowledge heightened performance expectations and had a phenomenal impact on nursing in general, leading to new and independent roles in many areas.

> Nursing has not been valued for its autonomous social contributions, independent decision-making, scholarly productivity, or collective striving for recognition, power and legitimization in professional policy-making and community circles. Feminists

have sometimes failed to look beyond the inaccurate sexist stereotypes of nurses and to acknowledge the multiple dimensions of professional nursing (Vance, Talbott, McBride, and Mason, 1985a, p. 281).

Chinn and Wheeler assert, "a major contribution of feminist thinking in relation to nursing is the basic tenet of feminist theory—that women are oppressed" (1985, p. 76). Persuasive arguments suggesting that nurses can be categorized as an oppressed group are provided by Roberts (1983). The discussion is an illuminating one and provides some intriguing explanations for characteristic behaviour observed in nurses. For example, of some interest is the low value some nurses place on participation in professional organizations. Emanating from a low degree of esteem for the profession, such behaviour is thought to be based on fear that associating with others who are oppressed may not be in one's best interest. Another example can be found in the struggle to legitimize midwifery in Canada, where many nurse midwives have supported a professional structure completely separate from nursing. Arguments put forward to explain this have tended to focus on the fact that nurse midwives do not wish to be associated with a profession perceived as having low status, despite its related phenomena of interest.

Systematic undervaluing of the contributions of the profession can be seen in an article in *Reader's Digest* (Schuyler, 1991). This story centred on efforts to save the life of a 5 year-old boy who had fallen through ice on Beaumaris Lake in a residential district in Edmonton, Alberta on April 16, 1989. The professional efforts of the paramedics and physicians were praised extensively while those of nurses were barely mentioned in this article. When the article was published even the paramedics who were involved were shocked to see how the writer had systematically ignored the extensive efforts of nurses to save the life of this child. The expertise and care given by a number of nurses to the care of this child were invisible to all but those who were principals in the events. The extension of this thinking explains the lack of attention to the history and accomplishments of the profession. "A feminist perspective would encourage us to embrace our rich cultural heritage within nursing and value our predecessors, who made brave and courageous strides in developing the foundation upon which nursing is built" (Chinn and Wheeler, 1985, p. 76).

The implications of a feminist view of practice, education, and research in nursing are important and require a shift in thinking and new approaches to care. The challenge to traditional patriarchal family structures represents an inherent challenge to nursing theories/conceptual frameworks as well because many of these have "underlying patriarchal assumptions about human experience" (Chinn and Wheeler, 1985). By advocating the same treatment for men and women in society, feminist consciousness-raising has been tremendously successful in challenging traditional roles of men and women in society. In health care, as in other areas, new approaches to care and treatment and to education in the health-care professions are resulting in a total restructuring because of the influence of new ideas from the women's movement. The change that is occurring is nothing short of revolutionary; the system that results will look very different from that that existed before feminist ideas were widely known and appreciated. Baer (1991) has sounded a note of caution however in terms of the directions of feminism. "Feminism will have succeeded not only when females have equal access to all fields but when traditionally female professions, such as nursing, gain the high value and solid respect they deserve"(p. 121).

■ ■ ■ ■

A FEMINIST APPROACH TO WOMEN'S HEALTH

The women's movement has had considerable impact on the ways that nurses have conceptualized health. This has been particularly true for women's health, as Baumgart commented in an interview.

> The health problems emphasized in most nursing curriculums are male-biased. We pay a great deal of attention to cardiac disease in our society. It's certainly important for women, but it's a major male medical problem. Why couldn't we concentrate as much on depression in women? What about elderly women? . . . We give a lot of time to the uterus and very little to the head. The implicit message is that cardiac disease is "normal" while depression is "deviant" (Allen, 1985, p. 21).

The areas of focus in health have arisen as an issue largely because of the women's movement. There is new attention to women's overall health problems (as opposed to reproductive health only), such as osteoporosis, depression, rape, premenstrual syndrome, and menopausal difficulties. The women's movement and the consumers' movement have jointly influenced the role of the health-care client and have legitimized an active role. Delineation of patients' rights in health care (see Chapter 20) has led to the consensus that a client has a right to information and should participate in decision making about care because there are often a number of options for treatment. Consumers, including women, are asking for clear statements of these options so they can be informed participants in the decision making process.

"Nurses are particularly well prepared to meet the health needs of women. Nurses have been schooled to build their assessments on clients' perceptions of their experience and to promote self-help, and that is exactly what women are demanding" (McBride, 1984, p. 66). For many years nursing curriculums have emphasized the importance of communication, interpersonal skills, and health assessment skills. Nurses "are health care providers best suited to meet consumer demands for self-determination, because their professional mandate has long been expressed in terms of helping the client" (McBride, 1984, p. 66), in the words of Virginia Henderson, "to gain independence as rapidly as possible" (Henderson, 1961, p. 42). Thus many of the directions the women's movement is taking coincide with those being taken by the nursing profession; women's health stands to benefit.

Radical changes in the structure of nursing practice in the United States have been taking place during the past decade. Because national health insurance does not exist in that country, nurses have been able to establish clinics or health collectives to serve the public. Vance et al. (1985) referred to the Loeb Center for Nursing and Rehabilitation in New York, the Erie Family Health Center in Chicago, and the Pennsylvania State Consultation Nursing Center as agencies doing important work with consumers, particularly those who have been "unserved and underserved" (p. 285). Also, nurses have been pushing for legislation that permits independent practice by nurses. "They want to promote the idea that the authority for nursing is based on a social contract, not on doctors' orders" (Vance et al, 1985, p. 285). Securing the authority to practise autonomously as a professional nurse has been a difficult struggle in the United States and is one that is only beginning in Canada.

The issues surrounding midwifery have been at the forefront of the movement in Canada. Despite the fact that midwifery has grown out of nursing (the large majority of midwives are nurses, and many believe that midwifery practice is nursing practice) midwives have chosen to separate from the nursing profession in terms of standards and control of their practice. Thus midwives are gaining the right to practise independently in several provinces. How their services will be funded is as yet unknown, but it is likely that it will be consistent with funding for all other health services delivered by professionals in the future. The machinery for direct federal funding for nursing services is in place with the provision for funding for "health practitioners" contained in Canada Health Act of 1984.

Provincial health plans may now include direct reimbursement for nursing services that can be funded under their plans, even though no province has yet chosen to implement into its health insurance plan the "health practitioner" clause introduced into the Canada Health Act of 1984. It is likely that, with the movement to community health centres, nurses will serve as entry points to the health system, and reimbursement for their services will be forthcoming through the health insurance system. "Today the women's movement has helped nurses to realize that their proper place includes not only protecting their right to practice, but reclaiming lost rights to work as independent professionals with consumers" (Vance et al, 1985a, p. 285).

▬ ▬ ▬ ▬

RESEARCH AND FEMINISM

Nursing research that focuses on women's issues may or may not take a feminist stance. A paradigm shift is necessary because previous theories and conceptual frameworks used in research did not view women's health from a female perspective and were therefore incomplete.

> These theories have a dual function: they offer descriptions of women's oppression and prescriptions for eliminating it. They are empirical insofar as they examine women's experience in the world, but they are political insofar as they characterize certain features of that experience as oppressive and offer new visions of justice and freedom for women (MacPherson, 1983, p. 19).

Feminist research is characterized more frequently as qualitative than quantitative. The emphasis on describing the meaning of women's health experiences leads frequently to the use of qualitative approaches. Such research tends to be exploratory and may encompass field studies. Qualitative approaches need to be used to gather basic data that has been unavailable in areas that have received little attention. "Because we have undervalued women's and nursing's 'ways of knowing,' we have unwittingly abrogated a powerful influence for change and in so doing deprived society of our strength" (Sohier, 1992, pp. 64-5).

While it is clear that both qualitative and quantitative approaches are likely to be useful in the long run, the problem for women's health is that there has been little exploratory work in some areas (Vance, Talbott, McBride, and Mason, 1985b). During the past decade nursing researchers have become increasingly conversant with qualitative methods, and many studies reported in journals use qualitative methods. Health problems of concern to women are receiving considerable attention from nursing researchers, as evidenced by publications in the nursing research journals (Chiarelli and Nadon, 1985).

The interpretation of results in research investigations has been the focus of attention by feminists. There is a concern that feminist values may bias the interpretation just as male values have historically biased the interpretation of previous research. "There needs to be an ongoing struggle to conduct research without allowing feminist values to become prisms that distort or bend the truth, or blinders that hide the truth entirely" (MacPherson, 1983, p. 24). Thus open and truly objective approaches are desirable for scholarly work. Undoubtedly, when the framework through which the data are viewed is broader and encompasses human values, the possibility that new interpretations will be derived is enhanced.

Concerns have been expressed about results of previous research investigations. Many studies have used only men as research subjects; results therefore are generalizable only to men. There is a need to broaden the subject base for investigations in general and to use women as well as men in a number of areas. There is also a need to communicate results of studies to consumers. "A feminist perspective also emphasizes the need to publish these future research findings in both professional and popular journals so that all women can benefit" (MacPherson, 1983, p. 24). Nursing research has much to offer in the area of women's health, and a feminist perspective can be very useful to nursing researchers to investigate "methods to get beyond the sex biases characterizing the existing research on women's health issues such as, for example, much of the biomedical research on menopause"(MacPherson, 1983, p. 24). There is much to be learned from research in the area of women's health. Nurses have just begun to recognize the challenges and to make a commitment to carry out meaningful work in these areas. Answers to some of the common and universal questions that concern women's health are vitally important to women. Approaches that incorporate a feminist perspective are essential in studying these problems, and nurses have leading roles to play in investigating topics of concern to women.

REFERENCES

Allen, M. (1985). Women, nursing and feminism: An interview with Alice J. Baumgart. *The Canadian Nurse, 81*(1), 20-22.

Baer, E.D. (1991). Even her feminist friends see her as 'only' a nurse. *International Nursing Review, 38*(4), 121.

Chiarelli, M., and Nadon, F. (1985). Women and mental health: A feminist view. *The Canadian Nurse, 81*(1), 23.

Chinn, P., and Wheeler, C.E. (1985). Feminism and nursing: Can nursing afford to remain aloof from the women's movement? *Nursing Outlook, 33*(2), 74-77.

Eisler, R. (1988). *The chalice and the blade.* San Francisco: Harper & Row.

Henderson, V. (1961). *Basic principles of nursing care.* London: International Council of Nurses.

Kleffel, D. (1991). An ecofeminist analysis of nursing knowledge. *Nursing Forum, 26*(4), 5-18.

MacPherson, K.I. (1983). Feminist methods: A new paradigm for nursing research. *Advances in Nursing Science, 5*(2), 17-25.

McBride, A.B. (1984). Nursing and the women's movement, *Image, 16*(3), 66.

Roberts, S.J. (1983). Oppressed group behaviour: Implications for nursing. *Advances in Nursing Science, 5*(4), 21-30.

Schuyler, L. (1991). Boy under the ice. *Reader's Digest. (Canadian edition), 139*(834), 54-58.

Sohier, R. (1992). Feminism and nursing knowledge: The power of the weak. *Nursing Outlook, 40*(2), 62-66,93.

Spender, D. (1982). *Women of ideas and what men have done to them.* Boston: Routledge & Kegan Paul.

Vance, C., Talbott, S., McBride, A., and Mason, D. (1985a). An uneasy alliance: Nursing and the women's movement. *Nursing Outlook, 33*(6), 281-285.

Vance, C., Talbott, S., McBride, A., and Mason, D. (1985b). Coming of age: The women's movement and nursing. In D.J. Mason and S.W. Talbott (Eds.), *Political action handbook for nurses* (pp. 23-37). Menlo Park, Calif: Addison-Wesley.

Warren, K. (1990). A critical social reconceptualization of environment in nursing: Implications for methodology. *Advances in Nursing Science, 11*(4),125-146.

CHAPTER SEVEN

Men in Nursing

JANNETTA MacPHAIL

Despite an increase in the number of men in nursing during the past two decades, men still constitute an insignificant proportion of the registered nurse population in Canada. This is remarkable at a time when the proportion of women in traditionally male-dominated professions has increased at a phenomenal rate. Areas now opened to women include business, dentistry, law, medicine, and pharmacy because of pressure from women's groups, whose allegations of sexism have led to changes in recruitment policies and affirmative action. Thus as many as one half of the admission placements in these disciplines are available to women. At the same time there have been notable increases in the number of men entering other traditionally female-dominated professions, such as teaching and librarianship.

Why has the proportion of men in nursing increased so slowly? What factors have influenced the entry of men into nursing? Will these factors continue to exert the same influence? What are the advantages of having more men in nursing? What has the nursing profession done or not done to change the proportion of men entering its ranks? What implications does the Charter of Rights have for the continuation of a predominance of women or men in any profession? These questions will be addressed in this chapter.

■ ■ ■ ■

HISTORICAL PERSPECTIVE

Historically nursing had its roots in the Roman matrons, such as Fabiola, who provided care and nurturance for the sick poor in their own homes. This was possible because of the matrons' wealth and arose from their desire to do "good" for others. Care of the sick continued to be female-dominated with the advent of female religious orders in Europe that assumed nursing as one of their responsibilities.

On the other hand, only men were allowed to tend the injured and sick during the Crusades in the eleventh century. This pattern was repeated when Canada was first explored and settled as New France by Jacques Cartier and Samuel de Champlain. As mentioned in Chapter 1 the first nurses were male attendants and Jesuit priests who were missionary immigrants. However, the impropriety of male priests caring for sick women soon brought about change, and three nuns were brought from France in 1639 to establish the first hospital at Quebec. This helped establish a pattern in Canada that continued for 4 centuries, whereby female religious orders, as one of their major missions, provided hospitals to care for the sick, prevent disease, and promote health. Later they took on the added responsibility of training nurses to staff the hospitals. After the middle of the twentieth century, religious orders began to withdraw from nursing education and management of hospitals, although today some orders, such as the Grey Nuns, continue to own hospitals that they influence as owners and members of the boards of directors.

Wars had a great influence on determining who attended the injured and sick men and who was recruited into nursing. Kus (1985) refers to antimale sexism as a major factor influencing attitudes in society that permitted only men to go to war. Not only was it considered appropriate, but men were rewarded for killing others and being killed in defense of their country. This was apparent in the battles against native peoples when Canada was first settled and in all subsequent wars, including World War I from 1914 to 1918 and World War II from 1939 to 1945. During World War I only men were permitted to join the Medical Corps to serve as stretcher bearers on the battlefield and to help the female nurses who staffed Canadian base hospitals prepare to care for the wounded. In both World Wars women were recruited in great numbers to staff civilian hospitals because many nurses left to enter the Nurse Corps of the three armed services divisions, and many men volunteered for, or were conscripted into, the services. This increased the number of women entering nursing even more and decreased the possibility of more men entering nursing because they had to fight.

During the Crimean War the attitude of having only male attendants care for the injured and sick prevailed until Florence Nightingale was asked by the British government to go to the Crimea with the small group of nurses she recruited. There she worked to improve the care provided for the soldiers and to decrease the loss of lives. Although Miss Nightingale was not easily accepted by the heads of the army, through her strong determination, expert knowledge, and nursing skill, the lives of many men were saved and their environmental conditions were vastly improved. She overcame barriers to women tending the wounded and sick during war, and later overrode Victorian barriers to women working outside the home. When she established the first nursing school at St. Thomas' Hospital in London in 1860, only women were accepted as applicants. The school was organized separately from the hospital, thus creating an opportunity for women to work outside the home and promoting "a measure of independence from men in the medical/hospital bureaucracy" (Halloran and Welton, 1994, p. 683). In the process of overcoming societal pressures for women to conform to Victorian beliefs and customs, Nightingale also excluded men from nursing.

■■ ■■ ■■ ■■

PROPORTION OF MEN IN NURSING

The proportion of men in nursing in Canada has increased very slowly over the past 26 years, as shown in Table 7.1.

TABLE 7.1 Comparison of Female and Male Nurses Employed in Canada, 1966 to 1992

Year	Total Number of RNs	Total Employed in Nursing	Female		Male	
			Number	(%)	Number	(%)
1966	Data not available	82,917	82,545	99.5	372	0.45
1975	182,828	144,193*	142,095	98.55	2,098	1.45
1986	236,993	204,571*	199,085	97.31	5,486	2.68
1988	249,673	210,506*	204,261	97.00	6,245	3.00
1992	263,683	234,128*	225,910	96.49	8,218	3.51

* Remainder employed in other than nursing or not employed or not stated.

Source: Statistics Canada. (1994). Registered Nurses Management Data, 1992. Ottawa: Health Statistics Division, Statistics Canada.

Even though the number of men employed in nursing in Canada increased by 546% from 1966 to 1975 and by 392% in 1992, that number still represents only 3.5% of the total nurse population, a slight increase over the 3.0% in 1988. If segregated by sex and compared with other health-care groups, the male registered nurse population is one of the smallest professional groups in the health-care system (Health Manpower Directorate, 1983). Okrainec (1986a) reported that the four provinces having the highest number of male nurses are Quebec, Ontario, British Columbia, and Alberta. In 1990 male nurses accounted for 7.5% of Quebec's registered nurse workforce and they represented 52% of the male nurses employed in Canada (CNA Connection, 1990).

A 1992 study of nurses in Canada, as shown in Table 7.2, indicates that of a total of 263,683 registered nurses, 91% of the men and 88% of the women, were employed in nursing. Both represent an increase from 90% and 84% respectively in 1988. The data also show that, of all of Canada's registered nurses, a slightly greater proportion of women than men were employed in fields other than nursing and that 5.55% of the female nurses and 1.95% of the male nurses were not employed at all. In 1988 the latter proportions were 6.11% for female nurses and 2.01% for male nurses. From these data it appears that fewer nurses are not employed for both sexes. There also was a decrease in the proportion of both male nurses (from 6.24% to 5.21%) and female nurses (from 7.98% to 3.13%) who failed to give any information about their employment status. The higher percentage of women not employed may reflect those temporarily out of the workforce for childbearing purposes, as well as the probability of a larger number of women retired because of their greater life expectancy. To consider gender differences in nursing one must examine factors that influence the entry of men into a traditionally female-dominated profession.

Comparison of Female and Male Nurses in Canada				
	Female		**Male**	
	Number	**(%)**	**Number**	**(%)**
RNs	254,666	100.00	9,017	100.00
Employed in Nursing	225,910	88.71	8,218	91.14
Employed in Other than Nursing	6,659	2.61	153	1.70
Not Employed	14,131	5.55	176	1.95
Not Stated	7,966	3.13	470	5.21

Source: Statistics Canada. (1994). Registered Nurses Management Data, 1992. Ottawa: Health Statistics Division, Statistics Canada.

■ ■ ■ ■

BARRIERS TO MEN ENTERING NURSING

One of the major barriers to men entering the nursing profession is societal attitudes about occupations appropriate for men and women. In general, nursing has not been considered an appropriate career choice for males because of its characteristics of nurturance, gentleness, and caring; males are supposed to be strong and powerful and not show emotions. Negative and discouraging reactions from others, including family members, have been reported by male nurses. Undoubtedly these young men had to be very determined and committed to persist in their efforts to pursue a career in nursing. They also reported implications that they might be "sissies" or "gay." Similar reactions from other health professionals, particularly physicians, have been encountered in years when medicine was predominantly male. Indeed, such reactions were not uncommon within the profession of nursing itself; some women nurses tended to regard men who selected nursing as not "real men."

Men were not accepted readily in nursing schools for many years. Initially, most of those accepted entered schools of nursing connected with mental hospitals, where they were accepted because of the belief that men were physically better able to deal with violence. Strength was considered so important in psychiatric nursing that this specialty did not become a required part of basic nursing education in Canada until the 1950s and even the 1960s in some schools. Until the 1960s and 1970s male nursing students were not permitted to study theory and practice in obstetric and gynecologic nursing; they devoted that time to urologic nursing, caring for male patients only.

Other evidence of resistance within nursing included the tendency of female instructors to assign male students to care primarily for male patients; negative reactions of female nursing staff to having male students in maternity and gynecologic nursing when these became a required part of their programs; resistance of female nursing staff to hiring male nurses, particularly for maternity nursing (although the majority of the obstetricians at that time were male); the tendenc to assign male nurses primarily to psychiatry and critical care units; and the te dency of nurse educators and nursing staff, even today, to refer to nursing st dents as "girls," a sexist label. When men began to enter nursing schools whe students were housed in dormitories there was no place for them because t buildings had been designed for women only.

For many years another barrier to men entering nursing was an econon.ic one; nurses were paid poorly. As a result men who may have been interested in nursing chose not to enter because of the societal expectation that they should be the "breadwinners." Male nurses have sometimes been criticized for aspiring to high positions as administrators in order to earn enough to support a family. In a study of British nursing, which has traditionally had a larger proportion of men than Canada or the United States, Nuttal (1983) reported that male nurses held half of the top nursing posts in the National Health Service, although they represented less than 10% of the state registered nurse population. In Canada about 15% of male nurses held management/administrative positions in 1992 while 11% of female nurses worked in this category. The percentage of male nurses in comparison with female nurses for three such positions is shown in Table 7.3.

With the advent of unionism in Canada in the 1960s, nursing salaries began to improve. Today they are much more adequate. In fact staff nurses' salaries in general are higher in Canada than in the United States, although one must consider differences in the cost of living when making comparisons. In his study of male nurses in Alberta, Okrainec (1986b, p. 17) reported that the respondents were satisfied with their salaries and that "married men, who represented 71% of the sample, were generally more dissatisfied with their income as compared to single men." To have sufficient income to support a family in the style many desire today requires moving to higher-level positions, which requires more education and therefore more investment of time and money. Male nurses who have high needs and aspirations will have to make such a commitment and investment, but the same requirements apply to female nurses who aspire to leadership positions.

TABLE 7.3 Male Nurses in Management/Administrative Positions Compared with Female Nurses 1992

Position	Male (%)	Female (%)
Director/Assistant Director	3.14	2.14
Supervisor/Coordinator	5.68	4.42
Head Nurse	5.90	4.10

Source: Statistics Canada. (1994). Registered Nurses Management Data, 1992. Ottawa: Health Statistics Division, Statistics Canada.

■■ ■■ ■■ ■■
EFFORTS TO SUPPORT MEN IN NURSING

Since there have been very few studies of men in nursing, little data exist to assess men's interest in and satisfaction with the profession. It is known that the number and proportion of men has increased, albeit very slowly. Okrainec (1986b) reported that the majority of the 163 respondents, who represented 62% of the male nurse population in Alberta, "were either satisfied or very satisfied with their choice of nursing as a career . . . ," and "only a small percentage (4.3%) expressed dissatisfaction with nursing" (p. 17). The three highest-ranked areas of satisfaction were "the attitude of male patients toward male nurses, acceptance as a nurse by female co-workers, and the attitude of female patients toward men in nursing" (Okrainec, 1986b, p. 17). Although it appears from these findings that attitudes toward male nurses are changing for the better, Okrainec cautions against generalizing his findings to the total population of male nurses because the sample was not a random one and was limited to one province. In addition, there is no evidence that the instrument developed by the investigator was pretested or that the validity and reliability of the instrument were established.

In the United States, where the proportion of male nurses is only slightly higher than in Canada, formalized mechanisms have been implemented to promote the integration of men into the total nursing population and to provide support for them in the process. These included the establishment of a Male Nurses Section within the American Nurses Association from 1941 to 1952, and legislation enacted in 1955 to permit male nurses to be commissioned as officers in the armed services, made possible through the efforts of the Honourable Frances Payne Bolton, the first woman in Congress. As a result nearly one third of the Army Nurse Corps was men, including medics and corpsmen from the Vietnam conflict who chose to enter nursing. Others chose to become physician's assistants, but found limited opportunity for advancement because assistants have no mobility beyond a specific physician. The physician's assistant concept did not develop in Canada; there was a deliberate decision against it by the medical and nursing professions.

Men in the United States interested in nursing became attracted to nursing programs designed specifically for university graduates, such as the program offered at Yale University, leading to a Master of Nursing (MN) degree, and the program at Case Western Reserve University, which offered the first and to date the only Doctor of Nursing (ND) Program in 1979. In the first 3 years of the ND program, the proportion of men in the program averaged 17% (MacPhail, Personal experience with ND program, 1979-1982). In addition, in the mid-1970s the nurse corps in the three US armed services divisions began to require a baccalaureate degree in nursing as an entrance requirement and offered generous support to nursing students to enroll in such programs. These students had to commit to a specific period of service after graduation.

Another formalized mechanism designed to provide support to men in nursing in the United States was the National Male Nurses Association, established in 1971; the name was changed in 1981 to the American Assembly of Men in

Nursing. The objectives of the organization were to encourage men to enter nursing programs, to support male nurses in their efforts to continue their education and professional development, and to assist them in demonstrating the contributions made by men to nursing and to society (Halloran, 1994). The organization also established an annual award, the Luther Christman Award, for outstanding leadership in nursing, which was not limited to men and was in fact given primarily to female nurses in the first 5 years of its existence.

Although no similar mechanisms for recognition and encouragement of male nurses have been developed in Canada, there has been an increase in the number of men attracted to and retained in nursing. In fact, the percentage of men in the total nurse population in Canada is only slightly less than that in the United States. Some speculate that the increase in Canada is related to the economy and unemployment. An increase in enrolment in postsecondary educational institutions can be expected because Canada has offered such generous subsidization of education. While some might decry admission under these circumstances, many excellent nurses, male and female, have chosen nursing as a second or third choice under such economic circumstances.

■ ■ ■ ■

RESEARCH ON MEN IN NURSING

In his review of research on men, Christman (1988) found a dearth of studies and identified many inadequacies in the methods of investigation used and interpretation of results. The research he reviewed included six survey studies, two studies using focused interview, and five studies using standardized test batteries to assess personality, intelligence, and attitudes. The questionnaires used in the survey research had not been tested adequately for validity and reliability. In general, study samples were small and not representative of the population being studied, which can "result in sampling bias and incomplete knowledge of the phenomenon under study" (Christman, 1988, p. 198). Christman (1988) concludes: "If clarification of the male role in the nursing profession was a goal of the research done so far, then there are major shortcomings in both the research and the outcomes of research" (p. 202). He questions the utility of studies that elicit opinion, and he does not support doing more of them. He suggests building on the beginnings of two studies by Brown and Stones (1972) and Holtzclaw (1981), both of which used standardized test batteries. He also emphasizes obtaining much larger samples that are from more than one site and representative of the population being studied. Other suggestions are:

> . . . (a) cohort studies over time; (b) controlled field experiments assessing competence in both academic and practice settings; (c) comparative studies of settings in which the presence of men nurses is noticeable with settings with none or only a few men; and (d) the nature and quality of interaction of male nurses with patients as well as physicians as compared with female nurses to ascertain whether or not any differences exist (Christman, 1988, pp. 203-204).

■ ■ ■ ■

CONCLUSION

There is no doubt that many factors have deterred men from entering and remaining in nursing and that some of the negative influences in society are finally beginning to change. Factors such as cultural influences may serve to attract or discourage young people, particularly men, from choosing nursing as a career. The increasing number of Canadian immigrants, coming from Oriental and Hispanic countries where men have not been a part of nursing, is one such factor. Another factor to be considered is that many fields, such as medicine, dentistry, business, law, and pharmacy, are now available to women. As more women are attracted to these fields, there may well be a reverse effect of attracting more men to nursing, particularly since there is increasing evidence that they are becoming better accepted.

There is little evidence that nursing programs have ever sought to attract and retain men in nursing. In contrast, efforts have been made by some traditionally male-dominated health professions to attract or at least encourage women. To attract more men to nursing, educators and administrators must work together to correct the myths and overcome barriers that deter them. Hospitals and other health-care agencies and nursing schools need to portray men in the role of nurse in their publicity materials to help change the public's perception of nursing. In addition, there has been no systematic effort to study the extent to which attitudes have changed in nursing or society about the acceptability of men as members of the nursing profession. To what extent have the advantages of having men in nursing been considered and propounded, such as increasing stability and continuity in practice settings, increasing longevity of service and commitment to a career in nursing, and perhaps to conducting research to improve practice and the care of patients? Men and women can offer such potential benefits if they are committed to and well prepared for a lifetime of service in the profession of nursing.

REFERENCES

Brown, R.G.S., and Stones, R.H.W. (1972). Personality and intelligence characteristics of male nurses. *International Journal of Nursing Studies, 9*(8), 167-177.

Christman, L.P. (1988). Men in nursing. In J.J. Fitzpatrick, R.L. Taunton, and J.Q. Benoliel (Eds.), *Annual review of nursing research, Vol. 6* (pp. 193-205). New York: Springer Publishing Co., Inc.

CNA Connection. (1990). Nursing in Canada. *The Canadian Nurse, 86*(2), 4.

Halloran, E.J. and Welton, J.M. (1994). Why aren't there more men in nursing? In J. McCloskey and H. Grace (Eds.), *Current issues in nursing* (4th ed.) (pp. 683-691). St. Louis: Mosby-Year Book, Inc.

Health Manpower Directorate. (1983). *Canada health manpower inventory*. Ottawa: Health and Welfare Canada.

Holtzclaw, B.J. (1981). The man in nursing: Relations between sex-type perceptions and locus of control. *Dissertation Abstracts International*, 4202A. (University Microfilms No. 81-16, 752).

Kus, R.J. (1985). A challenge to nursing: Eliminating anti-male sexism in American society. In J. McCloskey and H. Grace (Eds.), *Current issues in nursing* (2nd ed.) (pp. 979-989). London: Blackwell Scientific Publications.

Nuttal, P. (1983). British nursing: Beginning of a power struggle. *Nursing Outlook, 31*(3), 184-187.

Okrainec, G.D. (1986a). Trends in nursing for Alberta male nurses. *AARN Newsletter, 42*(5), 13-14.

Okrainec, G.D. (1986b). Men in nursing. *The Canadian Nurse, 82*(7), 16-18.

Statistics Canada. (1994). Registered Nurses Management Data, 1992. Ottawa: Health Statistics Division, Statistics Canada.

PART II

Nursing
Knowledge

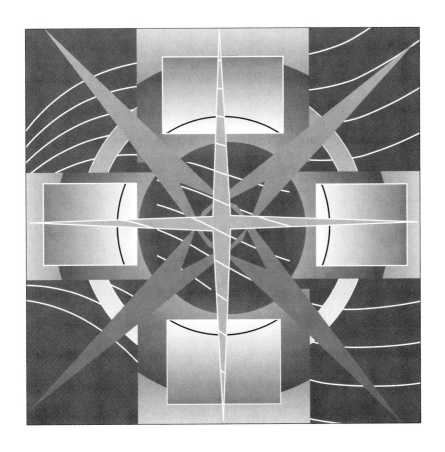

CHAPTER EIGHT

Knowledge Development in Nursing

MARION N. ALLEN
AND LOUISE A. JENSEN

Disciplines are centered primarily on knowledge development. Emphasis is placed on discovering, describing, extending, and modifying knowledge for the ultimate goal of the discipline. The aim of professional disciplines, such as nursing, is to know as well as deal with the actual implementation of knowledge in a practical sense (Donaldson and Crowley, 1978). Therefore the discipline of nursing provides the nursing knowledge that is the foundation for professional practice.

Since Florence Nightingale's time, nurses have been discussing and investigating the nature of knowing in nursing. That is, what do nurses need to know and what type of knowing is involved? Many nursing leaders, such as Harmer and Henderson, thought the way to answer these questions was to analyze the work or tasks that nurses do. Others felt that the way to answer these questions was to identify the concepts and phenomena that are of interest to nurses. Regardless of the answer, it was recognized that the knowledge needed in nursing was different than that of other health professions.

The discipline of nursing, as with all disciplines, can be viewed as comprising both a substantive and syntactical structure. The substantive structure, or subject matter of the discipline, is represented by its perspective and its domain or phenomena of interest. It consists of the body of ideas or concepts circumscribing the central subject matter and delineates boundaries of inquiry. The syntactical structure refers to the pattern of procedures by which the discipline applies concepts to achieve its results and the criteria used to justify the acceptance of truth of statements within the discipline (Donaldson and Crowley, 1978). As nursing evolves as a discipline, debates have occurred around the development of nursing knowledge.

■■ ■■ ■■ ■■

WORLD VIEW OF NURSING KNOWLEDGE

The perspective of a discipline includes the prevailing view held by most scholars in apprehending or perceiving phenomena within the domain (Algase and Whall, 1993). This perspective represents the belief system of the profession (Gortner, 1990), makes a set of assumptions regarding the nature of the world, and emphasizes some values over others (Algase and Whall, 1993). In addition, it defines the nature of inquiry in that discipline and the criteria for the credibility of knowledge (Kidd and Morrison, 1988). Nursing knowledge development is thus guided by philosophical claims about the nature of human beings and the human/environment relationship.

The essence of scientific truth is the most fundamental question pertaining to the development of nursing epistemology. Views of scientific truth provide a platform for appraisal of nursing theories and a way to understand methods of inquiry. Philosophic notions about scientific truth determine the research question as research questions in turn determine the method in nursing. Good science emanates from a solid philosophic base wherein the ends determine the means, rather than the other way around (Packard and Polifroni, 1992). According to Packard and Polifroni, the philosophical notions of truth that have influenced nursing may be stated as: (1) a stance based on realism wherein truth is larger than and different from human consciousness, an objective reality; (2) a metaphysical idealist stance that holds that truth is delineated by a consensus of scientists, (3) an epistemologic idealist stance whereby truth is no more and no less than that that may be reached through empirical means, and (4) a phenomenologic stance in which truth may be identified through the study of essential experience.

Nursing is a discipline in search of its philosophic foundation. Literature abounds in which various philosophies of science, from empiricism to critical theory, are proposed for nursing (Norbeck, 1987; Allen, 1985). In considering the growth and evolution of nursing knowledge, it is necessary to examine principal issues in the philosophy of science that have profoundly influenced knowledge-building approaches taken by the discipline. Basically three philosophies of science, i.e., rationalism, empiricism, and historicism, have been recognized as influencing views as to how knowledge develops. The epistemology of rationalism stresses the importance of a priori reasoning as the primary method of knowledge building. Empiricism as a world view of science embraces the notion that scientific knowledge is derived solely from sensory experiences. On the other hand, historicism recognizes science as a process of continuing research with knowledge evolving. However, currently there is much debate as to what the philosophic foundation of nursing should be, with emphasis being placed on achieving the "correct" view.

Another debate surrounds the question of whether a multiple or unitary philosophic perspective is required. Although several nurse scholars and philosophers call for an overriding or dominant philosophy of nursing, a current trend is toward greater exercise of pluralistic philosophic approaches (Meleis, 1987a; Fawcett, 1993). Drew (1988) cautions that the domain of nursing should not be viewed from a single philosophic stance. She believes that we are in danger of making similar errors as were done in the past when theorists battled for or against a single conceptual framework for nursing. She notes that when nursing knowledge is in its infancy the emphasis should be on theory expansion and tolerance of a wide variety of creative ideas. Uniformity of perspective is neither possible nor desirable.

There is therefore concern that nursing seems intent on finding an existing philosophy and adopting it as it stands as the philosophic foundation for the discipline. In contrast, others believe that development of a coherent and common philosophic orientation can lead to the development of a metaparadigm that can support a variety of nursing models. There is recognition on both sides that no single dominant philosophy has yet prevailed, which gives evidence that an appropriate philosophic foundation has not yet been found. It is argued that a philosophy for nursing must come from nurses (Reigel et al, 1992). The difference in opinion of whether pluralism is possible or desirable may stem from confusion over nursing philosophy versus philosophy of science. Nursing philosophy needs to be differentiated from science philosophy (Gortner, 1990), and science philosophy can be reframed according to the needs of the discipline. Currently the prevailing emphasis seems directed toward the development of a philosophy of nursing.

Also central to the perspective of nursing is the question regarding the nature of human beings and their relationship to the environment. Nursing's scientific development began with a reaction world view (humans are bio-psycho-social-spiritual beings) and evolved through the reciprocal interaction view of humans as holistic beings to the simultaneous action world view (unitary human beings identified by patterns) (Fawcett, 1993). The reciprocal and simultaneous paradigms have led to most of the contemporary nursing knowledge. Debate continues as to a correct view and/or the coexistence of multiple views for the development of nursing knowledge. Whatever world view evolves will hence dictate the substantive and syntactical structure of the discipline.

■ ■ ■ ■

SUBSTANTIVE STRUCTURE OF NURSING KNOWLEDGE

The nature and structure of nursing knowledge are addressed within the substantive structure of the discipline. The process of understanding and producing concepts essential to that body of knowledge comes from the theorizing activity of nurses. Theory development is the crucial element for the evolution of nursing into a professional discipline. The need for theory is no longer a matter of debate (Fawcett, 1984, Meleis, 1985); however, the specific content encompassing nursing knowledge, the source of that knowledge, and the kind of theory needed still lacks consensus. In addition, there is ongoing debate on how that knowledge should be structured.

Content Encompassing Nursing Knowledge

Recently nursing authors have been discussing nursing's substantive structure within the framework of a metaparadigm and paradigm (or disciplinary matrix) (Doheny, Cook, and Stopper, 1992; Fawcett, 1984). Paradigms or disciplinary matrices (nursing models) are more restrictive than the metaparadigm and represent a distinctive frame of reference within which the metaparadigm concepts and phenomena are viewed (Fawcett, 1984). The metaparadigm of a discipline defines what concepts are significant to a field.

Four main concepts, i.e., person, health, nursing, and environment, are perceived as central to the discipline. Although these concepts are accepted almost as a matter of fact (Conway, 1985), discussions still arise around such areas as the level of agreement on their meaning, whether nursing should be one of the metaparadigm concepts, and whether these four concepts include all concepts central to the discipline. The centrality of the four concepts in the discipline has been refuted by several nurse authors. Leininger (1984) states that human care is the critical and essential element of nursing and is the central concept of the metaparadigm. Meleis (1991) includes transitions, interaction, and nursing process with the concepts of person, health, nursing, and environment. Others believe the concept of person refers to the individual and as a consequence is too narrow. They believe the concept needs to be redefined to include pluralities of persons, such as families, groups, and communities (Schultz, 1987), or needs to view "person" both as human being and patient (Barnum, 1990). Whether nursing should be part of the metaparadigm is also questioned. For example, Conway states that nursing is the discipline, therefore nursing as action or activity of discipline members should not be a central concept. Leininger also rejects the idea that nursing can be a central concept because to her it is the phenomenon to be explained and predicted.

Other arguments seem to be not so much against the centrality of the four concepts but relate to the lack of consensus as to their meaning. Brodie (1984) exemplifies this position when she comments, "while congruence of concepts implies harmony and consensus, it does not assume common usage and universal acceptance of the meaning of each concept; nor does it establish the validity or testify to the usefulness of the concepts" (p. 88). The nursing literature abounds with varying definitions of health and environment. Similarly, as Hayne (1992) notes, the absence of a universally accepted definition of nursing is evidence of the lack of common meaning. Meleis (1987b) counters, noting that although agreement may not have been reached on definitions, a "territory for knowledge development" (p. 46) unique to nursing has been claimed. She further exhorts scholars to discontinue the debate and to engage in creating dynamic working definitions that are based on clinical and empirical examples. Maybe then, she notes, we will get consensus.

Following the identification and general agreement on the four major metaparadigm concepts, a literature debate ensued as to whether one, some, or all of these concepts needed to be included in nursing theory. Fawcett (1978) argued that theories including one or more of these concepts could be considered nursing theories, with the most sophisticated including all four. Flaskerud and Halloran (1980) suggest that in a nursing theory the concept of nursing as an activity must be included. They comment further that theories on person, health, illness, and environment, although helpful in explaining nursing's basic concepts and relationships, are also useful to other social and health sciences. Meleis (1991) asserts that theories developed to describe any of the central concepts are nursing theories when "the ultimate goal is related to the maintenance, promotion, or facilitation of health and well-being even though the theory may not specify the nursing actions" (p. 101). There is still lack of clarity as to what constitutes nursing theory and nursing questions. Crawford, Dufault, and Rudy (1979) suggest, however, that all theories and knowledge derived from nursing's unique perspective comprise nursing knowledge. From this perspective conceptual models are then derived that are useful guides to asking and answering nursing questions.

Each conceptual model presents a distinctive view of the phenomena of interest to the discipline and as a consequence outlines a comprehensive body of nursing knowledge (Fawcett, 1989). The proliferation of conceptual models during the last 25 years has consequently been linked with the interest in conceptualizing nursing as a discipline and to the concomitant introduction of ideas about nursing theory (Fawcett, 1989). While models were developed, debated, and discussed, a question arose: Should nursing have only a single conceptual model or many?

Riehl and Roy (1980) argued in their early writings that one conceptual model would lend stability to the discipline. It was also believed that one nursing model would not only guide our practice and education, but would help by posing all the pertinent questions and would provide a framework for all the pertinent answers. Yura and Walsh (1983) suggest that an eclectic combination of many of the different theories (models) could provide a rallying point for consensus that would make nursing more scientific, more rational, and more independently professional. Others contended, however, that one conceptual model would lead to premature closure on the options for the discipline (Stevens, 1985). In addition, the use of several models would permit viewing nursing from several perspectives and would increase our understanding of the scope and nature of the discipline (Feldman, 1980). There is some consensus that this is no longer an issue, and theoretic pluralism is accepted as important and desirable. However, Fawcett (1989) warns that the validity of the position supporting multiple models has not yet been established. In fact, Burney (1992) comments that there is a unifying theory developing in nursing vis-à-vis the theory of nursing diagnosis. She notes that various authors comment that the evolving theory of nursing diagnosis may make possible a clear and researchable definition of nursing's contribution and responsibility. Debate is now arising on how to use different models simultaneously to answer different questions. To aid in this process models are being classified according to their paradigmatic origins (developmental, interaction, systems) and philosophic underpinnings (totality versus simultaneity). This is proving to be a difficult task because the philosophical assumptions underlying the models are only beginning to be made more explicit.

Even though central concepts and their relationships with each other are beginning to be identified, discussions still ensue about whether nursing has a metaparadigm or is still at the preparadigm level. Hardy (1983), for example, states that until there is agreement on the concepts and one conceptual model of nursing, nursing will not have a metaparadigm. Conway (1985) also believes that whether nursing has a metaparadigm is debatable. She notes that in nursing there are divergent schools of thought concerning the phenomenon and no single set of rules to direct further theory building. In addition, there is lack of specificity in the usage of the word nursing. All this creates problems in attempts to arrive at a consensus, which is a prerequisite for a nursing metaparadigm. She concludes that nursing is in an evolutionary phase of development and continues to be at the preparadigm level.

The identification of the substance and phenomena for which the nursing discipline is accountable is far from complete. Even though there is broad consensus on the metaparadigm concepts, greater specificity is required for the knowledge to be useful in practice (Hinshaw, 1989). Various suggestions have been presented as a way to identify nursing's phenomena of interest. These include examining the questions in nursing studies and extracting underlying themes from them (Algase and Whall, 1993), examining the priority position papers of professional nursing organizations (Hinshaw, 1989), and analyzing models and exemplars (Meleis, 1991). Identification and attainment of agreement about the human phenomena that are of particular concern to nursing is one of the greatest tasks facing the discipline.

Sources of Knowledge in Nursing

Nursing practice has influenced the subject matter of knowledge development since Nightingale (Gortner, 1983). Should practice continue to be the major source of nursing knowledge? Various authors, such as Wald and Leonard (1964), declared that it should and they called for theories to be formulated from the realities of practice rather than from the perspective of other fields or disciplines. It is believed by others that nursing practice should not be the exclusive source. As Donaldson and Crowley (1978) point out, clinical practice deals with the person requiring immediate action. In contrast, the discipline encompasses a knowledge base relevant to all areas of practice and links past, present, and future. Its breadth goes beyond that required for nursing practice. This issue, as such, is no longer debated. It is recognized that the development of nursing knowledge requires a close relationship between theory, practice, and research (Meleis, 1991).

As nurses began to question the nature of knowledge required for nursing, the issue emerged as to whether the required knowledge and theory would be borrowed (theories for nursing) or unique (theories of nursing). Borrowed theory was knowledge developed by other disciplines and drawn upon by nursing, and unique theory was knowledge derived from observations of phenomena in nursing and asking questions unlike those that characterize other disciplines (Johnson, 1968). The case is made that there is value in using theory borrowed from or shared with other disciplines in that it allows for added and expanded opportunities in which nursing can interpret and utilize other perspectives that might be relevant to a given situation (Moore, 1990). It is argued that the use of adjunctive precepts, principles, and concepts is not only inevitable but essential. As Levine (1988) states, "this is not borrowed knowledge, but knowledge required for appropriate nursing decisions." She comments that nursing cannot stand apart within a body of knowledge it shares with other health-care disciplines. Adjunctive concepts are antecedent to all nursing theory. The emphasis is on refining and synthesizing the theory according to a nursing perspective (Cull-Wilby and Pepin, 1987).

In contrast, others contend that using frameworks and theories from other disciplines enlarges the knowledge base of that discipline, which is a contribution to knowledge but not nursing knowledge. They contend that borrowing means returning. Johnson (1968) and Donaldson and Crowley (1978), as well as others, point out that there may be no sense in this issue. Knowledge is part of the public domain and is not owned. Further, Donaldson and Crowley contend that knowledge can not be borrowed from other disciplines because each discipline's perspective is different and can not be understood if it is removed from the context in which it was generated. The borrowed concepts or theories are always redefined in the context of the borrowing discipline.

Confusion surrounding this issue may arise when talking about knowledge for the discipline and knowledge required by nurses for the practice of nursing. Some, such as Ellis (Algase and Whall, 1993), believe that disciplinary knowledge is just part of what nurses need in order to practise nursing. Thus the substantive structure of the discipline need not account for, encompass, or reformulate to a nursing view all the knowledge needed for practice. Confusion has also arisen from the use of terms. At the outset of the debate the issue centered around borrowed versus unique theory. But over time the issue centered around borrowed versus unique knowledge. R.E. Ellis (personal communication, 1982) commented that there may not necessarily be a need for uniqueness in talking about theory of a phenomenon. In talking about a body of knowledge, uniqueness or distinctiveness might be important. The uniqueness arises from the content and the way the knowledge is organized.

This issue has still not been resolved and, as Barrett (1991) contends, it has in fact become more complex. She believes the crux of the issue is what constitutes substantive knowledge in nursing: Is nursing primarily a basic or an applied science? As a basic science, knowledge original to the discipline (theories of nursing) is developed. In an applied science, knowledge is synthesized from other disciplines (theories for nursing) to do what is required in the practice of nursing. Rogers, Parse, and Newman, according to Barrett, state that nursing science doesn't derive from other basic or applied sciences but is an emergent basic science. Barrett comments that others, such as King and Johnson, have viewed nursing as an applied science in which reformulation of borrowed knowledge will lead to new concepts and theories of nursing intervention that will produce predictable results in clients. Hogan and DeSantis (1991) also note that the discipline has focused its attention primarily on applied research, leaving basic research to other disciplines. This lack of a comprehensive substantive base has led to continuation of borrowing theoretical assumptions and concepts from other disciplines. They contend that the result of this borrowing of and focus on applied research is a profession that has generally been unable to examine nursing phenomena grounded in nursing knowledge.

Implicit in this issue of unique versus borrowed is the question of whether nursing knowledge can and should be generated through the use of a nursing model. Models provide a frame of reference; they organize our thinking, observing, and interpreting. Their value lies in their ability to explain phenomena and to increase understanding or give a sense of what is going on and why (Lancaster and Lancaster, 1981). In a review of the use of nursing models in research, Silva (1987) and Allen and Hayes (1989) commented that their use has ranged from empirical validation of the models, to development of tools to measure concepts particular to the model, to inclusion by the researcher of a brief description of the relationship of the model to the study, however nebulous. These authors concluded that, although nursing models have been used to guide research, there are several gaps and weaknesses in their usefulness for generating nursing knowledge, particularly the lack of testing underlying assumptions of the model, proposed relationships between the concepts, and clarification of the concepts relevant to the model.

It is these gaps and weaknesses that have led nurses to argue that nursing models are inadequate for the development of knowledge needed in nursing. They are perceived as too abstract and general, even vague. Researchers argue that models are "envisioned ideals;" they outline the "oughts" and "shoulds" of nursing and are not testable scientific theories. The proponents for the use of nursing models counter with the argument that models outside the discipline also involve vague notions or ideals. They assert that only nursing conceptual models provide a framework for the development of nursing knowledge. They argue further that the model provides the focus by which decisions are made about the phenomena of interest to the discipline and the precise nature of the problem to be studied (Fawcett, 1989) and provides a means for organizing and guiding research. They comment that laws set forth in other nonnursing models and theories do not explain the phenomena of nursing (Phillips, 1988). Phillips comments that the use of models from other sciences as opposed to a nursing model leads one to still ask the question of whether nursing is a science.

Even though there are strong proponents for the use of nursing models to guide knowledge development in nursing, questions are beginning to arise about whether nursing conceptual models are needed any longer. It has been suggested that with the recognition of the uniqueness of what nursing can offer (Meleis, 1992), the work of developing knowledge within the structure of nursing conceptual models in favour of interdisciplinary theories for health care can be abandoned (Meleis, 1992; Smith, 1992b). The "quest for boundaries of domains is essential [only] when groups have no sense of identity" (Meleis, 1992, p.115). Smith states that the consequence of this position must be carefully considered; the survival of the discipline and the profession depend upon it. She believes that unless nursing has identifiable and distinctive knowledge integrated closely with practice, there is great danger that the disintegration of nursing as a distinct profession can and will occur. She calls for continued use of nursing models to provide the broad perspective within which knowledge is to be developed. In addition, Smith notes there is a need also for middle-range theories developed from this broad perspective in order to develop a coherent knowledge structure in the discipline.

Levels of Knowledge in Nursing

Closely aligned with the issues concerning the source of nursing knowledge is the debate centering around the kinds of theories needed in nursing. Should they be descriptive (basic and applied) or prescriptive? Should they be grand, middle-range or micro-theories? Dickoff, James, and Weidenbach (1968), along with others, called for theory beyond that of describing, explaining, and predicting behaviour. These authors believed that nursing theory should culminate in prescriptive or practice theory, which identifies practice goals and actions necessary for attaining these goals. Beckstrand (1978) countered, stating that there was no need for practice theory and, in fact, what Dickoff, James, and Weidenbach were proposing was not scientific theory but more beginning metatheory of nursing practice. Through an examination of the various aspects of practice knowledge (knowledge of how to control and make changes and knowledge of what is morally good) she concluded that practice theory is not distinct from science and ethics. Science seeks to develop the knowledge necessary to change and control, and meta-ethics and normative ethics provides knowledge about moral issues in nursing. Critics of Beckstrand's view (Meleis, 1991) comment that what Beckstrand was calling for was knowledge borrowed from other disciplines (applied theory). Confusion exists in this debate because many of the various authors did not join issue but rather took issue. For example, authors using one definition of theory critiqued the views of others who were using another definition. Prescriptive and practice theory were used interchangeably without a clear picture of whether they meant the same thing.

This debate has taken somewhat of a new twist and now centres around the kinds of knowledge, i.e., descriptive, explanatory, or prescriptive, most appropriate for nursing. Some theorists, using the parameters set by Dickoff, James, and Weidenbach assert that the ultimate aim of nursing science is to enable nurses to predict and control the phenomena of interest. Descriptive and explanatory knowledge are of concern only as a means to reach this more valued end (Moccia, 1988). Others believe that human phenomena are unique and unpredictable, therefore descriptive and explanatory knowledge is the ultimate goal. These concerns are transposed into the practice field, and questions are being asked about the nature of practice: Is nursing practice directed toward the control of human phenomena or toward assisting others in more fully understanding their realities and their positions within them (Allen, 1985)? Answers to these questions not only have major implications as to the phenomena of interest to the discipline and the kinds of knowledge developed but also have implications for the kind of practice that will ensue.

The debate around grand theories of nursing versus middle- and micro-range theories, referring to the scope of the theory, is comparable to the debate whether theories of, theories for, or theories in nursing are the most appropriate. The first part of the original debate on this issue focused on whether theory development should be directed toward a single unified nursing theory or diverse and multiple nursing theories. The second facet of the debate was whether one should begin by developing theories that delineate the scope and definition of or about nursing and the nursing process (Crawford, Dufault, and Rudy, 1979) or theories that will guide nursing action. The issue has been examined and re-examined and has been made more confusing through the use of differing definitions of theory and more recently redefining the issue as that of unique versus borrowed knowledge (Barrett, 1991). Theories of nursing are referred to as that knowledge original to the discipline, and theories for nursing as knowledge synthesized from other disciplines. Some refer to grand theories (theories of nursing) as synonymous with nursing models, while others refer to those theories derived from conceptual models (such as Newman's theory of health as expanding consciousness, which was derived from Roger's Science of Unitary Human Beings) as grand theories (Fawcett, 1989). When used interchangeably with a nursing model the consensus reached is, as stated earlier, that one theory or model of nursing may not be appropriate at this time. When grand theory is viewed as being derived from a nursing model then it is deemed appropriate because it is more circumscribed than the conceptual model, albeit still too broad for direct testing. However, it is generally accepted that middle-range theories, narrower in scope than grand theory, are extremely useful in nursing. These theories, suitable for testing, can guide nursing action and, as such, can be seen as theories for nursing "that would bring to bear a wider range of knowledge to bear on nursing problems" (Norris, 1969). Micro-range or partial theories, limited in scope, are frequently seen as trivial (Fawcett, 1989), though Fawcett notes that these can perhaps lead to middle-range theories with further research. Donaldson and Crowley (1978) offered a resolution to this issue by noting that what is important is not to identify a single theory of nursing, but to place theories within the context of the discipline.

Classification of Nursing Knowledge

"An organizing framework that permits scientists to impose order on the phenomena of interest is a necessary prerequisite for developing theories and theoretical models" (Kim, 1987). Such organizational schemes need to allow for the inclusion of key concepts and exclusions of those that are insignificant or no longer relevant. A variety of organizational schemes at various levels of abstraction have been proposed. Schlotfeldt (1988) conceptualized the discipline as an expandable and permeable sphere made up of segments of varying size, representing the kinds of professional knowledge (scientific, historical, philosophical, nursing strategies, approaches, and technologies) contained within the discipline. She suggests that this provides one approach to classifying and organizing the varying kinds of knowledge that constitute the nursing discipline. In a similar vein, Schultz and Meleis (1988) organize the knowledge specific to nursing around three types including clinical, conceptual, and empirical. Clinical knowledge is revealed primarily in the acts of practicing nurses and currently is the product of a combination of personal knowing and empiricism. Conceptual knowledge is the outgrowth of reflection on nursing phenomena, and empirical knowledge results from research. In contrast, Kim (1987), in an attempt to classify essential concepts in nursing, has proposed a typology organized around the major metaparadigm concepts. Her typology includes the four domains of client, client-nurse, practice, and the environment. Phenomena related to health are part of the client domain. Inclusive in each of these domains are the various efforts for knowledge generation.

Nursing diagnoses have also been proposed as useful ways to organize nursing knowledge. But of all the proposals put forth as organizational frameworks, it is this one that has led to the most debate. Roy (cited in Smith, 1988) notes that the "important long term potential of nursing diagnoses is in relation to ordering knowledge" (p. 83). Rasch (1987) also recognizes that the North American Nursing Diagnosis Association (NANDA) Taxonomy I might be useful for the discipline. Vincent and Coler (1990) remark that a taxonomy is useful in categorizing research needs and endeavours as well as assisting in theory development. They also note that theory developed in the context of the clinical area through the use of models of nursing diagnoses can be a viable guide for practice. Others in opposition comment that a taxonomy of nursing diagnoses is not appropriate because the body of knowledge to build the taxonomy is still too limited, and the identification of diagnostic categories leads to premature closure (Leininger, cited in Smith, 1988). Rogers (cited in Smith, 1988) comments that diagnosis is a static and outdated term and does not reflect the nature of nursing knowledge; she calls for new ways of organizing nursing knowledge.

Syntactical Structure of Nursing Knowledge

The syntactical structure of nursing knowledge refers to the methods of inquiry used by the discipline. Contemporary debate in nursing centres around such questions as: How is knowledge derived? What is the best way to obtain knowledge of nursing reality? What are the criteria of knowledge? The development of nursing theory is a relatively recent mandate in the discipline. The nature of knowledge required for nursing is closely related to and largely determined by the purpose and goals of nursing practice and the kinds of problems the discipline seeks to address (Carper, 1978). "What is nursing knowledge?" raises the concomitant question of "What is nursing research?" Nursing research has not had a long history. Much of the research reported in the 1960s described and evaluated nursing education and the personal and professional characteristics of nurses. In the 1970s the focus shifted to the development of concepts and models for describing, explaining, predicting, and prescribing nursing theory and practice. The 1980s were characterized by the acceptance and use of research. Research based on the existing diverse theoretical positions has developed slowly because of incomplete degrees of clarity among theoretical constructs, propositional linkages, and operational measures needed to test, verify, and expand theory.

Modes of Inquiry In Nursing

How do we know what we know? The complexity of nursing's epistemology was clearly demonstrated by Carper's (1978) delineation of four fundamental patterns of knowing in nursing: empirical, ethical, personal, and esthetic. Each way of knowing has a different purpose, expression, and process for development and evaluation. As nurses, our ways of knowing have not been fully articulated (Schultz and Meleis, 1988).

Empirics was originally based on the traditional notions of science in which reality is viewed as objective, verifiable phenomena, and knowledge is derived through a systematic collection of empirical data to validate hypotheses. However, the traditional approach to empiricism as the only way to acquire knowledge has been questioned. Nurses began to recognize the limitations of this view, such as the lack of tools to measure phenomena that concern nursing and the need for more than empirical facts when caring for people. As a result the view of what constitutes science has broadened to include evidence generated from naive inquiry (Reason and Rowan, 1981), such as phenomenology and other inductive methods. A sense of separation therefore has arisen among nurse inquirers who hold different epistemological positions and use different methods of inquiry (Schultz and Meleis, 1988). Some rely on reflection and reasoning, others select structured observation and hypothesis testing, while others prefer reflective interpretation. In the ongoing debate several camps may be identified. Some believe that empiricism, if not quantification, is the most appropriate avenue (Clarke and Yaros, 1988; Norbeck, 1987), while others maintain that qualitative methods hold the greatest promise (Field and Morse, 1985; Leininger, 1985). Others advocate triangulation of methods (Duffy, 1987; Gortner and Schultz, 1988), and finally, there is the stance that none of these are appropriate but rather the creation of new and different methods are favored (Moccia, 1988; Parse, 1987). These differing methods indicate that, if we do not know where we are going, how can we judge the means to get there? As Packard and Polifroni (1992) note, understanding the ends will inevitably clarify the means.

Esthetics refers to knowing about unique particulars as opposed to universals and comprehending the meaning that underlies an encounter with another person. Empathy serves as the main mode of this way of knowing. The truthfulness of this kind of knowledge is determined through criticism, seeking the relative truth in relation to the present and the future (Chinn and Jacobs, 1987). Little development of esthetic knowledge has taken place in nursing to date.

The third way of knowing, ethics, is knowledge that focuses on matters of obligation or what should be done. It involves understanding the different philosophical positions of what is right, what is good, and what should be desired. However, it also involves making judgments and carrying out actions that are deliberate and subject to interpretation of right and wrong. Because the practice of nursing is different from other health professions, debate is ensuing as to whether a separate nursing ethic based on the caring relationship between nurse and patient is needed as opposed to the traditional theories of bioethics (Fry, 1989, 1991). The method of determining the credibility of this kind of knowledge is justification, that is, determination of whether the particular theory, standard, or code is just and responsible (Chinn & Jacobs, 1987).

Personal knowledge was described by Carper (1978) as knowing the self and is concerned with the kind of knowing that promotes wholeness and integrity. Personal knowledge is primary to all knowing (Smith, 1992a). Unfortunately, we know very little about knowing the self and knowing how. The knowing how from practice may be enlightened through innovative methods of inquiry, such as grounded theory or phenomenologic research (Benner, 1983, 1985; Ray, 1987). Efforts to bring to understanding the self-knowledge and knowing how of nursing practice have begun to be aided by examination of women's ways of knowing. Belenky, Clinchy, Goldberger, and Tarule (1986) identified these as silence, received knowledge, subjective knowledge, procedural knowledge, and constructed knowledge. Nurses who subscribe to this view of knowing see theories as reality that is ongoing and always in process; their frames of reference are constructed and reconstructed (Visintainer, 1986). Reflection is the method for determining the credibility of personal knowledge (Chinn and Jacobs, 1987).

The use of one pattern of knowing does not preclude use of other epistemic approaches. Inquirers from differing and contradictory perspectives within the ways of knowing have a propensity to put forth the view that their way of knowing yields *the* truth rather than *a* truth. Perhaps it is not sufficient to speak of facts alone or to rely on research as the medium for knowledge development. Instead, some support that we should speak of experiences, intuition, and facts. Conceptualizations and expert knowledge from clinical practice may be equally powerful and credible (Schultz and Meleis, 1988). The type of knowledge used in practice has changed over the years, with a general trend toward increasing the scientific knowledge base (Chinn and Jacobs, 1987). The arguments for or the superiority of some methods over others has essentially boiled down to a recognition that basically different types of "problems" require different methods. All modes of inquiry are necessary to form a knowledge base in nursing, although efforts thus far have been mainly experimental. The nature of human experience requires openness to numerous ways of knowing. While the world view of nursing is clarified the essential questions in nursing will be asked, consistent with the practice of nursing. No a priori reason exists to suppose that one kind of knowledge is more authentic than another. Current nursing theory and research lack the rich knowledge embedded in expert clinical practice, which results from the use of all patterns of knowing (Benner, 1983, 1984). Central to the debate is nurse-scientists' limited view of inquiry that is incompatible with the philosophic orientation of holism to which nursing has subscribed. This overreliance on the reductionistic approach may have deterred theoretical progress. The increasing use of qualitative methods, such as ethnography and grounded theory, reflects the influence of historicism on our search to understand the complex responses to living with health-disease.

Nursing offers a plethora of research questions that arise from curiosity about phenomena in the field. Deciding on a mode of inquiry requires a full understanding of the nature of nursing phenomena. There are numerous rival hypotheses on how a science develops. Theory guides a researcher about what to observe but does not provide direction about suitable methods for making such observations. Methods for observing phenomena may differ depending on the nature of the phenomena, personal experience, and preference. The development and testing of a body of knowledge does not occur in a vacuum but reflects a specific disciplinary perspective (Hinshaw, 1989). Freedom and flexibility are necessary to choose attributes of prevailing paradigms that best describe or explain nursing phenomena. A pluralistic, eclectic approach is thus advocated by many theorists as opposed to an either/or approach or one grand approach to capture the entirety of the domain of nursing (Fitzpatrick and Whall, 1989; Fawcett, 1984: Meleis, 1985). Evolution of knowledge is consequently viewed as a process rather than a product. Rawnsley (1993) suggests dialectic reasoning may assist in the synthesis of multiple modes of inquiry to derive nursing knowledge.

Brown, Tanner, and Padrick (1984) noted a major limitation in nursing is the failure to build a cumulative science. With some exceptions, current nursing theory is usually arrived at rationally or deductively, with few empirical verifications. In the contemporary literature a tremendous profusion of studies can be found based on theoretical notions and predictions about events of importance and interest to the practicing nurse. To advance and integrate the findings of many studies that often appear to be disparate and unrelated, the nurse researcher needs to identify, understand, and synthesize the interrelationships among the studies. This is a difficult task due in part to the undefined domain of nursing that has led to ambiguous or competing definitions of nursing (Schlotfeldt, 1987). The use of pluralistic research methods, collaborative research teams, and multiple site studies are viewed as essential strategies to advance knowledge and build nursing science (Gortner, 1987).

Therefore the development of nursing theory requires a systematic process of inquiry. Components of that process include concept analysis, construction of theoretical relationships, testing of theoretical relationships, and practical validation of theory (Chinn and Jacobs, 1987). As a practice discipline nursing requires that the theoretical relationships be tested and the theory be validated in the real world. The purpose of evaluating theory is to determine whether the theory can guide research or practice and to determine which type of research is required to modify the theory in order to meet the criteria of clarifying phenomena of interest to nursing. The level of knowledge about the phenomena of interest directs the level of theory development and the type of questions asked in research. The approach used to develop theory will also depend on the researcher's view of the world. Consequently, the relationship among nursing theory, research, and practice is dialectic.

Criteria for Credibility of Nursing Knowledge

Literature abounds outlining ways that the adequacy and credibility of knowledge can and should be assessed. Central questions arise about what is truth and what criteria justify the acceptance of truth? Debates surround the question of which criteria are most valid.

Historically, clinical knowledge has been the product of a combination of personal knowing and empirics. It has usually involved intuition and subjective knowing, although these have tended to be ignored or denied. The esthetics and ethical patterns of knowing have also contributed to the development of clinical knowledge. Traditionally, clinical knowledge has been communicated through the retrospective publication of articles, and the credibility of clinical knowledge has been based on whether or not it works. Perhaps models of practice, the discovery of patterns within and across patients, might be appropiate criteria for the credibility of clinical knowledge (Schultz and Meleis, 1988).

The credibility of conceptual knowledge rests in part on the extent to which nurses find models and theories useful for communicating what they know (Schultz and Meleis, 1988). It is unclear as to why models outside the discipline as opposed to nursing models are so readily accepted to guide knowledge development in nursing. The terms model and theory used interchangeably when referring to these abstract conceptualizations has led to confusion about their purpose. Even though models have been identified as grand theory, it is perceived that they should be testable in the same way as other scientific theories. Whether or not a particular conceptual framework holds up to critical appraisal depends on its coherence and logical integrity (Meleis, 1985: Chinn and Jacobs, 1987). Empirics has largely influenced the development of conceptual knowledge in nursing. As a result, empirical criteria have largely been employed in justifying the adequacy of conceptual knowledge.

Empirical knowledge results from research. Induction and deduction are complementary and equally important processes for nursing science. The deductive method of theory development evaluates theory by testing empirical adequacy, ascertaining whether predictions are borne out by relevant data. Such testing relies on the null hypothesis test of significance. Another type of inference involved in generation of theory is retroductive. Certain observed phenomena come to the researcher's attention and are analyzed by detecting patterns. Once patterned, observations are explained by way of a retroductive theoretical reasoning process through the existence of an underlying causal mechanism. Theory appraisal is undertaken by comparing the hypothesized models rather than by comparing them with other competitive theories, as in theory testing. This method begins with problems, theories, or observations. Stability of patterns gained through exploratory analysis is critically examined through the use of confirmatory data analysis. The theory evoked explains the reason for the pattern of the data. Theories are created from and grounded in data (Glaser and Strauss, 1967); therefore data are not used solely for testing existing theories. A number of explanatory theories are generated to explain the data, with the most plausible theory receiving additional development and appraisal. This method encourages and demands that a plurality of research procedures be used, and that statistical inference will be used primarily to distinguish between systematic and haphazard trends in data. The credibility of empirical knowledge therefore rests on the degree to which the researcher has followed accepted procedures and on the logical derivation of conclusions from evidence without bias or prejudice (Gortner and Schultz, 1988). There is a growing consensus on what constitutes "good" science in nursing. Scientific inquiry is characterized by significance, observation, generalizability, reproducibility, and precision. In nursing science the units of analyses need specification, the technique with the best potential for explication of the phenomena should be selected, and the norms of intersubjectivity, understanding, generality, reproducibility, explanation, and precision should be defined and followed (Gortner and Schultz, 1988). In addition to the procedural criteria accompanying various research designs and methods, the credibility of empirical knowledge is assessed by systematic review and critique of research and by conferences geared to collaborating on what is known and clarifying the state of the art.

Ultimately, credibility criteria must be consistent with the various ways of knowing in nursing. Whether we debate about whether one or several sets of criteria are required as well as what the criteria should be, it seems possible that the criteria for accepting knowledge vary for each type of knowledge. Chinn and Jacobs (1983) view the theory validation process as the essence of the theory/practice relationship. If nursing theory relates to nursing practice then validation of theoretical propositions must take place in the practice setting. The practical validation of theory is accomplished through a deductive approach of translating theoretically derived propositions into hypotheses. In addition, abstract concepts are operationalized into observable facts. Fawcett (1978) similarily states that a theory in and of itself is irrelevant. The researcher finds data that support or refute the theorist's claims. The practitioner provides the ultimate test of relevance of the theorist's claims. Tension exists within this helix. Practicing nurses question the relevance to clinical practice of much of nursing research. Researchers are concerned about the diffusion of results into nursing practice. Findings should be used as concepts and principles, not as procedures or standardized rules. Although practical applications of theory are rarely possible, theory can be of immeasurable assistance at a practical level. Enhanced thinking and understanding of situations and events in the clinical setting and the resulting acquistion of new approaches or orientations to problems through research are two of the ways in which the interrelationship of theory and practice benefits clinical nursing practice. Also, practice benefits theory through the generation of ideas developed in the context of practice. The contribution of the basic sciences to the knowledge that underlies nursing practice cannot be denied. On the other hand, the body of knowledge needed for nursing practice will be incomplete unless questions about events specific to practice are asked.

Future Directions For Knowledge Development

The development of the discipline of nursing has gone through four stages including: theorizing, developing a syntax, concept development, and philosophical debate (Meleis, 1992). Debates that aid in the development of the discipline have ensued within these stages. Through the evolution of nursing knowledge, reliance on other disciplines is now lessening, and the ontological and epistemological questions grounded in nursing's central concepts can be seen. Critics of knowledge development in nursing suggest advancement of knowledge in the substantive area. Different paradigms or models of nursing are seen as both necessary and valuable. Maturation of a philosophy of nursing as a base for knowledge development has been offered as a means to end the debate over which method of inquiry is appropriate. All modes of inquiry are viewed as necessary to form a knowledge base in nursing. The nature of human experience requires openness to numerous ways of knowing and scientific inquiry. As the world view of nursing is clarified, the essential questions in nursing will be asked, consistent with the practice of nursing. The development of systematic knowledge should be and will continue to be a priority in planning the future of the discipline of nursing (Schlotfeldt, 1988).

REFERENCES

Algase, D.L., and Whall, A.F. (1993). Rosemary Ellis' views of the substantive structure of nursing. *Image, 25*, 69-72.

Allen, D.G. (1985). Nursing research and social control: Alternative models of science that emphasize understanding and emancipation. *Image, 17*, 58-64.

Allen, M.N., and Hayes, P. (1989). Models of nursing: Implications for research in nursing. *Recent Advances in Nursing, 24*, 77-92.

Barnum, B. (1990). *Nursing theory: Analysis, application, evaluation*, (3rd ed.). Boston: Little, Brown & Co.

Barrett, E.A.M. (1991). Theory: Of or for nursing? *Nursing Science Quarterly, 4*, 48-49.

Beckstrand, J. (1978). The notion of practice theory and the relationship of scientific and ethical knowledge to practice. *Research in Nursing and Health, 1*, 131-136.

Belenky, M.F., Clinchy, B.M., Goldberger, N.R., and Tarule, J. M. (1986). *Women's ways of knowing: The development of self, voice, and mind*. New York : Basic Books.

Benner, P. (1983). Uncovering the knowledge embedded in clinical practice. *Image, 15*, 36-41.

Benner, P. (1984). *From novice to expert: Excellence and power in clincial nursing practice*. Menlo Park, CA: Addison-Wesley.

Benner, P. (1985). Quality of life: A phenomenological perspective on explanation, prediction, and understanding in nursing science. *Advances in Nursing Science, 8* (1), 1-14.

Brodie, J.N. (1984). A response to Dr. J. Fawcett's paper: "The metaparadigm of nursing: Present status and future refinements". *Image, 16*, 87-88.

Brown, J.S., Tanner, C.A., and Padrick, K.P. (1984). Nursing's search for scientific knowledge. *Nursing Research, 33*, 26-33.

Burney, M.A. (1992). King and Neuman: in search of the nursing paradigm. *Journal of Advanced Nursing, 17*, 601-603.

Carper, B.A. (1978). Fundamental patterns of knowing in nursing. *Advances in Nursing Science, 1*(1), 13-23.

Chinn, P.L., and Jacobs, M.K. (1983). *Theory and nursing: A systematic approach*. St Louis: C. V. Mosby.

Chinn, P.L., and Jacobs, M.K. (1987). *Theory and nursing: A systematic approach* (2nd ed.). St Louis: C. V. Mosby.

Clarke, P.N., and Yaros, P.S. (1988). Commentary: Transitions to new methodologies in nursing science. *Nursing Science Quarterly, 3*, 147-151.

Conway, M.E. (1985). Toward greater specificity in defining nursing's metaparadigm. *Advances in Nursing Science, 7*(4), 73-81.

Crawford, G., Dufault, Sr. K., and Rudy, E. (1979). Evolving issues in theory development. *Nursing Outlook, 27*, 346-351.

Cull-Wilby, B.L., and Pepin, J.I. (1987). Towards a coexistence of paradigms in nursing knowledge development. *Journal of Advanced Nursing, 12*, 515-521.

Dickoff, J., James, P., and Weidenbach, E. (1968). Theory in a practice discipline. Part I: Practice oriented theory. *Nursing Research, 17*, 415-435.

Doheny, M., Cook, C.: and Stopper, C. (1992). *The discipline of nursing: An introduction* (3rd ed.). Norwalk, CT: Appleton & Lange.

Donaldson, S.K., and Crowley, D.M. (1978). The discipline of nursing. *Nursing Outlook, 26*, 113-120.

Drew, B.J. (1988). Devaluation of biological knowledge. *Image, 20*, 25-27.

Duffy, M.E. (1987). Methodological triangulation: A vehicle for merging quantitative and qualitative research methods. *Image, 19*, 130-133.

Fawcett, J. (1978). The relationship between theory and research: A double helix. *Advances in Nursing Science. 3*, 49-62.

Fawcett, J. (1984). The metaparadigm of nursing: Present status and future refinements. *Image, 16*, 84-87.

Fawcett, J. (1989). *Analysis and evaluation of conceptual models of nursing* (2nd ed.). Philadelphia: F.A. Davis.

Fawcett, J. (1993). From a plethora of paradigms to parsimony in worldviews. *Nursing Science Quarterly, 6*, 56-58.

Feldman, H.R. (1980). Nursing research in the 80's: Issues and implications. *Advances in Nursing Science, 3*(1), 85-92.

Field, P.A., and Morse, J.M. (1985). *Nursing research: The application of qualitative approaches*. Rockville, MD: Aspen.

Fitzpatrick, J.J., and Whall, A.L. (1989). *Conceptual models of nursing: Analysis and application*. Norwalk, CT: Appleton & Lange.

Flaskerud, J.H., and Halloran, E.J. (1980). Areas of agreement in nursing theory development. *Advances in Nursing Science, 3*(1), 1-7.

Fry, S.T. (1989). Toward a theory of nursing ethics. *Advances in Nursing Science, 11*(4), 9-22.

Fry, S.T. (1991). A theory of caring: Pitfalls and promises. In D.A. Gaut & M.M. Leininger (Eds.). *Caring: The compassionate healer* (pp. 161-172). New York: National League for Nursing Press.

Glaser, B.G., and Strauss, A.L. (1967). *The discovery of grounded theory*. New York: Aldine Publishing Company.

Gortner, S.R. (1983). The history and philosophy of nursing science and research. *Advances in Nursing Science, 5*(2), 1-8.

Gortner, S. (1987). To build the science. In S.R. Gortner (Ed.), *Nursing science methods: A reader*. (pp 5-15). San Francisco: University of California.

Gortner, S.R. (1990). Nursing values and science: Toward a science philosophy. *Image, 22,* 101-105.

Gortner, S.R., and Schultz, P.R. (1988). Approaches to nursing science methods. *Image, 20,* 22-24.

Hardy, M. (1983). Metaparadigms and theory development. In N.L. Chaska (Ed.). *The nursing profession: A time to speak out* (pp. 427-437). New York: McGraw-Hill.

Hayne, Y. (1992). The current status and future significance of nursing as a discipline. *Journal of Advanced Nursing, 17,* 104-107.

Hinshaw, A.S. (1989). Nursing science: The challenge to develop knowledge. *Nursing Science Quarterly, 2,* 162-171.

Hogan, N., and DeSantis, L. (1991). Development of substantive theory in nursing, *Nurse Education Today, 11,* 167-171.

Johnson, D.E. (1968). Theory in nursing: Borrowed and unique. *Nursing Research, 17,* 206-209.

Kidd, P., and Morrison, E.F. (1988). The progression of knowledge in nursing: A search for meaning. *Image, 20,* 222-224.

Kim, H.S. (1987). Structuring the nursing knowledge system: A typology of four domains. *Scholarly Inquiry for Nursing Practice, 1,* 99-110.

Lancaster, W., and Lancaster, J. (1981). Models and model building in nursing. *Advances in Nursing Science, 3*(3), 31-42.

Leininger, M.M. (1984). *Care: The essence of nursing.* Thorofare, NJ: Charles B. Slack.

Leininger, M.M. (1985). *Qualitative research methods in nursing.* Orlando: Grune and Stratton.

Levine, M.E. (1988). Antecedents from adjunctive disciplines: Creation of nursing theory. *Nursing Science Quarterly, 1,* 16-21.

Meleis, A.I. (1985). *Theortical nursing: Development and progress.* New York: J.B. Lippincott.

Meleis, A.I. (1987a). Revisions in knowledge development: A passion for substance. *Scholarly Inquiry for Nursing Practice, 1,* 5-19.

Meleis, A.I. (1987b). Theoretical nursing: Today's challenges, tomorrow's bridges. *Nursing Papers, 19,* 45-57.

Meleis, A.I. (1991). *Theoretical nursing: Development and progress* (2nd ed.). Philadelphia: J.B. Lippincott.

Meleis, A. (1992). Directions for nursing theory development in the 21st century. *Nursing Science Quarterly, 5,* 112-117.

Moccia, P. (1988). A critique of compromise: Beyond the methods debate. *Advances in Nursing Science, 10*(4), 1-9.

Moore, S. (1990). Thoughts on the discipline of nursing as we approach the year 2000. *Journal of Advanced Nursing, 15,* 825-828.

Norbeck, J.S. (1987). In defense of empiricism. *Image, 19,* 28-30.

Norris, C. (1969). Introduction. In C.M. Norris (Ed.), *Proceedings, First Nursing Theory Conference.* Kansas City, KS: Department of Nursing Education, University of Kansas Medical Center.

Packard, S.A., and Polifroni, E.C. (1992). The nature of scientific truth. *Nursing Science Quarterly, 5,* 158-163.

Parse, R.R. (1987). *Nursing science: Major paradigms, theories and critiques.* Philadelphia: Saunders.

Phillips, J.R. (1988). The reality of nursing research. *Nursing Science Quarterly, 1,* 48-49.

Rasch, R.F.R. (1987). The nature of taxonomy. *Image, 19,* 147-149.

Rawnsley, M.M. (1993). Dialectics and the diverse discourse in nursing sciece. *Nursing Science Quarterly, 6,* 2-4.

Ray, M.A. (1987). Technological caring: A new model in critical care. *Dimensions of Critical Care Nursing, 6,* 166-173.

Reason, P., and Rowan, J. (1981). *Human inquiry. A sourcebook of new paradigm research.* New York: John Wiley & Sons.

Reigel, B., Omery, A., Calvillo, E., Elsayed, N., Lee, P., Shuler, P., Siegal, B. (1992). Moving beyond: A generative philosophy of science. *Image, 24,* 115-120.

Riehl, J.P., and Roy, C. (1980). *Conceptual models for nursing practice* (2nd ed.). New York: Appleton-Century-Crofts.

Schultz, P. (1987). When clients mean more than one: Extending the foundational concept of person. *Advances in Nursing Science, 10*(1), 71-86.

Schultz, P.R., and Meleis, A.I. (1988). Nursing epistemology: Traditions, insights, questions. *Image, 20,* 217-221.

Schlotfeldt, R.M. (1987). Defining nursing: A historic controversy. *Nursing Research, 36*(1), 64-67.

Schlotfeldt, R.M. (1988). Structuring nursing knowledge: A priority for creating nursing's future. *Nursing Science Quarterly, 1,* 35-38.

Silva, M.C. (1987). Conceptual models of nursing. In J.J. Fitzpatrick and R.L. Taunton (eds.), *Annual review of nursing research* (Vol 5, pp. 229-246). New York: Springer Publishing.

Smith, M.C. (1988). Perspectives on nursing science. *Nursing Science Quarterly, 1,* 80-85.

Smith, M.C. (1992a). Is all knowing personal knowing? *Nursing Science Quarterly, 5,* 2-3.

Smith, M.C. (1992b). The distinctiveness of nursing knowledge. *Nursing Science Quarterly, 5,* 148-148.

Vincent, K.G., and Coler, M.S. (1990). A unified nursing diagnostic model. *Image, 22,* 93-95.

Visintainer, M.A. (1986). The nature of theory and knowledge in nursing. *Image, 18,* 32-38.

Wald, F.S., and Leonard, R.C. (1964). Towards development of nursing practice theory. *Nursing Research, 13,* 309-313.

Yura, H., and Walsh, M.B. (1983). *The nursing process.* Norwalk, CT: Appleton-Century Crofts.

CHAPTER NINE

Theory Testing and Theory Building: Research in Nursing

HEATHER F. CLARKE

During the past 20 years theory building in nursing has focused on the development of theories of, for, and in nursing. Some nurse theorists, such as Martha E. Rogers, Sister Callista Roy, and Imogene M. King, have been concerned with grand theories of nursing. Other nurses have developed theories and conceptual frameworks related to specific approaches for nursing care; Dorothea Orem's selfcare and Madeleine Leininger's transcultural care are two such examples. Still other theorists have given their attention to the generation and testing of constructs and concepts used in nursing, such as vulnerability, resilience, social support, and uncertainty. Regardless of the magnitude of the theory, nurse theorists seek to solve both ill-defined and acknowledged problems. Their aim is to clearly explain phenomena of concern to the practice of nursing therapeutics. Theory development and research aimed at generating and testing nursing theory attempts to ground the theory in observations for the purposes of adding breadth and depth to nursing knowledge, discovering nursing truths, and ensuring that the theory is socially and scientifically relevant.

A variety of research designs, using both qualitative and quantitative research methodologies, are required to ensure that data collection and analysis in knowledge and theory development goes beyond logical empiricism and deductive reasoning. If the gap between research and practice is to be reduced, inductive approaches of theory generation and testing are as essential as deductive methods.

This chapter will explore research issues involved in theory development, including the generation and testing of theory. Issues relevant to the research process in theory development include deciding on research designs appropriate to the theory development purpose, choosing qualitative and/or quantitative methods, and evaluating research reports.

■ ■ ■ ■

PURPOSES AND OBJECTIVES

The purposes of this chapter are to discuss the appropriateness of various research designs for the generation and testing of nursing theory, discuss the application of qualitative and quantitative methods to those research designs, and present criteria for evaluating the scientific merit of research reports. The major elements of various approaches to nursing research will be discussed, and careful study will enable students to identify research methods for four theory levels, generate research questions, suggest research designs, and critique a research report.

■ ■ ■ ■

NURSING PARADIGM
Definition of Nursing

From the time of Florence Nightingale, nurses have been charged with caring for the sick and the well, emphasizing restoration, promotion, and maintenance of health (Nightingale, 1969). Today nurse scientists are deeply involved in developing their discipline's own unique knowledge base about individuals, families, groups, and communities, as well as the environment, health, and transactions among these core elements of nursing. They are expanding the definitions of these elements of nursing, examining the therapeutics of nursing care, and understanding in greater depth and breadth the determinants of health, behaviours of individuals and populations, and qualities of the changing environment.

In Nightingale's *Notes on Nursing: What It Is and What It Is Not* (1969), originally published in 1859, nursing was defined as having "charge of the personal health of somebody and what nursing has to do is to put the patient in the best condition for nature to act upon him" (p. 133). A century later Henderson (1961) defined nursing as

> . . . assisting the individual, sick or well, in the performance of those activities contributing to health or its recovery (or to a peaceful death) that he would perform unaided if he had the necessary strength, will or knowledge. And to do this in such a way as to help him gain independence as rapidly as possible (p. 42).

Although these definitions illustrate the consistent orientation of nursing to the provision of care that promotes well-being in the people served, they do not reflect the influence of contemporary nursing theories and changing paradigms. For this chapter the American Nurses Association's (ANA) definition of nursing will be used because it reflects the evolution of nursing. It also makes explicit the phenomena that are of concern to nurses. "Nursing is the diagnosis and treatment of human responses to actual or potential health problems" (ANA, 1980, p. 9).

Based on this definition, nurses are concerned with two types of human response:

1. reactions of individuals, groups, and communities to *actual* health problems; and
2. reactions of individuals, groups, and communities to *potential* health problems.

They are concerned with the health-restoring and health-supporting behaviors of both the well and the ill and how these behaviours may vary with environmental influences. Nurses are concerned with characteristics of phenomena such as single or multiple occurrences and episodic or continuous responses. The phenomena of concern to nurses, including assessment, diagnosis, and therapeutic care, are complex and multifaceted, requiring an understanding from both inductive and deductive perspectives.

Foundations of Nursing

Information as a basis for knowledge development and a determinant of nursing actions comes from various sources including the individual nurse, the environment, nursing theory, and nursing research. Carper (1978) proposed that practice requires four patterns of knowing: empiricism, ethics, personal knowledge, and esthetics. Each way of knowing is an essential component of the knowledge base for professional practice, and no one kind should be used in isolation from the others. The emphasis in this chapter, however, is on building knowledge through research—the empirics of knowing.

The basic function of research is to generate or test theory. It is a vehicle for theory development—identifying a phenomenon, discovering its dimensions or characteristics, specifying relationships between the dimensions, or developing evidence about hypotheses derived from the theory. Although there are many definitions of research, the one proposed by Waltz and Bausell (1981) is used in this chapter: "Research is a systematic, formal, rigorous and precise process employed to gain solutions to problems and/or to discover and interpret new facts and relationships" (p. 1). This definition allows for various modes of inquiry and neither requires nor precludes that the study be totally empirical, based solely on experimental findings (Fawcett and Downs, 1992).

Barnum (1990) defines a theory as ". . . a statement that purports to account for or characterize some phenomenon" (p. 1). This is the least restrictive of the many definitions of theory and permits descriptions of one concept to be considered theory (Fawcett and Downs, 1992). Thus it allows for descriptions, explanations, and predictions to be considered theory. This is consistent with the function of theories, which describe, explain, or predict phenomena.

Shifting the Paradigm

Because nursing is a practice discipline concerned with the delivery of caring services to humans, it has a professional obligation to contribute to theory development—particularly to prescriptive or "situation-producing" theories that address nursing therapeutics and systems of care (Dickoff, James, and Wiedenbach, 1968). Prescriptive theories are developed to control, promote, and change phenomena (Meleis, 1985). Therefore research for theory-building and theory-testing must move beyond defining concepts and their relationships to predicting their correlational and causal relationships and testing hypotheses. Further development of nursing theory must continue to address nursing's interventions or therapeutics within the complexities of care systems, human behaviour, and health and disease processes.

Although nurse scholars have developed a nursing paradigm that includes theories and applications of nursing therapeutic care consistent with the ANA definition of nursing, there is a paucity of research aimed at theory testing that includes prescribing and controlling. Kuhn (1970) defines paradigms as "universally recognized scientific achievements that for a time provide(s) model problems and solutions to a community of practitioners" (p. viii). Evaluation of our current nursing paradigm suggests that a shift is required and is in its early stages. The shift involves incorporating both subjective and objective perspectives into theory-generating and theory-testing research, using both inductive and deductive reasoning, critically evaluating the appropriateness of both qualitative and quantitative methods and considering new or modified research designs. This shifting paradigm will require nurse scientists to pursue programs of research collaboratively and among multiple sites. In concert with knowledge and theory development and the nursing paradigm shift, there is a need to encourage and facilitate diffusion and acceptance of such within the discipline of nursing.

■ ■ ■ ■

DEVELOPING NURSING THEORY

Nursing Science and Knowledge

Several years ago Donaldson and Crowley (1978) drew a distinction between the discipline of nursing and the profession of nursing. The latter refers to the activities of practitioners in the field; the former refers to the body of systematic knowledge. Later Benoliel (1984) suggested, ". . . the substance of the discipline of nursing needs to incorporate at least two broad components: professional foundations and nursing science" (p. 2). What is consistent in these two perspectives is the need for knowledge and theory development that is prescriptive and that addresses both professional practice and the phenomena of concern within the professional practice of nursing.

The goal of knowledge development for professional foundations is the creation of prescriptive theories that direct the implementation of professional practice (e.g., code of ethics, practice principles), while the ultimate goal of knowledge and theory development in nursing science is ". . . the creation of descriptive and prescriptive theories that incorporate knowledge about the conditions necessary and sufficient for the promotion, maintenance and restoration of states of health in human beings" (Benoliel, 1984, p. 3). The focus of this chapter is nursing science. Fawcett (1983) states that this nursing knowledge must be derived from a combination of humanitarian and scientific inquiries within the context of the wholeness of human beings interacting with their environments and with a focus on nurses' therapeutic care-giving.

Research and Theory

"Theory without research and research without theory do little to advance knowledge in a meaningful way" (Fawcett and Downs, 1992, p. v). Because theory development and research influence one another, they broaden the boundaries of knowledge. Woods (1988) described the relationship between theory development and research as ". . . a spiral with research refining theory and theory refining research" (p. 118).

Like other practice professions, nurses use knowledge and explanations invented by members of other disciplines as well as those they develop themselves. The goal of manipulating this information is different from other practice professions, and nursing must separate the knowledge that is important to nursing from the knowledge that is not (Visintainer, 1986). Knowledge specific to the nursing perspective, as well as that generated within nursing, should drive future investigations and continue to provide the basis for the practice of nursing.

It is the work of nurse scientists to conduct research and build theory that: (1) is stimulated by questions derived from practice; (2) recognizes the need for new information; (3) integrates borrowed knowledge; (4) creates or builds new perspectives; and (5) tests and validates proposed nursing theories. In the shifting paradigm nurses must use and develop knowledge from many sources; create new ways of investigating and testing concepts, constructs, and theories; and explain the results and applications to others within and beyond the nursing discipline.

■ ■ ■ ■

RESEARCH DESIGN AND THEORY DEVELOPMENT
Research Choices
Research contributes to theory development by generating theory and by testing theory. Multiple and varied research designs are required to accomplish this. "Designing a nursing study is the creative process of planning the empirical aspects of an investigation. Research designs link the investigator's abstract thinking about a topic with the realities of studying a topic" (Woods, 1988, p. 117). Designs guide investigation and thus deserve considerable attention by the investigator. The use of complementary qualitative and quantitative research methods creates a variety of options that have the potential to provide different information about the nature of the phenomena.

Major determinants of the design and methods to be used are: 1) the purpose of the inquiry, 2) research question(s), 3) the nature of the phenomenon to be studied, and 4) practical and ethical considerations. Investigators weigh these considerations when selecting a research design. Of paramount importance is the question posed. In turn, the question depends on the current state of knowledge as expressed in theory (Fawcett and Downs, 1992). When little is known about a phenomenon, the investigator may undertake a careful description of a single concept rather than attempt to determine the relationship of several factors. When considerable knowledge exists upon which to base hypotheses, investigators control the phenomena and measure outcomes to explain or predict the phenomena. Theory-testing studies usually address only some of the relationships included in a theory—that is, they may test a few hypotheses instead of the entire theory. As the results of many studies accumulate, the theory can be revised or discarded.

Theory-generating and Theory-testing Research

Theory-generating research is designed to discover and describe phenomena and their observed relationships (Woods, 1988). It often employs inductive reasoning, descriptive and exploratory research designs, and qualitative methods. Theory-testing research, on the other hand, attempts to determine how accurately a theory accounts for observed facts by empirically testing hypotheses about theoretical relationships. Deductive reasoning is usually employed with predictive and explanatory research designs and quantitative methods.

Dickoff, James, and Wiedenbach (1968) identified four levels of nursing theory based on the relative maturity of the scientific base involved. Research approaches must match the level and the scientific base. Table 9.1 outlines salient research considerations with respect to theory development. For further descriptions the reader is encouraged to explore texts and articles on both theory development and research.

Qualitative methods are applicable for initial theory development. In levels I and II of theory development it is common for the investigator (1) to have only a conceptual orientation as a guide, (2) to be looking for descriptions of concepts and their relationships, (3) to test for correlational and predictive relationships among concepts and their variables, and (4) to wish to understand the situation from the client(s)' perspective(s). Although some quantitative methods may be helpful in defining concept relationships, qualitative methodology must be applied as well.

Quantitative research methods are primarily applied to theory-testing and further development (level III). Research designs for quantitative methods can be more rigorous in specifying assumptions and ruling out or specifying and measuring error sources than can qualitative methods. Woods (1988) notes that despite the fact that nursing is a practice discipline, relatively little discussion about designs for testing prescriptive theory appear in our literature, an area certainly requiring critical attention.

■■ ■■ ■■ ■■

METHODS ISSUES

Qualitative/Quantitative Controversy

Historically there has been a clash between advocates of quantitative and qualitative methods for generation and verification of theory. Initially, qualitative data was used in a nonsystematic, nonrigorous way (Glaser and Strauss, 1967). However, later methodologic advances demonstrated that accurate evidence could be produced, and qualitative research was employed to get surveys started. After this, quantitative research—discovering facts and testing current theory—was to take over.

The qualitative/quantitative dichotomy was perpetuated by many of the nursing scholars who addressed research methodologies in published works during the early 1980's (Porter, 1989). Some, recognizing the preeminent influence of quantitative research, sharply criticized its deficiencies and strongly promoted qualitative methods as being more congruent with the philosophic and practical traditions of nursing. Others took a less popular stance, suggesting that both

TABLE 9.1 Theory Development and Research

Theory Development	Theory Level	Research Design	Methods	Uses
Theory Generating	I. Naming	Descriptive ▪grounded theory ▪ethnography ▪phenomenology	Qualitative	Identify concepts Define concepts or phenomena
		▪survey ▪case studies	Quantitative Qualitative	Describe prevalence, incidence, value of phenomena in population
	II. Situation Depicting	Exploratory ▪comparative ▪correlational ▪case studies	Qualitative and Quantitative	Define concepts relationships
Theory Testing	III. Situation Relating	Predictive ▪naturalistic ▪cross-sectional ▪prospective ▪retrospective ▪experimental and quasi-experimental	Qualitative Quantitative	Predict correlational and causal relationships Test hypotheses Manipulate phenomena and measure its effects

methods could be useful to nurse scientists. More recently both methods have been recognized as being potentially valuable for adding breadth and depth to the analysis, enhancing external validity and bolstering internal validity (Porter, 1989). Nurse scientists have suggested that qualitative and quantitative methods might be combined, used sequentially, or used concurrently.

Myers and Haase (1989) suggested that the integration of quantitative and qualitative research approaches is inevitable and essential in furthering nursing science and they proposed guidelines for doing so. They believe that the consequences of method integration may be reflected in more unified investigative approaches, broader questions, different team compositions, and cost savings at the personal and organizational levels.

This paradigm shift in the methods controversy is consistent with the position taken by Glaser and Strauss (1967) that there is no fundamental clash between the purposes and the capacities of qualitative and quantitative methods or data.

> . . . We believe that each form of data is useful for both verification and generation of theory . . . In many instances, both forms of data are necessary . . . as supplements, as mutual verification, and . . . as different forms of data on the same subject, which when compared will generate theory (pp. 17-18).

Chinn (1985) examined myths, persisting in the traditional male-defined scientific enterprise, that influence the methods used in nursing's search for new knowledge. Particularly significant are the myths related to "scientific supremacy," "empirical evidence," "objectivity," and "the perfect method." These myths can be "debunked" by (1) insisting on integration of all patterns of knowing (scientific, esthetics, ethical, and experimental) into the whole of knowing (Benoliel, 1984; Chinn, 1985); (2) recognizing the limitation of empirical evidence and integrating other methods of justification, criticism, and introspection into the knowledge base for understanding (Chinn, 1985); (3) acknowledging the nurse(s) responsible for the knowledge search, thus exposing underlying assumptions and views of their reality (Chinn, 1985); and (4) valuing alternative qualitative and quantitative methods in a fundamental way and not merely as stepping stones to the "perfect method" (Chinn, 1985; Benoliel, 1984; Atwood, 1984).

Maximizing the research

Methods of data collection most suited to qualitative and quantitative methods are summarized in Table 9.2. Regardless of the methodologic perspective, selection of the methods must be congruent with the theoretic framework of research and bear directly on the question being asked or hypothesis being tested.

In addition to qualitative/quantitative issues in research and the development of nursing knowledge and theory, consideration should be given to multiple triangulation, collaborative research, and secondary analysis of data.

Triangulation integrates both qualitative and quantitative methods and theoretical perspectives salient to the discipline of nursing (Mitchell, 1986). A triangulated study combines different theoretical perspectives, different data sources, different investigators, and different methods within a single study. It supports the study of the complex and dynamic phenomena of human behavior.

TABLE 9.2 Data Collection Methods

Data Collection Method	Qualitative	Quantitative
▪ Unstructured observation	X	
▪ Structured observation	X	X
▪ Open-ended interviews and questionnaires	X	
▪ Closed and mixed interviews and questionnaires		X
▪ Participant observation	X	
▪ Unwritten available data	X	
▪ Written available data	X	
▪ Projective tests		X
▪ Other structured methods, e.g., physiological measurements	X	

Multiple triangulation, a complex form of triangulation, combines more than one type of triangulation into a study design (Denzin, 1970). This may be accomplished by including in the research design (Mitchell, 1986) two or more of the following factors:

1. Data sources that differ by person, place, or time
2. Two or more data collection methods that relate to qualitative and quantitative methods
3. Multiple questions to be answered or competing hypotheses to be tested
4. Multiple investigators

Collaborative research involves multiple investigators who study the same question, hypothesis, or theory in different populations, different aspects of the research problem in the same population, or a combination of the two. The use of multiple investigators helps to expand the generalizability of the results, to reduce the potential bias (impossible when only a single investigator is involved), and to improve the reliability of data collection and analysis (Denzin, 1970). The probability that a holistic approach to human behavior will be taken is increased when investigators with differing expertise collaborate on the entire research process, from problem identification to report writing.

Secondary analysis of data collected for purposes other than the research problem currently being investigated can be valuable in research related to both the generation and testing of nursing theory. It provides another data source for triangulation. However, when deciding whether to use data collected for other purposes, a number of factors must be considered including: (1) whether the unit of analysis differs between original and proposed methods, (2) whether the lapse in time since the original collection of data makes the data obsolete or poses immense problems in interpretation, and (3) whether sufficient information is available on the methods of the primary study to make reliable interpretations of the data in secondary analysis.

▬ ▬ ▬ ▬

CRITICALLY EVALUATING THE RESEARCH REPORTS

The close connection between theory and research mandates evaluation of the theoretical elements of a research report as well as the methods used to generate or test the theory (Fawcett and Downs, 1992). Nurses should be able to critically evaluate reports of theory-generating and theory-testing research to judge the applicability and significance of the results to their practice. The evaluation must be a critical, objective, and systematic analysis of the report based on specific criteria. It should include examination of the investigator's interest, purposes, or goals for the study; the research problems or questions and significance of these; the theoretical or conceptual framework in relation to the questions, hypotheses, and purposes of the investigation; the methods, including design, sampling, instruments, data collection, and analysis; and results and discussion.

The following questions can be used as a basis for critical evaluation of both theoretical and research elements. An attempt has been made to develop the questions so that they are appropriate for evaluation of both theory-generating and theory-testing studies and all types of research designs.

1. PROBLEM
    a. Are the questions to be answered stated precisely and clearly?
    b. Is the significance of the problem discussed?
    c. If a theory-generating study, is the theoretical and social significance explained?
    d. If a theory-testing study, is the theoretical basis for the hypotheses discussed?
    e. Is the relevance of the problem convincing?
    f. Is the problem researchable?
    g. Are the variables and concepts identified and defined?
    h. Is the scope of the study identified?
2. THEORETIC or CONCEPTUAL FRAMEWORK
    a. Are the investigator's assumptions stated? Are they valid and logical?
    b. Is the literature review comprehensive and pertinent to the research problem?
    c. Does the review include implications for the research problem under study?
    d. Is it apparent how this study will fill gaps in current knowledge or extend developed theory?
    e. If a theory-testing study, are the theory components identified, e.g., concepts and propositions?
    f. Are other competing or alternative theories, models, or concepts presented?

3. METHODS
   a. Sample
      1. Is the subject population described? Is it appropriate for the theory development and research purpose?
      2. Is the described sampling method logical?
      3. Does it have the potential for generalizability?
      4. Are sources of bias identified?
      5. Are the principles of human subject protection followed?
   b. Data collection
      1. Are the measures and/or instruments sensitive and meaningful for the problem and the subjects?
      2. Is there evidence of instrument validity and reliability?
      3. Have data collection methods and instruments been pretested?
      4. Are major sources of bias recognized?
      5. Are procedures described?
   c. Data analysis
      1. Are the selected procedures appropriate for the theory being developed and data obtained?
      2. Is the level of significance discussed?
   d. Design
      1. Is the design appropriate to the research question(s)?
      2. Is the description explicit enough to permit replication?
4. FINDINGS and DISCUSSION
   a. Are the limitations clearly specified?
   b. Are the results presented with clarity and precision and organized logically?
   c. Is there sufficient information presented to answer the research questions?
   d. If a theory-generating study, do the concepts and propositions that emerged from the data analysis clearly reflect the raw data?
   e. If a theory-testing study, how well do the empirical data conform to the hypothesized expectation? Are appropriate conclusions drawn to reject or accept the hypotheses?
   f. Are the tabular and graphic presentations self-explanatory, supplementary to the text, easy to understand and complete?
   g. Are the conclusions warranted by the study results? Are both statistical and clinical significance addressed?
   h. Does the discussion compare the results to those of previous studies and present possible explanations for differences? Do the explanations indicate the extent to which objectives were achieved, questions answered or hypotheses supported?
   i. Were the empirical indicators appropriate proxies for the concepts under study?
   j. Were the procedures appropriate methods to observe the phenomena proposed by the investigator?
   k. Are the implications for theory, practice, education, or further research generative, innovative, and creative?

l. If a theory-generating study, are the major concepts and propositions identified, classified, and summarized?

m. If a theory-testing study, are conclusions drawn regarding the support or refutation of hypotheses and the empirical adequacy of the theory?

n. Do the conclusions go beyond what was demonstrated by the data?

Despite lack of complete precision, systematic evaluation of research is a necessary process for any nurse. With thoughtful practice one can soon identify major problems, shortcomings, omissions, strengths, and weaknesses of a study. The questions suggested above are by no means exhaustive but they address important aspects of any study. It is up to individuals to draw their own conclusions and consider these in relation to knowledge development and its use.

■■ ■■ ■■ ■■

KNOWLEDGE AND RESEARCH UTILIZATION

Issues in knowledge and research utilization have been of concern to most disciplines (Loomis, 1985). Brett (1987) and Coyle and Sokop (1990) believe that the influence of theory is slow to occur because a theory and its related research findings do not tell clinicians what to do. Rather, research findings gradually influence thinking and doing over the long periods of time required to first disseminate the information and then change fixed sets of beliefs. Understanding, accepting, reorienting, adopting, and applying the results of research and theory development to the world of practice are all required. Throughout these processes nurses must consider the validity, reliability, and generalizability of the knowledge base and research findings; the relevance to clinical practice; the context and readiness of situations in which adoption of these principles is to take place; interests, values, awareness, and perceptions of relevant policy makers and practitioners; communication networks; and means of evaluating theory application (Glaser, Abelson, and Garrison, 1983; Loomis, 1985). Is it any wonder that shifts in paradigms are slow and sometimes painful? Utilization of theory and research findings will be further discussed in chapter 13.

REFERENCES

American Nurses Association. (1980). *Nursing: A social policy statement*. Kansas City, MO: Author.

Atwood, J.R. (1984). Advancing nursing science: Quantitative approaches. *Communicating nursing research: Vol. 17. Advancing nursing science: Qualitative and quantitative approaches.* Boulder: Western Interstate Commission for Higher Education.

Barnum, B.J.S. (1990). *Nursing theory: Analysis, application, evaluation* (3rd ed.). Glenview, IL: Scott, Foresman/Little, Brown Higher Education.

Benoliel, J.Q. (1984). Advancing nursing science: Qualitative approaches. *Communicating nursing research: Vol. 17. Advancing nursing science: Qualitative and quantitative approaches.* Boulder:

Western Interstate Commission for Higher Education.

Brett, J.L. (1987). Use of nursing practice research findings. *Nursing Research, 36,* 344-349.

Carper, B.A. (1978). Fundamental patterns of knowing in nursing. *Advances in Nursing Science, 1*(1), 13-23.

Chinn, P.L. (1985). Debunking myths in nursing theory and research. *Image: The Journal of Nursing Scholarship, 17*(2), 45-49.

Coyle, L.A. and Sokop, A.G. (1990). Innovation adoption behavior among nurses. *Nursing Research, 39,* 176-180.

Denzin, N. (1970). Strategies of multiple triangulation. In N. Denzin (Ed.), *The research act* (pp. 297-313). New York: McGraw-Hill.

Dickoff, J., James, P., and Wiedenbach, E. (1968). Theory in a practice discipline: Parts I & II. Practice-oriented research. *Nursing Research, 17*(5 and 6), 415-435 and 545-554.

Donaldson, S.K., and Crowley, D.M. (1978). The discipline of nursing. *Nursing Outlook, 26*(2), 113-120.

Fawcett, J. (1983). Hallmarks of success in nursing theory development. In P.L. Chinn (Ed.), *Advances in nursing theory development* (pp. 3-17). Baltimore: Aspen Publications.

Fawcett, J. and Downs, F.S. (1992). *The relationship of theory and research* (2nd ed.). Philadelphia: F. A. Davis Co.

Glaser, B.G., and Strauss, A.L. (1967). *The discovery of grounded theory: Strategies for qualitative research*. Hawthorn, NY: Aldine Publishing.

Glaser, E.M., Abelson, H.H., and Garrison, K.H. (1983). *Putting knowledge to use*. San Francisco: Jossey-Bass.

Henderson, V. (1961). *Basic principles of nursing care*. London: International Council of Nurses.

Kuhn, T.S. (1970). *The structure of scientific revolutions*. Chicago: University of Chicago Press.

Loomis, M.E. (1985). Knowledge utilization and research utilization in nursing. *Image: The Journal of Nursing Scholarship, 17*(2), 35-39.

Meleis, A. (1985). *Theoretical nursing: Development and progress*. Philadelphia: Lippincott.

Mitchell, E.S. (1986). Multiple triangulation: A methodology for nursing science. *Advances in Nursing Science, 8*(3), 18-26.

Myers, S.T. and Haase, J.E. (1989). Guidelines for integration of quantitative and qualitative approaches. *Nursing Research, 38*, 5, 299 -301.

Nightingale, F. (1969). *Notes on nursing: What it is, and what it is not*. New York: Dover Publications.

Porter, E.J. (1989). That qualitative-quantitative dualism. *Image: Journal of Nursing Scholarship, 21*, (2), 98-102.

Visintainer, M.A. (1986). The nature of knowledge and theory in nursing. *Image: Journal of Nursing Scholarship, 18*(2), 32-38.

Waltz, C. and Bausell, R. B. (1981). *Nursing Research: Design, statistics and computer analysis*. Philadelphia: F. A. Davis Co.

Woods, N.F. (1988). Designing nursing research. In N.F. Woods and M. Catanzaro (Eds.). *Nursing research: Theory and practice*. Washington, DC: The C. V. Mosby Co.

CHAPTER TEN

Research-Mindedness in the Profession

JANNETTA MacPHAIL

T he term *research-mindedness* was first coined in relation to nursing research by Sir John Brotherston (1960). It is a useful term that conveys both awareness of and openness to nursing research. In recent years much has been written about the importance of increasing research in nursing practice because research is needed to advance knowledge and improve practice. Considerable attention also has been given to problems and inadequacies related to the dissemination and application of research findings in practice. Although the amount of research in nursing practice has increased in recent years, the process of research development in nursing has been slow. Even slower has been the incorporation of research findings into practice. Many factors contribute to this state of affairs, some of which can be identified as deterrents to the development of nursing. On the other hand, there are changes in nursing that facilitate research in practice and make it more relevant for all nurses.

∎ ∎ ∎ ∎

RESEARCH-BASED NURSING PRACTICE

Research-based practice means nursing practice based on valid and reliable research findings obtained from scientific investigation of nursing practice problems. Much of nursing practice today is still based on opinion and experience—that is, on knowledge derived from trial and error or based on opinions and methods passed from generation to generation through books, articles, papers, conferences, workshops, and even educational programs in nursing. Nonetheless, an increasing number of nurses are recognizing the importance of research and are developing skills for critically evaluating research reports that are relevant to their practice. Johnson (1979) states: "Research, as a basis for practice, is increasingly necessary as a professional nurse becomes less content with past reliance on instinct and tradition and wants hard data for planning nursing care" (p. 1).

Schlotfeldt (1971) states: "Thus for nursing, as for any practice discipline, investigators must identify the central focus of practice and delineate the phenomena about which theories need to be developed" (p. 140). The central focus of nursing practice is helping people, whether sick or well, to attain, maintain, or regain their optimal level of health and functioning. Nursing practice encompasses a variety of strategies or interventions, such as comfort measures, teaching, anticipatory guidance, support, and compensatory activities. Compensatory activities are actions taken by the nurse to compensate for what the patient cannot or will not do for himself or herself. They may include such activities as suctioning to maintain a clear airway, assisting with ambulation to maintain circulation and joint and muscle function, and assisting with feeding to maintain nutritional status and elimination. All such strategies are designed to enhance the individual's health-seeking behaviours, to stimulate avoidance of disease and disability, to promote maximum use of the person's own resources in coping with disease or dysfunction, and to help persons cope with family responsibilities and crises. A holistic conception of human beings is appropriate for nurses because their interventions or strategies are designed to improve an individual's functioning as a total being (Schlotfeldt, 1971).

The nature of nursing practice makes it evident that nurses should study individual or group behaviour in relation to attaining, maintaining, or regaining health. The focus of research—to develop a scientific base for practice—involves the person's behaviour in relation to motivation to be healthy, as well as behaviour in coping with life crises. Life crises include such normal events as birth, developmental stages, and decline, as well as genetic failure, disease, and disability. Nursing research may also include behavioural responses to a wide variety of diagnostic and therapeutic interventions ordered by physicians. The feature that distinguishes nursing research from other research about human beings is the type of knowledge about persons that nurses need and use in practice. Consequently research to advance knowledge and improve practice is concerned with people's behaviour in response to circumstances that require nursing action and their behaviour in response to that action (Schlotfeldt, 1971).

Schlotfeldt (1987) states: "Nursing scholars should address pertinent questions that will guide observations and stimulate the generation of theoretical constructs about phenomena that are of particular concern to nurses and worthy of testing" (p. 66). She then poses six questions that pertain to identification and investigation of "innate human health-seeking mechanisms and innate and learned health-seeking behaviours [that] are of particular concern to nurses" (p. 66). Her questions concern naming, classifying, and characterizing mechanisms and behaviours, and testing nursing strategies to enhance them.

It is evident that scientific investigation of nursing practice has great potential for improving practice. Why then is there not more research, and why are the research findings that exist not applied to improve practice? Identifying some of the deterrents to doing research and having a research base for nursing practice will help answer these questions.

■ ■ ■ ■

DETERRENTS TO CONDUCTING RESEARCH

Before translating research into practice, research must be conducted. One of the major deterrents to research is the limited number of nurses prepared to conduct research. Although the number of nurses prepared at the doctoral and master's degree levels has increased considerably in the past decade in Canada and the United States, the proportion of nurses actually conducting research to strengthen the scientific base of practice is still limited. The number of nurses in Canada holding an earned doctorate increased from 81 in 1980 to 124 in 1982 to 193 in 1986 and to 257 in 1989, and the number of nurses involved in doctoral preparation increased from 72 in 1980 to 121 in 1982 to 224 in 1986 and to 265 in 1989 (Stinson, Larsen, and MacPhail, 1984; Stinson, MacPhail, and Larsen, 1988; Lamb and Stinson, 1990). Thus the number of nurses with an earned doctorate increased by 53% from 1980 to 1982, by 56% from 1982 to 1986, and by 33% from 1986 to 1989. The number of nurses engaged in doctoral study increased by 68% from 1980 to 1982, by 85% from 1982 to 1986, and by 18% from 1986 to 1989. However, the increments have decreased markedly, particularly in the number of nurses engaged in doctoral study. The reasons for the latter decrease are not known but may be related to insufficient funding for graduate study and the lack of doctoral programs in nursing in Canada in 1989. The establishment of four doctoral programs in nursing since then (University of Alberta, January 1991; University of British Columbia, September 1991; University of Toronto, September 1993; and a joint doctoral program by McGill University and Université de Montréal, September, 1993) should help to increase the number of Canadian nurses pursuing doctoral education. Also needed are more funds for doctoral study and greater expectations on the part of employers in universities, colleges, and health-care agencies, that a greater proportion of the nurses involved in teaching and leadership in health-care agencies have doctoral preparation.

In spite of the increased numbers, many nurses still study the nurse—that is, the roles, relationships, and functions of the nurse; education in nursing; or organization and management of nursing services. Although functional studies in nursing are important, they do not help strengthen the scientific base of nursing practice. Perhaps one of the reasons many nurses have studied functional aspects is that they were prepared at the graduate level in disciplines other than nursing and have studied phenomena with the orientation of disciplines such as education or administration. Nonetheless, nurse researchers have made remarkable progress in the past few years since the introduction of the idea that nurses should systematically investigate their strategies or interventions as do other professionals in practice fields. As discussed in Chapter 12, there has been an encouraging increase in clinical research reported at national conferences over the past 7 years. This change is representative of ongoing trends in nursing research in Canada.

A second deterrent to increasing research in nursing practice is that many nurse researchers are not involved in or knowledgeable about nursing practice. Ellis (1974) states "One cannot formulate significant research questions in any field without knowledge of that field. No amount of knowledge of research methods can overcome lack of knowledge of nursing if one seeks to ask significant questions in the field of nursing" (p. 32). This does not imply that some nurse researchers have no knowledge of nursing practice, but that they have insufficient knowledge of current practice to ask meaningful research questions. Thus we may see nurses prepared in other disciplines and out of touch with current practice studying phenomena from the perspective of those disciplines rather than from a nursing perspective. Insufficient knowledge of nursing may be displayed in the assumptions made, variables selected, instrumentation used, or any facet of the research process. Fortunately, ignorance or insufficient knowledge of nursing practice can be overcome, but only if recognized and acknowledged by the nurse investigator (Ellis, 1974).

A third deterrent to conducting research in practice is difficulty in *asking* the research question, which is the most complex and the most important task of any investigator. It is important to remember that research can solve problems, but not all problems are research questions. The question, "Why don't staff nurses use the medication cart as it was designed?" reflects a problem. It may imply the question of how to get them to do it. The problem may be a management or morale problem, but as stated, is not a research problem (Ellis, 1974).

There are two major types of questions that are not researchable. These are value, or "should", questions and yes/no questions. Types of researchable questions as identified by Wilson (1985) are:

1. Why are things this way? For example, why do cancer patients without hope participate in painful experiments?
2. What would happen if? For example, what would happen if sex education were taught in all schools?
3. Which approach would work better? For example, is group or individual counselling more effective with clients who abuse alcohol?
4. Who might benefit from this? For example, would hospitalized children have faster recovery if parents were permitted and taught to participate in their care (p. 117)?

Another categorization of types of research questions, as developed by Dickoff, James, and Wiedenbach (1968) is:

1. Factor-isolating or "naming." For example, what are the stages of the grieving process?
2. Factor-relating or "what is happening here?" For example, what is the relationship of parents' own childhood experiences to engaging in subsequent child abuse or neglect?
3. Situation-relating or "what will happen if?" For example, will feedback training decrease suffering among chronic pain patients?
4. Situation-producing or "how can I make it happen?" For example, how can I intervene to prevent postoperative vomiting (p. 420)?

Bush (1985) believes that anything that can be described, quantified, or measured is potentially researchable. Brink and Wood (1983) define a researchable question as one that yields problem-solving information, produces new research, adds to theory, or improves practice. Lindeman and Schantz (1982) define it more narrowly as a question that can be answered by collecting observable data, that includes reference to the relationship between two or more variables, and that emanates from what is known about the phenomenon.

Defining researchable questions requires time and thought and a thorough search of literature to determine what is known about the phenomenon being considered. Only in this way can one decide if a question is worth investigating. Other factors that apply to the feasibility of studying the question are time, availability of subjects, cooperation of others, facilities and equipment, money, experience, and ethical considerations.

A fourth impediment to the conduct of meaningful research is what Willems and Rausch (1969) identified as a lack of congruence between research purposes and research methods. Sometimes questions or problems are distorted to fit a method when the nature of the problem should determine the method. Although disjunction between purpose and method is not peculiar to nurses undertaking research, it may be a greater problem if the researchers are remote from practice and are trying to fit questions with research methods learned in another discipline.

Insufficient time has been identified by many authors as another impediment to conducting research. Lack of time is a concern to faculty members who devote much time to teaching, curriculum development, committee work, and professional activities. Time for research may be limited because of the orientation in nursing to "doing" and "being busy" and a tendency to want immediate results. A number of writers have indicated that practitioners may have difficulty understanding what investigators are doing with their time as they proceed through the research process. They have also indicated that nurses tend to want immediate results and fast action and have difficulty understanding that a hunch may not be borne out by research. On the other hand, educators may have difficulty using their time for research when they are accustomed to devoting it to teaching, curriculum study and revision, and committee work. This might also be related to lagging commitment, as termed by Werley (1972).

Another deterrent to research in practice may be lack of access to patients. Access may be limited by physicians who have certain prerogatives in relation to their patients, whether hospitalized, in clinics, or in offices. Access may also be limited by nurses who do not support or understand nursing research; nurses are in key positions to influence physicians, other nurses, and patients by educating them about the importance of research in nursing practice. This is not to suggest that patients' rights should not be protected, or that research proposals should not be subject to rigorous review for ethics and quality. Rather, it is to urge nurses to think about their influence on access to patients and promoting nursing research.

Insufficient funds to support research is an obstacle for all types of nursing research. It is a major problem in Canada because separate funding for nursing research has never been provided on the federal level. In the United States separate funding has helped investigators gain experience in research design and grant writing that is needed to be able to compete in the larger arena (Gortner, 1986). On the federal level the Canadian government provides research funds for the humanities and social sciences through the Social Sciences and Humanities Research Council (SSHRC), for the natural sciences and engineering through the Natural Sciences and Engineering Research Council (NSERC), and for medicine and other health-related disciplines through the Medical Research Council (MRC). Although MRC funds are supposed to be available to health sciences other than medicine, the majority of the funds are awarded to medicine. Moreover, nursing has lobbied vigorously for representation on the MRC for a number of years, through individual nurse leaders and researchers and nursing organizations such as the Canadian Nurses Association (CNA) and the Canadian Association of University Schools of Nursing (CAUSN). Because of discussions held in 1982 the MRC established a "Working Group on Nursing Research," composed of nursing leaders and researchers. They proposed separate funding for nursing research that would include funds for doctoral study for nurses, but no action was taken by the MRC on these recommendations. In 1986 the MRC finally appointed a nurse—the Executive Director of the CNA—to the Council and appointed an ad hoc committee to recommend modifications in funding policy for nursing research. In 1987 nursing leaders and researchers in universities were encouraged by a new initiative announced by the MRC: separate funding would be available for programmatic research in nursing. Nursing faculties/schools in universities were invited to send a letter of intent to submit a full proposal for research funding organized around a central theme. Seventeen universities responded from which the MRC selected six to submit a full grant proposal (Alberta, British Columbia, McGill, McMaster, Montreal, and Toronto). After much concentrated work and eager anticipation on the part of those writing the proposals, the outcome was very disappointing: no programmatic research grants were awarded. Only three individual faculty members in different institutions were awarded funds to support research that was part of the programmatic research proposals. Moreover, when the term of the nurse on the MRC ended in 1989, she was replaced by a physiotherapist. CNA and CAUSN continued to lobby for nurse representation on the MRC, and early in 1991 a nurse, Ursula Verstraetes, was appointed to the MRC Council. Nursing is the largest health profession and desperately needs funds to support research and research development. Since 1989 the number of nursing career investigators funded by the National Health Research and Development Program (NHRDP)/MRC increased from three to six. In addition, six other nurses have been awarded *Career Scientist* grants by the Ontario Ministry of Health and the Research Division of the British Columbia Children's Hospital, which require that the recipients devote 75% of their time to research and other scholarly activities.

On the national level, nurses have had access to small research grants through the Canadian Nurses Foundation (CNF) since 1985 when a small research grants program was first established by CNF. Until that time the Foundation's funds had been awarded for education to nurses studying at the graduate and undergraduate levels. The amount of the research grants, however, was limited to $2500 or less, which would require investigators to have access to other funds to support their research endeavours or obtain released time from other responsibilities. As more funds were raised by the CNF through nurses' contributions and some external funding, the maximum amount of a research grant was raised to $5000 in 1993. In 1990 two new research grants were established to be administered through the CNF: the Dr. Dorothy J. Kergin Research Grant in Primary Care in the amount of $15,000 and the Pharmaceutical Manufacturers Association of Canada-Health Research Foundation/CNF Research Grant for $10,000 (CNA Connection, 1991). Since both are limited to designated areas of research, there may not be suitable applicants every year. Two more research grants of $15,000 each were made available in 1994 for research in any area of nursing practice (Personal communication with Beverly Campbell, Executive Director of CNF, January 27, 1994). Although the research grants available from CNF are still relatively small, they have increased to $5000 and four are for larger amounts. In addition, there is evidence of progress in the number of grant proposals received and the total amount awarded annually: $9602 in 1989, $21,582 in 1990, $37,500 in 1991, $75,823 in 1992, and $56,720 in 1993. The number of grant proposals received increased from 23 in 1990 to 33 in 1992, as did the number of grants awarded, from 7 in 1990 to 15 in 1992 (CNF, 1990, 1992). The decrease in funds awarded in 1993 is related to the quality of the grant proposals received, which reflects the need for better preparation in grant writing through graduate education and grant-writing workshops.

Some provincial nursing associations offer small research grants as well, but again the amounts of funding available are limited. Nurses may apply for research funding through disease-oriented specialty organizations, such as heart, lung, diabetes, and cancer, but they are competing with medicine and other health disciplines.

The Alberta Foundation for Nursing Research (AFNR), another source of separate research funding for nursing, was established by ministerial order in 1982 as a response to lobbying by the Alberta Association of Registered Nurses (AARN) and nursing leaders of the University of Alberta and the University of Calgary. A fund of $1 million was allocated for use over a 5-year period and a board of directors was appointed to establish research categories, guidelines, and a review process and to award and administer the funds. Support services to administer the fund were provided by the Alberta Department of Advanced Education. At the end of the 5-year period, negotiations and political pressure once again succeeded in obtaining a $1 million award for another 5-year period (to 1993). The first awards were made in the 1983-84 fiscal year, and a total of $2,163,806 had been awarded to Alberta nurses by the end of the 1991-92 fiscal year. The amounts awarded per year and the number of awards made reflect remarkable progress, as evidenced by the allocation of $19,015 to seven recipients for 1983-84; $280,404 for 33 awards in 1988-89; $392,675 for 29 awards in 1990-91; and $314,499 for 26 awards in 1991-92 (Alberta Foundation for Nursing Research, 1991, 1992). Also encouraging is that a significant number of the studies funded by AFNR are being published and presented at national and international research conferences. With the establishment of the AFNR, Alberta became the first and only province or state worldwide to designate funds exclusively for nursing research. It is also the first research funding endeavour in Canada in which nurses have had a primary role in reviewing proposals and awarding funds. Regrettably, with severe cutbacks in funding for education, research and health care by the Alberta government, the AFNR annual grant was reduced to zero for 1994-95. In her 1993-94 Chairman's Report, Sheila Embury states: "One of the major challenges facing the [AFNR] Board will be to ensure continued financial support for nursing research in Alberta. The March 1994 [grant] competition will be the last funded from current sources" (p. 1)

■ ■ ■ ■

DETERRENTS TO DISSEMINATING AND APPLYING RESEARCH FINDINGS

Another type of deterrent to research pertains to impediments in the dissemination and application of research findings. The majority of practising nurses cannot understand research reports or critically evaluate research results. This impediment is related to the fact that the majority of nurses are still prepared at less than a baccalaureate level and their programs did not include a research course or research-based teaching. In addition, nursing education has tended to nurture values other than those that foster inquiry, intellectualism, scientific investigation, and respect for "thinkers" as well as "doers."

Most nursing education takes place in institutions, such as hospital schools of nursing and community colleges, that do not expect faculty to be involved in research. Many of these institutions do not even require faculty to have a master's degree. They have been oriented to education as a value system that is reflected in expectations held for faculty and in the status and rewards systems, which are known to strongly influence faculty behaviour. Research must become an integral part of the faculty role; it is essential that faculty use research in teaching and help students evaluate research findings, applying those that are valid and reliable to practice. Because the majority of nurse educators have not been prepared for research and are not expected to conduct research and use it in teaching, it is not surprising that only a small proportion of nursing educators are using research in teaching.

Johnson (1979) identifies inadequacies in publishing policies and practice in nursing literature as another barrier to research-based teaching in nursing-education programs.

> It is not universally accepted in nursing that authors of textbooks and articles for practitioners should rely heavily on scientific investigations to substantiate the knowledge transmitted and recommendations for activities. In some textbooks the documentation of the pronouncements is inadequate. One cannot determine if the information is the author's opinion, derived from theory, gained from experience, dictated by authority, or based on scientific investigation (p. 128).

Johnson (1979) points out another problem, that should concern all nurses because of the possible consequences. She notes that several journals "published primarily for practitioners discourage authors from citing the sources of information they are conveying. In fact, some journals have editorial policies that prohibit citation of sources" (p. 128). Such policies, developed by entrepreneurs taking advantage of nurses unaware of the importance of a scientific base for practice, do not help nursing in its effort to develop research or research-based teaching and practice.

Inadequate preparation is a deterrent to both the development of research and the dissemination of research findings. This inadequacy may result in poor conceptualization of the problem, improper choice of research methods, inadequate attention to the validity and reliability of instruments, selection of an inadequate population from which to generalize findings, and other inadequacies in design. One of the consequences of poor research is results that are not worth disseminating. Fortunately, some reports are rejected by journals and by those who review abstracts for research conferences, although it may be difficult to assess the methods used from a brief abstract. Downs (1983a) noted that the quality of research submitted to the journal *Nursing Research* had improved over the previous 4 years, but the rejection rate still stood at 85%. She also noted that poor methods, which were once the greatest problem, are now secondary to poor logic in the formulation of research design. Another inadequacy she identified was a severe discrepancy between the concepts selected and their measurement; descriptive studies should be completed before proceeding with measurement.

Investigators have alleged that some journals give preference to quantitative research over qualitative research. Instead of dichotomizing the two research methods, investigators need to base selection of the method used on what is known about the phenomena being studied. Downs (1983b) states that qualitative researchers criticize the work of quantitative researchers because it tries "to prove what is already known, has no meaning for nursing practice, and is generally of limited scope because the objective is to produce statistics." Meanwhile, quantitative researchers allege that "qualitative research is unscientific and soft because it cannot be numerically categorized" (Downs, 1983b, p. 259). She asserts that the allegation that quantitative research supporters are hindering the publication of qualitative studies is nonsense. She also identifies some of the inadequacies in reporting qualitative research that she perceives as problems, such as not explaining how conclusions are reached, why a sample was inadequate, or why the particular sample was appropriate. Some specification is necessary and must be supported by proper documentation. (Downs, 1983b). Qualitative research methods are appropriate for studying some of the phenomena in nursing because we know so little about them. Before quantifying a phenomenon, much has to be learned about it through descriptive and exploratory studies. Investigators using this method must apply proper rigour and interpret methods and findings clearly in relation to the conclusions that can be drawn.

Nursing leaders' insufficient support for research in nursing service and nursing education may be another deterrent to conducting research and applying research findings. McClure (1981) has noted that, in order to be supportive of research, the nurse executive needs substantial knowledge of research methods and research literature, not only to provide a climate supportive of research but also to sponsor a study through various review committees and make the arrangements necessary for the investigation to proceed. She believes that commitment of time and energy is essential to promoting and facilitating research and applying the findings to practice.

■■   ■■   ■■   ■■

STRATEGIES TO PROMOTE RESEARCH AND RESEARCH-BASED PRACTICE

The deterrents identified in relation to the development of research and the promotion of research-based practice suggest possible solutions in themselves; however, the solutions may be difficult to institute and will require strong commitment and determination on the part of nurses involved in research, education, and practice.

A basic, self-evident requirement for furthering research is to increase the proportion of nurses prepared at the baccalaureate level, which is the first level of nursing education in which students obtain an appreciation of the importance of research, an introduction to research methods, and beginning ability to critically evaluate research reports. Although in recent years there has been a remarkable increase in commitment to the goal of a baccalaureate degree requirement for entry to nursing practice by the year 2000, there is still resistance among some nurses and other groups. Careful attention should be given to this resistance while designing mechanisms and models for increasing the opportunities for persons entering nursing and registered nurses to earn a baccalaureate degree. In addition to increasing the proportion of baccalaureate-prepared nurses, there is need to evaluate the nature of research preparation included in baccalaureate programs to ensure that it is not directed toward teaching people to do research, but rather increasing awareness of and openness to research and developing beginning ability to critique research and differentiate the findings that merit application.

A second strategy is to increase the proportion of nurses prepared at the master's and doctoral levels. To increase enrolments more funding is needed, for which all nurses should lobby. Funding for research training has been provided to other disciplines through NSERC, SSHRC, MRC, and the National Health Research and Development Program (NHRDP), a program within the Health Promotion Directorate of Health and Welfare Canada. Over the past 2 decades, a number of nurses have been awarded fellowships from NHRDP for doctoral study in nursing in the United States and in other disciplines. In addition, a few nurses have been granted Health Research Scholar Awards, which provide funding to the university to support 75% of the recipient's time in research and other scholarly activities. For the nine recipients to date, this has resulted in a tremendous investment in furthering their research endeavours. Thus some nursing faculty have competed successfully for NHRDP funds to support research training and the actual conduct of research; however, the number has been small and the proportion almost infinitesimal when compared with funding for medicine and other disciplines.

In addition to increasing enrolments, attention must be given to the quality of graduate programs and the quality of research preparation within them. Nurses must be made aware of the importance of obtaining good research preparation in graduate study and not opt for the easiest and fastest route to a master's degree, which is the rationale given by some for selecting graduate programs. It is also important to ensure quality in nursing research and have faculty involved in their own research. Leaders in nursing education need to develop a climate that supports and rewards research, obtain resources to help faculty increase their research competence and grantsmanship skills, and hold faculty accountable for conducting research and disseminating findings. It is important to encourage nurses to pursue graduate study in nursing rather than in other disciplines so they will focus attention on studying nursing problems from a nursing perspective. This possibility has become more feasible with the establishment of four doctoral programs in nursing since January 1991, although funding limits the number of doctoral students admitted. Nurses should demand sound preparation in research and be helped to understand the importance of doing a thesis or independent investigation under expert guidance. Doctoral education in nursing, which has recently been instituted in Canada after the development of a sound research program by university faculty, implies the availability of faculty expertise in conducting research and guiding students in their research.

In recent years nursing literature has reflected increased efforts to promote, facilitate and implement collaborative strategies between nursing education and nursing practice in the interests of clinical nursing research (Bowman, Alvarez, Evans, Smith, and O'Brien, 1992; Davies and Drake, 1992; Henderson and Brouse, 1992; Kipnis, Turner, and Vander Wal, 1992; McKiel and Dawe, 1991; Tierney and Taylor, 1991). While some strategies are facilitated by collaboration models or a system of joint appointments, others are much less formalized. More information on collaborative models or strategies is presented in Chapter 25. All are based on basic principles of having a mutual sense of purpose; mutual commitment to common goals and ideals; maintaining open and frequent communication to engender trust and readiness for joint endeavours at the operational level as well as at higher levels in the organizations; being flexible and patient; anticipating resistance that is normal in any new endeavour, and being prepared to deal with it; and ensuring that both organizations benefit and gain recognition and visibility through research presentations, press releases, and publications.

Pepler (1992) describes the strategies used in a major teaching hospital to promote research-based practice. A consultant in nursing research, Pepler has designed a 24-hour educational program presented over a 12-week period that is available to nursing staff from other hospitals as well. It has "helped nurses gain the knowledge and skills to find, interpret and judge research findings and to change their world of practice" (p. 27). Other outcomes reported were greater use of research consultation services, ability to understand research presentations at conferences, and increased support for nursing research and research-based practice.

Janken, Dufault, and Yeaw (1988) selected unit-based, research roundtable discussions undertaken jointly by faculty and nursing service, as an approach to increase awareness of the relevancy of research to practice and to disseminate research findings among nursing staff and nursing students. They report that the process required time, patience, and persistence but resulted in more favourable attitudes toward research, increased application of research findings in practice, enhanced communications, and the development of a new respect between students and staff.

Another strategy to promote and facilitate research in service settings is the appointment of a clinical nurse researcher, who plays an active role in identifying study topics and demonstrating involvement in and commitment to nursing research. The very presence of such a person increases the visibility of research and research activities. It is important to note that a clinical nurse researcher requires doctoral preparation with sound knowledge of research design and methods. The challenge is to create a research climate that encourages questioning and an awareness of the importance and potential of research. The clinical nurse researcher in an agency may have a problem of isolation. One solution to this problem is to involve the researcher in a joint appointment with the cost shared by the health-care agency and a university faculty of nursing. This is an approach that has been and is being applied effectively by several universities (Alberta, British Columbia, Calgary, Dalhousie, Manitoba, McGill, McMaster, Ottawa, and Toronto) in collaboration with hospitals and other health-care agencies. A study conducted by the Western Interstate Commission for Higher Education in Nursing in the United States from 1973 to 1976 included 219 hospitals and 217 health-care agencies. Of the 219 hospitals, 8% had a full-time clinical nurse researcher and 31% had a part-time clinical nurse researcher. The percentage in community health agencies was 2% full-time and 22% part-time clinical nurse researchers (Krueger, 1978). A similar trend occurred in Canada in the 1980s and 1990s.

The role of the clinical nurse researcher, or faculty member in a joint appointment as part-time clinical nurse researcher, is to educate the staff about nursing research, increase awareness of research and its importance and potential for improving practice, and establish a proper research review process for screening nursing research proposals before they go to the agency review committee. The clinical nurse researcher also helps nursing staff interpret research findings, identify researchable problems, and assist in the conduct of research. Other important responsibilities are to serve as a role model by conducting research; to interpret nursing research to other disciplines, notably medicine; and to serve as a reviewer of medical research proposals. It is important to ensure that the research review process is rigourous within the institution and to assist in the application of valid and reliable research findings in practice. The enactment of such a role requires a nurse who is skilled in communication, is sensitive to the reactions of others, applies theories of planned change, and is competent in research methods. It also requires strong administrative support.

Knafl, Bevis, and Kirchhoff (1987) conducted a telephone survey of clinical nurse researchers in the United States to document the range of activities and responsibilities associated with the role and explore perceptions of how the role was developed and enacted. Despite considerable diversity in perceptions of enactment, most clinical nurse researchers reported devoting most of their time to research activities focused primarily on nursing practice studies and involving nursing staff in the identification of problems and conduct of research. Almost 50% of the research pertained to patient care and understanding patient behaviour, and more than 25% had been initiated by staff nurses. The clinical nurse researchers "view themselves and are viewed by their chief nurse executives as making a significant contribution to the hospital" (Knafl, Bevis, and Kirchhoff, 1987, p. 252).

Providing research consultation is another strategy employed to promote and enhance development of nursing research. Consultation in research design is usually available in universities; however, such resources are not usually provided in health-care agencies except through joint appointments. Thurston, Tenove, Church, and Bach-Peterson (1989), in their 1986 survey of nursing research being conducted in Canadian hospitals, found that 170 research projects were ongoing. The report does not specify what proportion of the projects were being conducted by graduate students in nursing or by nursing faculty; however, it is encouraging to find so much research activity. They also identified administrative commitment and support as the most important facilitator of nursing research and research-based practice. Also important are consultation services, library resources, educationally prepared nurses, funding, and time to be involved in research (Thurston, Tenove, and Church, 1990). These findings are supported by Fitch (1992) and Rosswurm (1992). Research consultation has been provided to nurses in Saskatchewan through the Saskatchewan Nursing Research Unit (established in 1983 under the directorship of Norma Stewart, jointly sponsored by the College of Nursing at the University of Saskatchewan and the Saskatchewan Registered Nurses Association, and since September 1984, the Saskatchewan Union of Nurses). A similar model was established in Manitoba in 1985 with the appointment of Lesley Degner as Director of the Manitoba Nursing Research Unit (jointly funded by the School of Nursing of the University of Manitoba and the Manitoba Association of Registered Nurses). For the 1986-87 fiscal year the AFNR provided research consultation to the nurses of Alberta through the secondment of Mary Renfrew Houston from the University of Lethbridge. This service was made possible by a one-time grant from the Alberta Department of Advanced Education. Extensive communication and publicity were used to advertise and interpret the research consultation services to nurses throughout the province. In the first 6 months consultation was provided to more than 100 nurses; 36% were from hospitals and nursing homes, 26% from colleges and universities, and 12% from professional associations and committees (AFNR, 1987). The response was gratifying and clearly reflected a great need for research consultation in Alberta. This need still exists in Alberta, as identified by the AFNR Board of Directors who asked the Alberta Association of Registered Nurses (AARN) "to explore the possibility of creating a Nursing Research Consultant position" (AFNR, 1990-1991, p. 2). Such a position has not been created to date, but the universities provide some consultation and support through joint appointees and other collaborative endeavours.

A strategy proposed and supported by some nurse investigators is to have researchers provide an interpretation of results in understandable form on a systematic basis. Kirchhoff (1983) raises the question: When staff nurses "need data base sources, should they struggle with the reported research journal or should they be satisfied with the short summaries provided by some of the clinically-oriented journals" (p. 246)? Although the answer to this question may seem obvious, there is need to provide those informational sources through an intermediate step. One strategy, developed by Haller, Reynolds, and Horsley (1979) in Michigan, was to provide research-based protocols for the nursing staff in several hospitals. This was a collaborative endeavour between education and service.

Another strategy was used by the American Association of Critical Care Nurses; reviews of studies in critical-care nursing with suggestions for practice were provided through their clinical journal, *Focus*. A similar approach was employed by the *Western Journal of Nursing Research* through their column "Using Research in Practice." However, it is essential to provide a scholarly critique of the original research and ensure that staff nurses realize that such protocols and suggestions cannot be applied without an interim step of interpretation by a competent investigator. Kirchhoff (1983) also suggests that research conferences include a response to a research presentation entitled "Clinical Application," which should be presented by a skilled researcher-clinician. Such an approach might encourage more practitioners to attend conferences.

Another strategy to facilitate the development of research is to organize research interest groups within the professional organization or within a health-care agency or group of agencies. It is important to have leaders with research expertise in such groups and to clearly define the purpose of the group. Is the purpose to learn to read and apply research findings, to conduct research, or both? Should there be one general research group or should there be smaller groups focused around particular clinical interests? Experience with such interest groups has demonstrated great potential when leadership is provided by nurses knowledgeable about research methods and able to utilize their knowledge in studying practice problems. Other approaches, in health-care agencies, are organizing research rounds, having research presentations at noon, and forming journal clubs in which discussion of research is led by a competent investigator. Another technique is to involve staff in data collection so they have a sense of what is involved in research and learn that research results are not immediately forthcoming.

Participation in the process of research review and ethical clearance is a strategy to be used under the direction and guidance of a competent researcher who works with staff to help them understand all factors that must be considered. The problem is that one must assess the quality of a research proposal in order to give ethical clearance; if the study is not designed well it is not ethical to take the subjects' time. This means that the clinical nurse researcher or faculty member giving the leadership has to select a committee and educate the members in the review process. They must be introduced to nursing research and the requirements for reviewing and interpreting nursing research, which implies having at least a baccalaureate degree. Guidelines for such a research review process have been developed in some health-care agencies, such as the University of Alberta Hospitals, where a clinical nurse researcher provided leadership in the process.

These guidelines are made available to others who are involved in promoting and facilitating research in other agencies.

Opportunities to share research findings can be provided through written media as well. Initially this may be through the health-care agency's monthly communique. Many, such as professional association newsletters, have a communication mechanism of some type where a column can be devoted to research in nursing. This should only be done under the guidance of a capable researcher to ensure that quality is maintained and that the terminology is appropriate for research neophytes.

A final strategy to increase the dissemination of research findings is to increase opportunities for publishing nursing research in Canada, such as through a journal devoted to nursing research that will have an adequate readership to make it economically feasible. *Nursing Papers*, now the *Canadian Journal of Nursing Research*, has been edited and published through McGill University since 1968, with Laurie Gottleib currently serving as senior editor. Although its readership has been limited, it is increasing with more doctorally prepared nurses conducting research and sharing their findings. Since 1987 the *Western Journal of Nursing Research*, published in the United States, has been edited at the University of Alberta by Pamela Brink and Marilynn Wood of the Faculty of Nursing. In 1991 a new research journal, *Clinical Nursing Research: An International Journal*, was launched with the first issue published in January 1992. It also is edited at the University of Alberta by Marilynn Wood and Patricia Hayes. As the title implies, this new refereed journal focuses on clinical practice problems. "It provides an international forum to encourage discussion among clinical practitioners, to enhance clinical practice by pinpointing potential clinical applications of the latest scholarly research, and to disseminate research findings of particular interest to practicing nurses" (Wood and Hayes, 1992, p. 2). Thus there has been considerable progress recently in increasing opportunities to publish nursing research. These are in addition to the United States research journals *Nursing Research, Research in Nursing and Health, Advances in Nursing Science,* and *Image: Journal of Nursing Scholarship*, which have a wider readership but also more competition for publication.

■ ■ ■ ■

CONCLUSION

Increasing the quantity and quality of research endeavours in nursing and applying research results to practice will require strong commitment on the part of nursing educators and leaders in health-care agencies. Leadership is crucial to effecting changes in organizations or professions, but in this instance there must also be competent nurse investigators to interpret knowledge of research and research findings in terms that can be understood by practising nurses. All must have the determination and commitment to pursue these goals and the ability to effect change in people and systems. Of utmost importance is that all nurses accept the challenge and take advantage of opportunities to commit themselves to increasing research endeavours, extending the scientific foundation for nursing practice, and ultimately improving practice through research.

REFERENCES

Alberta Foundation for Nursing Research. (1986-1987). *Annual Report.* Edmonton, Alberta: Author.

Alberta Foundation for Nursing Research. (1990-1991). *Annual Report.* Edmonton, Alberta: Author.

Alberta Foundation for Nursing Research. (1991-1992). *Annual Report.* Edmonton, Alberta: Author.

Bowman, J., Alvarez, L., Evans, M., Smith, R., and O'Brien, B. (1992). Taking the first step. *The Canadian Nurse, 88*(1), 22-24.

Brink, P.J., and Wood, M.J. (1983). *Basic steps in planning nursing research: From question to proposal* (2nd ed.) Belmont, CA: Wadsworth Health Services.

Brotherston, J.A.F. (1960). Research-mindedness and the health professions. In *Learning to investigate nursing,* (p. 4). Geneva, Switzerland: International Council of Nurses and Florence Nightingale Fund.

Bush, C.T. (1985). *Nursing research.* Reston, VA: Reston Publishing.

Canadian Nurses Foundation. (1990). *1990 Annual Report.* Ottawa, Ontario: Author.

Canadian Nurses Foundation. (1992). *1992 Annual Report.* Ottawa, Ontario: Author.

CNA Connection. (1991). Research grants. *The Canadian Nurse, 87*(6), 4.

Davies, B. and Drake, E. (1992). Student-staff collaborative power for Nursing Research. *The Canadian Nurse, 88*(1), 30-32.

Dickoff, J., James, P., and Wiedenbach, E. (1968). Theory in a practice discipline: Part I. Practice oriented theory. *Nursing Research, 17*(5), 415-435.

Downs, F. (1983a). Oz revisited [Editorial]. *Nursing Research, 32*(1), 3.

Downs, F. (1983b). One dark and stormy night [Editorial]. *Nursing Research, 32*(5), 259.

Ellis, R. (1974). Asking the research question. In *Issues in research: Social, professional and methodological* (pp. 31-35). Kansas City, MO: American Nurses Association.

Fitch, M. (1992). Five years in the life of a nursing research and professional development division. *Canadian Journal of Nursing Administration, 5*(2), 20-26.

Gortner, S.R. (1986). Impact of the Division of Nursing on research development in the United States. In S.M. Stinson and J.C. Kerr (Eds.) *International issues in nursing research* (pp. 113-130). London: Croon Helm.

Haller, K.B., Reynolds, M.A., and Horsley, J.A. (1979). Developing research-based innovation protocols: Process, criteria and issues. *Research in Nursing and Health, 2*(2), 45-51.

Henderson, A. and Brouse, J. (1992). Development of a research committee at a community hospital. *Canadian Journal of Nursing Administration, 5*(2), 17-19.

Janken, J.K., Dufault, M.A., and Yeaw, E.M. (1988). Research round tables: Increasing student/staff awareness of the relevancy of research to practice. *Journal of Professional Nursing, 4*(3), 186-191.

Johnson, J.E. (1979). Translating research into practice. In *Power: Nursing's challenge for change* (pp. 125-133). Kansas City, MO: American Nurses Association.

Kipnis, T., Turner, L. and Vander Wal, R. (1992). Promoting the spirit of inquiry. *The Canadian Nurse, 88*(1), 36-38.

Kirchhoff, K.T. (1983). Using research in practice: Should staff nurses be expected to use research? *Western Journal of Nursing Research, 5*(3), 245-247.

Knafl, K.A., Bevis, M.E. and Kirchhoff, K.T. (1987). Research activities of clinical nurse researchers. *Nursing Research, 36*(4), 249-252.

Krueger, J. (1978). Utilization of nursing research: The planning process. *Journal of Nursing Administration, 8*(1), 6-9.

Lamb, M. and Stinson, S.M. (1990). *Canadian nursing doctoral statistics: 1989 update.* Ottawa: Canadian Nurses Association.

Lindeman, C.A., and Schantz, D. (1982). The research question. *Journal of Nursing Administration, 12*(1), 6-10.

McClure, M.L. (1981). Promoting practice-based research: A critical need. *Journal of Nursing Administration, 11*(11 & 12), 66-70.

McKiel, E. and Dawe, U. (1991). Hospital-based nursing research programs: A requirement for progress. *Canadian Journal of Nursing Administration, 4*(3), 26-28.

Pepler, C. (1992). Fostering change through education. *The Canadian Nurse, 88*(1), 25-27.

Rosswurm, M.A. (1992). A research-based practice model in a hospital setting. *The Journal of Nursing Administration, 22*(3), 57-59.

Schlotfeldt, R.M., (1971). The significance of empirical research for nursing. *Nursing Research, 20*(2), 140-142.

Schlotfeldt, R.M. (1987). Defining nursing: A historic controversy. *Nursing Research, 36*(1), 64-67.

Stinson, S.M., Larsen, J., and MacPhail, J. (1984). *Canadian nursing doctoral statistics: 1982 update.* Ottawa: Canadian Nurses Association.

Stinson, S.M., MacPhail, J., and Larsen, J. (1988). *Canadian nursing doctoral statistics: 1986 update.* Ottawa: Canadian Nurses Association.

Thurston, N., Tenove, S., Church, J., and Bach-Paterson, K. (1989). Nursing research in Canadian hospitals. *Canadian Journal of Nursing Administration,* 2(1), 8-10.

Thurston, N., Tenove, S. and Church, J. (1990). Hospital nursing research is alive and flourishing. *Nursing Management,* 21(5), 50-54.

Tierney, A. and Taylor, J. (1991). Research in practice: An 'experiment' in researcher- practitioner collaboration. *Journal of Advanced Nursing,* 16, 506-510.

Werley, H. (1972). This I believe about clinical nursing research. *Nursing Outlook,* 20(11), 718-722.

Willems, E.P., and Rausch, H.L. (1969). *Naturalistic viewpoints in psychological research.* New York: Holt, Rinehart & Winston, Inc.

Wilson, H.S. (1985). *Research in nursing.* Don Mills, Ontario: Addison-Wesley Publishing Company.

Wood, M.J., and Hayes, P. (Eds.). (January 1992). Frontispiece. *Clinical Nursing Research: An International Journal,* 1(1), 2.

CHAPTER ELEVEN

The Financing of Nursing Research in Canada

JANET ROSS KERR

Nursing research has become an important sphere of activity, with growing recognition of the importance of nursing research to practice, accompanied by increased availability of research support and the appointment of individuals to conduct research. However, development of research activity in nursing has occurred gradually as a result of a slowly enlarging pool of nurses with research expertise. This development parallels the evolution of graduate education in nursing because teaching research methods and conducting research investigations to fulfill thesis requirements are important aspects of graduate education in nursing. Understandably, most research in any field takes place in university settings.

Since graduate education in nursing was established little more than a quarter of a century ago, nursing research activities have increased in scope and number. Opportunities in master's degree programs in nursing are now available across the country, and although admission is still very competitive, accessibility presents less of a problem than it once did. Master's degree programs provide the background in research to enable capable students to undertake doctoral work. Doctoral programs in nursing have begun in earnest with the funding of the first program at the Faculty of Nursing, University of Alberta, in January of 1991, when the first four students were admitted to the program. Four more such programs have followed in rapid succession. The University of British Columbia School of Nursing admitted its first students in September 1991, while approval of program funding for the the University of Toronto Faculty of Nursing program and the joint program between McGill University and the University of Montreal occurred in time for admission of students in September 1993. McMaster University has been the latest university to grant PhD degrees in nursing with the commencement of its program in September 1994.

The establishment of the entire range of university programs in nursing, from baccalaureate through doctoral degree levels, is a process that is well underway but by no means completed. Rationalizing the process rests on the view of the university as "a social institution, the specific mission of which is the transmission and the advancement of higher learning" (Hurburtise and Rowat, 1970, p. 37). The association between teaching and research has been described as a natural one, albeit complex. "Some kinds of research and some features of the research enterprise, are vital for good teaching: every university teacher should be involved in these kinds of features, and supported in them under the teaching budget" (Bonneau and Corry, 1972, p. 23).

At the conclusion of the stormy decade of the 1960s, Canadian universities began responding to the challenges and issues raised. One criticism of that period of rapid growth and student unrest was that too much time and energy were being expended on the research endeavour and too little on identifying and encouraging excellence in teaching. It is somewhat curious that universities came under fire for supposedly being preoccupied with research at precisely the same time as the nursing profession was engaged in the difficult struggle to establish its first graduate programs. During this process, the need for nursing's development of its research potential was underscored. Symons (1975) commented: "The slowness in developing graduate schools of nursing in Canada has, in turn, adversely affected the amount of research undertaken in this field. Little support has been available for publication, or for investigating problems in nursing and health care of particular interest to Canadians" (p. 212).

In her exploration of the meaning of the concepts of professionalization and deprofessionalization, Stinson (1969) postulates that the development of the research function is a vital component of professionalization:

> Supplying professional services inheres in the principle that initiating research, training various kinds of research workers, and `marketing' findings must not be left to the whims of chance or at the entire mercy of commercial interests. This means evolving not only intraprofessional mechanisms for the development and application of substantive knowledge but articulating these devices with those of other professions and those of the broader society (p. 167).

Although the need and concomitant timeliness of research in nursing has been recognized both inside and outside the nursing field, there have been problems in effecting change. It is likely that these problems will continue to be stumbling blocks for some time. The social reality of the last quarter of the twentieth century is that limits to growth of universities have appeared in the form of greatly decreased numbers of learners from the 18- to 22-year-old age group. This situation has occurred simultaneously with adverse and unstable world economic circumstances leading to shaky national economies and, subsequently, to financial stringency in all public institutions. However slow the basic development of research and graduate study in nursing is, there is little doubt that the process will continue. Stinson (1969) asserted that successful delivery of nursing services to society would ultimately require "that three simultaneous processes be going on: (1) accumulation of the K-S (knowledge-skill) component, (2) transmission of it, and (3) extension of it, mainly through systematic research" (pp. 156-157).

Concerted efforts to develop organizational support for nursing began in earnest in the early 1970s, when attention had been drawn to the crucial nature of that support: "A paradox of modern day research is that it is at once an intensely individual, personal endeavour, yet, if it is to be brought about, much less constitute benefits for society, it is immensely dependent upon organization—and highly complex organization at that" (Stinson, 1977, p. 10).

The first national conference on nursing research in Canada was held in Ottawa in 1971 under the auspices of the University of British Columbia, with federal assistance from the National Health Research and Development Program (NHRDP). As this was a "first" for the nursing profession in Canada, historical overviews were presented on the kinds of nursing research projects conducted over the years by governments, service agencies, professional associations, and universities (Griffin, 1971; Imai, 1971; Poole, 1971). These overviews documented that most studies had been undertaken since 1965, and some were funded by a variety of sponsoring agencies. In relation to university based projects, Griffin (1971) commented:

> Funds for either faculty or graduate students' research have not been obtained for many projects. Of those reported, only 22 faculty and 23 students indicated some sponsorship. A few respondents indicated funds had not been obtained "yet" and doubtlessly the graduate students were indirectly funded for their research through funding during all or part of their graduate education programs (p. 96).

▬ ▬ ▬ ▬

FEDERAL SUPPORT FOR RESEARCH

The federal government first recognized a need for improved research and development because of the war effort, and as a result, the National Research Council (NRC) was formed in 1916. Its role was "undertaking, assisting and promoting scientific and industrial research in Canada" in certain specified areas (Secretary of State, 1975, p. 2). The Canada Council was established in 1957 to support research in the humanities and social sciences. The Medical Research Council (MRC) and the National Sciences and Engineering Research Council (NSERC) originally operated within the framework of the NRC of Canada, but the MRC became fully autonomous in 1969, as did the NSERC in 1978. The Social Sciences and Humanities Research Council (SSHRC), established in 1978, encompasses programs administered originally by the Canada Council. These three granting councils (MRC, NSERC, SSHRC) do not conduct intramural research programs of their own. Each is dedicated entirely to provision of grants and awards to support extramural research, conducted primarily in universities and their affiliated institutions. Each council is responsible for the areas of research indicated by its name. In addition, other agencies and departments of the federal government have always been involved in granting smaller amounts to support research. The NHRDP of Health and Welfare Canada is one such research-funding unit with particular relevance to nursing research support (Peitchinis, 1971).

Three categories of federal research support provide funds: research grants, research fellowships, and auxiliary grants, the latter providing only indirect support for research. Funds may be awarded directly to faculty members and institutions "to assist them in the performance of projects initiated and controlled by the grant recipients" (Secretary of State, 1975, p. 35). Fellowships are funds that are channelled directly to faculty members or graduate students for research training. Historically, NRC received the largest share of federal research funds; this is still evident in the amounts allocated to NSERC and MRC, which were originally encompassed within NRC. For the 1987-88 fiscal year, research funding was provided through grants and fellowships: 52% to NSERC, 27% to MRC, 10% to SSHRC, and 11% to the Health Protection Program, which includes NHRDP (Statistics Canada, 1987). Since the early 1970s, there has been public conflict and debate over the levels of federal support available for research. From 1971 to 1974, federal research funding in Canada experienced a period of no growth, and in December 1975, the funds of the MRC were temporarily frozen. The result was that research teams across the country had to curtail or discontinue research activities. The "hard line" taken by the federal government toward medical research was vigorously denounced by the medical community at the time:

> Those who downplay research show little inclination to give up its practical benefits. Only the cost is shunned, not the fruits. If Canadians want the high quality of health care they deserve, they must be prepared to pay for it. And a reasonable tab for medical research must remain prominently displayed on the invoice (Osmond, 1976, p. 10).

Since then, public debate has continued on the issue of federal research funding. Powerful lobbies for science and engineering research and for medical research appear to have been successful. Undoubtedly, federal research-funding policy will continue to be the subject of considerable debate as the social merit of its decisions is weighed against the need for spending in other areas. More recent developments, which may eventually have some impact on federal funding for health research, centre on provincial research-funding activities. In Ontario the proceeds of lottery funds have been targeted for health research, and in Alberta in 1980, the provincial government created the Alberta Heritage Foundation for Medical Research (AHFMR), a research-granting agency, using $300 million from the Heritage Savings Trust Fund. The interest accrued on this principal is the source of medical research funding by the AHFMR.

■ ■ ■ ■

SOURCES OF FUNDING FOR NURSING RESEARCH

The three primary areas for which external research support is sought are research projects, research training, and space and equipment for conducting nursing research. Discussion is limited to the first two sources because they precede and condition the eventual development of the third. However, it should be noted that the first Center for Nursing Research in Canada was established at McGill University in 1971 with federal support from Health and Welfare Canada. Until funding for nursing research became readily available as an integral part of the terms of reference of the NHRDP of Health and Welfare Canada, there were few sources of funds other than the limited resources of the Canadian Nurses Foundation (CNF) and those of private foundations and voluntary organizations.

The 1971 documentation provided by Griffin reveals that research funding was not secured for many projects:

> It must be underlined that, to date, a substantial portion of Canadian nursing research has been done by graduate students at their own expense, and by nursing faculty and health agency members, often on their own time, and on a non-funded basis. As such, direct cost figures give us only a hint of the time, equipment, supplies and publication costs of all the nursing research being done (p. 22).

Slowly, almost imperceptibly, new sources of funding for nursing research have been opening up for nurses since the 1970s. Some of these sources are provincial organizations, whereas others are national ones. Notable among some of the organizations that include nursing in their mandates are the British Columbia Health Care Research Foundation, the Canadian Cancer Society, the Canadian Heart Foundation, the Hospital for Sick Children Foundation, the Kidney Foundation of Canada, the Manitoba Health Research Board, the Ontario Ministry of Health, the Quebec Ministry of Health, and the Saskatchewan Health Research Board.

One agency established by the Government of Alberta, the Alberta Foundation for Nursing Research (AFNR), is unique in that funding was exclusively directed to nursing research. This Foundation was created in 1982 by ministerial order and was designed to administer a grant of $1 million for nursing research over the next 5 years. This occurred in response to direct lobbying by members of the Provincial Council and Executive of the Alberta Association of Registered Nurses and by other nurses who became involved in making the case for a funding organization that would be a part of or parallel to the AHFMR that was being established at the same point in time. Since 1987, a $200,000 annual grant has continued to be designated for nursing research. In 1990, this amount was increased to $300,000 annually. The continued mandate of AFNR has made Alberta nurses a leading force in nursing research development in Canada. Although the 1994-95 budget of the Foundation was eliminated in the provincial thrust to eliminate deficit financing, the $150,000 allocated for 1995-96 restored it to about one-half of the previous level. Efforts to restore these funds for nursing research are ongoing. Emphasis has been placed upon nursing practice research, but all types of nursing research projects have been considered to fall within the mandate of this funding organization. Funding categories include research projects, demonstration/evaluation projects, facilitation projects, research support for graduate students at the master's and doctoral levels, conferences on nursing research, and postdoctoral fellowships. The number of research proposals to AFNR have increased over the more than 10 years the fund has been in existence. Since the 1991 granting year, the number of projects approved by the Foundation exceeded available funds.

■ ■ ■ ■

FUNDING FOR RESEARCH PROJECTS IN NURSING AT THE FEDERAL LEVEL

A review of federal research grants for projects relating to health care between 1949 and 1963 revealed that no funding was awarded for research projects in university schools of nursing (Defence Research Board, 1963).

TABLE 11.1   Research Project Grants to Nurses From Federal Sources: 1964 to 1968 and 1972 to 1976*

Year	Amount Awarded
1964-65	$ 11,300
1965-66	25,074
1966-67	27,414
1967-68	28,415
1972-73	48,840
1973-74	88,709
1974-75	318,002
1975-76	555,168

*Historical information was reported for all individual nurses receiving research grants.

From Good, S.R. *Support of research in universities,* 1964-68, p. 12; *Directory of federally supported research in universities (1971-73 to 1975-76).* Ottawa: Canada Institute for Scientific and Technical Information, National Research Council.

Beginning in 1963, support became available for nursing research in progressively incremental amounts (see Table 11.1). Although these funds were reported as allocated for nursing research between 1964 and 1968, funding for only one investigation, conducted by a nursing co-principal investigator from a university school of nursing, could be identified from a review of lists of all health science projects funded in those years (Good, 1969). The nurse who served as co-principal investigator was Helen M. Carpenter of the University of Toronto, whose cooperative project with an East York/ Leaside health unit investigator received a federal grant of $7100 (Defence Research Board, 1967, p. 18). A review of Table 11.1 reveals that funding began to increase dramatically after 1968. During the 1975-76 fiscal year, $572,005 was awarded for nursing research projects in university schools of nursing, providing funding for 15 research projects under the direction of 10 nursing principal investigators across the country. Not only was there a substantial increase in funding from 1964 to 1976, but the increase between the 1974-75 fiscal year and the 1975-76 fiscal year was a substantial 38% (Kerr, 1978).

Research Project Grants to Nurses From Federal Sources: 1964 to 1968 and 1972 to 1976

It became clear to nurses that even with the level of support provided by the NHRDP during the 1985-86 fiscal year and funds awarded by other organizations, there was a critical need for funding from the federal government that was specifically designated for nursing. Of the three major granting councils, both the MRC and the SSHRC included nursing among the disciplines eligible for funding. Nevertheless, nursing researchers found it difficult to get either council to review proposals. Grant applications were often sent from one agency to another; many ended up being considered by NHRDP. Few nursing research project proposals were funded by either the MRC or the SSHRC. In response to the

Canadian Nurses Association's (CNA) efforts to communicate nurses' concerns about this process and the resulting low level of federal funding for nursing research, the MRC established the Working Group on Nursing Research in 1982. Final recommendations in the Report of the Working Group in 1985 referred to the need to designate funds for nursing research within the MRC's structure and the need to assist in creating opportunities for the establishment of PhD in Nursing programs across the country. No federal action was taken on the recommendations until early 1988, when the MRC announced its decision to collaborate with NHRDP to make separate funding available for nursing research on a competitive basis. University nursing programs were invited to submit proposals, to be considered in the same manner as current development grants and program grants of MRC, for funding over approximately 3 years. This resulted in the funding of a small number of nursing researchers across the country, a result that did not please the nursing community. Lobbying efforts have continued, and in 1994 it was announced that the mandate of the MRC would be broadened to include health science research. In that the new guidelines published by the MRC are in the process of implementation, it remains to be seen whether nursing research will be well-served by the new approach to be taken in the MRC.

■ ■ ■ ■

RESEARCH SUPPORTED BY UNIVERSITY SCHOOLS OF NURSING

Table 11.2 documents the results of an investigation of research support to university schools of nursing, including funds expended by schools for nursing research as reported by the individual universities (Kerr, 1978, 1986). The significance of the change in the extent of the research in university schools of nursing over time may be readily appreciated. From a very small endeavour in just a few schools, nursing research has become a more broadly based and better financed undertaking. Although the figures reported are aggregate sums that may include funds received from external granting agencies for program development, they give some indication of the "state of the art." It is interesting to note that all universities with graduate programs received funds for research in the 1980-81 fiscal year, as well as one institution that had not yet initiated a graduate program.

From the rather bleak levels of research funding reported for the 1965-66 fiscal year to the vastly increased amounts reported in later years, it is evident that funding for nursing research in university schools of nursing has entered a new era. Undoubtedly, this change has been predicated on new expectations for faculty performance in research; without the development of research expertise among faculty it would not have been possible. Essential to the transition was the appointment of members of faculty qualified at the doctoral level who were prepared to undertake research. The lack of availability of a funded doctoral program in nursing in Canada until 1991 forced nurses to be resourceful and to find alternatives that enabled them to develop research skills. These alternatives included entering doctoral programs in nursing in other countries, most notably the United States, and seeking admission to doctoral programs in other disciplines. The development of funded doctoral programs in nursing in Canada since 1991 has increased access to doctoral programs for nurses, even though

TABLE 11.2 Funds Expended for Nursing Research Reported for Canadian Association of University Schools of Nursing, 1965-66 to 1990-91

	1990-91	1985-86	1980-81	1975-76		1970-71		1965-66	
	Assisted Research: Nursing	Assisted Research: Nursing	Assissted Research: Nursing	Assisted Research: Nursing	Total University Research Funds (%)	Assisted Research: Nursing	Total University Research Funds (%)	Assisted Research: Nursing	Total University Research Funds (%)
University of British Columbia	135,657	81,290	13,074	104,333	2.95	19,805	0.27	1,519	0.03
University of Alberta	396,871	19,862	0	18,366	0.14	13,126	0.17	NA	NA
University of Calgary	0	20,280	0	NA	NA	NA	NA	NA	NA
University of Saskatchewan	33,410	35,712	7,135	NA	NA	NA	NA	NA	NA
University of Manitoba	0	6,140	0	88,728	0.10	0	0	NA	NA
University of Western Ontario	50,000	0	0	7,232	0.06	6,711	0.10	0	0
University of Toronto	212,377	32,643	89,070	171,574	0.58	84,723	0.44	12,091	0.14
McMaster University	382,181	78,887	101,517	145,825	1.12	80,613	1.13	NA	NA
Université de Montréal	195,690	18,669	0	61,363	0.32	0	0	NA	NA
McGill University	129,084	20,300	61,663	170,892	0.81	35,242	0.23	NA	NA
Queens University	39,269	10,644	0	NA	NA	NA	NA	NA	NA
Dalhousie University	85,034	0	0	0	0	92,606	2.69	37,063	NA
University of Ottawa	51,073	NA	NA	NA	NA	NA	NA	NA	NA

All data prior to 1980 from financial statements, accountants' records and records of the schools of nursing of the above universities; *Reference list of health science research in Canada, 1980-81* (source for 1980-81 information), *1985-86* (source for 1985-86 information), and *1990-91* (source for 1990-91 information).

enrollments have been somewhat limited in most schools in the early years of development of programs. In Table 11.2, funds for nursing research grants reported in the *Reference List of Health Science Research in Canada, 1990-91* were used as the source of information. Table 11.3 provides information on funds for research initiatives reported by the institutions to the Canadian Association of University Schools of Nursing. These figures are higher than those presented in Table 11.2 in almost all cases, undoubtedly because they include internal funding and sources of funds other than those reported in the Reference List.

■ ■ ■ ■

NURSING RESEARCH IN HEALTH-CARE AGENCIES

In the 1980s nursing research became a growth activity in health-care agencies with increasing recognition of the importance of nursing research to health care and the availability of research support. In many large teaching hospitals nursing researchers were appointed to formulate and conduct research within the nursing department initially. These individuals often toiled alone in their pursuit of research activities. By the end of the decade, research activities were having a significant impact on nursing practice, and the research programs and spirit of inquiry that had evolved were the envy of many, including other disciplines. Collaboration between nursing researchers in health-care agencies and those in university schools of nursing were mutually beneficial. Joint appointments between these organizations thrived and facilitated the investigation of nursing research problems. This collaborative work undoubtedly resulted in important outcomes in terms of the nature of research questions asked and the

TABLE 11.3	Funds Expended for Nursing Research Reported for Canadian Association of University Schools of Nursing: 1990-91	
Institution	All Operating Maintenance and Travel Grants	All Grants/Faculty-Principal Investigators
University of British Columbia	271,104	271,104
University of Alberta	786,361	542,861
University of Calgary	31,047	31,047
University of Saskatchewan	70,299	43,653
University of Manitoba	173,252	90,709
University of Western Ontario	317,117	60,237
University of Toronto	795,495	745,495
McMaster University	1,927,883	1,000,636
Université de Montréal	889,821	869,121
McGill University	439,666	287,132
Queens University	256,906	206,008
Dalhousie University	17,610	17,610
University of Ottawa	796,687	226,724

Source: Canadian Association of University Schools of Nursing, Personal Communication, March 1994.

quality of the research effort. By the early 1990s many of the hospital-based nursing research positions were being phased out or significantly changed in response to a perceived need for fiscal restraint. Remaining positions were reconfigured to emphasize responsibilities for measurement and evaluation on a hospital-wide basis. The impact on nursing research is as yet unclear, but undoubtedly a diluted emphasis on research-based practice will result.

In a unique, state-of-the-art study of nursing research activities in Canadian teaching hospitals in 1985, 84 institutions were surveyed (Thurston, Tenove, and Church, 1987). The study documented completion of 170 investigations: 118 focused on nursing care, 44 focused on nursing-care delivery, and 8 focused on other areas. Almost one third of the 59 projects identified were funded externally, and administrative commitment and support were underscored as the most important factors in facilitating nursing research. The authors concluded: "Nursing research, although in an early state of development, had become a visible and credible activity in teaching hospitals" (Thurston et al, 1987, p. i). In a later study conducted in 1990, 45 Canadian teaching hospitals were surveyed to determine the extent of nursing research within these organizations (Thurston, Tenove, and Church, 1990). The majority had a process for reviewing research proposals by a committee. Results again indicated that the presence of a position for a nursing researcher and the establishment of research review committees provided encouragement for the development of nursing research in the institution (Thurston, Tenove, and Church, 1990). *The Reference List of Health Science Research in Canada* for 1985-86 documented the provision of $55,982 in research funds to nursing researchers in health-care agencies (Canada Institute for Scientific and Technical Information, 1985-1986). Health-care agencies have a special interest in ascertaining the efficacy of methods of care as well as in exploring management questions that may lead to improved care. It is likely that there will be considerable expansion of nursing research in the future as health-care administrators observe the benefits of increased knowledge about nursing care and the most effective means of providing it in health-care environments.

REFERENCES

Bonneau, L.P. and Corry, J.A. (1972). *Quest for the optimum: Research policy in the universities of Canada.* Ottawa: Association of Universities and Colleges of Canada.

Canada Institute for Scientific and Technical Information. (1980-81, 1985-86, 1990-91). *Reference list of health science research in Canada.* Ottawa: The Institute.

Defence Research Board. (1963). *Medical research projects completed in Canada, 1949-1963.* Ottawa: Author.

Defence Research Board. (1967). *Reference list of medical research projects in Canada.* Ottawa: Author.

Good, S.R. (1969). *Submission to the study of support of research in universities for the Science Secretariat of the Privy Council.* Ottawa: Canadian Nurses Association and Canadian Nurses Foundation.

Griffin, A. (1971). Nursing research in Canadian universities. In *National conference on research in nursing practice.* Ottawa: School of Nursing, University of British Columbia.

Hurburtise, R. and Rowat, D.C. (1970). *The university, society and government: The report of the commission on the relations between universities and governments.* Ottawa: University of Ottawa Press.

Imai, R. (1971). Associations and research activities. In *National conference on research in nursing practice.* Ottawa: School of Nursing, University of British Columbia.

Kerr, J.C.R. (1978). *Financing university nursing education in Canada: 1919-1976.* PhD dissertation, University of Michigan: Ann Arbor, MI.

Kerr, J.C.R. (1986). Structure and funding of nursing research in Canada. In S.M. Stinson and J.C. Kerr (Eds.), *International issues in nursing research* (pp. 97-112). London: Croom Helm.

Osmond, D.H. (1976). Sickness in Canada's health system. *The University of Toronto Graduate,* Spring, 10.

Peitchinis, S.H. (1971). *Financing post-secondary education in Canada.* Toronto: Council of Ministers of Education in Canada.

Poole, P.E. (1971). Research activities conducted or sponsored by government or service agencies. In *National conference on research in nursing practice.* Ottawa: School of Nursing, University of British Columbia.

Secretary of State. (1975). *Review of educational policies in Canada: Government of Canada report.* Toronto: Council of Ministers of Education in Canada.

Statistics Canada. (1987). *Federal science expenditures and personnel. 1987-88.* Ottawa: Statistics Canada.

Stinson, S.M. (1969). Deprofessionalization in nursing? Ed.D. dissertation. Teachers' College, Columbia University: New York.

Stinson, S.M. (1977). Central issues in Canadian nursing research. In B. LaSor and M.R. Elliot (Eds.), *Issues in Canadian nursing* (pp. 3-42). Scarborough: Prentice-Hall Canada Ltd.

Symons, T.H.B. (1975). *To know ourselves: The report of the Commission on Canadian Studies (Vols. I-II).* Ottawa: Association of Universities and Colleges of Canada.

Thurston, N.E., Tenove, S., and Church, J. (1987). *Nursing research in Canadian teaching hospitals.* Calgary, Alberta: Department of Nursing, Foothills Provincial General Hospital and Faculty of Nursing, University of Calgary.

Thurston, N., Tenove, S. and Church, J. (1990). Hospital nursing research is alive and flourishing. *Nursing Management, 21*(5), 50-54.

CHAPTER TWELVE

Scope of Research in Nursing Practice

JANNETTA MacPHAIL

T he scope of research in nursing practice is influenced by one's philosophy of nursing practice. For most nurses nursing practice pertains to the direct care of individuals or groups, with a view to helping them attain, maintain, and regain their optimal level of health and functioning. For other nurses practice includes educating nurses, conducting nursing research, and administering nursing services or nursing education. In general, nurse researchers classify nursing practice research as that involving studies of direct care.

■ ■ ■ ■

DEVELOPMENT OF NURSING RESEARCH IN CANADA

The pattern of development of nursing research in Canada was similar to that of nursing education in universities; the initial focus was on functional nursing— that is, teaching and administration—as opposed to clinical nursing. This was also the trend in the development of nursing research in the United States (Gortner and Nahm, 1977; O'Connell and Duffey, 1978) and in the United Kingdom (Hockey, 1986). Cahoon (1986) points out that pressures to improve nursing education in Canada promoted a focus on nursing education studies until the mid-century and that clinical nursing studies were relatively infrequent until the late 1960s. Stinson (1986) notes that the focus shifted from nursing education to nursing service administration by the late 1960s and to research in nursing practice by the mid-1970s. Cahoon (1986) observed that "the majority of studies were conducted by university nursing faculty members and/or, as of the late 1960s, their graduate students" (p. 164). This trend continued into the 1970s and 1980s, even though some large health-care agencies had established a position for a clinical nurse researcher. Thurston, Tenove, and Church (1987) found, in a survey of Canadian teaching hospitals, that 150 nursing research projects were ongoing. The current trend emphasizes research in nursing practice designed to improve practice; there is less emphasis on research pertaining to nursing education and administration. This trend is probably due to the increasing number of

146

nurses prepared at the doctoral level in nursing and to the importance attached to nursing practice among the general population of nurses today.

■ ■ ■ ■

CLASSIFICATION OF NURSING RESEARCH

A number of analyses have classified nursing research into categories (O'Connell and Duffey, 1978; Gortner, Bloch, and Phillips, 1976; Gortner and Nahm, 1977; Loomis, 1985; Hayter and Knafl, 1986). These analyses have been of nursing research in the United States, of nursing research published in nursing research journals in the United States, or in the case of Loomis (1985), of dissertation titles and abstracts. No similar classification of nursing research has been conducted and reported by Canadians.

The major avenue for Canadian nurses to report their research findings and share ongoing research projects has been primarily National Nursing Research Conferences, which were initiated in 1971 by the Canadian universities that offered graduate programs in nursing (Alberta, British Columbia, Calgary, Dalhousie, Manitoba, McGill, Montreal, Newfoundland, Saskatchewan, Toronto, and Western Ontario) and were held approximately every 18 months. The proceedings of the first 10 conferences, held between 1971 and 1985, were published and served as the information source for the author to analyze the scope of research in nursing practice and to identify trends or themes that will be reported in this chapter.

Another source of Canadian nursing research is the journal *Nursing Papers*, which was first published in 1968 by McGill University School of Nursing under the editorship of Dr. Moyra Allen, who is recognized for her vision and leadership in the development of nursing research in Canada. Although preference was given to articles based on research, *Nursing Papers* was not devoted entirely to nursing research. Beginning in 1986, the journal bore the added title of *The Canadian Journal of Nursing Research*, and then *Nursing Papers* was deleted from the title in 1988. Because the journal had not been devoted completely to research and because it was difficult to differentiate research articles from others, it was not used in analyzing nursing research for the purposes of this chapter.

A further source of Canadian nursing research is identified by Stinson (1986), who states that the *Index of Canadian Studies*, initiated in 1964 by the Canadian Nurses Association (CNA), is the most extensive cataloguing of Canadian nursing research; however, there is not yet a comprehensive repository of all Canadian nursing research.

■ ■ ■ ■

ORGANIZATION AND FUNDING OF NATIONAL NURSING RESEARCH CONFERENCES

The First National Nursing Research Conference was held in 1971 in Ottawa; it was organized and sponsored by the University of British Columbia School of Nursing and supported by the Department of National Health and Welfare. Speakers were invited to address problems of research in professional practice. Only one of the invited speakers was a nurse—not an unexpected situation at this early stage in the development of nursing research. The nurse speaker was

Dr. Faye Abdellah, an eminent leader in the development of nursing research, who presented a historical perspective of nursing research in the United States. A symposium followed by discussion groups led by selected nurse leaders focused on current nursing research activities in Canada, as conducted or sponsored by government and service agencies, professional associations, and Canadian universities. In the introduction the project director, Dr. Floris King (1971), stated:

> Prior to 1960 there were few significant research studies in nursing practice reported in Canadian nursing literature. Research studies which appeared were primarily reports of surveys conducted to establish facts about activities in which nurses were engaged, income and employment conditions of nurses, supply and demand for nurses in particular geographic areas, and content of educational programmes. These were important starts in nursing research in Canada (p. 1).

At the end of the conference the 380 participants presented resolutions that pertained to education of researchers, facilitation of nursing research in healthcare agencies, and the need to hold research conferences on a regular basis to present research findings and share research ideas.

Table 12.1 presents the years of the first 10 national nursing research conferences (1971 through 1985), the host universities, and the sources of funding as reported in the proceedings of each conference.

The conferences were all organized by Canadian universities on a volunteer basis, and an offer to host the next conference was usually made at the end of each conference. The first five conferences were invitational and all obtained external funding, initially from the Department of Health and Welfare and subsequently from the National Health Research and Development Program (NHRDP), which is part of the Department of Health and Welfare. The sixth conference was the first that was open to all persons; it was also the first to be supported solely by nurses through registration fees and contributions from the provincial nurses' associations of the two host provinces, Manitoba and Saskatchewan. Subsequent conferences were also supported by registration fees and a contribution from the provincial nurses' association of the host province or of the provinces involved in sponsorship and organization. In addition, continued federal funding through NHRDP or the Department of Health and Welfare were apparent, although the amount was reduced. The conferences held in 1983 and 1985 sought and received funding from the Secretary of State for simultaneous translation.

The 1985 National Nursing Research Conference in Toronto closed with a decision that no national nursing research conference would be planned for 1986 because the University of Alberta had announced in 1983 that the second International Nursing Research Conference would be hosted by the University of Alberta in May 1986. Because plans had not been made for another national nursing research conference, the Executive Committee of the Canadian Association of University Schools of Nursing decided in the fall of 1986 to ask McMaster University to host a research conference in conjunction with the annual meeting of the Learned Societies in June 1987.

After 1978, the published proceedings of the 10 National Nursing Research Conferences were printed and provided to all participants. The cost was included

TABLE 12.1 Host Universities and Sources of Funding for National Nursing Research Conferences

Year of Conference	Host Universities	Site	Sources of Funding	Reference
1971	British Columbia	Ottawa	Department of Nat'l Health and Welfare	King (1971)
1973	McGill & Montreal	Montreal	DHW	Allen, Thibaudeau (1973)
1974	McMaster, Toronto, & Western Ontario	Toronto	DHW	Godden, Cahoon (1974)
1975	Alberta, Calgary, Manitoba, & Saskatchewan	Edmonton	DHW	Zilm, Stinson Steed, Overton (1975)
1977	Ottawa & Canadian Nurses Association	Ottawa	DHW	CNA (1977)
1978	Manitoba & Saskatchewan	Winnipeg	Registration fees and the two provincial nurses' associations	Crawford, Kyle (1978)
1980	Dalhousie & four Atlantic Nurses' Associations	Halifax	Registration fees, four nurses' associations, and NHRDP	McKay, Zilm (1980)
1982	British Columbia & Victoria	Victoria	Registration fees, RNABC, NHRDP, and BC Goverment	Zilm, Hilton, Richmond (1982)
1983	McGill, Montreal, & Laval	Montreal	Registration fees, Quebec Nurses' Association, NHRDP, Secretary of State	Kravitz, Laurin (1983)
1985	Toronto	Toronto	Registration fees, MRC, NHRDP, Secretary of State	King, Prodrick, Bauer (1985)

in the registration fee initiated in 1978; however, as the cost of printing increased it became difficult to publish proceedings. Additional funding to continue this process was sought by the host universities.

■ ■ ■ ■

DEMOGRAPHIC DATA AND FOCUS OF NATIONAL NURSING RESEARCH CONFERENCES

Demographic data for nine national nursing research conferences are presented in Table 12.2. These data indicate remarkable increases in the number of participants, the number of papers presented, and the number of investigators involved in the projects, particularly in later years. The first conference (1971) is not included in the analysis because it did not involve the presentation of research papers. The number of participants was low in the early years, when

TABLE 12.2 Demographic Data on National Nursing Research Conferences, 1973-1985

Data	1973	1974	1975	1977	1978	1980	1982	1983	1985
No. of participants	40	57	68	105	101	145	200+	354	300
No. of research papers presented	11	12	13	11	14	18	26	29	49
No. of authors –1	11	6	12	10	6	10	15	14	26
–2	–	3	1	1	8	4	7	6	10
–3	–	3	–	–	–	2	2	7	5
–more	–	–	–	–	–	2	2	2	8
Discipline of –Nursing	11	17	15	13	20	27	40	51	83
Investigators –Other	–	4	–	–	–	8	4	10	15
Highest degree of researchers									
Nurses: Doctorate –Nursing	0	0	0	0	0	2	2	6	12
–Other	1	4	3	3	6	9	12	9	13
Master's –Nursing	7	10	6	6	9	11	19	21	39
–Other	3	2	2	3	3	2	6	5	10
Baccalaureate	0	0	1	0	1	2	1	1	8
No degree	0	1	1	0	1	0	0	1	1
Other									
disciplines: Doctorate – PhD	0	2	0	0	0	7	4	3	8
Doctorate – MD	0	2	0	0	0	0	0	1	5
Baccaulareate	0	0	0	0	0	1	0	0	2

attendance was by invitation only. Although the number of participants did not increase in 1978, the first year that invitation was not required, a steady increase is evident in subsequent years. There has also been a significant increase in the number of abstracts submitted, from 38 in 1982, from which 26 papers were selected, to 110 in 1985, from which 49 papers were selected.

The number of papers presented increased in 1985 because this was the year that a standard procedure, a critique of each research paper given by a discussant, was eliminated. The increase in number of papers and abstracts reflects the augmentation in nurses' involvement in research over a period of 14 years and the standardization of presentation to research conferences in other disciplines. The trend has been to provide more opportunity for investigators to share their research findings and allow time for discussion by all attendees instead of limiting the discussion of a paper to a planned discussant.

Two items of interest are the change in number of authors involved in preparing papers and the increase in the number of nurses involved as investigators as compared with the number of investigators from other disciplines. Also interesting is the change in the involvement of investigators from other disciplines versus nurses from 1980 to 1985. In 1980, 23% of the investigators were from other disciplines and two served as principal investigator. In 1982, only 9% were from other disciplines, and none served as a principal investigator. In 1983 and 1985, the percentage of investigators from other disciplines was 16% and 15%, respectively, with none serving as principal investigator or co-principal investigator.

The change in the educational preparation of nurse investigators over the years is illustrated in Table 12.2. It is interesting to note that the number of nurses with doctoral preparation increased from one in 1973 to 25 in 1985. There were no nurse investigators with doctorates in nursing until 1980, when there were two; that number increased to 12 in a 5-year period. Through the years, the number of nurses who held a master's degree in nursing and were involved in research exceeded the number with preparation in a field other than nursing; of the 49 who held master's degrees in 1985, 39 had earned the degree in nursing. The nurses with baccalaureate degrees or diplomas were few, and their involvement in research was as assistants. The difference in the level of education between nurses and investigators from other disciplines demonstrates that in disciplines other than nursing, most of those involved in research are educated at the doctoral level.

■ ■ ■ ■

ANALYSIS OF CONTENT OF THE NATIONAL NURSING RESEARCH CONFERENCES

Originally the first two conferences did not have titles, and titles were adopted later to reflect a focus on nursing practice research and on particular concerns related to the preparation of investigators and problems to be addressed in developing nursing research. The 1974 conference was entitled *Decision Making in Nursing Research*; however, the research presented was not all clinical in nature. The primary purpose of that conference, as stated by Cahoon (1974), "was to enable Canadian nurse-researchers to share ideas about on-going research activities and to analyze determinants which influence decision-making in nursing research" (p. 1). The title of the 1975 conference was *Development and Use of Indicators in Nursing Research,* and its goal was to address physical, psychological, and social indicators. Hockey (1975) defined indicators as tools that attempt to extend knowledge and "help to focus disciplined attention to key issues and encourage logical thought progression" (p. 8).

The 1977 conference, a workshop on research methods in nursing care, was designed to help nurse participants identify problems in methods of investigation and to share solutions to these problems. The 1978 conference focused on issues, innovations, and problems related to methods of nursing-care research. The focus on research in nursing practice was continued in subsequent conferences, as indicated by their titles. They were designed to focus attention on use of the research process in nursing practice, with the goal of advancing nursing knowledge to improve nursing care.

Several reviews of nursing research have appeared in the literature, and each has developed a method of categorization suited to the particular purposes of that review. Hayter (1984) developed 10 coding categories for review of research published in four research journals (*Nursing Research, Research in Nursing and Health, Advances in Nursing Science, Western Journal of Nursing Research*). The categories are as follows: nurses, nursing process, delivery systems, research activities, nursing education, theory and conceptual frameworks, historical studies and chronologies, patients/clients/consumers, basic research, and literature review. An attempt was made to use all of the categories but the last two to analyze the research reported in the proceedings of the 10 national nursing research conferences; however, after careful consideration, the categories used to organize the research papers presented at the 10th National Nursing Research Conference were deemed more appropriate for this review. The categories are as follows: practice differentiated into seven subcategories; health-care delivery, including nursing administration; research methods/instruments; nurse and nurse role; clinical decisions/diagnosis; nursing education; philosophical/theoretical; and historical studies (Table 12.3).

The number of research studies pertaining to practice increased dramatically from 5 in 1973 to 39 in 1985; however, the number should be compared with the total number of studies because practice represented almost half of the studies in 1973, 1974, and 1975. The proportion increased to 64% in 1977, decreased to 29% in 1978, and increased again to 66% in 1980. The percentage of practice studies continued at a high level, with 68% in 1982, 64% in 1983, and 79.5% in 1985. Whether these percentages reflect the proportion of nursing research that focused on practice from 1973 to 1985 is not known. The figures indicate the high emphasis placed on nursing practice research by the organizers of the national nursing research conferences. This trend reflects nurses' efforts to establish a scientific base for practice and to extend and advance nursing knowledge.

Note the decreased interest in studies of the nurse, nursing roles, and nursing education, all of which dominated nursing research activities from the early part of the century into the 1950s. The analysis reflects limited interest or involvement

TABLE 12.3   Categories of Nursing Studies Reported at National Nursing Research Conferences, 1973 to 1985

Categories	1973	1974	1975	1977	1978	1980	1982	1983	1985
PRACTICE	5	6	6	7	4	12	15	18	39
Aging	–	–	–	1	–	2	2	3	4
Chronicity and meaning of illness	2	–	1	–	–	–	1	1	5
Pain	–	–	–	1	–	1	–	2	6
Personal/environmental interaction	1	5	4	2	2	5	5	3	4
Stress/adaptation/ social support	–	–	–	1	–	–	–	3	8
Parenting	–	–	–	–	–	1	–	4	5
Parent and child	2	1	1	2	2	3	7	2	7
OTHER									
Health-care delivery (including nursing administration)	1	2	1	3	2	2	4	3	4
Research methods/instruments	–	–	4	–	3	1	2	4	4
Nurse and nurse roles	3	3	1	1	–	1	2	1	–
Clinical decisions/diagnosis	–	–	1	–	–	–	1	1	–
Nursing education	–	1	–	–	4	2	2	–	–
Philosophical/theoretical	–	–	–	–	–	–	–	1	2
Historical	2	–	–	–	1	–	–	–	–
TOTAL	11	12	13	11	14	18	26	28	49

in historical research and philosophical research, which should be a cause of concern to nurse researchers and leaders in Canadian nursing. This analysis of the content of research presentations at the 10 national nursing research conferences indicates that, in Canada, there has been interest and emphasis on research in nursing practice and on problems pertaining to design and methods for the past 16 years. This trend, which has continued over the years, should be a source of pride for Canadian nurses. It reflects concern for the quality of nursing care because it is only through research that knowledge is advanced and care is improved.

■ ■ ■ ■

ORGANIZATION OF ANNUAL NURSING RESEARCH CONFERENCES

The Canadian Association of University Schools of Nursing (CAUSN) began sponsoring an annual nursing research conference to be held in early June in connection with the annual meeting of the Learned Societies, because of their commitment to the development of nursing research in Canada. (CAUSN had sponsored annual conferences in conjunction with the Learned Societies before, but the papers presented were not necessarily research reports.) The host university prepared for the review of abstracts by reviewers from other universities

TABLE 12.4   Categories of nursing studies reported at annual nursing research conferences, 1987 to 1992

Categories	1987	1988	1989	1990	1991	1992
PRACTICE	22	45	70	54	52	25
Aging/Elderly	3	8	6	6	8	1
Chronicity and meaning of illness	2	4	8	8	6	8
Pain	1	–	5	5	3	1
Personal/environmental interaction	1	8	11	2	6	3
Stress/adaptation/social support	3	9	13	10	11	1
Parenting	6	12	15	5	3	3
Parent and child	3	1	8	4	5	3
Family	3	3	4	2	2	3
Health promotion	–	–	–	12	8	2
OTHER						
Health-care delivery	5	2	12	13	1	4
(including nursing administration)						
Research methods/instruments	2	–	10	14	10	7
Nurse and nurse roles	8	1	1	12	4	5
Clinical decisions/diagnosis	1	1	1	2	2	-
Nursing education	16	6	11	15	8	8
Philosophical/theoretical	1	–	–	3	1	2
Historical	1	1	1	–	–	–
Research networking	1	–	–	4	–	–
Ethics/values	–	–	–	1	1	3
TOTAL	57	56	106	118	79	54

and assumed responsibility for organizing the conference and obtaining funds, in addition to registration fees, to cover expenses.

The first CAUSN-sponsored Annual Nursing Research Conference was hosted by McMaster University in 1987, the second by the University of Windsor in 1988, the third by Université Laval in 1989, the fourth by the University of Victoria in 1990, the fifth by Queen's University in 1991, and the sixth by the University of Prince Edward Island in 1992. There have been no reports of the annual conferences, but the programs given to participants in each of the conferences were used to analyze the nature of the research presented as a means of assessing the continued development of nursing research in Canada. Information about the number of participants was not available, nor was it possible to determine the educational credentials of the principal investigators or others involved in the research. This information could easily have been made available by requesting that academic credentials be included on the abstracts submitted. Credentials *were* included in the abstracts of papers presented at the University of Windsor.

Table 12.4 identifies the categories of research studies presented at the six annual nursing research conferences sponsored by CAUSN. The categories are those used for analysis of the 10 national nursing research conferences plus four others—Family and Research Networking, added when the first three conferences were analyzed in 1990, and Health Promotion and Ethics/Values added when the last three conferences were added to the analysis in 1993. The topic for the 1987 conference, "Innovations in Nursing Education and Practice: The Role of Research," may have been the reason for the higher percentage of nursing education studies reported at this conference (28% as compared with 11% in 1988, 10% in 1989 and 1991, 13% in 1990, and 15% in 1992). There were also more studies pertaining to the nurse and nursing role in 1987 than in the next 2 years, 14% as compared with 2% and 1%, respectively, but the proportion increased again to 10% in 1990, 5% in 1991, and 9% in 1992. These two factors and the fact that 9% of the studies reported in 1987 were related to health-care delivery questions, resulted in nursing practice research representing only 39% of the studies in 1987, as compared with 82% in 1988, 66% in 1989 and 1991, and 46% in 1990 and 1992. The high proportion of practice studies in 1988 and 1991 may have been influenced by the conference themes, "Women and Health" and "Lifestyles and Health: Nursing Research in the 1990s," respectively. It is interesting and encouraging to note the increase in attention to instrument development and testing for validity and reliability, because critiques of nursing research in recent years have identified inadequacy in these areas in many studies. This inadequacy has been evident at research conferences and in editorials in the major nursing research journals (see Chapter 10), especially in *Annual Reviews of Nursing Research*, volumes 1 through 8, edited by Werley, Fitzpatrick, and others. Such inadequacies merit serious consideration by researchers and reviewers of abstracts for research conferences, as does the need for adequate sampling from which to generalize findings and the need for more replication of nursing research studies. As discussed in Chapter 10, there is a tendency to generalize findings, even though researchers caution against it. Moreover, the consumers of research may not be aware of inadequacies in sampling procedures and the size of samples used.

Although for the most part it was not possible to examine the educational and research preparation of the researchers who shared their methods and findings at the three conferences, in instances where this information was provided, it caused some concern. For example, of the 33 principal investigators presenting papers at the 1988 conference, 24 were prepared at the master's level, 2 at the baccalaureate level, and only 7 at the doctoral level. This leads one to question whether the gradually increasing proportion of nurses in Canada with doctoral degrees, as reported by Stinson, MacPhail, and Larsen (1988), were fulfilling their responsibility to conduct research and provide leadership to others in designing and conducting quality research. Perhaps the focus of this particular research conference influenced those who submitted abstracts; however, many persons are usually interested in studying women's health issues.

The number of abstracts submitted for the research conferences decreased from 109 in 1987 to 72 in 1988, followed by marked increases to 174 in 1989 and 195 in 1990 and subsequent decrements to 109 in 1991 and 75 in 1992. In speculating about factors that may have contributed to the fluctuations, it may not be reasonable to expect a high level of participation every year when one considers the time required to design and conduct research, the cost of travel across the country, and the limited availability of funding to support nursing research and travel to share findings.

It is interesting to observe the variability in research pertaining to health-care delivery from 9% in 1987 to 3% in 1988 to 11% in the next 2 years, followed by a marked decrease to 1% in 1991 and an increase to 7% in 1992. Nurses in practice settings are studying important problems in the organization and administration of these settings, as well as clinical problems. Also interesting is the decreased attention to studies of the nurse and nursing roles and, to some extent, nursing education, which dominated nursing research in the first half of the century and even into the 1950s. The analysis reflects very limited interest and/or involvement in historical research and philosophical/theoretical research; this should be a cause of concern to nurse researchers and leaders in Canadian nursing. Interest in historical research may be augmented through the organization of the Canadian Association for the History of Nursing, a group that has been meeting annually, in conjunction with other national nursing meetings, since 1987. Interest could also be stimulated through the development of doctoral education in nursing with the establishment of the programs at the University of Alberta in January 1991, the University of British Columbia in September 1991, the University of Toronto in 1993, and the conjoint program at McGill University and l'Université de Montréal in 1993.

Planning for future research conferences is becoming a collaborative endeavour by CAUSN, CNA, and the Canadian Nursing Research Group (CNRG), which is an Interest Group within the CNA organizational structure along with 19 other interest groups that have met the criteria for membership to date. Both CAUSN and CNRG have a representative on the CNA Research Committee and the focus is on strengthening relationships among the three organizations and the CNF to facilitate the continuing advancement of nursing research in Canada, including co-sponsorship of national nursing research conferences to be held biennially.

Two international nursing research conferences have been organized by Canadian nurses in Alberta in the past decade. The first was the 1986 International Nursing Research Conference sponsored by the University of Alberta Faculty of Nursing, which was attended by 800 nurses from 38 countries. The second was the 1993 International Conference on Community Health Nursing Research co-sponsored by the University of Alberta Faculty of Nursing and the Edmonton Board of Health, which attracted 900 nurses from 40 countries (AARN Staff, 1993). Both featured outstanding speakers from many countries for plenary sessions and the presentation of many hundreds of research reports by nurse researchers from the countries attending. Both conferences contributed greatly to the advancement of nursing research, to increasing the visibility of Canadian nurse researchers on the international scene, and to enhancing international relations in nursing.

■ ■ ■ ■

INFLUENCE OF A FOUNDATION ON RESEARCH IN NURSING PRACTICE

The Alberta Foundation for Nursing Research (AFNR), established by ministerial order in October, 1982, began funding research in December 1983 after developing a process for receiving and reviewing grant applications and granting funds, giving visibility to the foundation's objectives and research funding opportunities, and developing a self-evaluation mechanism to enable the Board of Directors to assess performance on an annual basis. Grants were provided in accordance with the Board's assessment of areas of greatest importance in meeting AFNR's objectives, which included "research investigations which have relevance for nursing practice in any setting; educational training of researchers; and the communication of nursing research" (AFNR, 1984, p. 5). The six categories designated originally were:

1. a Research Project category for investigations that apply to the solution or management of problems pertaining to nursing practice
2. a Demonstration/Evaluation Project category for projects that involve the implementation and evaluation of innovations in the organization or delivery of nursing care
3. a Research Fellowship category, which provides nurses with paid salary time solely for the purpose of conducting research investigations
4. a Facilitation Grant category, which provides funds to nurses who wish to develop innovative ideas into feasible research grant proposals
5. a Student Research Allowance category, which provides students with funds to help meet research related expenses
6. a Conference and Workshop category for conferences or workshops designed to facilitate and/or communicate the development of nursing research

The AFNR Board of Directors made changes in the categories and in the amounts awarded as new ideas evolved and experience indicated that some of the amounts designated were insufficient to achieve the research objectives. For example, the maximum award for the Research Project category was increased from $25,000 to $50,000 and to $85,000, the maximum duration was increased from 2 to 3 years in the 1989-90 fiscal year, and a Research Trainee award was established but discarded in 1986 after 2 years (AFNR 1989, 1990). In the 1990-91 fiscal year two new awards were introduced: a Postdoctoral Grant at a maximum of $50,000 for a 2-year period, designed to support a nurse with a recently earned doctorate in establishing a research program, or to help an established academician in obtaining specialized research training under an established scholar; and a Postmaster's Grant at a maximum of $10,000 for 1 year, designed to help a master's-prepared nurse in becoming involved in clinical research and fostering research utilization (AFNR, 1990, 1991, 1992).

Table 12.5 lists the grants awarded by the AFNR from the inception in 1983 through March 31, 1992. Analysis of the report of awards made each year (AFNR, 1984, 1985, 1986, 1987, 1989, 1990, 1991, 1992) indicated that priority has been given to funding research in nursing practice, in keeping with the Board's original objectives. Priority has also been given to research training through student research bursaries and research support services, and to the communication of nursing research through support of research conferences. For the first time in the history of the AFNR, the number of projects recommended by the Scientific

TABLE 12.5 AFNR Grants Funds Awarded 1984 to March 31, 1992

Category of Award	1983/84 ($)	1984/85 ($)	1985/86 ($)	1986/87 ($)	1987/88 ($)	1988/89 ($)	1989/90 ($)	1990/91 ($)	1991/92 ($)	TOTAL
Research Project	13,216	25,000	188,090	239,745	129,538	200,469	229,423	294,824	195,982	1,516,287
Demonstration Project	1,379	0	0	0	0	22,519	0	0	0	23,898
Facilitation	1,420	9,296	17,075	17,450	29,130	9,333	10,000	20,000	10,000	123,704
Conference	0	25,000	5,860	10,000	28,180	0	0	64,850	25,000	158,890
Student bursaries	3,000	5,000	7,500	7,500	23,000	24,000	17,000	13,000	21,000	121,000
Research support services	0	0	61,314	0	0	24,083	0	0	27,517	112,914
Research trainee*	0	0	25,000	47,113	0	0	0	0	0	72,113
Postdoctoral grant**	0	0	0	0	0	0	0	0	25,000	25,000
Postmaster's grant**	0	0	0	0	0	0	0	0	10,000	10,000
	19,015	64,296	304,839	321,808	209,848	280,404	256,423	392,674	314,499	2,163,806

* Research Trainee category discontinued at end of 1986

** Postdoctoral and Postmaster's categories added in 1991-92.

Source: AFNR (1990, 1991, and 1992). Annual reports. Edmonton, Alberta: The Foundation

Review Committee and approved by the Board of Directors as fundable, exceeded available funds in the 1991-92 fiscal year (AFNR 1991, 1992). The majority of the awards were for investigation of nursing practice problems, but a few grants supported development and testing of research instruments, studies of the nursing work environment, investigation of nursing administration problems with direct relevance to nursing practice, and studies pertaining to evaluation of nursing practice. All of the studies were pertinent to nursing practice and the climate in which practice and research take place.

Regrettably, with severe cutbacks in funding for research, education, and health care in Alberta, funding for the AFNR was totally eliminated from the 1994-95 budget of the Alberta government. This was unexpected by the Board of Directors who were ready to recommend that funding be increased based on their assessment of the outcomes of research funded over the past 12 years. The Board will administer the committed research funds for the next 3 years, even though no administrative funds were provided for this purpose. One of their major challenges will be to continue to seek financial support for nursing research in Alberta. This will continue as a challenge for the nurses of Alberta who lobbied vigourously in the 1970s to secure the initial funding for the Alberta Foundation for Nursing Research, a remarkable achievement.

■ ■ ■ ■

CONCLUSION

Analysis of the content of research presentations at the national nursing research conferences and the annual nursing research conferences and research endeavours funded by the AFNR indicates that in Canada there has been continued interest in and emphasis on research in nursing practice and problems pertaining to design and methods for the past 2 decades. This trend reflects concern for quality of nursing care and for advancing knowledge to improve care. Canadian nurses recognize the need to increase and enhance nursing research and are giving priority to lobbying for funding for research and doctoral education in nursing to attain their goals.

REFERENCES

AARN Staff. (1993). First international conference—Community health nursing research. AARN Newsletter, 49(10), p. 5.

Alberta Foundation for Nursing Research, (1984). *Annual Report*. Edmonton, Alberta: Author.

Alberta Foundation for Nursing Research. (1985). *Annual Report*. Edmonton, Alberta: Author.

Alberta Foundation for Nursing Research. (1986). *Annual Report*. Edmonton, Alberta: Author.

Alberta Foundation for Nursing Research. (1987). *Annual Report*. Edmonton, Alberta: Author.

Alberta Foundation for Nursing Research. (1989). *Annual Report*. Edmonton, Alberta: Author.

Alberta Foundation for Nursing Research. (1990). *Annual Report*. Edmonton, Alberta: Author.

Alberta Foundation for Nursing Research. (1991). *Annual Report*. Edmonton, Alberta: Author.

Alberta Foundation for Nursing Research. (1992). *Annual Report*. Edmonton, Alberta: Author.

Allen, M., and Thibaudeau, M-F. (Eds.), (1973). *Proceedings of the Colloquium on Nursing Research*. Montreal, Quebec: McGill University

School of Nursing and l'Université de Montréal Faculté des sciences infirmieres. Parts 1, 2, and 3.

Cahoon, M. (1974). Foreword. In J. Godden, and M. Cahoon, (Eds.), *Decision making in nursing research: Proceedings of the Third National Conference on Research in Nursing*. Toronto, Ontario: The University of Toronto Faculty of Nursing.

Cahoon, M. (1986). Research developments in clinical settings: A Canadian perspective. In S.M. Stinson and J.C. Kerr (Eds.), *International issues in nursing research* (pp. 182-204). London and Sydney: Croom Helm.

Canadian Nurses Association. (1977). *Research methodology in nursing care: Proceedings of the Workshop on Research Methodology in Nursing Care*. Ottawa, Ontario: Author.

Crawford M., and Kyle, M. (Eds.). (1978). *Methodology in nursing care research: Issues, innovations, problems: Proceedings of the National Nursing Research Conference*. Saskatoon, Saskatchewan: University of Saskatchewan College of Nursing.

Godden, J., and Cahoon, M. (Eds.). (1974). *Decision making in nursing research. Proceedings of the Third National Conference on Research in Nursing*. Toronto, Ontario: The University of Toronto Faculty of Nursing.

Gortner, S.R., Bloch, D., and Phillips, T.P. (1976). Contributions of nursing research to patient care. *Journal of Nursing Administration, 6*(3), 23-28.

Gortner, S.R., and Nahm, H. (1977). An overview of nursing research in the United States. *Nursing Research, 26*(1), 10-33.

Hayter, J. (1984). Institutional sources of articles published in thirteen nursing journals, 1978 to 1982. *Nursing Research, 33*(6), 357-362.

Hockey, L. (1975). Indicators in Nursing Research with Emphasis on Social Indicators. In J. Zilm, S. Stinson, M. Steed, and P. Overton (Eds.), *Development and Use of Indicators in Nursing Research: Proceedings of the 1975 National Nursing Research Conference*. Edmonton, Alberta: University of Alberta School of Nursing.

Hockey, L. (1986). Nursing research in the United Kingdom: The state of the art. In S.M. Stinson and J.C. Kerr (Eds.), *International Issues in Nursing Research* (pp. 216-235). London and Sydney: Croom Helm.

King, F. (Ed.). (1971). *National Conference on Research in Nursing Practice: Proceedings of the First National Nursing Research Conference.*

Vancouver, British Columbia: University of British Columbia School of Nursing.

King, K., Prodrick, E. and Bauer, B. (Eds.). (1985). *Nursing research: Science for quality care. Proceedings of the 10th National Nursing Research Conference*. Toronto, Ontario: University of Toronto Faculty of Nursing.

Kravitz, M., and Laurin, J. (Eds.). (1983). *Nursing research: A base for practice: Proceedings of the 9th National Nursing Research Conference*. Montreal, Quebec: McGill University School of Nursing and l'Université de Montréal Faculté des sciences infirmières.

Loomis, M.E. (1985). Emerging content in nursing: An analysis of dissertation abstracts and titles: 1976 to 1982. *Nursing Research, 34*(2), 113-119.

McKay, R., and Zilm, G. (Eds.). (1980). *Research for practice: Proceedings of the National Nursing Research Conference*. Dalhousie, Nova Scotia: Dalhousie University School of Nursing.

McMaster University School of Nursing and the Canadian Association of University Schools of Nursing/The Learned Societies. (1987). *National Nursing Research Conference: Innovations in Nursing Education and Practice: The Role of Research*. (Available from McMaster University School of Nursing, Hamilton, Ontario L8N 3Z5.)

O'Connell, K. and Duffey, M. (1978). Research in nursing practice: Its present scope. In N.L. Chaska (Ed.), *The nursing profession: Views through the mist*. (pp. 161-174). New York: McGraw-Hill Book Co.

Queen's University School of Nursing and the Canadian Association of University Schools of Nursing/The Learned Societies. (1991). *National Nursing Research Conference. Lifestyles and Health: Nursing Research in the 1990s* (pp. 6-8). (Available from Queen's Univesity School of Nursing, Kingston, Ontario K7L 3N6.)

Stinson, S. (1986). Nursing research in Canada. In S. Stinson and J. Kerr (Eds.), *International issues in nursing research*. (pp. 236-258). London and Sydney: Croom Helm.

Stinson, S., MacPhail, J., and Larsen, J. (1988). *Canadian nursing doctoral statistics: 1986 update*. Ottawa: Canadian Nurses Association.

Thurston N., Tenove S., and Church, J. (1987). *Nursing Research in Canadian Teaching Hospitals*. Calgary: Foothills Provincial General Hospital and University of Calgary Faculty of Nursing.

University of Windsor School of Nursing and the Canadian Association of University Schools of Nursing/The Learned Societies. (1988).

National Nursing Research Conference. Women and Health. (Available from University of Windsor School of Nursing, Windsor, Ontario.)

Université Laval, École des Sciences Infirmières and Association Canadienne des Écoles Universitaires de Nursing/Congrès des Sociétés Savantes 1989. (1989). Colloque Annuel de Recherche en Sciences Infirmères. (Available from l'Université Laval, Ecole des Sciences Infirmiéres, Laval, Quebec.)

University of Prince Edward Island and the Canadian Association of University Schools of Nursing/The Learned Societies. (1992). Canadian health care by the year 2000: Multicultural and multidisciplinary issues. (Available from the University of Prince Edward Island School of Nursing, Charlottetown, PEI.)

University of Victoria School of Nursing and the Canadian Association of University Schools of Nursing/The Learned Societies. (1990). Innovations in nursing education and practice: The role of research. (Available from University of Victoria School of Nursing, Victoria, British Columbia V8W 2Y2.)

Zilm G., Stinson, S., Steed, M., and Overton, P. (Eds.). (1975). Development and use of indicators in nursing research: Proceedings of the 1975 National Nursing Research Conference. Edmonton, Alberta: University of Alberta School of Nursing.

Zilm, G., Hilton, A., and Richmond, M. (Eds.). (1982). Nursing research: A base for practice, service and education. Proceedings of the National Nursing Research Conference. Vancouver, British Columbia: University of British Columbia School of Nursing.

CHAPTER THIRTEEN

Utilizing Research Findings in Practice: Issues and Strategies[1]

HEATHER F. CLARKE

A s health-care funds diminish and nurses participate more in shaping health-care reform, public demands for accountability in nursing increase. To meet this demand the nursing profession must demonstrate how nursing care makes a difference—that is, how health-care resources and therapeutic nursing interventions are effectively and efficiently used to improve the health status of clients of the health-care system. There is substantial evidence to support the claim that practice-based research yields reliable and valid information upon which to base crucial decisions about optimum client care and wise use of scarce health-care resources. The health-care system can no longer afford health care that is not supported by research findings. Thus it is essential that the practice of nursing move at a more rapid pace from a system that has been largely based on tradition and ritual to one based on research.

Important issues related to the promotion and implementation of research-based nursing practice as well as strategies to meet the challenges, are discussed in this chapter. Issues pertaining to cost benefits and infrastructures will be identified, and guiding principles for development of strategies will be discussed. Issues related more specifically to nursing practice, partnerships, and adoption of innovative approaches will be explored, and utilization frameworks will be presented as a powerful strategy to promote research-based nursing practice. Principles and questions related to each issue are posed to stimulate critical examination of one's own work environment and practice, and discussion of such with colleagues.

---

[1]The author wishes to acknowledge the contribution of Ann McKintock, RN, MSN. The document she prepared for RNABC on research-based nursing practice has formed the basis of several sections of this chapter.

THE PURPOSE OF RESEARCH-BASED NURSING PRACTICE

The everyday decisions nurses make are complex and require accurate, reliable information upon which to predict the patient, family, and health system outcomes of specific nursing interventions. Research is the means by which this vital nursing knowledge is generated and validated, but the research process cannot stop with the conduct of research. The process also includes dissemination of findings and their use and evaluation. Research utilization is the "use of research as a means of verifying or as a basis for changing nursing practice . . . the purpose of such . . . is to substantiate or improve the quality of nursing practice" (Horsley, 1985, p. 135). Research-based nursing includes research utilization, as well as the conduct of research to study clinical questions or test hypotheses. Although not addressed in this chapter, research-based practice in nursing administration should also be valued and considered essential, especially in today's rapidly changing environment in which fiscal restraints have created new problems and stresses for both nursing administrators and their colleagues.

The suggestion that nursing practice should be research-based is not a new one. Florence Nightingale viewed research as an integral part of nursing and believed that nursing practice should be generated from confirmed facts and epidemiological data (Nutting and Dock, 1907). One hundred years later the issue of research-based practice is receiving attention from the nursing profession, with more nurses questioning whether their nursing practices are based on ritual, tradition, intuition, or outdated teachings.

Rational choices for nursing practice can only be made when nurses possess the necessary facts. Professional nursing requires discarding unsubstantiated tradition and allowing research evidence to challenge practice. If the discipline of nursing is to meet current and future health-care needs, nursing practice must not be based purely on beliefs, traditions, and rituals but rather on rational, humanistic knowledge that is susceptible to change as a result of new research findings and ideas. Promoting and implementing research-based nursing practice is not a simple task, nor does it only rely on nurses in the clinical area. There are forces hindering its advancement in the discipline, as well as potential forces for moving ahead. At the health-care system level there are both macro- and micro-level hindrances—costs to the system and agency, and lack of supportive infrastructures—particularly within health-care agencies. Within the profession of nursing there are perceived, if not real, barriers to the development of collaborative partnerships within and across agencies and to the acceptance and integration of innovations in clinical practice.

HEALTH-CARE SYSTEM ISSUES
Costs and Benefits

One of the reasons it has been difficult to sway decision makers, especially those in health-care agencies, about investing in nurses and the research process, is that the over-riding perspective of "worth" or "pay-off" has been one of cost-benefit analysis rather than cost-effectiveness analysis. Focusing solely on monetary aspects neglects the essential human and social costs and benefits. Cost-benefit analysis weighs the inherent worth of a program in costs and benefits that are expressed in numerical terms, especially dollars (Fordyce, Mooney, and Russell, 1982). It is the "whether" of decision-making: whether the costs are justified by the benefits. Cost-effectiveness analysis is the "how" of decision-making; it weighs the relative merit of one program against another, given an already established objective. Outcomes or consequences are not always measured in monetary terms and can include considerations such as preventing death, reducing disability, and improving client activity levels (Fordyce, Mooney, and Russell, 1982).

In promoting research-based nursing practice, it is imperative that the cost-effectiveness of the process be considered, rather than merely its cost-benefit. Recent attention to outcomes research, both in nursing and health care in general, supports a cost-effectiveness perspective that includes measures of effectiveness (degree to which an action can accomplish a purpose or help bring about an expected outcome) and efficiency (ability to accomplish a task within a minimum expenditure of time and effort).

Measuring Outcomes

In the past nursing has experienced limitations in clearly defining and measuring outcomes, monetary or otherwise. A review of the literature reveals that research that evaluates nursing interventions rarely addresses the efficacy of a given intervention—that is, its capacity to produce effects. Also there is confusion over the term *nursing outcome* as it has been used as process, endpoint, patterning and program evaluation (Shamian, 1992). Debate about this and the development of *nursing sensitive outcome* measures has centred on the issue of the impact of other disciplines' interventions on nursing interventions and client and system outcomes. Marek and Lang (1992) support Shamian's (1992) caution that any single discipline's approach is too narrow and limited to address the wide variety of structures and interventions that influence outcomes. It is contradictory for nurses to advocate a holistic perspective while practising from an exclusionist point of view. Undoubtedly there is a need to move into multidisciplinary, holistic effort where the impact of multiple interventions and providers can be studied. Nursing must be part of that move; however, before nurses can participate as equal partners the relationship of outcomes to process and structure variables requires naming and categorizing these variables from a nursing perspective. Consensus about naming of variables is needed among nurses in practice, in research, and in organized nursing (Marek and Lang, 1992). In Canada attention to building such a consensus is reflected in papers given at the conference sponsored by the Canadian Nurses Association (CNA), the Nursing Minimum Data Set Conference in 1992, and further strategic planning on nursing components of health information by the Alberta Association of Registered Nurses (Wendy Duggleby and Kathryn Hannah, personal communication, 1994).

Despite the limitations nursing research has demonstrated the effectiveness of nursing care in terms of improved client care and satisfaction with that care. It has also demonstrated that high-quality, research-based care can be delivered at reduced cost to an agency even though an explicit cost-benefit analysis was not done. Three major categories of effectiveness outcome indicators have been used in nursing research: 1) patient related indicators—physiological, psychosocial, and functional measures; behaviour, knowledge, symptom control, and resolution of nursing diagnoses or nursing problems; 2) consumer/environment related indicators—quality of life, home functioning, family and care-giver strain, goal attainment, and patient satisfaction; and 3) organization related indicators—utilization of service, and safety (Marek and Lang, 1992; Shamian, 1992).

Examples of Cost-effectiveness

A frequently cited meta-analysis that compared patient outcomes resulting from research-based nursing care with those resulting from routine, procedural nursing care validated the effectiveness of research-based nursing care. The analysis showed that not only did more patients in the research-based intervention group have better outcomes than those who received routine nursing care, but also the magnitude of improvement was greater. The results were both statistically and clinically significant. (Heater, Becker, and Olson, 1988). Patient-related outcomes measured included changes in observed behaviour; changes in cognitive level of understanding; changes in health or normal functioning, such as heart or respiratory rate as compared with a baseline measure; and changes in the manner of relating to self and to others.

A second meta-analysis undertaken by Olson, Heater, and Becker (1990) evaluated the effectiveness of research-based nursing interventions used with children and their parents. Once more it was found that subjects receiving specified research-based nursing interventions benefited more often and to a greater extent than did those receiving standard or routine nursing care. Better patient outcomes in this study included improvement in self-care practices, reduction in anxiety for children and their parents, and increased clinical improvement for premature infants.

Although neither of the meta-analyses included monetary outcomes, it can be argued that these positive patient outcomes resulted in monetary gains. For example, improved clinical outcomes for premature infants would lead to reduced acuity of illness and lower levels of required staffing; increased self-reliance in health behaviours of clients would eventually lead to reduced reliance on costly episodic or emergent care; psychosocial gains could be shown to lead to reduced need for mental illness interventions as well as reduction in social problems, such as family violence and substance abuse. These short- and long-term outcomes could be translated into cost savings for the health-care system and clients.

A landmark study by Brooten and her colleagues (1986) demonstrated that, with the care provided by a nurse specialist, low birth-weight infants could be safely discharged home an average of 11 days earlier, at a cost savings to the health-care system of $18,560 (US) for each infant. Another study, a clinical trial involving peripheral vascular disease patients, showed that the group who received "traditional" nursing care had more in-patient days at a higher cost per day than did the experimental group who were on a research-based exercise plan (Ventura et al, 1984). At the end of the 26-week data-collection period, the combined cost of the experimental intervention plus the research project costs was found to be significantly lower than the cost of traditional care.

Agencies that support research-based nursing practice improve nurses' work satisfaction (Kenneth and Stiesmeyer, 1991). Smeltzer and Hinshaw (1988) believe that creation of a research environment serves as a major retention strategy in the clinical setting because it involves nurses. According to Gortner (1986), research-based practitioners learn "the joy of discovery" in their everyday practice (p. 554). When asked which elements were most significant to quality work-life, nurses indicated that intellectually challenging work, creative problem-solving, and an opportunity to grow and be in touch with new ideas were essential (Attridge and Callahan, 1987). Additionally Attridge and Callahan found that nurses tend to equate power with their ability to apply knowledge. Research becomes powerful when the knowledge generated is utilized. Enhanced power increases nurses' credibility, supports their autonomy, and ideally encourages a more balanced relationship between nurses and physicians. If research-based nursing practice improves satisfaction, and thereby reduces turnover, it reduces costs for the institution and improves the efficiency of the health-care system.

Costs of Research-Based Nursing Practice

There are both hidden and visible costs associated with research-based nursing practice. Visible costs include salary for nurse-researchers, computers or other equipment costs, computer time, and consultation fees. Hidden costs are associated with time of researchers, staff and secretaries applied to reviewing the literature, developing a research proposal or nursing protocol, analyzing the data or evaluating patient outcomes, writing reports, and disseminating results. As well, there are hidden costs of professional development and change implementation. Findings from the evaluation of the Research Consultation Services of the RNABC (1990b), revealed that nurse researchers and participating staff were unable to carry out research activities within the work day.

These findings suggest that the real costs of nursing research may be invisible to nurse administrators and not included in agency budgets. Sasmor (1986) states that, like nursing staff education, "nursing research costs have often been hidden in the bundled services known as nursing" (p. 4). She suggests that once nursing costs are "unbundled," nursing research will be more likely to survive and thrive because nursing research enables nurses to decrease costs and improve quality of care.

Research-Based Nursing Practice: An Investment

In her review of the economic value of conducting and applying nursing research, Fagin (1982) found that the return on investment from nursing research far exceeded what she cited as acceptable to the investment community. The review demonstrated the cost-effectiveness of primary nursing, innovative staffing plans, research-based patient teaching plans, and nurse-delivered primary care to both home-care clients and public school client populations. Fagin concluded that nursing research is severely underfunded by any measure commonly accepted in the marketplace, and that investment in nursing research and research-based practice leads to "a terrific economic payoff" (p. 1849). Ten years later the same conclusions are apparent.

Overall, the benefits of implementing research-based nursing practice can be shown to far outweigh the visible and invisible costs. In a research-friendly environment, staff will begin to question their practice and systematically document the problems of greatest concern. This fosters a sense of accountability and professionalism, which itself leads to increased job satisfaction and lower staff turnover (Smeltzer and Hinshaw, 1988). For nurse managers and administrators, research-based nursing practice provides reliable data to describe the effectiveness and significance of nursing interventions or programs, to allocate or reallocate their resources, and to participate in health policy formulation. Research-based nursing practice ensures that the quality and cost-effectiveness of nursing care will be the best possible.

Principles

The following principles can be derived as a basis for practice:
1. Commitment beyond verbal support by managers and administration provides the recognition necessary for valuing research-based nursing practice.
2. Analysis of monetary and non-monetary costs and benefits in nursing research and utilization studies provides necessary data for effective decision-making.
3. Research and evaluation studies in clinical practice can no longer ignore issues of cost-benefit, effectiveness, efficiency, and efficacy.
4. Naming and categorizing nursing-sensitive outcome measures as well as other nursing components is critical to the development of health information databases and research.

Questions

In identifying issues of importance in strengthening the utilization of nursing research in an agency, the following are some questions that could be asked:
1. What value does your agency place on nursing research and research-based nursing practice? How is this demonstrated?
2. What steps can be taken to reinforce the value placed on nursing research and research-based nursing practice?
3. How would you measure the effectiveness of employing personnel differently in order to facilitate research utilization? What data would you collect? What tools would you need?
4. How are the nursing components of health information databases being developed in your area? How are you contributing?
5. What other key points do you think should be stated as principles of costs and benefits?

Infrastructures

When respondents of the RNABC (1990b) evaluation study were asked about the resources required to facilitate their research efforts, they indicated that other consultants (statisticians and other nurse consultants), libraries, release time, administrative support, collegial support, and seed money were all essential but often missing. Other authors concur and add that access to research reports, time to read and critique them, clearly demonstrated support by administration, start-up and maintenance funding, educational preparation or relevant in-service education, and autonomy to implement research findings in practice are resources requisite to the utilization of research findings (Champion and Leach, 1989; Funk, Tornquist, and Champagne, 1989b; and Sayner, 1984). Research-based nursing practice requires a supportive infrastructure.

Infrastructure can be defined as those structures, policies, and facilities in a health-care agency that support specific activities, such as research and utilization of findings in practice. Basic organizational elements supportive of research activities include a nursing research committee (NRC) and key administrative positions that include responsibility for research leadership within the agency (Clinical Nurse Researcher or Director of Nursing Research). Other essential elements include services (space, secretarial, computers), time (release time), communication (channels and a climate to facilitate two-way dialogue between researchers and consumers), and consultation (methods, design, and grantsmanship).

Essential Infrastructure Elements

Six essential infrastructure elements have been identified:

1) *Nursing Research Committees* constitute a visible endorsement of nursing research and serve as a powerful means of facilitating nursing research utilization (Stetler, 1983). Their structures and processes vary with the needs, interests, and membership of the organization. Generally, however, their functions include the promotion of activities to generate interest and participation in research internally and the coordination of policies and procedures for qualified external nursing researchers to access agency resources and clients (Kenneth and Stiesmeyer, 1991). Research promotion activities may include presenting research findings, publishing a research newsletter, consulting on research proposal writing, promoting or providing research education, and liaising between the staff and the research program (Edwards-Beckett, 1990; Thurston, Tenove, and Church, 1990; Kenneth and Stiesmeyer, 1991; RNABC, 1993a, 1993b).

2) *Clinical Nursing Researchers* (CNRs), along with senior nurse administrators and nursing unit managers, are responsible for creating an organizational environment supportive of conducting and using nursing research. According to Knafl, Bevis, and Kirchhoff (1987), the CNR is a doctorally prepared nurse employed by a health-care agency to foster and coordinate nursing research using research and grantsmanship skills, an astute understanding of nursing practice, and leadership abilities. The role has been created to bring nursing research and practice into closer alignment. In some agencies the CNR role is assumed by the Director of Nursing Research. Eagle, Fortnum, Price, and Scruton (1990) describe the CNR's responsibilities as: (1) education of general staff, educators, and management nurses in the areas of research design, methodology, data analysis, critical appraisal of research studies, and the value of translating valid research findings into new clinical practice; (2) leadership of the Nursing

Research Committee and implementation of its terms of reference; (3) consultation on all phases of the development of educational research, clinical research, administrative research, internal projects, grant proposals for external funding, and on the development of nurses' skills in the areas of design, measurement, data analysis, and research finding reports (written or oral); and (4) liaison with appropriate groups (senior nursing administrators, nursing unit managers, and clinicians) to discuss current nursing issues and develop potential research questions.

3) *Services* include making available to nurses space and resources (e.g. computers, libraries, secretarial services, etc.) required to conduct or use research.

4) *Release time* is an important element. Even motivated nurses have difficulty engaging in research activities when doing so is primarily in their off-hours. Although lack of motivation has been cited as a barrier to utilizing nursing research (Varricchio and Mikos, 1987; Hunt, 1981; Sayner, 1984; Kramer, Albrecht, and Miller, 1985; Funk, Champagne, Wiese, and Tornquist, 1991), recent surveys have found that lack of time, recognition and meaningful rewards are equally, if not more, significant barriers (Davies and Eng, 1991; RNABC, 1993a, 1993b).

5) *Communication* has been cited as a major barrier to research utilization (King, Barnard, and Hoehn, 1981; Chambers, 1989; Bock, 1990; Repko, 1990). Clinical nurses have difficulty finding relevant studies (Pank, Rostron, and Stenhouse, 1984; Haughey, 1988; Funk, Champagne, Wiese, and Tornquist, 1991). They find that much of the literature includes findings with little relevance to the clinical situation, or if relevant, studies are presented in an unusable form (Pank, Rostron, and Stenhouse, 1984). Researchers often present findings in tentative terms in response to hypothetical inquiries and discuss results as they relate to theory and the need for further inquiry. While appropriate among researchers, this style of communication provides little on which nurse practitioners can base their care (King, Barnard, and Hoehn, 1981). To overcome this barrier it is suggested that researchers make the practice setting the focus of their scientific inquiry and disseminate their findings in a comprehensible and relevant manner to the practitioner.

6) *Consultation* within an agency relies upon all other elements being in place. Consultants and their services may be required in the practice content area, statistics, research design, grantsmanship, or utilization. Access to both nurse and non-nurse consultants is desirable, as is knowledge about the type, location, availability, and name of the consultant.

A recent survey of all clinical agencies (hospitals, public health units, and home-care departments) in British Columbia found very few of these infrastructure elements in place, particularly in public health units and home-care departments (RNABC, 1993b). If research-based nursing practice was part of the nursing department's philosophy and goals, the most common and often only form of infrastructure support was an NRC. To date, little attention has been paid to nurses' job descriptions and responsibilities for research-based nursing practice; however, most of the health-care agencies expected staff nurses to question practice and use research findings. This suggests that even though nurses might be involved in research activities and might change practice based on research findings, it is unlikely they will receive support or recognition for such in performance appraisals.

Approaches to Infrastructure Development

Two approaches have been suggested for establishing an infrastructure for nursing research within organizations: decentralized and centralized (MacKay, Grantham, and Ross, 1984). In the decentralized or program model, research projects or the examination and application of research findings are conducted under specific unit budgets, using resources of that particular unit. In the centralized or department model, all nursing research efforts are coordinated within one centralized department. The advantage of the decentralized approach is that control of the research remains very close to those who will eventually use the findings. The advantages of the centralized approach are that a department head with clearly structured authority and accountability assumes responsibility. Centralized resources can be shared and can support several on-going projects, yet the department serves as a central cost centre, doing the accounting for each project. A departmental structure gives visibility for nursing research, both within the hospital and the community.

With changing administrative approaches, it is unlikely that either a centralized or decentralized approach will be taken but rather one that uses both approaches and possibly combines them with a quality assurance program. Shared decision-making approaches to management necessitates and fosters both centralized and decentralized approaches where research-based practice is a goal of the nursing department. Allocating scarce resources for greatest effectiveness will encourage the combining of programs. There are advantages and disadvantages of combining nursing research with a quality assurance program. The primary advantage is that linking research with a mandated process increases its viability. It also increases the probability that research will be related to patient care and that successful quality assurance approaches will be shared with others outside the institution. The major disadvantage is that confusion may arise regarding definitions and functions of quality assurance and research, and that territorial issues may surface (Larson, 1983). Watson, Bulecheck, and McCloskey (1987) suggest that, if quality assurance can be conceptualized as a form of nursing research that contributes to better patient care and better practices for the profession of nursing, advances in nursing practice will be dramatic.

The approach chosen to develop research infrastructures will depend upon several factors, but most importantly the organizational structure and philosophy of the agency. To facilitate research-based nursing and maintain practice standards for consumer safety, it is vital that formal recognition of nursing research be given within the organizational structure. This entails establishing an infrastructure that provides the support, visibility, and credibility necessary when seeking funding and other resources.

Experiences

A survey of 45 Canadian teaching hospitals was conducted to determine the extent of nursing research within these organizations (Thurston, Tenhove, and

Church, 1989). Fifty-five percent had a written protocol or policy for approving and conducting research and had a committee responsible for project approval and direction. Most of these committees were entitled Nursing Research Committees (NRCs). Findings supported previous reports that the establishment of both NRCs and nursing research program director positions have a positive effect on nursing research and research utilization.

A survey of 174 British Columbia health-care agencies was undertaken to assess the development of agency-based nursing research (RNABC, 1993b). Results from a response rate of 56.3% indicated that only 31.6% of the agencies had a mission statement that included research. Fewer than 43.9% reported having a nursing philosophy that explicitly referred to research. Very few nursing departments (15.1%) had a definition of nursing research to guide the development of their nursing research programs. NRCs existed in less than one quarter (17.3%) of the hospitals, with their presence related to a greater number of research activities. If research-based nursing practice is to become a reality, urgent attention must be paid to developing supportive infrastructures.

Principles

1. A climate that promotes and supports inquiry facilitates research-based nursing practice.
2. The advancement of research-based practice in nursing depends upon a supportive administrative infrastructure.
3. Infrastructures that support research-based nursing practice include organizational structures, support services, time, communication systems, and consultation.

Questions

1. Does your agency have supportive infrastructures for nursing research?
    - If so, what do they look like, and how might they be strengthened?
    - If not, what would be the best structure for your agency to adopt?
2. What would you need to consider when creating or maintaining a nursing research infrastructure (ie. support, resources, barriers)?
3. What other key points do you think should be stated as principles of infrastructures?

■ ■ ■ ■

PROFESSIONAL PRACTICE OF NURSING
Partnerships

The research process does not end with completion of the study or dissemination of results. It also involves assessment of findings for clinical application, utilization of findings to improve nursing care, and evaluation of the clinical outcomes of research-based practice. Who is responsible for this complex set of activities? In addition to researchers, there is need for nurses in administration, education, and clinical practice roles to have specific and critical responsibilities that may be best actualized in collaborative partnerships. Although interdisciplinary collaboration is often desirable, harmonious partnerships within nursing are the crucial first steps.

Administrative Roles

At the senior management level, nursing administrators are responsible for ensuring that the corporate philosophy is integrated into the nursing department philosophy and daily operations. They actualize a philosophy that places value on research-based nursing practice by setting nursing policies and procedures that are based on nursing research findings, developing job descriptions for unit managers and clinicians that include research responsibilities, and making infrastructure support available within and beyond the agency.

At the operational level nursing unit managers anchor the organizational efforts for research utilization. They are responsible for establishing a climate that encourages inquiry and change. Such a climate is established by identifying clinical problems, organizing release time for staff nurses to read and critique research, assisting with the selection and critique of studies, and encouraging application and evaluation of valid and reliable findings. Other supportive nurse manager activities include managing resources, appraising staff performance, networking, and collaborating.

Nurse administrators and nursing unit managers must work together to create a research environment. Their collaborative efforts can ensure that nurses feel free to question practice, that consultation is available to support their efforts, that time is provided for research activities and professional development, that agency resources are allocated to research-based nursing practice, that opportunities are provided to incorporate research findings into practice and evaluate clinical outcomes, and that staff members who undertake nursing research receive due recognition for their endeavours. Many staff nurses do not perceive that they have a supportive research climate in their agencies (Alcock, Carroll, and Goodman, 1990), but identify such support and commitment as critical to facilitating nursing research (Thurston, Tenove, and Church, 1989).

Education Roles

Other partners in research-based nursing practice are nursing educators, those who teach in academia and those who instruct in the clinical area. It has been observed that developments in nursing practice have been hampered by the formal separation of teachers, researchers, and practitioners (Wilson-Barnett, Corner, and DeCarle, 1990). Ross (1985) states that educators often feel uncomfortable in their role as "guests" of the agency because they perceive that they are in the way and that their presence and that of their students are a burden to an already hard-pressed nursing staff. Consequently, they do as little as possible to "interfere" with unit routines, minimizing their disruptiveness while at the same time reducing their potential to provide insightful input. This is supported by survey results that indicate that agency staff do not perceive faculty who are in their agency for education or research purposes as potential consultants (RNABC, 1993b). Some educators who undertake research as part of their required scholarly activities may choose to conduct non-clinical research as a means of avoiding this uncomfortable atmosphere (Wilson-Barnett, Corner, and DeCarle, 1990).

Alcock, Carroll, and Goodman (1990) suggest that university nursing faculty examine their approach to clinical practice research. In their study, staff nurses perceived from university faculty a lack of appreciation of the potential contribution they have to make to research projects. One way to facilitate faculty/clinician appreciation is through joint appointments between schools of nursing and health-care agencies and by having a faculty member on the agency NRC.

Unit-based clinical instructors, whose responsibility is continuing and in-service education for nursing staff, may not share the same sense of alienation that faculty educators experience. However, they do face the challenge of encouraging staff nurses to incorporate nursing research into their practice. How can this be accomplished? It has been noted that the major reason nurses do not apply research findings in clinical practice is because they do not possess the skills to utilize the findings. They either do not understand the relevance of the findings, or they are unable to actually apply the findings to nursing decisions or nursing actions (Hunt, 1981; Kramer, Albrecht, and Miller, 1985). Clinical educators have a significant role in in-service programs designed to enhance or impart the framework and skills required to utilize nursing research and support the nursing department's philosophy and objectives.

Clinical Nurse Specialist Roles

Clinical nurse specialists (CNSs) should be leaders in the research utilization process. They strive to deliver quality health care to a specific population of patients by assuming the roles of consultant and change agent in clinical practice, education, and research (Hamilton et al, 1990). Hickey (1990) described five essential steps in research utilization for which the CNS is responsible: 1) Assessment of system readiness for research utilization; 2) design of the research utilization plan; 3) implementation of a research utilization process; 4) evaluation of the innovation, with revisions as necessary; and 5) report of findings for utilization, replication and further research to clinical nurses and nursing researchers.

The difficulties that CNSs experience in meeting the research expectations of their roles are well documented. Their greatest constraint is time. Gortner (1986) identifies the need for a high degree of organizational support for research and fulfillment of the nursing research responsibilities of the CNS role as well as developing partnerships with staff nurses and managers.

A vitally important player in the research partnership is the staff nurse. Staff nurses may raise questions from practice that provide impetus for research studies (Kirchhoff, 1991). They are in an excellent position to collaborate with researchers in nursing and other disciplines and implement changes in practice that will have a positive impact on the quality, efficacy, and cost of health care (Alcock, Carroll, and Goodman, 1990). Successful collaboration between nursing researchers and staff nurses requires that they meet on common ground to establish research priorities leading to meaningful and applicable outcomes.

Brett's (1987) study of the use of nursing research findings suggests that there is some optimism about the state of research dissemination and use at least among staff nurses. In the study the majority of nurses (61%) who were aware of research-based innovations were persuaded to use the innovation and did use it at least sometimes in their practice. Although no relationship existed among levels of educational preparation, exposure to research courses or activities and reading professional journals did correlate with adoption of the innovations by administrators, educators/researchers, and clinicians.

Principles

1. Collaboration is enhanced when agencies identify specific research-related responsibilities for nurse administrators, educators, researchers, and clinicians.
2. Researcher-practitioner collaborative partnerships help reduce the gap between what caregivers need to know and the information that researchers provide—that is, between knowledge development and knowledge utilization.
3. Nursing administrators play an important role in promoting the partnership between nursing research and practice.

Questions

1. What policies need to be in place to promote a collaborative approach to research utilization and research-based nursing practice?
2. How would your agency's job descriptions need to be revised to involve all nurses more directly in research utilization?
3. What resources are available in your agency to support collaborative research-utilization efforts to promote research-based nursing practice?
4. What other key points do you think should be stated as principles of partnerships?

■■ ■■ ■■ ■■

INNOVATION ADOPTION BEHAVIOR

In an era when nursing research is becoming more visible to practising nurses because clinical agencies are setting up nursing research departments and employing nursing researchers, why are the results of research so seldom reflected in nursing practice? Part of the problem may be that most nurses are unsure about the applicability of published research findings in their practice. They do not know when research findings are ready to be used in their particular setting. Nurses are perfectionists, with a tendency to look for absolute proof of the facts before research findings are usable (Wood, 1992). Using research findings in nursing practice usually requires adopting an innovation such as a new idea, a different way of thinking about an issue, and a change in behaviour.

The process of adopting innovations

Rogers (1983) conceptualizes the diffusion and adoption of innovations as occurring in a time-ordered sequence of stages through which all individuals, including nurses, must pass. The knowledge stage occurs as nurses become aware of the innovation. In the persuasion stage, nurses form a favourable or unfavourable attitude toward the innovation and then decide whether to adopt or reject the innovation on a trial basis. Finally, in the implementation stage, nurses use the practice on a regular basis. If a new practice is mandated without the practitioners moving through the appropriate stages, it is unlikely to be implemented consistently or as intended, or it may be rejected.

Factors Affecting the Process

Several factors influence the process of adopting a new practice. Coyle and Sokop (1990) and Brett (1987) found the major influences on adopting innovations were professional nursing literature (especially *Nursing Research*), research-oriented conferences and in-services, and role models. However, only a small percentage of nurses is exposed to these sources. Factors influencing nurses in the persuasion stage are hospital policy, policy and procedure manuals, and the opinions of other professionals. Brett (1987) found that it was perceived rather than actual hospital policy about research-based nursing practice that influenced the adoption of innovations among her sample of nurses. Policy and procedure manuals that support the use of research findings are reviewed and revised frequently and substantiated with research references. Negative opinions or perceptions from other health-care colleagues deter nurses' passing through the persuasion stage (Alcock, Carroll, and Goodman, 1990; RNABC, 1993b). In the last two stages, decision and implementation, the most common barriers identified by clinicians are organizational barriers. Nurses perceive that they lack authority and do not have the administrative support to change nursing practice. Whether or not this is the case, it is the perception that inhibits adoption of innovations.

Based on a review of approaches to the diffusion and adoption of technology, Romano (1990) identified factors affecting the rate of moving through the stages: the relative advantage to the patient and the system, compatibility with existing values and experiences, complexity of the approach or the complexity of the situation, opportunity for the innovation to be tested, and the visibility of results. When only one or two of these factors are addressed, movement through the stages of adoption is adversely affected.

Using knowledge generated from research is generally not a natural element of everyday nursing practice. Nurses with responsibility for promoting research-based nursing practice may find it helpful to address issues concerning the availability of research-based knowledge to practising nurses, the ability of nurses to read and interpret research findings, credibility of the research, relevance of the findings to practice, and support for applying the findings in practice.

Example: Implementing Patient-Controlled Analgesia

In 1992 nurses from a number of different hospitals in British Columbia observed that staff on their units were having some difficulty with the introduction of patient-controlled analgesia (PCA) pumps. The staff nurses expressed concern about the pump's safety and appropriateness for patients with certain characteristics or histories. Subsequently a collaborative research project was undertaken in 11 hospitals with 14 nurse co-investigators. After reviewing and analyzing the literature about PCA according to Romano's five factors affecting the rate of adoption of innovations, it was agreed that the most likely factor affecting the adoption of PCA was the compatibility of the innovation with existing values and experiences of nurses. The effectiveness of PCA had been extensively studied and advantages well documented in published research articles. The complexity of the approach was not considered to be different from other technology-based nursing care provided by staff nurses.

Through focus group interviews with nurses from each of the 11 agencies, data were collected about their perceptions and understanding of the philosophy of patient-controlled analgesia, with or without use of the pump; their experiences in implementing a PCA approach; and their introduction to PCA. A preliminary analysis of the data identified four factors as influencing the integration of the PCA approach into their practice. First the nurses were given no explanation or information about the new practice; rather they were told to implement it. Secondly, there were some misconceptions or misinformation among the nurses about pain management, the side effects of some analgesics, and the possibility of interaction between addictive drugs and analgesics. Thirdly, staff nurses felt isolated from the decision-making process. Fourthly, the nurses identified very clearly that in-service education support and practice time are critical to the adoption of an innovation. These preliminary results have already led to changes in some of the hospitals and to plans for systematic introduction of PCA in non-study hospitals, giving attention to the stages nurses must go through as well as their need for knowledge.

Research-Utilization Frameworks.

Strategies to promote and facilitate the adoption of innovations include the use of a research-utilization framework. Frameworks assist with movement through the identified phases and provide a structure for making research the foundation for nursing practice. The most well-known frameworks are those developed by the Western Interstate Commission for Higher Education in Nursing (WICHEN) (Krueger, Nelson, and Wolanin, 1978); the Conduct and Utilization of Research in Nursing (CURN) (Horsley, Crane, and Bingle, 1978); the Nursing Child Assessment Satellite Training (NCAST) (King, Barnard, and Hoehn, 1981); and the framework elaborated by Stetler (Stettler, 1976). These four frameworks demonstrate some common elements and essential differences. In theoretical terms, the WICHEN and CURN frameworks are both based on the concepts of diffusion of innovation and planned change (Stetler, 1985). NCAST focuses solely on diffusion of innovation. The Stetler framework differs in that it was inductively developed. Change is not the focus; rather the framework encourages a problem-solving approach that assumes the nurse is a knowledge-oriented, critical thinker (Stetler, 1985).

How well a given framework will serve a situation or agency depends on the framework's efficacy, the type of problem or situation that the user wants to address, and how congruent each framework's theoretical basis is with how nurses make decisions, solve problems and/or generally use knowledge as caregivers, managers and educators (Stetler, 1985). In addition, the framework must fit with the organization's structure, philosophy of nursing practice, and available resources. Based on the work of Stetler (1985) and the expressed needs of nurses and health-care agencies in British Columbia, a decision-making model for utilization of research findings in practice was developed and published in the workbook, *Nursing Research: From Question to Funding* (RNABC, 1990a). Four phases of the model with decision outcomes are: 1) articulation or definition of the problem and location of research reports; 2) evaluation or critical review of research findings for scientific merit and clinical significance; 3) comparison of findings to the practice setting; and 4) application or definition of the contribution to practice and evaluation if implemented. Application of this framework requires partnerships among nurses with clinical expertise, research experience, and administrative responsibilities. Each phase requires particular nurses to be involved, decisions to be made, and resources to be accessed. The framework can be modified and explained in greater detail by individual agencies, thus making it relevant to both staff needs and the organizational structure.

As an example of a framework's usefulness, one health-care agency in British Columbia has adopted the RNABC research utilization framework as a strategy to promote research-based nursing practice. The nursing research committee with staff, administrative, and educator representation, has worked on explicating the objectives of and responsibilities for each phase, changing terminology to fit the agency's mission and setting and identifying resources required for each phase. The committee's work has been discussed at general nursing council meetings and with staff. Refinements based on their input have resulted in an agency-specific, research-utilization framework that maintains the integrity of the original and addresses the needs of the agency. The intent is to decentralize further work with the framework to areas of practice where it will be used and evaluated against the process of recommending and adopting research-based nursing practices. Regardless of the research-utilization framework used, the importance of the strategy is that it fosters an inquiring, curious attitude that results in problem identification and resolution and facilitates adoption of innovations into research-based nursing practice.

Principles

1. Research utilization depends upon the interest, commitment, and expertise of nurses in all areas and cannot be achieved by any one individual working in isolation.
2. Success of research utilization requires that it be proactive, deliberate, and systematic, addressing the process of adopting innovation.
3. Research utilization frameworks provide guides for nursing practice, research, and educational and administrative systems.
4. Relevant research utilization frameworks include phases aimed at identifying the problem, critically reviewing the literature, translating findings to practice, implementing the new practice, and evaluating the outcome.

Questions

1. What are the pros and cons of using a framework to promote research-based nursing practice? What problems could be anticipated? What benefits?
2. Which, if any, of these frameworks would you choose for your agency? What criteria would you use to direct your selection?
3. How does the philosophy underlying your chosen framework meet with your organization's philosophy and department of nursing's practice of decision making, problem solving, education, and nursing-care delivery?
4. What other key points do you think should be stated as principles of utilization frameworks?

■■ ■■ ■■ ■■

FUTURE CHALLENGES

Facilitating the process of research utilization in nursing practice is not an easy task, but neither is it an impossible dream. Some activities suggested that might facilitate the research process include funding key research positions, creating institutional infrastructures, encouraging and assisting nurses to attend practice-based research workshops and conferences, providing continuing education courses to assist nurses in critiquing research, creating a reward system within the agency for research utilization in practice, promoting collaborative efforts between agency personnel and other health-care agencies or educational institutions, establishing a means for nurses to access research reports relevant to their practice, promoting demonstration projects that illustrate the cost-effectiveness of changing from a traditional, intuitively-based practice to one that is research-based, and ensuring that research utilization is a role expectation for all nursing positions (management, educational, and clinical) and that it is reinforced in job descriptions, agency policy, and the institution's philosophy of nursing.

Diagnosing barriers and planning and implementing strategies to overcome them are challenges. The first challenge is to demonstrate the cost-effectiveness of nursing research and to justify the allocation of resources and personnel to create the necessary infrastructures. The second challenge is to reduce the time gap between when knowledge is developed and when it is used. The third challenge is to create agency infrastructures. Agency support "in principle" is not sufficient to transform nursing practice from a ritual base to a research base. Efforts to address these challenges require partnerships within and among agencies and among agencies and professional groups.

REFERENCES

Alcock, D., Carroll, G., and Goodman, M. (1990). Staff nurses' perceptions of factors influencing their role in research. *The Canadian Journal of Nursing Research, 22*(4), 7-18.

Attridge, C., and Callahan, M. (1987). *Women in women's work: An exploratory study of nurses' perspective of quality work environments.* University of Victoria, Faculty of Human and Social Development.

Bock, L. (1990). From research to utilization: Bridging the gap. *Nursing Management, 21*(3), 50-1.

Brett, J.L. (1987). Use of nursing practice research findings. *Nursing Research, 36*(6), 344-349.

Brooten, D., Kumar, S., Brown, L., Butts, P., Finkler, S., Bakewell-Sachs, S., Gibbons, A., and Delivoria-Papadopoulos, M. (1986). A randomized clinical trial and home follow-up of very-low-birth-weight infants. *The New England Journal of Medicine, 315*(15), 934-939.

Chambers, C. (1989). Barriers to the dissemination and use of research in nursing practice. *NRIG Newsletter, 8*(2), 2-3.

Champion, V., and Leach, A. (1989). Variables related to research utilization in nursing: An empirical investigation. *Journal of Advanced Nursing, 14,* 705-710.

Coyle, L.A., and Sokop, A.G. (1990). Innovation adoption behavior among nurses. *Nursing Research, 39*(3), 176-180.

Davies, B., and Eng, B. (1991). *Final Report: Survey of nursing research programs in children's hospitals.* Vancouver, BC: BC's Children's Hospital

Eagle, J., Fortnum, D., Price, P., and Scruton, J. (1990). Developing a rationale and recruitment plan for a nurse researcher. *Canadian Journal of Nursing Administration, 3*(2), 5-10.

Edwards-Beckett, J. (1990). Nursing research utilization techniques. *Journal of Nursing Administration, 20*(11), 25-30.

Fagin, C. (1982). The economic value of nursing research. *American Journal of Nursing, 12*(12), 1844-1849.

Fordyce, J.D., Mooney, G.H., and Russell, E.M. (1982). Economic analysis in health care. *Health Bulletin, 39*(10), 21-38.

Funk, S.G., Champagne, M.T., Wiese, R.A., and Tornquist, E.M. (1991). Barriers: The barriers to research utilization scales. *Applied Nursing Research,* 4(1), 39-45.

Funk, S.G., Tornquist, E.M., Champagne, M.T. (1989). Application and evaluation of the dissemination model. *Western Journal of Nursing Research, 11*(4), 486-991.

Gortner, S. (1986). Research for a practice profession. In L. Nichols (Ed.), *Perspectives on nursing theory,* (pp. 549-555). Toronto: Little, Brown & Co.

Hamilton, L., Vincent, L., Goode, R., Moorhouse, A., Hawker Worden, R., Jones, H., Close, M., and DuFour, S. (1990). Organizational support of the clinical nurse specialist role: A nursing research and professional development directorate. *Canadian Journal of Nursing Administration, 5*(3), 9-13.

Haughey, B. (1988). Utilizing research findings in nursing. *Clinical Nurse Specialist, 2*(4), 184.

Heater, B., Becker, A., and Olson, R. (1988). Nursing interventions and patient outcomes: A meta-analysis of studies. *Nursing Research,* 37(5), 303-307.

Hickey, M. (1990). The role of the clinical nurse specialist in the research utilization process. *Clinical Nurse Specialist, 4*(2), 93-96.

Horsley, J. (1985). Using research to practice: The current context. *Western Journal of Nursing Research, 7*(1), 135-139.

Horsley, J., Crane, J., and Bingle, J. (1978). Research utilization as an organization process. *Journal of Nursing Administration, 8*(7), 4-6.

Hunt, J. (1981). Indicators for nursing practice: The use of research findings. *Journal of Advanced Nursing, 6*(5), 189-194.

Kenneth, H., and Stiesmeyer, J. (1991). Strategies for involving staff in nursing research. *Applied Nursing Research, 10*(2), 103-107.

King, D., Barnard, K., and Hoehn, R. (1981). Disseminating the results of nursing research. *Nursing Outlook, 29*(3), 164-169.

Kirchoff, K. (1991). Who is responsible for research utilization? *Heart and Lung, 20*(3), 308-309.

Knafl, K., Bevis, M., and Kirchhoff, K. (1987). Research activities of clinical nurse researchers. *Nursing Research, 36*(4), 249-252.

Kramer, M., Albrecht, S., and Miller, R. (1985). A team approach to nursing research. *Nursing Forum, 22*(1), 19-21.

Krueger, J., Nelson, A., and Wolanin, M. (1978). *Nursing research: Development, collaboration, and utilization.* Germantown, MD: Aspen.

Larson, E. (1983). Combining nursing quality assurance and research programs. *The Journal of Nursing Administration,* 32-38.

MacKay, R.C., Grantham, M.A., and Ross, E.M. (1984). Building a hospital nursing research department. *Journal of Nursing Administration,* 14(7/8), 23-27.

Marek, K.D., and Lang, N.M. (1992). Nursing sensitive outcomes. In *Papers from the Nursing Minimum Data Set Conference* (pp. 100-120) Ottawa: Canadian Nurses Association.

Nutting M.A., and Dock, L.L. (1907). *A history of nursing.* New York: Putnam & Sons.

Olson, R., Heater, B., and Becker, A. (1990). A meta-analysis of the effects of nursing interventions on children and parents. *Maternal Child Nursing, 15*(2), 104-108.

Pank, P., Rostron, W., and Stenhouse, M. (1984). Using research in nursing. *Nursing Times,* 80(11), 44-45.

Repko, L. (1990). Turn research reports into an assessment challenge. *RN, 53*(8), 56-61.

Rogers, E.M. (1983). *Diffusion of innovations.*(3rd ed.). New York: The Free Press.

Romano, C.A. (1990). Diffusion of technology innovation. *Advances in Nursing Science, 13*(2), 11-21.

Ross, F. (1985). Uneasy bedfellows. *Nursing Times, 81*(44), 38-39.

RNABC (1990a). *Nursing research: From question to funding.* Vancouver, BC: Author.

RNABC (1990b). *Report on the evaluation of member services of the Research Consultation Services.* Unpublished report. Vancouver, BC.

RNABC (1993a). *Nursing and research in undergraduate education programs: A BC survey.* Vancouver, BC: Author.

RNABC (1993b). *Nursing and research in clinical agencies: A BC survey.* Vancouver, BC: Author.

Sasmor, J.L. (1986). Cost and research. *NAACOG Newsletter, 13,* 4.

Sayner, N. (1984). Research in the clinical setting: Potential barriers to implementation. *Journal of Neurosurgical Nursing, 16*(5), 279-281.

Shamian, J. (1992). Response to K. D. Marek's and N. M. Lang's paper on nursing sensitive outcomes. In *Papers from the Nursing Minimum Data Set Conference* (pp. 121-126) Ottawa: Canadian Nurses Association.

Smeltzer, C., and Hinshaw, A. (1988). Research: Clinical integration for excellent patient care. *Nursing Management, 19*(1), 38-44.

Stetler, C. (1976). Nurses and research: Responsibility and involvement. *National Intravenous Therapy Association, 6*(3), 207-212.

Stetler, C. (1985). Research utilization: Defining the concept. *Image: The Journal of Nursing Scholarship, 17*(2), 40-44.

Thurston, N., Tenove, S., and Church, J.(1989). Nursing research in Canadian Hospitals. *Canadian Journal of Nursing Administration, 2*(1), 8-10.

Thurston, N., Tenove, S., and Church, J. (1990). Hospital nursing is alive and flourishing. *Nursing Management, 21*(5), 50-54.

Varricchio, C., and Mikos, K. (1987). Research: Determining feasibility in a clinical setting. *Oncology Nursing Forum, 14*(1), 89-90.

Ventura, M., Young, D., Feldman, M., Pastore, P., Pikula, S., and Yates, M. (1984). Cost savings as an indicator of successful nursing intervention. *Nursing Research, 34*(1), 50-53.

Watson, C.A., Bulecheck, G.M., and McCloskey, J.C. (1987). QAMUR: A quality assurance model using research. *Journal of Nursing Qaulity Assurance, 2*(1), 21-27.

Wilson-Barnett, J., Corner, J., and DeCarle, B. (1990). Integrating nursing research and practice—the role of the researcher as teacher. *Journal of Advanced Nursing, 15*(5), 621-625.

Wood, M. (1992). Shaping practice through research. *Clinical Nursing Research,* 1(2), 123-126.

PART III

Nursing Care Delivery

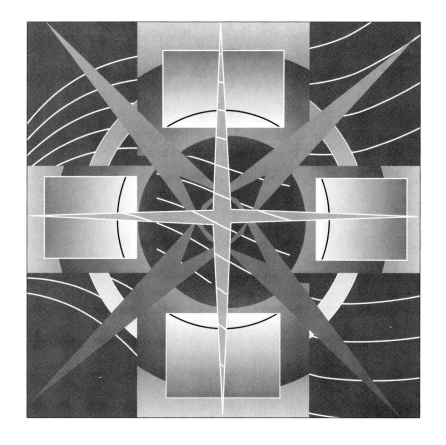

Quality of Care: Where Have We Come From— Where Are We Going?

JANET ROSS KERR AND DOREEN REID

I ncreasing diversification and sophistication in the health-care field have been accompanied by steady increases in national expenditures for health care. Concomitant changing social values about health characterize the general population. Better informed health consumers are demanding increased accountability in health care. Investigative and consciousness-raising activities of consumer rights groups have resulted in a high media profile; health lobbyists have argued for environmental protection, health promotion, and provision of health-care services that are available, effective, and appropriate. As a result, North American attitudes toward health care and health-care professionals have undergone a significant transition. Health care is considered a right rather than a privilege, and health-care professionals are expected not just to provide care, but to provide quality care.

The relationship between accessible, cost-effective, high-quality patient care and institutional excellence has been explored in several studies on magnet hospitals (Kramer and Schmalenberg, 1988; McClure, Poulin, Sovie, and Wandelt, 1982). In identifying hospital organizations that had developed a reputation for vitality and innovation, other factors of considerable interest to the nursing department emerged. These included low turnover, less frequent need for orientation of new staff, high commitment and identification with institutional values on the part of staff, more infrequent use of inexperienced staff or agency personnel, and cooperative working relationships among staff members (Kramer and Schmalenberg, 1988). The highly desirable nature of these variables and the fact that they are associated with excellence in care underscores the importance and relevance of efforts to ensure quality patient care.

Historically, quality assurance in health care was defined as the self-regulating activities of the various professions. The prevailing view that only relevant health-care professionals could describe the nature of competent practice meant that physicians, nurses, and other professionals were not challenged in the way that they dealt with matters of professional misconduct. Today the situation is very different. While professional groups granted the privilege of autonomously conducting regulatory functions still have those privileges, there is more public scrutiny of the process. In many provinces, lay members of professional governing boards and their disciplinary committees are appointed by the Lieutenant-Governor-in-Council to represent the interests of the public in professional deliberations. Professional groups are constantly pressured by the media for full and open disclosure of the results of disciplinary operations. Thus the professional conduct of physicians, nurses, and other health-care professionals is a subject for public discussion and debate, something that was unheard of in the past.

■ ■ ■ ■

HISTORICAL DEVELOPMENTS IN QUALITY ASSURANCE

The assessment of the quality of nursing care is believed to be an important and essential strategy for monitoring and stimulating excellence in nursing practice, administration, education, and research. Credit for the first documented study in health care and nursing, based on the use of standards, is attributed to Florence Nightingale, who in 1858 investigated the quality of care rendered to military personnel (Nightingale, 1858). In the United States the idea of developing standards for health care was formalized in 1918. The American standards were subsequently adopted in Canadian hospitals and applied to all disciplines and services. In 1952 the Joint Committee on Accreditation of Hospitals (JCAH) was formed, and until 1958 this organization assumed responsibility for accrediting Canadian hospitals. In 1958 the Canadian Council on Hospital Accreditation (CCHA) was formed for accrediting health-care agencies in Canada. Since that time the CCHA has provided the external stimulus for quality assurance programs in nursing. Accreditation standards and requirements have been revised on a regular basis and reflect increasingly strenuous monitoring. Beginning in the 1970s, the CCHA standards required the presence of a quality assurance program in hospitals across Canada.

Over the next decade, considerable effort was made to develop formal programs for assessing, monitoring, and improving care. Although quality assurance activities were visible in all disciplines, the primary focus was directed toward developing quality-monitoring, programs in nursing, undoubtedly because nursing is the largest and most critically important service in health-care agencies. Provincial professional associations in nursing have instituted quality assurance activities. Guidelines for implementing quality assurance programs and nursing practice standards have been developed by these organizations. Nursing consultants with quality assurance expertise have been retained by the professional associations to provide assistance to nursing service departments in provincial health-care agencies in developing programs or ongoing activities in quality assurance. Many hospitals have established a quality assurance department within the division of nursing with the responsibility to implement and monitor quality-related activities. Nursing expertise has also been important in developing standards at the level of the Board of Directors of the

CCHA, where the Canadian Nurses Association (CNA) has been represented with two seats on the governing board.

The common denominator of quality assurance programs has been standards. Donabedian (1980) proposed three levels for assessing quality: structure, process, and outcome. Structural standards focused on the human and material resources available and their organization in a health-care setting. Examples included the philosophy of the institution, resources and supplies, staffing patterns, and characteristics of the environment of care. Process standards focused on the role of the nurse and on nursing activities performed in the interest of meeting patient care goals. Examples of process standards are the nursing process, communication between nurses and clients, and nursing activities. Outcome standards were mainly client oriented, and described the anticipated results of the care process. Outcomes generally refer to the results of health care. It has been difficult to attribute outcomes to any one health-care profession because a team effort is necessary to achieve results.

The majority of the effort in quality assurance programs has been directed at the process level of care because the activities of a health-care profession can be assessed and measured directly at this level. The assessment has been concurrent or, more frequently, retrospective. If concurrent, nursing care was reviewed or measured at the same time the care was delivered; if retrospective, the review took place at some time after the provision of care. The advantages of the concurrent method included the potential for collecting more and better information and the availability of direct information from clients. Because the information was gathered sooner, changes could be made more quickly. Disadvantages included increased cost implications and possible disruption to the activities of the nursing unit. Retrospective reviews were attractive because cost implications tended to be lower. There was less disruption to the nursing unit because the client's record was usually the focus of this review. However, with this type of review it was not usually possible to collect information directly from the client, and nurses responsible for the data on the chart were not available to elaborate on it or to answer questions that arose. Because there was evidence that both concurrent and retrospective reviews provided valuable and unique information about the process of care, many agencies implemented both types in their quality assurance programs.

In many agencies, staff nurses have been asked to assist with the implementation process as data collectors. Those responsible for the program felt this involvement was important because it allowed nurses to be a part of the monitoring process; it was generally believed that involvement enhanced commitment to the program. It also allowed nurses to become involved in a peer review process for evaluating nursing care. Some hospitals chose to have quality audits carried out by nurses as part of their day-to-day practice. Others chose to assign audit responsibilities to a small group of nurses who rotated on an annual basis. Researchers noted that there were disadvantages in random involvement of untrained and inexperienced observers in the data collection process, indicating that the quality of the information collected was less than adequate in terms of reliability and validity. The quality of the process itself was dependent on the program manager having an understanding of measurement and statistical issues in order to combine appropriate methods and involve staff members.

The literature on quality assurance is plentiful. Most publications can be described as descriptive, covering areas such as the nature of quality; the components of a quality assurance model/framework; the categorizations of quality; the rationale for developing quality assurance techniques and programs; and establishing, maintaining, and improving quality assurance programs. The sector of the literature that deals with research on quality assessment is limited, focusing primarily on instrument development. Although there has been a great deal of research in the area of instrument development, there has been little attention to the type of testing that should be an integral part of the process. Most instruments have demonstrated little more than face validity, raising questions about the value of results in quality assessment programs using inadequately tested instruments. It has also posed problems for the interpretation of research that uses instruments purporting to measure the quality of nursing care.

Ventura tested instruments to measure quality that were commonly used in tertiary care institutions. Studies were conducted at the Veterans Administration Medical Center in Buffalo, New York, to investigate the relationship between QualPacs and the Phaneuf nursing audit. A Pearson product-moment correlation of coefficient 0.01 was obtained for total scale scores using 97 patients (Ventura, Hageman, Slakter, and Fox, 1980). In another study in which the scales of QualPacs and the Rush-Medicus instrument were correlated, it was found that some subscales were related whereas others bore little relationship to each other. This led to the conclusion that different dimensions of quality were addressed in each instrument and further exploration of the nature of the concept of quality was necessary (Ventura, Hageman, Slakter, and Fox, 1982). Results support those of an earlier investigation by Trussel and Strand (1978), which identified differences between concurrent and retrospective reviews of the same patients.

Examination of interrater reliability of these same instruments also identified difficulties with the QualPacs and the Rush-Medicus instruments. Minimal standards for evaluating results were not met by the QualPacs instrument; the Rush-Medicus instrument only met them in testing situations where the test conditions were carefully controlled. Ventura, Hageman, Slakter, and Fox (1980) recommended that interrater reliability be calculated on a regular basis, using the intraclass correlation coefficient (ICC) before and after data collection, and that a minimum standard for measuring results should be an ICC of at least 0.75.

A study conducted at the University of Alberta in Edmonton, Alberta, assessed the reliability and validity of the Rush-Medicus process audit—an in-house tool for measuring quality developed by one hospital—the Process Chart Audit, and the MAPS Outcome Audit—an instrument developed by the Alberta Hospital Association (Alberta Hospital Association, 1983). ICCs in two data collection periods were calculated for each instrument. On the Rush-Medicus instrument, ICCs were 0.76 in the first period and 0.93 in the second; on the Process Chart Audit, ICCs were 0.77 and 0.75; and on the MAPS Outcome Audit, ICCs were 0.94 and 0.89. No significant differences were noted between the ratings of the two observers; ICCs that were greater than the recommended standard of 0.75 were obtained for all three instruments in both testing periods based on total scale scores. A discrepancy was noted in the ICC obtained for the Rush-Medicus instrument in both testing periods that could not be explained. In terms of subscale results, improvement from the first data set to the second was noted. For the Rush-Medicus process audit, all subscales of the second data set were above the 0.75 ICC standard. Results of the MAPS Outcome Audit, in terms of the ICC values for subscales, also met the 0.75 standard and were the most impressive, suggesting a high level of reliability. ICC values for the subscales of the Process Chart Audit varied widely in both data collection periods, a finding that might be expected considering the lack of testing of this instrument. These investigators concluded that the recommended 0.75 ICC level for interrater reliability may be too low and should be closer to 0.85 (Giovannetti, Kerr, Bay, and Buchan 1986).

The validity-testing portion of the study assessed the relationship between the instruments being tested using Pearson correlations. The coefficient for Rush-Medicus and MAPS was 0.27; for Rush-Medicus and the Process Chart Audit, 0.23; for MAPS and the Chart Audit, 0.29. It was obvious that correlations were very low; in fact, none explained more than 9% of the variance. Based on Ventura's earlier findings these results were not unexpected. The conclusions of these researchers were consistent with Ventura's; the three instruments measured different dimensions of quality (Giovannetti et al, 1986).

Because of the limitations in using existing instruments to measure quality, a number of hospitals purchased pre-packaged quality assurance programs. A variety of consulting firms that have international recognition in quality assurance have used vigourous marketing strategies, offering to provide a quality assurance program tailored to the institution. Their assistance came at considerable cost and included both positive features and limitations. Many nursing departments chose to employ external consultants to work with hospital-based staff. Ultimately the department assumed responsibility for the operation of the program.

■ ■ ■ ■

LIMITATIONS OF QUALITY ASSURANCE PROGRAMS

Reference has been made to problems with quality assurance programs and monitoring. A major challenge facing all executive officers of agencies in times of diminishing financial resources is the cost-effectiveness of all programs, including quality assurance programs. As the number of professionals required for successful operation of quality-monitoring programs has increased, so have costs associated with programs implemented by external consultants. Funds expended have been considerable, and some suggest, disproportionate to the results achieved.

A second area of concern is whether those responsible for designing and implementing programs are knowledgeable in research and quality assessment. Knowledge about the research literature is important, as is the ability to assess the strengths and weaknesses of various approaches to quality in order to maximize the former and minimize the latter in programs selected for implementation. Many nurses who have been responsible for in–service education are now also responsible for managing quality assurance activities in health-care agencies. While this has been an expedient way for agencies to implement quality monitoring, it has been based on the assumption that those responsible have the time, interest, background, and expertise to function effectively in both spheres. The limited testing of the reliability and validity of instruments used for quality monitoring has continued to be a major concern for nursing departments. Many instruments do not measure dimensions of quality consistently and therefore provide little value to those who wish to judge performance within the institution from the results obtained. Also, the low correlation between instruments used to measure the same dimensions of quality has raised concerns about what is ultimately being measured.

Ventura et al (1980) and Giovannetti et al (1986) have noted that measurement must be made carefully so that the quality-monitoring process yields reliable findings. Controlled conditions have required that raters be carefully trained and monitored. This may mean that certain nurses are designated as quality auditors and seconded to the program for a period of time. While this system supports the principles of good data collection, the process has been seen as delegating the responsibility for quality care to a few individuals whose role is primarily inspection. Another limitation of quality assurance programs has been the retrospective focus on the achievement of standards. Much of the emphasis of quality-monitoring activities has occurred after the fact when it is least possible to make the necessary changes. Also, minimum standards of achievement have been acceptable in determining whether criteria have been met or not met.

Finally, perhaps the greatest limitation has been the focus of quality assurance programs. Quality assurance activities have been largely department specific, thus limiting the resolution of interdisciplinary issues. Many of these issues, such as processes of admission, transfer, discharge, consultation, and materials distribution, have been resistant to change despite a variety of quality-monitoring techniques. Non-elective patients still wait for 2 to 3 hours to be seen by a nurse or physician in the emergency department. Patients continue to be sent home without adequate instructions. Wheelchairs continue to go missing and elderly patients continue to fall. These events are not confined to individual departments; improvement in the quality of care requires the concerted efforts of all disciplines working together.

Quality assurance has, for the last two decades, provided the focus for improving the care given to patients. Many of the activities related to monitoring, evaluating, problem analysis, and auditing will continue to be applied with a shift in emphasis to what is being referred to as Total Quality Management, which assumes a corporate approach to quality through a process of continuous improvement.

■ ■ ■ ■

THE TRANSITION TO TOTAL QUALITY MANAGEMENT

Total Quality Management (TQM) is a "structured, systematic process for creating organization-wide participation in planning and implementing continuous improvement in quality" (Whetsell, 1990, p. 16). The origins of TQM date back to the 1930s, when Dr. Edward Deming, a graduate from Yale University and a consultant in statistical studies, put forward his theory of continuous improvement as a consultant to Western Electric Laboratories (later AT&T Bell Laboratories) and other U.S. industries. He believed that problems, and therefore opportunities to improve quality, were built into the complex production processes and that defects in quality could rarely be attributed to the people involved with the process. Problems were generally not caused by poor motivation or effort but rather job design. In his theory of continuous improvement, Deming advocated a strong and long-term commitment by management including the need for clearly defined mission and vision statements. He believed quality should be the central focus of the organization and that emphasis needed to shift from inspection to prevention. Preventing defects before they occur and improving processes so that defects do not occur are the goals for which all organizations should be striving. Long-term relationships with suppliers were essential rather than accepting the lowest bid. He believed that the training and retraining of employees was critical to the success of the organization and that management's role was to coach employees. Finally, he believed that reducing variability in processes would ultimately lead to sustaining improvements in these processes. For the next 50 years, Deming's philosophies lay dormant in the United States and did not appear again until a now-famous documentary titled *If Japan Can . . . Why Can't We?* aired on a national U.S. television network in 1980. This program profiled Dr. Deming and his theory, which affected Japanese industry and was to change the focus of American business industries, health and educational organizations as well as public and private services forever (Sahney and Warden, 1991).

Largely ignored in America, in 1950 Deming accepted an invitation from the Union of Japanese Scientists and Plant Managers to lecture on his ideas of quality control and improvement. Deming's ideas sparked the interest and enthusiasm of Japanese management and workers. As a result of his teachings, over the next 20 years the Japanese made enormous strides in improving the quality of their products and services. They rapidly acquired an international reputation for high-quality, low-cost products and captured alarming U.S. market shares in the automobile, camera, television, and electronic industries. The loss of market share for major U.S. industries provided the stimulus and urgency to focus attention on the quality of products and customer service. This movement was made by such industrial giants as Ford Motor Company, Motorola, Xerox, Campbell Soup, IBM, 3-M, Hewlett Packard, and Federal Express, which became the flagship organizations in the transition to quality management practices in both private and public organizations (Deming, 1986).

In the 1980s, many leaders in hospitals across both Canada and the United States were facing significant pressures previously experienced in industry to improve the quality of services while addressing the need to reduce the rate of steadily increasing costs. Quality assurance programs in hospitals were not providing the foundation on which to make the significant changes thought to be necessary and the culture of quality, so much a part of the fabric of successful industries, was not identifiable in the health-care industry. The successes that industries had made in improving quality and reducing costs caught the attention of hospital managers. Could the quality improvement principles that had proven to be successful in industry have any applicability in hospitals? Many were sceptical of any relationships to be found between manufacturing products and the highly complex, people-focused hospital milieu.

Donald Berwick (1990), a professor of pediatrics at the Harvard Medical School and a pediatrician with the Harvard Community Health Plan, disagreed with this view. Although steps being taken in both Canada and the United States to control costs and improve health were unsuccessful, he believed the challenges facing industries over the previous two decades were no different than those facing health care. In 1987 he launched the National Demonstration Project on Quality Improvement in Health Care (NDP), which was an exploratory study designed to answer the question: Can the tools of modern quality improvement with which industries have achieved breakthroughs in performance, improve health care as well? This landmark study described in the book *Healing Health Care*, documents the efforts of 21 health-care organizations paired with an equal number of industrial quality management experts to use the principles of quality management in the implementation of hospital-based pilot projects. During the 8-month demonstration study, 17 hospitals completed projects that improved processes such as transport of critically ill neonates, use of portable x-rays, appointment waiting times, patient discharge, and hiring nurses. At least 15 of the projects were considered successful. These pioneer teams made several discoveries during the projects. They found that quality improvement methods and tools were applicable to health care. Cross-functional teams were valuable in improving health-care processes. Data useful for quality improvement abounded and it was established that costs of poor quality were high. Involving physicians in the quality improvement process was difficult but essential, and quality transformation was dependent on leadership. This work was the first documented evidence that the use of quality management principles initially implemented in industry could be applied to processes used in hospitals. Many of these hospitals have continued to make profound changes and provide a model for the successful implementation of a quality management philosophy in Canadian hospitals.

■■ ■■ ■■ ■■

TEN KEY CONCEPTS OF TOTAL QUALITY MANAGEMENT

There are a number of key concepts that are central to the quality management process. Many of these concepts reflect a significant shift in thinking and focus. The development of these concepts was guided by successful implementation in industry as well as health care (Sahney and Warden, 1991; McLaughlin and Kaluzny, 1990; Thompson, 1991; Walton, 1986).

1. **Management from the top**
   Leadership and commitment of senior management is a key factor in the implementation of quality management. The need for management to drive the quality improvement process and to actively participate is critical to the success of TQM.

2. **Transformation of the corporate culture**

   The process of cultural transformation is a long-term commitment that may take from 5 to 10 years in most hospitals. Leaders consistently encourage, nurture, support, and reward continuous quality improvement activities. A successful transformation requires both logical direction and emotional commitment.

3. **Customer focus**

   Patients and staff are viewed as customers. A customer is anyone who receives or is affected by a product or a process, and therefore patients, families, hospital visitors, hospital employees, physicians, volunteers, and suppliers are included in that category. Meeting and exceeding the needs of patients and staff is a priority goal and involves not only an evaluation of current services but expectations and ideas for improvement.

4. **Process focus**

   Quality management focuses on key processes rather than on the people involved in the process. This approach is based on the premise that 85% of the problems encountered in organizations are the result of cumbersome or poorly defined processes. Problems are attributable to staff performance only 15% of the time. There are frequent complaints about hospital admitting departments, where patients can experience long waits before they are taken to their assigned room. A traditional reaction is to chide the supervisor, and in turn the staff, for not doing a good job. However, admitting patients to hospitals is a complex process that crosses various departmental lines. Only after analysis of the process can changes be made that will improve the process. Staff are dedicated to providing high-quality care; it is the process that requires improvement.

5. **Employee involvement**

   Everyone in the organization is involved in continuous quality improvement. Working within the guidelines and boundaries established by managers, staff are empowered by receiving information, resources, and authority to improve work processes that will benefit patients and themselves. Problem resolution occurs at the lowest possible level of the organization, where staff have the greatest knowledge about potential causes and solutions.

6. **Education**

   Staff education and training at all levels of the organization are central to a motivated and contributing workforce. Education programs include an awareness of TQM principles, the steps in quality improvement, the use of quality improvement tools, just-in-time training, and teamwork skills.

7. **Preventive systems**

   Quality management is a continuous cycle of improving processes before errors are made or complaints are received. Doing the right things right the first time and all the time is considered much more cost-effective than redoing work. Responsibility for improving processes rests with those directly involved in the process.

8. **Teamwork**

   Teamwork is a collaborative, interdisciplinary function with decision-making and authority occurring at the lowest possible levels in the organization. Most processes flow across the organization and between departments rather than up and down the hierarchy. Therefore quality teams are comprised of those people who are most knowledgeable about the process. The team leader could be anyone in the organization who is knowledgeable about the process under review and who has demonstrated group leadership skills, knowledge of the quality improvement process and skill in the use of quality tools.

9. **Measurement and process improvement**

   Quality management is data driven. Decisions are made based on fact, not opinions. Quality improvement tools and techniques are used by teams to create a systematic approach to problem analysis, resolution, and evaluation. The process of improvement adapted by the organization provides a consistent proactive approach to problem solving that is used by all teams. Approximately 50 to 70% of the time spent on a quality improvement process is focused on collecting and analyzing data. Team members frequently report that data analysis revealed information about root causes that differed from opinion.

10. **Recognition and reward**

    A central theme in quality management is the recognition of teams as they make process improvements. Rewards are provided for team functioning in preference to individual performance. Participation in quality improvement processes is considered an essential component of day-to-day activities and therefore regular attendance at team meetings is required and rewarded.

■ ■ ■ ■

THE PROCESS OF QUALITY MANAGEMENT

The steps in the quality improvement process are generic and reflect a basic scientific approach. These steps are:

1. select a problem on which to work
2. organize a team to work on the project
3. gather data to identify root causes of the problem
4. implement a plan of action based on the data analysis
5. continuously monitor results

Two more formalized methodologies are now being widely used to standardize the process of improvement. In the box on page 192, the sequence of steps designed by Juran (1989), a student of Deming, are shown. This model conceptualizes the process as a journey having four phases: project definition and organization, a diagnostic journey, a remedial journey, and holding the gains.

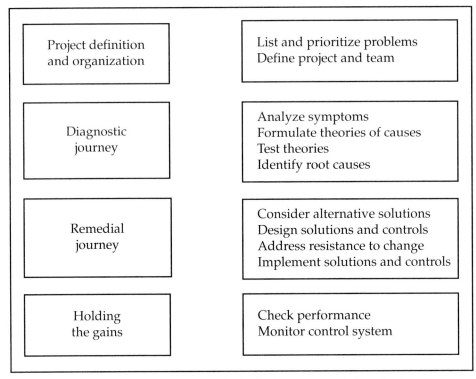

Steps in the QIP (*Source:* Plsek, Onnias, and Early. *Quality improvement tools.* Juran Institute, Inc., 1988, p. 1.)

A second commonly used model involves nine-step methodology called FOCUS-PDCA (James, 1989):

- **F**ind a process to improve.
- **O**rganize a team familiar with the process.
- **C**larify current knowledge of the process.
- **U**nderstand sources of variation.
- **S**elect the process improvement.
- **P**lan a change.
- **D**o carry out the change.
- **C**heck and observe the effects of the change.
- **A**ct, adapt or modify the plan (p. 33).

These two methodologies, and others less commonly used, are cyclical. As a process is improved the cycle begins again, either to achieve a new level of performance or to address a new quality improvement opportunity. The goal is prevention, not detection, of errors through continuous improvement.

THE TOOLS OF QUALITY MANAGEMENT

There are seven tools that are used to identify and analyze work processes and to assess outcomes (Plsek, 1990). The use of these quality tools and other techniques have gradually replaced the practice of routine auditing associated with quality assurance programs.

- A **flow chart** provides a pictorial representation of the steps in a process and how they relate to each. For example, flow-charting the process of patient admission provides each team member with a common understanding—and is usually enlightening.
- A **check sheet** is a form used to show the frequency of events and is particularly useful in showing patterns and translating opinions into facts. Recording the number of times equipment is unavailable or broken provides factual data.
- A **Pareto chart** uses data derived from a check sheet and shows the frequency of occurrence. Using the data, the Pareto, or 20-80 rule, is applied, which states that 20% of the issues account for 80% of occurrences. If a team is studying the reasons for delays in patient transport to radiology, a check sheet will identify the factors contributing to delays and a Pareto chart will determine the specific factors that are causing delays 80% of the time.
- A **cause-and-effect diagram** or **fish-bone diagram** is used to record contributing causes (methods, materials, people, equipment) of a problem. A check sheet and Pareto chart are then used to determine the "vital few" that require improvement.
- A **histogram** is a bar graph that displays the distribution of data within a category. If a team were studying the response time of the hospital's pharmacy to a narcotic order, this instrument would show the frequency with which the response time fell within a time interval.
- A **run chart** is used to display data over time, such as the length of time a nonemergent patient waits to be seen by a nurse in the emergency area.
- A **scatter diagram** is used to plot two variables to determine if a correlation exists. For example, the number of patient days per month could be plotted with the number of nursing hours to see if staffing is efficient.

FUTURE DIRECTIONS ENSURING QUALITY OF CARE

The 1990s have been and will continue to be times of rapid and unprecedented change in health care. All of the structures, functions, roles, and expectations that have defined delivery and consumption of health-care services are being challenged. Traditional hierarchical models are being reconfigured, and functions historically organized by department (such as nursing, medicine, pharmacy, laboratory) are being redefined. Concepts, such as cross-functional teams, seamless organizations, clinical treatment teams, functional work groups, empowerment, coaching, and continuous quality improvement, are central to what is being called a paradigm shift from traditional management processes to a system-wide quality management philosophy.

Total quality management is beginning to establish a foothold in the Canadian health-care system. Many hospitals have made a commitment to the initial steps of implementation and are several years into its development.

Recent revisions to the Canadian Council of Hospitals and Facilities Accreditation Survey Standards reflect a quality management focus and the consequent elimination of separate standards for departments providing patient-care services. The proposed 1994 standards focus on the facility-wide integration of clinical and support processes across departmental boundaries and the team functioning that is essential for effective and efficient implementation. Nursing has and will continue to direct quality monitoring of nursing care, thus ensuring that professional standards are maintained. Quality-monitoring instruments, which have been the underpinnings of nursing quality assurance programs, continue to be used to monitor standards of nursing practice; however, the audit process is being replaced by new methodologies associated with a total quality management philosophy. A number of information networks (organizations established for the purpose of sharing information electronically) and distance education programs are beginning to appear on a national level. The Canadian Hospital Association has developed a distance program on TQM. In Ontario a Canadian Quality Improvement (CQI) Network is being developed through which experiences, best practices, successes, and failures can be shared. Deputy ministers of health across Canada have addressed the development of a national strategy for quality in a recent draft proposal.

Notwithstanding these exciting developments, there continue to be doubts raised about the significance and applicability of quality management principles from industry to health care. Over the years many programs carried out in the name of quality, most notably guest relations initiatives,[1] have not achieved intended outcomes. Such programs failed because they were too simplistic and too narrowly focused. In the case of guest relations programs, simply telling staff to be nice to people glossed over the fact that interpersonal understanding and interaction is exceedingly complex and must be addressed in more appropriate ways. TQM has not been successfully implemented in some organizations. Lack of recognition of the cultural change that is required within the organization is frequently cited as a major barrier to change. Impatience, lack of consistency, intolerance of failure, crowded organizational agendas, and retreating to old ways of doing things are also among the many reasons for the failure of TQM in organizations. There are many factors that determine successful TQM, all of which must be addressed by leaders in the organization. These include a true cultural transformation, a well-developed quality strategy, ongoing educational programs available to all staff regardless of level in the organization, well-prepared team leaders, empowerment of front-line staff, and a quality improvement council charged with prioritizing quality issues, developing policy, and identifying a process for the identification of projects and teams. The TQM movement has occurred in the context of recessionary times that have necessitated deep cuts in health and social service spending with resultant major shifts in roles and functions of all health team members. The projected movement of the focus of care from the acute care setting to the community also is a factor influencing the future development of TQM programs.

---

[1]Guest relations initiatives were programs in the late 1980s designed to ensure that the "workers" or the staff of an organization were sensitive to the "customers" or patients. The intent was to improve patient satisfaction.

The shift from quality assurance programs to a hospital-wide quality management philosophy has shown promising results in the pursuit of cost-effective, quality care. Nurses have been at the forefront in developing and monitoring standards of practice that have provided the foundation for the future. Efforts by the nursing profession to improve patient care and public accountability by refining and enhancing quality processes will continue to be instrumental in the redesign of health care. However, it must be recognized that the management of staff and delivery of care in an acute or long-term care facility are highly complex processes involving continuous judgement calls. Such leadership cannot be reduced to a list of objectives or be captured by step-by-step, assembly-line, rigidly-applied methods. Front-line and management nurses have been victims as well as champions in the radical shifts in philosophy and approaches in the health-care environment of the 1990s, including the assessment of the quality of care.

REFERENCES

Alberta Hospital Association. (1983). *Management analysis and planning systems.* Edmonton, Alberta: Unpublished materials.

Berwick, D., Godfrey, A.B., and Roessner, J. (1990). *Curing health care: New strategies for quality improvement.* San Francisco: Jossey-Bass, Inc., Publishers.

Deming, W.E. (1986). *Out Of Crisis.* Cambridge, MA: MIT Press.

Donabedian, A. (1980). *Explorations in quality assessment and monitoring* (Vol. 1). Ann Arbor, MI: Health Administration Press.

Giovannetti, P., Kerr, J.C., Bay, K., and Buchan, J. (1986). *Measuring quality of nursing care: Analysis of reliability and validity of selected instruments—file report.* Edmonton, Alberta: Faculty of Nursing, University of Alberta.

James, B.C. (1989). *Quality management of health care delivery.* Chicago: American Hospital Association.

Juran, J.M. (1989). *Juran on planning for quality.* New York: The Free Press.

Kramer, M., and Schmalenberg, C. (1988). Magnet hospitals: Part I - Institutions of excellence. *Journal of Nursing Administration, 18*(1), 13-24.

McClure, M., Poulin, M., Sovie, M., and Wandelt, M. (1982). *Magnet hospitals: Attraction and retention of professional nurses.* Kansas City, MO: American Nurses Association.

McLaughlin, C., and Kaluzny, A. (1990). Total quality management in health: Making it work. *Health Care Management Review, 15*(3), 7-14.

Nightingale, F. (1858). *Notes on matters affecting the health, efficiency and hospital administration of the British army.* London: Harrison & Sons.

Plsek, P. (1990). A primer on quality improvement tools. In D. Berwick, A. Godfrey, and J. Roessner, *Curing health care.* (pp. 177-220). San Francisco: Jossey-Bass, Inc., Publishers.

Sahney, V., and Warden, G. (1991). The quest for quality and productivity in health services. *Frontiers of Health Service Management, 7*(4), 2-40.

Thompson, R. (1991). The six faces of quality. *Health Care Executive, 6*(2), 26-27.

Trussel, P.M., and Strand, N. (1978). A comparison of concurrent and retrospective audits of the same patients. *Journal of Nursing Administration, 8*(5), 33-38.

Ventura, M., Hageman, P.T., Slakter, M.J., and Fox, R.N. (1980). Interrater reliabilities for two measures of nursing care quality. *Research in Nursing and Health, 3*(1), 25-32.

Ventura, M., Hageman, P.T., Slakter, M.J., and Fox, R.N. (1982). Correlations of two quality of nursing care measures. *Research in Nursing and Health, 5,* 37-43.

Walton, M. (1986). *The Deming Management Method.* New York: Dodd, Mead & Company.

Whetsell, G. (1990). Total quality management. *Health Progress, 71*(8), 16-19.

CHAPTER FIFTEEN

From Shortage to Oversupply: The Nursing Workforce Pendulum

ELEANOR ROSS

The health-care system is in the midst of major reforms in Canada and internationally. The Canadian health-care system is shifting from an acute care medical model to a health-focused and community-oriented model. Total quality management, continuous quality improvement, customer-oriented or patient-focused care, cost-effectiveness, efficiency, appropriate care by appropriate health providers, decentralization and regionalization, joint ventures, and strategic alliances are the buzz words. Hospitals have downsized, closed, and\or amalgamated. Home care programs have expanded to include the concept of "hospital in the home." Nurses have lost jobs but nurses have also opened store-front clinics and nurse-run community health centres (Canadian Nurses Association [CNA], 1993a). The nurse practitioner role is being seen as an effective way to deliver high-quality health-care services in primary, secondary, and tertiary centres (CNA, 1993c; Quality of Worklife Research Unit, 1993).

Within this rapidly changing environment, nurses continue to play a major role in delivering health services and to be recognized as invaluable to the health of Canadians. The importance of recruiting and retaining nurses cannot be overemphasized. Canadians recognize that "nursing manpower shortages . . . have serious, negative repercussions on the availability of, access to and scope of health services—precisely those attributes of the Canadian Health system on which we pride ourselves" (Canadian Hospital Association [CHA], 1988). One of the most challenging tasks for nursing, hospital administrators, governments, and society is to ensure that enough nurses are available to provide care now and in the future. Many studies in Canada (Alberta Association of Registered Nurses [AARN], 1988; Hospital Council of Metro Toronto, 1988; Meltz and Marzetti,

1988; Ontario Nurses Association, 1988; Ordre des Infirmières et Infirmièrs du Québec [OIIQ], 1989; Newfoundland Ministry of Health, 1988) and in the United States (American Organization of Nurse Executives, 1988; Government of the United States, 1988) have indicated that "the remedies for the difficulties of recruitment of nurses and for the problems in salaries and working conditions depend on the recognition of the nursing profession, on the autonomy of nursing practice, on their educational requirements and on their enormous and distinctive contribution to the health system" (Ordre des Infirmières et Infirmiers du Québec, 1989).

This chapter describes trends in the employment of nurses, the supply of nurses, supply imbalances, challenges facing the profession, and recommendations for change. The discussion is based on available data, with the recognition that certain data have limitations due to a variance in definitions over time and among sources of data collection.

■■ ■■ ■■ ■■

TRENDS IN EMPLOYMENT OF NURSES

Registered nurses (RNs) continue to form the largest occupational group in Canada. The RN workforce has increased rapidly: the number of RNs increased by 33% from 1961 to 1971 and by 68% from 1971 to 1981 (see Table 15.1). A review of Registered Nurses Management Data (Statistics Canada, 1990, 1993) indicated that there were 249,673 RNs in Canada in 1988 with an estimated 227,213 employed in nursing, while in 1992 there were an estimated 263,683 registered nurses with an estimated 234,128 working in Canada.

Nurses and others believe that a large number of RNs are either inactive or working at jobs outside health care; however, studies in Canada (Meltz and Marzetti, 1988) and the United States (Aiken and Mullinix, 1987) have demonstrated that the profession of nursing has one of the highest rates of participation and retention of predominantly female occupations. Eighty percent or more are actively employed either full- or part-time. Because the profession of nursing is predominantly female, and women continue to be primarily responsible for child rearing and other household duties, an employment rate of 80% may be as high as can be anticipated. Thus it is doubtful that unemployed nurses are a potential resource for hospital employment if shortages exist.

Table 15.1 presents census data for 1971, 1981, and 1986 for occupations in nursing. While the number of RNs increased rapidly, the number of registered nurse assistants (RNAs), aides, and orderlies increased slowly and actually decreased in the 1980s. Change in the number of nursing supervisors exhibited a similar pattern. The percentage of increase for therapists and those employed in unclassified nursing and therapy occupations was higher than that of RNs.

The rapid increase in the number of RNs was due to at least four factors. The first factor was the increase in nurse employment in and out of hospitals. Some observers suggested that there was a shortage of hospital RNs, possibly due to the increased demand for nursing in home and ambulatory care. However, studies indicated that, although the number of RNs employed in the community had increased, the number employed in hospitals had also increased.

TABLE 15.1   Nurses and Other Selected Occupations in the Labour Force

	Number			Percentage Change		
	1971	1981	1986	1971 to 1981 (%)	1981 to 1986 (%)	1971 to 1986 (%)
CANADA						
Nurses, registered, graduate, and nurses-in-training	104,635	175,825	221,980	68.0	26.3	112.1
Supervisors, nursing	14,550	21,270	19,700	46.2	−7.4	35.4
Nursing assistants	27,285	44,900	35,470	64.6	−21.0	30.0
Nursing aides and orderlies	70,940	85,670	81,465	20.8	−4.9	14.8
Physical, occupational, and other therapists	6,250	13,680	18,680	118.9	36.5	198.9
Nursing and therapy occupations not otherwise classified	9,480	14,180	27,415	49.6	93.3	189.2

From Meltz, N. and Marzetti, J. (1988). *The shortage of registered nurses: An analysis in labour market context.* Toronto: Registered Nurses Association of Ontario.

Table 15.2 presents data about where nurses work; the categories are standard Statistics Canada classifications. Despite small decreases in the proportion of RNs working in hospitals over the 15 years presented, 73% of RNs were still working in hospitals in 1986. Although the proportion for related health-care institutions (nursing homes and homes for the aged) was small, the number of RNs working in this category has increased from 10,585 in 1981 to 26,790 in 1986. The number of RNs in the diagnostic and therapeutic services group (visiting home nurses) has almost tripled from 1981 to 1986. In summary, two thirds of the increase in the number of nurses employed was in hospitals and one third was outside, particularly in related health-care institutions, such as nursing homes, and in diagnostic and therapeutic services, such as visiting home nurses.

The second factor in the increase of employed RNs was the trend of reduction in the bed to RN ratio; over the years there have been increasing numbers of RNs per bed (Meltz and Marzetti, 1988). In 1977 the ratio in Ontario was 1:88; by 1985, the ratio had dropped to 1:45. This trend may have been due to the increased acuity and complexity of patient care, which required more RNs around the clock, and the shorter average length of stay. However, there is a paucity of research to support this explanation.

The third factor, which can be seen in Table 15.1, was the reduced number of assistants, aides, and orderlies. In 1971 the number of RNs (104,635) was slightly smaller than the total number of supervisors, assistants, aides, and orderlies (112,775). By 1986, however, the number of RNs (221,980) was almost double that of the other three groups (136,635). In Ontario the shift was even more dramatic: 42,740 RNs compared with 39,780 supervisors, assistants, aides, and orderlies in

TABLE 15.2 Where Nurses Work in Canada

	Number			Percentage		
	1971	1981	1986	1971 (%)	1981 (%)	1986 (%)
Community, business and personal service industries	–	–	–	–	–	–
Health and welfare services	–	–	–	–	–	–
Hospitals	75,405	133,295	162,515	79.5	75.9	73.2
Related health-care institutions	1,880	10,585	26,790	2.0	6.0	12.1
Welfare organizations	2,410	6,815	–	2.5	3.9	
Offices of physicians and surgeons	3,565	5,280	6,480	3.8	3.0	2.9
Diagnositic and therapeutic services (not elsewhere specified)	*	2,625	7,105	–	1.5	3.2
All other health and welfare	3,600*	5,090	4,075	3.8	2.9	1.8
TOTAL	86,860	163,690	206,975	91.6	93.2	93.2
Education and related services	1,390	1,900	1,895	1.5	1.1	0.9
All other community and business service	1,120	2,730	3,290	1.2	1.6	1.5
TOTAL	89,370	168,320	212,160	94.3	95.9	95.6
Manufacturing	980	1,335	1,390	1.0	0.8	0.8
Construction	40	80	15	0.0	0.0	0.0
Transportation, communication, and other utilities	90	175	295	0.1	0.1	0.1
Trade	245	425	440	0.3	0.2	0.2
Finance, insurance, and real estate	155	300	320	0.2	0.2	0.2
Public administration and defense	3,820	4,770	6,360	4.0	2.7	2.9
Agriculture, forestry, fishing, trapping, and mining	95	160	225	0.1	0.1	0.1
All industries (TOTAL)	94,795†	175,575‡	221,980§	100.0	100.0	100.0

From Meltz, N. and Marzetti, J. (1988). *The shortage of registered nurses: An analysis in a labour market context.* Toronto: Registered Nurses Association of Ontario.
*1971 data include "Diagnostic and therapeutic service" in "All other health and welfare."
†Excludes 9,835 nurses in training (because the data does not provide anything to compare them with in future years).
‡Figure differs form the total of above because of rounding.
§Includes 775 industry unspecified.

1971; 84,415 RNs compared with 33,145 in the other three groups in 1986. The number of RNs was two-and-one-half times the total number of the other three groups in Ontario (Meltz and Marzetti, 1988). RNs increased from 21.3% to 32.7% of the total employees in hospitals, whereas assistants, aides, and orderlies decreased from 20.3% to 11.87% (Meltz and Marzetti, 1988). Although this trend was explained by the fact that hospitalized patients were sicker and required more care than in years past, in reality RNs were paid a relatively low wage and were very adaptable. As Aiken and Mullinex (1987) stated:

> Registered Nurses, as versatile employees, can provide all the services for which hospitals sometimes employ nurses' aides and licensed practical nurses, and they can also often perform a wide range of other functions, including those assigned at other times to secretarial and clerical personnel, laboratory technicians, pharmacists, physical therapists, and social workers. Nurses substitute for physicians under some circumstances, and commonly assume hospital management roles after regular work hours. Thus, when nurses' relative wages are low as compared with other workers', it is advantageous for hospitals to employ them in greater numbers and in lieu of other kinds of workers. Even if nurses' wages are 20 to 30 percent higher than those of licensed practical nurses or secretaries, it may still be more economical to hire nurses, because they require little supervision and can assume responsibility for a wide range of duties. The increased demand for nurses created by low relative wages can lead to shortages . . . (p. 643).

By 1993, however, nurses salaries in Canada had increased because of pay equity legislation and negotiated salary increases. At the same time, hospitals began downsizing and a number of layoffs occurred. Layoffs included middle-management nurses, staff nurses, and registered practical nurses. Discussions began about a nurse extender, or a "generic worker", and the use of auxiliary staff to support the registered nurse. In particular, discussions began about reducing the inappropriate utilization of nurses (Aiken, 1990; Miller, 1992). The nurse practitioner role is being discussed by governments and the media as a cost-effective way of delivering health care. The implications of these changes remain unclear at this time.

The fourth factor in the increase of employed RNs was the increase in the proportion working part-time. The increase from 27% in 1970 to 43% in 1985 of the number of RNs working mostly part-time is illustrated in Table 15.3. Almost half of the RNs in Canada were working part-time in 1985. Undoubtedly, a change in the number of hours worked by almost 100,000 nurses could substantially affect the number of full-time equivalent nurses.

▬ ▬ ▬ ▬

TRENDS IN SUPPLY

The sources of RNs in Canada are recent graduates from hospital programs, community colleges, and university programs; immigrants from other countries who have had nursing education; and former RNs returning to the workforce. Because there are few studies of the career patterns of Canadian RNs, it is difficult to estimate the number that are returning to nursing (Baumgart, 1988).

TABLE 15.3   Percentage of Canadian Nurses Working Part-time*

	Females (%)			Males (%)		
	1970	1980	1985	1970	1980	1985
Nurses, registered, graduate, and nurses in training	27.6	38.9	43.4	10.6	15.8	18.2
Supervisors, nursing	13.2	23.2	26.2	3.2	8.5	7.3
Nursing assistants	17.4	38.0	45.9	6.0	18.2	20.2
Nursing aids and orderlies	23.6	39.0	45.4	8.8	21.1	31.2

From Census of Canada.
*Based on persons who worked mostly part-time during each year, by self-declaration or basic data-gathering instrument.

In 1986 87.5% of the employed RNs had graduated from Canadian schools of nursing; 9.1% had graduated from schools in other countries. Whereas nursing school programs in Canada have continued to achieve maximum enrolment, enrolment in nursing programs in the United States has dropped by 20% since 1983 (Aiken and Mullinix, 1987). However, observers in Canada indicate that a decrease in the number of applicants for nursing programs is occurring, a trend similar to that in the United States. Moreover, in the United States the shrinking applicant pools have forced nursing programs to lower admission standards (Rosenfeld, 1988). High school students interested in nursing scored lower than the national average on university entrance exams.

Interest in nursing as a career may be declining for a number of reasons, including increased career opportunities for women, rigid and capped salary structures for staff nurses, and lack of economic return for degrees in nursing. Also, the number of nursing students is decreasing due to a declining number of 18-year-olds and fewer young adults entering the workforce.

■■ ■■ ■■ ■■

SUPPLY-DEMAND IMBALANCES

Imbalances in a labour market can occur through unfilled vacancies or unemployment and underemployment (Meltz and Marzetti, 1988). Vacancies indicate an inability to recruit people for or retain them in a particular position. The vacancy rate is calculated by dividing the number of positions vacant for some period of time (e.g., 42 days) by the average number of positions and multiplying by 100 to obtain a percentage.

Although vacancy rates had been reported in some areas across Canada in the 1980s, the rates had varied tremendously. For example, in October 1989, Ontario vacancy rates varied depending on the area of specialty and the type and location of the hospital. Whereas the provincial RN vacancy rate in Ontario was 4.1%, the vacancy rate in metro Toronto was 9.1%, and the average provincial vacancy rate excluding metro Toronto was 1.7% (Ontario Ministry of Health, 1988, 1990). Critical and long-term care nursing had the highest vacancy rates at 6.3% and 6.1%, respectively. Meltz and Marzetti (1988) found that critical and long-term care consistently had high vacancy rates, and vacancy rates for chronic care, psychiatric, and active teaching hospitals were also well above the provincial average. By 1993 the vacancy rate was virtually zero because of the funding cutbacks and downsizing that occurred in the 1990s. As a result, the number of nurses entering the workforce or relocating was minimal or in casual or part-time positions only. Lack of consistent reliable data and research about unemployment of nurses makes it difficult to determine the rate of unemployment.

A low unemployment rate can indicate a shortage; a high rate can indicate a potential supply source of RNs. The data available on unemployment of nurses in Canada show consistently low rates and rates that are 50% or less of the overall unemployment rates across Canada. The data also suggest that unemployed nurses do not form a large untapped pool of workers. In 1993 7.46% of Canadians were collecting unemployment insurance benefits vs. 1.25% of Canadian nurses (CNA, 1994). The actual numbers of nurses collecting unemployment benefits were 3192 in 1991, 3862 in 1992, and 3445 in 1993 (CNA, 1994).

■ ■ ■ ■

CHALLENGES FACING THE PROFESSION

Our health-care system depends overwhelmingly on the work of women. Four out of five workers in health-related occupations are women; 4 out of 10 workers overall are women (Ryten, 1988). Because of the large number of women in health care, part-time work is more prevalent in health care than in the general economy (33% vs. 21%); part-time work is also more prevalent among women health providers than among women in the rest of the economy (39% vs. 33%) (Ryten, 1988). In 1985 only 57% of employed women graduate nurses worked full-time; 43% worked part-time (see Table 15.3).

Work patterns have continued to vary between men and women and between different health-care occupations. For example, 88% of male pharmacists and 70% of female pharmacists worked full-time, but 82% of female physicians worked full-time, and 57% of registered nurses worked full-time (Ryten, 1988). Ryten questioned whether the "proportion of women working full-time is almost an indicator of the social and economic status of its practitioners" (p. 7).

During the past 25 years women have entered traditionally male occupations, such as medicine and engineering; however, men have not entered traditionally female occupations, such as nursing, at the same rate. In the past 10 years more women than men have graduated from universities. Women have made great strides in pursuing higher education, but their participation has benefited fields of study that are not predominantly female (Ryten, 1988). Fagin and Maraldo (1988) state: "The nursing shortage will worsen, because little girls do not want to grow up to be nurses anymore. Nursing is considered women's work, and despite the strides made by the women's movement, women's work is as undervalued as ever" (p. 365).

A key characteristic of the Canadian labour market in the 1980s and the 1990s is the continually increasing demand for well-educated and skilled workers. "This trend reflects both changes in the occupational `mix' of employment toward managerial and professional jobs, which require higher levels of education and skills, as well as increases in the skill content and educational requirements of most occupations" (Feature, 1988, p. 19). This trend in the labour market is also evident in the health-care industry, in hospitals, and in the nursing profession. Nevertheless, the health-care system and hospitals have been slow to recognize and support the RNs' need for additional skills and knowledge. Campbell (1987) described nursing's challenge in today's cost-containment environment:

> Nurses provide today, as they always have, an essential element of health care. Organizational support for their work, however, remains as low as it has been in past decades. Sophisticated new management methods systematically devalue nurses' knowledge and displace their professional judgment in the process of organizing funding restraint in health care institutions. Being required to absorb a disproportionately heavy burden of cost containment must be seen as a gender-specific form of oppression of nurses. The contemporary approach to cost containment looks uncomfortably like the solution to hospital funding problems of an earlier era when nursing students provided unpaid labour (p. 463).

A review of the Canadian labour market in general and the female workforce in health care specifically identifies two trends: women are pursuing higher education but are choosing to different work patterns than men after entering the workforce. The profession of nursing has been in the forefront of these trends.

The 1990s have witnessed a more turbulent, more chaotic, and more challenging economic and health-care environment. Reorganization and decentralization are key principles in the many institutional changes. Program management (Monaghan, Alton, and Allen, 1992), case management (Lamb, Deber, Naylor, and Hastings, 1991), and patient-focused care (Moffitt, Daly, Tracey, Galloway, and Tinstman, 1993) are the trends. Although many studies have highlighted that the nursing issues are related to lack of recognition, lack of professionalism, and lack of authority for responsibility, these new management structures have not necessarily addressed the empowerment of nurses or the need for the nurse to be a professional knowledgable worker. In some structures the lack of a chief executive nurse, who articulates a vision for nursing and excellent patient care, can be seen as a continuum of the devaluing of nurses' work.

A review of the data in 1990 suggested that nurses had not been leaving the profession as often suggested, but were actually working and attempting to make changes in the system. The profession of nursing had become more vocal; illegal strikes had occurred in the 1980s. Although there was much anger and unrest among nurses causing salaries to improve, systemic change that would empower nurses has not resulted.

Every study in the 1980s in Canada (AARN, 1988; Meltz and Marzetti, 1988; Ontario Ministry of Health, 1988; Ontario Nurses Association, 1988; Ordre des Infirmières et Infirmiers du Québec, 1989; Newfoundland Ministry of Health,

1988; Registered Nurses Association of Ontario, 1988) and in the United States (American Organization of Nurse Executives, 1988; Government of the United States, 1988; Wandelt et al, 1986) had recommended structural changes that would address unsatisfactory conditions of nursing work. As a result of the nursing shortage in 1989, the Ontario Ministry of Health funded a 5-year "Quality of Worklife Unit" established jointly at the University of Toronto and McMaster University.

■■ ■■ ■■ ■■

RECOMMENDATIONS FOR CHANGE

A review of trends in the employment of nurses, supply of nurses, and supply imbalances indicates that Canada does not have a "shortage" of RNs and the level of "surplus" is difficult to assess due to a lack of consistent and reliable nursing unemployment data. In 1989 there were specialties, hospitals, and other nursing areas in Canada that had high vacancy rates; in 1993, there were no vacancies and an undetermined level of unemployment. More than 50% of RNs in Canada worked part-time. At the time of the myth of a nursing shortage, nursing leaders knew that increasing the number of nurses was not a solution. The "nursing shortage" phenomenon was acknowledged as being complex and requiring a comprehensive and collaborative approach to address the various issues. The need for government officials, hospital administrators, and nurses to collaborate was identified.

Because health care is a provincial matter in Canada, the provincial governments, in planning for health care, should have a coordinated health-care human resource strategy to address the imbalances in supply and demand for RNs. The World Health Organization and others (Bankowski and Fulop, 1987; Edmonstone, 1988; Hall, 1988; Hsu and Lovelace, 1986; Terris, 1988) have highlighted the health-care, human resource issues and have provided guidelines for human resource planning, but Canada and the provincial governments have continued to focus on single-profession and limited human resource planning. The need for a coordinated health-care, human resource plan based on the health needs of Canadian citizens cannot be overemphasized.

Governments have a responsibility to review and update legislation that will enact structural changes that give nurses the authority to participate in decision making. This legislation is needed to ensure that nurses' participation in decision making is not simply by virtue of invitation, as it is at present in most provinces. Administrators of health-care delivery organizations should preserve the RN's time for direct care of patients and families. Staffing affects quality and cost of patient care (Flood and Diers, 1988). Organizations should design and implement innovative, cost-effective staffing methods that include job restructuring, use of support personnel, flexible scheduling plans, and labour-saving technology (Aiken and Mullinix, 1987; Glandon, Colbert, and Thomasma, 1989; Donnelly, Yarbrough, and Jaffe, 1989). Also, administrators should consider nursing as a revenue centre rather than a cost centre and thus begin to value and recognize nursing's contribution to the organization (Johnson, 1989).

Management should introduce incentives to encourage experienced nurses to remain in clinical care. Wage structures and benefit packages that recognize experience and advanced education are urgently needed. As Benner and Wrubel (1989) stated:

> Like other professional groups made up predominantly of women, nurses have been viewed as short-term workers rather than career workers. . . . Nursing administrators have not uniformly treated the nurse as a knowledge worker. To cope with high turnover rates, they often set up extensive rules, guidelines, and protocols inappropriate to the level of discretionary decision making required of the professional nurse. . . . Empowering the practicing nurse is the best remedial action for the organization (pp. 387-388).

The health-care system has been a hierarchical and bureaucratically managed sytem. "The essence of a bureaucratic way of doing business is the choice for safety, caution, and control" (Block, 1990, p. 5).

As a result of the rapidity of the changes within the government's cost-cutting initiatives, many agencies have downsized not only in numbers of beds but in numbers of nurses. Meanwhile, these agencies and units are continuing to deliver care in the same traditional way of the past 30 and more years. The need for innovation, creativity, and entrepreneurial acts has never been greater. The need to maximize every nurse's skill and knowledge is paramount. To do this, the way in which nurses deliver care must be redesigned. Every unit or agency likely requires a different system of delivering care based on the needs of a specific population of patients or clients.

Nurses also have a part to play in addressing some of the issues. Each nurse must value and recognize the importance of nursing care and be able to articulate that value. Nurses should realize the strength of nursing; it includes many different groups, organizations, and specialties. External groups have suggested that a major problem in nursing is a lack of unity or unified voice. However, this may be a "blame the victim" phenomenon similar to those seen in other women's issues. Such comments by government and administrators maintain the status quo; they need not do anything about the nursing problems since they are "nursing's problem." Therefore systemic and legislative changes that would deal with worklife issues are not addressed. Nurses should take pride in their differences and recognize that some among their number perceive the "shortage" issue to be a result of worklife and workplace problems common to nurses everywhere.

Nursing must also become more politically aware. Legislation and policies that direct how decisions are made and who makes them need to be fully appreciated by all nurses. Hayes and Fritsch (1988) state:

> Nurses are part of a large, potentially powerful group, yet they often complain that they feel powerless to effect changes either in health care or in their daily practice. They are uncomfortable with the notion of power, especially political power and despite their political potential, traditionally have remained inactive. Some of this discomfort arises from nurses' socialization as women, with their inability to control their personal and professional life space, as well as from their socialization into the nursing profession itself with its affective ideals of uniformity and docility (p. 33).

▬ ▬ ▬ ▬

CONCLUSION

Data have shown that Canada does not have a shortage of RNs but there is possibly a surplus, the size and nature of which has not yet been determined. However, there are a number of problems related to working conditions, especially in hospitals, where the majority of nurses still work. The problems include inadequate financial reward, limited autonomy in clinical situations, and inability to participate in management decisions about resource allocation, which affects support services and staffing. New and expanded roles for nurses are being discussed and implemented. Collaboration between government, administrators, and nurses continues to be a priority in order to deal adequately and comprehensively with the various quality of worklife issues facing nurses in Canada today.

REFERENCES

Aiken, L. (1990). Charting the future of hospital nursing. *Image, 22*(2), 72-78.

Aiken, L., and Mullinix, C. (1987). Special report: The nurse shortage—myth or reality? *New England Journal of Medicine, 317*(10), 641-646.

Alberta Association of Registered Nurses. (1988). *Brief on concerns of registered nurses employed in Alberta hospitals and nursing homes to the Premier's Commission on Future Health Care for Albertans.* Edmonton, Alberta: The Association.

American Organization of Nurse Executives. (1988). *Proceedings of the invitational conference on the nursing shortage: Issues and strategies, October 7, 1988.* Chicago: American Hospital Association.

Bankowski, Z. and Fulop, T. (Eds). (1987). Health manpower out of balance: Conflicts and prospects. *Highlights of the XXth CIOMS Conference, Acapulco, Mexico, September 7-12, 1986.* Geneva: Council for International Organizations of Medical Sciences.

Baumgart, A.J. (1988). The nursing workforce in Canada. In A.J. Baumgart and J. Larsen (Eds.), *Canadian nursing faces the future: Development and change* (pp. 45-70). Toronto: CV Mosby Co.

Benner, P., and Wrubel, J. (1989). *The primacy of caring.* Menlo Park, CA: Addison-Wesley.

Block, P. (1990). *The Empowered Manager: Positive Political Skills at Work.* San Francisco: Jossey-Bass Publishers.

Campbell, M. (1987). Productivity in Canadian nursing: Administering cuts. In Coburn, D'Arcy, Torrance, and New (Eds.), *Health and Canadian society: Sociological perspectives* (pp. 463-475). Markham: Fitzhenry & Whiteside.

Canadian Hospital Association. (1988). *Issues concerning the Canadian health care system and its funding.* Submission to the Standing Committee on National Health and Welfare. Ottawa: Author.

Canadian Nurses Association. (1993a). *Nurses make the difference: A brief on cost-effective nursing alternatives.* Ottawa: Author.

Canadian Nurses Association. (1993b). *Leading in a time of change: The challenge for the nursing profession: A discussion paper.* Ottawa: Author.

Canadian Nurses Association. (1993c). *The nurse practitioner: A discussion paper.* Ottawa: Author.

Canadian Nurses Association. (1994). Get active! Ensuring employment in the midst of change. *CNA Today, 4*(1), 1.

Donnelly, L.J., Yarbrough, D., and Jaffe, H. (1989). Organizational management systems decrease nursing costs. *Nursing Management, 20*(7), 20-21.

Edmonstone, J. (1988). Managing the manpower resource: The nature of the problem. *Hospital and Health Services Review, 84*(1), 13-15.

Fagin, C.M., and Maraldo, P.J. (1988). Feminism and the nursing shortage: Do women have a choice? *Nursing and Health Care, 9*(7), 364-367.

The changing nature of the Canadian labour market: The increased importance of education and training (1988). *Quarterly Labour Market and Productivity Review,* Winter, 17-23.

Flood, S.D., and Diers, D. (1988). Nurse staffing, patient outcomes and cost. *Nursing Management, 19*(5), 34-43.

Glandon, G.L., Colbert, K.W., and Thomasma, M. (1989). Nursing delivery models and RN mix: Cost implications. *Nursing Management, 20*(5), 30-33.

Government of the United States. (1988). *Secretary's Commission on Nursing: Final report.* 1(12).

Hall, T. (1988). Guidelines for health workforce planners. *World Health Forum, 9*, 409-413.

Hayes, E., and Fritsch, R. (1988). An untapped resource: The political potential of nurses. *Nursing Administration Quarterly, 13*(1), 33-39.

Hospital Council of Metro Toronto. (1988). *Report of the HCMT Nursing Manpower Task Force.* Toronto: The Council.

Hsu, D., and Lovelace, J.C. (1986). Health human resources in Canada. *Educ Med Salud, 20*(3), 351-362.

Johnson, M. (1989). Perspectives on costing nursing. *Nursing Administration Quarterly, 14*(1), 65-71.

Lamb, M., Deber, R., Naylor, C.D., and Hastings, J. (1991). *Managed care in Canada: The Toronto Hospital's proposed Comprehensive Health Organization.* Ottawa: Canadian Hospital Association Press.

Meltz, N., and Marzetti, J. (1988). *The shortage of registered nurses: An analysis in a labour market context.* Toronto: Registered Nurses Association of Ontario.

Miller, J. (1992). Use of unlicensed assistive personnel in acute care settings. *Journal of Nursing Administration, 22*(12), 12-13.

Moffitt, G.K., Daly, P.R., Tracey, L., Galloway, M., and Tinstman, T.C. (1993). Patient-focused care: Key principles to restructuring. *Hospital and Health Services Administration, 38*(4), 509-521.

Monaghan,B.J., Alton, L., and Allen, D. (1992). Transition to program management. *Leadership in health services, 1*(5), 33-37.

Newfoundland Ministry of Health. (1988). *Report of the Advisory Committee on Nursing Workforce.* St. John's, Newfoundland: The Ministry.

Ontario Ministry of Health. (1988). *Report on nursing manpower.* Toronto: Advisory Committee on Nursing Manpower.

Ontario Ministry of Health. (1990). *Report of the hospital nurse staffing survey: October, 1989.* Toronto: Health Manpower Planning Section/Policy Development and Coordination Division.

Ontario Nurses Association. (1988). *The nursing shortage in Ontario.* Toronto: The Goldfarb Corporation.

Ordre des Infirmières et Infirmiers du Québec. (1989). *Hypertension: An urgent need for action.* Montreal: The Ordre.

Quality of Worklife Research Unit (September, 1993). *Utilization of nurse practitioners in Ontario: A discussion paper requested by the Ontario Ministry of Health;* (Working paper series 93-4). McMaster University and the University of Toronto, Hamilton, Ontario: Author.

Registered Nurses Association of Ontario. (1988). *Sorry no care available due to nursing shortage: A prescription for reforming human resource planning in health care.* Toronto: The Association.

Rosenfeld, P. (1988). *Nursing student census with policy implications.* New York: National League for Nursing.

Ryten, E. (1988). *Women as deliverers of health care.* Unpublished speech presented at the Canadian Association of University Schools of Nursing Annual Conference, University of Windsor, Windsor, Ontario: June, 1988.

Statistics Canada. (1993). *Registered nurses management data, 1992.* Health Ottawa: Health Manpower Statistics Section, Health Division.

Statistics Canada. (1990). *Registered nurses management data, 1988.* Health Ottawa: Health Manpower Statistics Section, Health Division.

Terris, M. (1988). Meeting the needs for health workers: Proportions, prerogatives, and priorities. *Journal of Public Health Policy, 9*(3), 309-318.

Wandelt, M. et al. (1986). Why nurses leave nursing and what can be done about it. *American Journal of Nursing, 81*(1), 72-77.

CHAPTER SIXTEEN

Political Awareness in Nursing

JANET ROSS KERR

A lthough most Canadians report that they place great value upon the health-care system that has developed over the past half century as a result of federal enabling legislation, the philosophic bases of the system are being widely questioned, spurred along by a mounting federal/provincial debt as a result of continuous budget deficits. The system is thus undergoing extensive review and changes are being implemented rapidly in some parts of the country. More sophisticated methods of care and treatment, high technology solutions to previously unsolvable problems, and increased specialization in the health professions have led to a need to prioritize health-care needs and identify the nature and types of health-care services that are and can be made available. The fact that physicians have continued to be the sole gatekeepers to the health-care system has led to continuing problems for those who wish to access the system, and to higher costs than would be incurred if nonphysician health-care professionals were used more effectively in the system. Nurses in particular have historically been underused; a number of Canadian studies have demonstrated the effectiveness of services provided by nurses (Chambers, Bruce-Lockhart, Balck, Sampson, and Burke, 1977; Hoey, McCallum, and LePage, 1982; Ramsay, McKenzie, and Fish, 1982). Compensation for physicians on a fee-for-service basis is considered to be an important issue in the underutilization of nurses.

The health-care system is "big business" in Canada, with more than 9.9% of the Gross Domestic Product expended for health (Health Canada, 1994). Health expenditures are almost entirely in the public sector due to the institution of national health insurance operated by provincial governments under public auspices. Any public sector activity that involves substantial expenditure of tax dollars engenders considerable debate and competition among providers of the service. This is obvious in the health-care arena, where the various health-care professions are competing to increase their "share of the pie." Physicians have been extraordinarily successful in increasing income earned for services provided. Physicians' incomes have increased considerably over the past half century; the substantial increase attests to the success physicians have had in the political arena. Nurses have been demonstrating increasing ability to argue for proportionately increased compensation for their services, and significant gains have been made in the past 15 years.

The fact that nursing is and has been a sex-segregated profession since its inception in Canada must be considered a factor. Historically members of the profession have had to struggle to gain appropriate recognition, respect, and remuneration for their services. Increased awareness of the need for respect for women's rights has occurred gradually over the past century; important gains have been made in the past 3 decades. The parallel rise of the women's movement and unionism in nursing, which began in the 1960s, has been a significant development; members of the profession are challenging the status quo assiduously and assertively, striving for higher salaries and better working conditions. Nurses have gradually gained understanding of the processes and skills involved in influencing others, becoming more powerful and exercising more control over the factors that influence their working lives.

Although nurses are commonly thought of as political novices, Krampitz (1985) has noted, "the actions of nurses as political activists are well recorded in the profession's proud history" (p. 10). In the early history of Canadian nursing, Jeanne Mance could be considered a political activist *par excellence;* she raised and sustained support for her hospital in New France. Florence Nightingale's accomplishments as well are legendary and, "as a reformer and political activist she helped establish a new attitude toward the contributions of nurses in a military environment and the education of women" (Dock [cited in Krampitz, 1985, p. 10]). Florence Nightingale's skill as a researcher was impressive, and her interpretation of the statistics she collected led to important and lasting changes in the organization of the health services of the British Army (Nightingale, 1858). She demonstrated the positive effect of good nursing on the health of soldiers; the principles apply to health care in general. There were important offshoots from her work, for the British populace and indeed for people in other nations, as the Nightingale model of nursing was carried far afield.

Nurses in Canada argued strongly between 1900 and 1922 for legislation encompassing registration for nurses. This campaign was successful and every province had such legislation by the end of 1922. More recent political activity by nurses was also successful; the lobbying carried out by the Canadian Nurses Association (CNA) for the Canada Health Act of 1984 resulted in an amendment to the Act, after it was tabled in Parliament, that permitted federal funding for "health practitioners." This legislation also made it possible for a provincial health plan to fund services of nurses or other health professionals on a direct reimbursement basis, as the services of physicians and dental surgeons had been financed since the Medical Care Act of 1968 was passed.

■■ ■■ ■■ ■■

THE IMPORTANCE OF DEVELOPING POLITICAL AWARENESS

The term *politics* is used in many different ways. For some it may stimulate images of smoke-filled rooms, devious dealings, or power in the hands of a few.

For others the images have a different and more generic meaning. Maraldo (1985) noted, "politics is ubiquitous, occurring wherever two or more people are gathered" (p. 81). Among the earliest philosophers who attempted to understand the relationship between politics and people were Aristotle and Plato. Plato discussed the development of political leaders in some depth in *The Republic*, describing the qualities of leadership. Maraldo (1985) observes, "Aristotle's and Plato's views of politics as intrinsic to human behaviour have not been heeded over the years" (p. 82); neither the ways that political leaders worked nor the factors that shaped political behaviour have been studied to any extent.

Politics can be viewed as the art of influencing another person. In practical terms, political activity means influencing for the purpose of allocating scarce resources wisely. In the health-care arena, there is new realization of the limits to growth; this effectively means limits placed on care and treatment. Expensive, high-technology health care for all is not affordable in the Western World. Developed countries are learning what developing countries have known all along—that decisions must be made about health-care priorities, and that not everyone can be the recipient of expensive care and treatment. Certain individuals will be responsible for deciding how to allocate the available resources, and others will have a political responsibility to provide the reasons for allocating resources in one way or another. As Maraldo (1985) noted, "the truth of the matter, however, is that everyone who functions in society must be, to some extent, a political animal. There is no escaping politics in any arena" (p. 81).

Many nurses recognize the importance of developing political skills, realizing that these skills are as important on the nursing unit as they are in other spheres of social activity where decisions must be made. As Mason and McCarthy (1985) have stated, "the ultimate reason for enhancing the nurse's political power, be it in the workplace, community, government, or professional organization, is to improve the health care that patients receive" (p. 38). There tends to be more awareness of the importance of political factors in the development of policy than in working or other everyday situations. Where service is the primary activity, the politics of patient care may be less visible, but they are important and essential to good care.

Nurses as a group have sometimes expressed a sense of powerlessness. Many nurses believe that nursing is low in the health-care hierarchy in terms of power and influence. They adopt an indifferent approach believing that expressing their views will not be useful because they will not be heard. A nurse who adopts such an approach will not be able to argue for the needs of patients. These negative attitudes are based on false assumptions about society; fortunately, more nurses are taking an active interest in political activity and in learning how to influence others. Although professional groups have always recognized the value of lobbying for their objectives and using political skills to advantage, they are now attempting to educate members about developing political skills to enhance success in achieving objectives.

Nurses may have to work harder than other professional groups to establish a power base. There is strength in numbers, and that is an important factor where nursing is concerned because nurses are the largest group of health-care professionals. However, nurses also have the lowest level of academic preparation among the health-care professions. Less than 15% of practising nurses in Canada hold a baccalaureate degree; in other health professions the baccalaureate degree is usually a minimum requirement for entry to practice. In addition, nurses have struggled with an image of subservience, partially because nursing has been sex stereotyped. Currently the proportion of the profession that is female is greater than 96.9% (Canadian Centre for Health Information, 1992). The medical profession on the other hand has historically been male dominated, but this is rapidly changing. In some medical schools more than 50% of the students are women; however, the sex-stereotype in nursing is deeper, and men are not yet entering the nursing profession in increased proportions—certainly not at the rate women are entering traditionally male-dominated professions. Nevertheless, many changes are occurring because of the women's movement, increased recognition of human rights, and increased recognition of nursing's contribution to health care. These factors bode well for nursing in the future, as arguments for restructuring and policy change within the health-care system are likely to engender considerable interest and support.

▬ ▬ ▬ ▬

CREATING POLITICAL AWARENESS: UNDERSTANDING THE FUNDAMENTALS OF POLITICAL ACTION

Understanding the formal and informal systems in the workplace is a basic necessity for effective political action. By learning how to work within these systems, nurses can greatly enhance the achievement of their goals. Although it is essential to understand both, comprehending the informal structures and processes of an organization is a more difficult and less defined task than understanding formal ones. It is also important to develop good communication skills, working with other individuals in the organization to understand their roles and functions and the problems they face. Those wielding a substantial amount of power within the organization should be identified as key individuals, and the development of working relationships with these individuals is essential. Informal groups within the organization may also be important; although they may be organized around activities unrelated to the organization, they may represent networks for exchange of information. Social contacts may also be helpful in developing useful channels for political activity.

Talbott and Nichols (1985) have referred to some principles for political action:

- Look at the big picture
- Do your homework
- Nothing ventured, nothing gained
- Get a toe in the door
- Quid pro quo
- Walk a mile in another's moccasins
- Strike while the iron is hot
- Read between the lines
- Half a loaf is better than none
- Rome was not built in a day (p. 157)

There is no substitute for understanding how an organization works or for thinking carefully about the nature and scope of problems and how they might be solved. Nurses must be risk takers; no gains will be made if no action is taken. Timing is essential to achieving a goal. It is necessary to understand all sides of the question to develop a more effective strategy, and negotiation and compromise may be required in the final solution. A high degree of communication skill is required.

▬ ▬ ▬ ▬

INTERPERSONAL COMMUNICATION

The most important factor in the political arena is effective interpersonal communication. Because politics involves influencing others, effective relationships are essential. It is impossible to influence others if interpersonal activity is not positive and dynamic. Vance (1985) has stated, "the exercise of influence involves three components, or the 'three C's' of political influence: communication, collectivity, and collegiality" (p. 166). In this hierarchy, communication is the fundamental skill, as all of the other techniques build upon it. By communicating effectively with others, goals may be enhanced and attained. Joining with others in pursuit of common goals is a very effective technique and is also recognized as an effective political strategy. It is important to work cooperatively and willingly with others in pursuing collective goals. Approaching others with respect and understanding increases the possibility that political activity will be enhanced and more effective.

Although communication is important on every level, its fundamental tenets remain the same. Attention has recently focused on networking, or joining together with others to achieve common goals. This can be accomplished in many ways. Networking is an important political strategy and it may be personally rewarding. Nursing curricula usually contain courses designed to enhance interpersonal effectiveness. Because nurses are in close contact with patients, preparation in the area of interpersonal communication is essential to good patient care. This is a subject that is emphasized in baccalaureate degree programs.

▬ ▬ ▬ ▬

DEVELOPING A BASE OF SUPPORT

Consolidating and developing a base of support often takes considerable skill and time. Credibility must be established, and the desire to work in the best interests of the organization and its goals must be demonstrated. In professional associations this means working with the public interest in mind. It is important to demonstrate that clear and careful thought preceded the development of a campaign for support on a particular issue, as this may be a powerful factor in convincing potential supporters that the issue is worth supporting. As noted previously, there is power in numbers and nursing has a great advantage in this respect. The campaign is more likely to be successful if many people are committed to working toward the goal. Nurses have not always recognized the strength in their numbers; they have only mobilized group support on the most crucial of issues. Many nursing organizations now recognize this potent force and are using its power to advantage.

■ ■ ■ ■

THE PURSUIT OF GOALS

Effective political strategy is a labour-intensive process that requires clear thinking and the ability to recognize factors, processes, and actors of importance. Identifying an issue or problem is important. Its relative importance must be measured against that of other issues or problems that arise. Action cannot be taken in all matters, so it is important to *choose one's issues*. There is always some cost in pursuing a problem to its conclusion in the political sphere, and the possible negative consequences must be weighed against the positive benefits that may result. Bowman (1985) has referred to this process as "risk analysis. The risks and payoff of challenging an issue must be measured in the goal-setting process. What will be lost if the issue is not pursued? What will be gained if it is? How certain are those losses or gains? What are the short term and long term effects of either choice?" (p. 202). Analysis of the issue is essential to determine if pursuing the issue is reasonable. Once a decision has been made to pursue a particular goal, additional analysis determines what other resources might be helpful.

The CNA has historically taken courses of action designed to result in maximum benefit to the health of consumers. Recently the CNA addressed the Standing Committee on Social Affairs, Science and Technology of the Senate of Canada, urging them to "refocus the system to a better balance of illness care, rehabilitation, prevention and promotion" and discussing "effective utilization of all our resources" (CNA Connection, 1990, pp. 8, 10). The action the CNA took relative to offensive advertising before the opening of Expo '86 in Vancouver is an example of an organization identifying a specific issue, then moving quickly toward effecting some change. A federal government advertisement encouraging attendance portrayed a group of nurses in chorus-girl-type roles expressing the merits of attending the Exposition. The CNA, on receiving complaints from nurses as the first ads were aired, moved swiftly through the Executive to protest the negative portrayal of nursing. The protest was made at the federal cabinet level, the matter was dealt with quickly, and the controversial ads were swiftly withdrawn.

Because every issue is different, a plan of action must be outlined for the benefit of all those involved in the campaign. It is important to determine how the issue will be dealt with, both formally and informally. It is possible that many avenues will need to be taken to argue for or against the issue of concern; these need to be outlined at the outset and revised as necessary. One person alone may be able to make the case for change, or it may be necessary for an entire organization to be involved. This was the case in 1982 and 1983, when the Alberta Association of Registered Nurses lobbied for the passage of a new Registered Nurses Act incorporating mandatory registration. The entire membership was asked to send letters of support to members of the Legislative Assembly and the Cabinet. Ultimately, the fact that so many of the members got involved influenced the legislators to decide to move forward with the Act.

Bowman (1985) refers to professional strategies, public strategies, and procedural strategies as categories that can be considered when plans are being developed to pursue an issue. A contemporary issue of interest across the country is legalization of midwifery in Canada. Although midwifery developed from its roots in nursing and currently the vast majority of midwives are nurses, midwives have, through extensive lobbying, been able to convince legislators and the general public that a separate and independent profession is in the public interest. Legislation to legalize midwifery has been passed in Ontario, British Columbia, and Alberta, and an infrastructure is emerging to support the regulation of the profession and the development of educational programs to prepare midwives.

■ ■ ■ ■

BENEFITS OF ENHANCED POLITICAL AWARENESS

Much can be gained by developing a cadre of politically skilled, professional nurses. Rodger (1993) has stated that, "Our challenge is to exercise our power and influence and use the political process to help bring about a major change in the delivery of nursing services to the society" (p. 25). There are important public implications for such activity, both at the individual and collective levels. The priorities of patient care are subject to politics at all levels. Nurses spend more time with patients than any other group of health-care professionals and are in an excellent position to understand, appreciate, and argue for consideration of their needs and concerns. Nurses must also continue to work for optimum conditions in the workplace because the quality of nursing care will be enhanced through the pursuit of such a goal. In collective bargaining, political skills are essential tools that will make the process a smoother and more satisfying one for all concerned. Collaboration between nurses and other health-care professionals can do much to enhance the effectiveness of nurses. Most important of all, understanding the political process and recognizing political strategy is an important first step in developing the ability to influence others. Zander (1985) has summed this up: "Application of the tools of organizational analysis, . . . together with change strategies, including heightened political sensitivity, will enable nurses to create magnetic environments" (p. 239).

REFERENCES

Bowman, R.A. (1985). Recognizing, developing, and pursuing an issue. In D.J. Mason and S.W. Talbott (Eds.). *Political action handbook for nurses* (pp. 196-204). Menlo Park, CA: Addison-Wesley.

Canadian Centre for Health Information. (1992). *Registered Nurses Management Data*. Ottawa: Statistics Canada, pp. 18, 20.

CNA Connection. (1990). *The Canadian Nurse, 86*(4), 8-10.

Chambers, L.W., Bruce-Lockhart, P., Balck, D.P., Sampson, E., and Burke, M. (1977). A controlled trial of the impact of the family practice nurse on volume, quality, and cost of rural health service. *Medical Care, 15*(12), 971-981.

Health Canada. (1994). Preliminary estimates of health expenditures in Canada. *Provincial-Territorial Summary Report, 1987-1991*. Ottawa: Health Information Division, Policy and Consultation Branch, Health Canada.

Hoey, J.R., McCallum, H.P., and LePage, E.M. (1982). Expanding the nurse's role to improve preventive service in an outpatient clinic. *Canadian Medical Association Journal, 127*(1), 27-28.

Krampitz, S.D. (1985). Historical overview of nursing and politics. In D.J. Mason and S.W. Talbott (Eds.). *Political action handbook for nurses* (pp. 10-22). Menlo Park, CA: Addison-Wesley.

Maraldo, P. (1985). Politics is people. In D.J. Mason and S.W. Talbott (Eds.). *Political action handbook for nurses* (pp. 81-87). Menlo Park, CA: Addison-Wesley.

Mason, D.J., and McCarthy, A.M. (1985). Politics of patient care. In D.J. Mason and S.W. Talbott (Eds.). *Political action handbook for nurses* (pp. 38-52). Menlo Park, CA: Addison-Wesley.

Nightingale, F. (1858). *Notes on matters affecting the health, efficiency and hospital administration of the British Army.* London: Harrison & Sons.

Ramsay, J.A., McKenzie, J.K., and Fish, D.G. (1982). Physicians and nurse practitioners: Do they provide equivalent health care? *American Journal of Public Health, 72*(1), 55-57.

Rodger, G.L. (1993). Nurses and the political process. *AARN Newsletter, 49*(2), 24-25.

Talbott, S.W., and Nichols, B. (1985). Political analysis: structures and processes. In D.J. Mason and S.W. Talbott (Eds.). *Political action handbook for nurses* (pp. 143-164). Menlo Park, CA: Addison-Wesley.

Vance, C.N. (1985). Political influence: Building effective interpersonal skills. In D.J. Mason and S.W. Talbott (Eds.). *Political action handbook for nurses* (pp. 165-180). Menlo Park, CA: Addison-Wesley.

Zander, K. (1985) Analyzing your workplace. In D.J. Mason and S.W. Talbott (Eds.). *Political action handbook for nurses* (pp. 227-239). Menlo Park, CA: Addison-Wesley.

CHAPTER SEVENTEEN

The Organization and Financing of Health Care: Issues for Nursing

JANET ROSS KERR

A lthough nursing is an essential health-care service and represents one of the largest professional components of the health-care budget, health-care financing is an area that is generally not well understood by nurses. The study of health-care financing, including the financing of nursing services, is generally left to the health-care economists and health administrators, and few curricula in schools of nursing have attempted to address the subject. However, it is important for nurses to understand how the system operates, because health-care financing can affect the nature of nursing services and the form in which they can be offered. Comprehending the complex system of arrangements for federal-provincial cost-sharing and knowing how nursing is affected is necessary if nurses are to exercise their professional responsibility to interact with and influence government, the public, and other health professions in areas of practice, education, and research. It also provides essential background for nurses in arguing for health-care reform.

■ ■ ■ ■

THE HEALTH-CARE SYSTEM: A COMPARATIVE VIEW

Health-care financing in Canada shifted from the private to the public sector in 1957. Since the 1867 passage of the British North America Act at the time of Confederation, responsibility for health has rested with the provinces. The Constitution Act of 1982 confirmed the historical division of powers between the federal government and the provinces. Canada's arrangement is different from that of other nations with centralized health-care systems where authority for health-care is vested in the federal government. The United Kingdom (UK), France, and Sweden are examples of countries where responsibility for health care is vested in the federal government. Wallace (1980) observed that:

The fathers of Confederation clearly thought they were assigning the provinces the less important and inexpensive functions of government, among which education, hospitals, charities and municipal institutions were then reasonably numbered. They could scarcely have foreseen the way in which time would reverse their expectations, so that the costliness of the responsibilities laid upon the provinces subsequently increased to the point where it was financially impossible to defray them. Within thirty years after Confederation social and economic conditions had so altered that public opinion was demanding government action on matters held in 1867 to be primarily personal and of no concern to the state (p. 27).

The constitutional division of authority and responsibility for health care also provides a partial explanation for the length of time it took to implement a national health insurance program. Because jurisdictional responsibility for health lies within the provinces, achievement of uniform changes to benefit the entire country is a difficult task. Over the years, federal interest in this sector of provincial responsibility has been high because of the value placed on health and its importance in the life of society. The greater taxing power of the federal government in a publicly funded system has led the provinces to look to the government for help in financing the operation of the system.

The United States has not yet implemented a national health insurance program, although as a campaign platform in the 1992 election, President Bill Clinton pledged to bring in health legislation so the U.S. population would be covered by universal health-care insurance. The U.S. health reform debate is underway. However, the passage of legislation does not promise to be easily accomplished. Although the division of powers between federal and state/provincial governments in relation to health are similar in the U.S. and Canada, members of one party are not required to vote as a block in the U.S. House of Representatives and the U.S. Senate. This means that lobbying by interested individuals and groups must be directed toward individual members of these bodies as well as those who hold the reins of party power. The achievement of unanimity on a matter of national importance, such as a national plan of health insurance, is clearly more difficult because of the power held by individual elected members. These considerations, along with a value system centred on individual responsibility and free enterprise, explain why a form of Medicare in the United States had only been achieved for those over 65 years of age prior to the Clinton initiatives.

In contrast, the United Kingdom introduced its National Health Service in 1948, providing a model of health-care financing for Commonwealth countries in particular. There were differences, however, in the national health plan adopted by the United Kingdom and that introduced in Canada. When legislation to establish Medicare in Canada was introduced, the approach was not to restructure the existing health-care system. The legislation simply was an overlay on the existing system, providing a framework for financing it. A two-tiered system of health-care financing has emerged more recently in the United Kingdom, the inefficiencies and shortcomings of the public system giving rise to a private one for those of means, complete with third-party insurance.

■ ■ ■ ■

THE DEVELOPMENT OF A NATIONAL SYSTEM OF MEDICARE: A HISTORICAL PERSPECTIVE

Although universal health insurance was first suggested in 1919, it took a long time to implement the system. Taylor (1978) has commented that:

> Our heritage of the Elizabethan Poor Law had placed responsibility for the sick poor on local government, but many cities, towns and especially rural municipalities in Canada quickly reached the point of near or actual bankruptcy from the combination of declining revenues and expanding relief payments for food, clothing and shelter. Medical care, except in the direst emergency conditions, was a luxury that only few individuals or municipalities could afford (p. 4).

The continuing financial problems facing hospitals during the early decades of this century have been reported and analyzed. The struggle was greater in the voluntary hospital, but even among municipally owned institutions, the reluctance to provide adequate funds made financing a continuing nightmare for trustees and administrators (Agnew, 1974, p. 149). During the Depression years, a difficult situation deteriorated further until many hospitals had large deficits. In the 1930s, only 40% to 50% of the patient days in public hospitals had been paid in full by 55% to 60% of the patients. Eight percent of patients paid for part of their hospital stay, and one third of those remaining were unable to pay their bill (Agnew, 1974, p. 151). In addition, "a fairly sharp division was usually drawn between paying and non-paying patients" (Agnew, 1974, p. 153), and extra payment for private accommodation was used to help offset deficits.

Physicians and professional nurses also experienced difficulties during this period. Since the proportion of patients unable to pay medical bills had escalated, many physicians had a difficult time financially. In Saskatchewan "many in the medical profession . . . had suffered economic disaster along with the crest of the population during the 1930s, and many physicians received payments of $50 or $75 per month from the Saskatchewan Relief Commision" (Report of the Saskatchewan Department of Public Health, 1933, p. 7 [as cited in Taylor, 1978, p. 83]). Nurses also felt the pinch, and graduate nurses' positions in private duty nursing evaporated with the stock market crash. In Calgary,

> General Hospital graduates, unable to get positions as special nurses, were glad to be taken on the hospital staff at a monthly salary of thirty dollars in addition to room and board. Many supervisory nurses, already on staff, had to take substantial salary reductions as the city slashed and re-slashed its hospital budget in a desperate attempt to make ends meet with the reduced taxes it was able to collect (Agnew, 1974, p. 150).

Beginning in the 1920s, a number of small prepayment plans for hospital care were developed to provide for hospital services. Care was prepaid for all who were covered by the plan. There were many factors that encouraged thinking about using a system of insurance on a wider scale to create a health-care system that would eliminate hardships for persons who became ill, allow hospitals to operate on other than a hand-to-mouth basis, and ensure that health-care professionals received remuneration for services provided. The Depression, as well as the World War II years, were difficult for Canadians; in 1937, Canada ranked seventeenth in infant mortality among developed nations (Advisory Committee on Health Insurance, 1943, [as cited in Taylor, 1978, p. 5]). The views of politicians were also an important factor, particularly those of the party leader. Taylor (1978) commented on this reference to the views of Prime Minister MacKenzie King:

> In the initiation of any government proposal, the personal objectives and commitment of the party leader who occupies the position of premier or prime minister at a particular juncture in history is frequently the most crucial factor in the decision to act or not to act . . . . But that his views were a powerful force in incorporating health insurance and other social security measures in the post-war reconstruction proposals is clear (pp. 9-10).

EARLY HEALTH INSURANCE PLANS

Commercial insurance companies began developing plans in the 1930s, and publicly sponsored arrangements for prepaid care were initiated by municipalities, hospitals, and regional groups soon after. The first known voluntary plan for prepayment of hospital care in Canada was the Edmonton Group Hospitalization Plan, introduced by the four major general hospitals in that city in 1934. Initial efforts to establish a Blue Cross Plan in the province had met resistance from some institutions, so the four hospitals started their own small plan. This plan was extended to the rest of Alberta in 1948 as a Blue Cross Plan under the sponsorship of the provincial hospital association. Hospitalization benefits were provided when needed as prepaid fees for those who enrolled (Agnew, 1974). The first province-wide Blue Cross Plan in Canada, initiated in 1937, was created by an act of the Manitoba Legislature and administered by the Manitoba Hospital Service Association. Similar plans were implemented in other provinces: Ontario (1941), Quebec (1942), and Nova Scotia, New Brunswick, Prince Edward Island, and British Columbia (1943) (Agnew, 1974). Many of the plans eventually added medical and surgical services to the plans they offered. Because different authorities were responsible for developing and maintaining plans offered in different provinces, there was considerable variation in benefits from plan to plan. The basis of most of the plans was payment of premiums by enrolees. A substantial segment of the Canadian population was not covered by any form of prepaid insurance due to ineligibility for plans limited to specific groups of people, or inability to pay the required premium.

THE ROAD TO NATIONAL HEALTH INSURANCE

Federal involvement in financing health care had been discussed since the Honourable W.L. MacKenzie King developed a proposal for health insurance in the platform of the Liberal Party in the election of 1919. In 1929 the standing committee on industrial and international relations of the House of Commons recommended that, "with regard to sickness insurance, the Department of Pensions and National Health be requested to initiate a comprehensive survey of the field of public health, with special reference to a national health programme"

(Agnew, 1974, p. 165). The report was approved in 1933, and in 1935 the Employment and Social Insurance Act provided for collecting information and advising groups in provinces planning a health insurance program. Because the Act was declared unconstitutional in the courts, it was not until 1942 that a federal committee on health insurance was established to study the issues. At that time the Canadian Medical Association (CMA) endorsed the principles of health insurance, and although it preferred fee for service as the method of payment for medical services, it indicated that a capitation, or salary method of remunerating physicians, might also be needed.

A federal-provincial conference, convened in 1945, "proposed universal health insurance with federal-provincial cost sharing" and "produced a model draft health-care bill for the provinces" (Vayda, Evans, and Mindell, 1979, p. 218). Due to concern that such legislation would interfere with provincial autonomy and that Canada's health-care facilities and personnel were inadequate to carry the load that health insurance would bring, the legislation failed. The province of Saskatchewan, under the leadership of Premier T.C. Douglas, instituted a hospital insurance plan financed entirely by the province in 1947. Payment of premiums was basic to this plan and every Saskatchewan resident was required to register for it. The plan was subsidized from general revenues, and in 1948 the provincial sales tax was increased to help finance it. In 1949 a similar program was established in British Columbia.

■■ ■■ ■■ ■■

FEDERAL LEGISLATION FOR HEALTH-CARE FINANCING

The federal government's first foray into health-care financing occurred in 1948 through the National Health Grants Program. Assistance was provided for hospital construction, public and mental health programs, and professional training to "gear up" for hospital insurance. At a federal-provincial conference held in 1955, an agreement was reached about the details of a national hospital insurance plan; the details were translated into legislation in the form of the Hospital Insurance and Diagnostic Services Act of 1957. Provinces were given the option to join, with the federal government paying "an amount equal to 25% of its own per capita cost (less authorized charges) plus 25% of the national per capita cost multiplied by the number of insured persons" (Brown, 1980, p. 523). Programs were required to provide universal coverage, portability of coverage from province to province, comprehensive coverage for all in-hospital care in general and certain other designated care services, and public, nonprofit administration of plans was mandatory (LeClair, 1975). Administration of the plans was to be carried out by the individual provinces. All provinces had accepted the terms of the Act by 1961 (Vayda, Evans, and Mindell, 1979).

The next struggle was to include medical care in the insurance plan. The Royal Commission on Health Services of 1964 emphasized the importance of including medical care in the national health insurance program. Again it took many years to reach agreement on the nature and form of the legislation, and the federal program was preceded by a program developed by the province of Saskatchewan (1962). Physicians opposed the Saskatchewan plan, and the 1962

Saskatchewan physicians' strike of 23 days will long be remembered. In 1968 the federal Medical Care Act was established to provide reimbursement to provincial health insurance plans for physicians' services. This was provided under the same cost-sharing conditions as assistance for hospital services. Again there was opposition from physicians, who feared interference in the physician/patient relationship and the possibility that the fee-for-service system of remuneration for physicians would be abandoned as the plan was implemented. New Brunswick joined in 1971 and the provisions of the Act then applied to all provinces.

In the 1970s the federal government became concerned about escalation in health-care costs. With the unlimited 50/50 cost-sharing arrangement, there was no ceiling on the federal share of health-care cost reimbursement. As the federal deficit increased, the government passed the Fiscal Arrangements and Established Programs Financing Act of 1977. The provisions of this Act, which applied to hospital care, medical care, and postsecondary education, provided for block funding, reducing the federal contribution to health care to 25%, with additional federal contributions based on increases in the Gross National Product. Federal income taxes were decreased to allow the provinces to increase their taxes to offset the federal reductions. For the first time funding was provided for extended and home care. In 1982 the federal government changed the method of calculating contributions through amendments to the health-care financing legislation of 1977. This meant that provinces received considerably less federal assistance than before. The federal government responded to provincial objections to decreased funding by reiterating that decreases in federal income taxes had left room for increases in provincial income taxes.

The federal government was disturbed by the increasing incidence of extra-billing and user fees in the provinces and by the premiums charged in some provinces. Brown (1980) commented that, after the passage of the 1977 act, "user charges have increased both in prevalence and in amount. Extrabilling by physicians over medicare payments increased markedly during 1978 and 1979" (p. 522). Provinces had considerably more flexibility under the new rules for federal financing of health care: they could reduce their contributions to health care; to compensate, user charges for various health-care services could be instituted. If provinces decreased funding of medical services relative to the fee schedule, the practice of extrabilling was stimulated. According to Brown (1980):

> Allowing doctors to extra bill not only thwarts the social objective of free care, but also promotes a system under which total costs (public costs plus private costs) will be higher than they would be either under completely socialized medicine or under an unregulated market. Hospital user charges, on the other hand, suggest fewer problems because their development would not suggest a corresponding loss in government control over prices (p. 531).

■ ■ ■ ■

THE CANADA HEALTH ACT OF 1984

Another confrontation between the federal government and the provinces occurred over the way health-care dollars would be expended. The federal government took the position that extrabilling and user fees were eroding Medicare, and further that if those practices were allowed to continue and increase, a two-tiered system of health care would develop, one for the rich and another for the poor. There was a great deal of variation among the provinces in the extent to which user charges and extrabilling were practised. Quebec had the most restrictive rules on extrabilling: physicians who extrabilled were required to opt out of the plan and bill patients directly, and their patients could not seek reimbursement from the plan. A number of provinces, including New Brunswick, Nova Scotia, Prince Edward Island, Saskatchewan, and Alberta, allowed physicians to extrabill and remain in the plan. At the time the legislation was introduced, two provinces, British Columbia and Newfoundland, had user charges for daily stays in acute care beds, but Alberta had an admission charge. Chronic care patients were assessed a daily charge in some provinces: British Columbia, Alberta, Manitoba, Ontario, Quebec, and New Brunswick. Only British Columbia, Alberta, and Ontario charged premiums.

The Canadian Nurses Association (CNA) was strong in its representation to the federal government on its position on provisions in the proposed legislation. This position was very clear: health care should be provided regardless of ability to pay; extrabilling by physicians and user charges by health-care agencies should be disallowed; health professionals should be remunerated on a salary-based system; and insured services should be extended to include community, home care, and long-term care services provided by qualified health-care professionals (CNA, 1983a). The CNA also supported the idea of financial incentives for provinces that developed lower-cost health programs and services by using the skills of health-care professionals more effectively.

> We need to develop alternatives to our high cost, high tech health care service and begin to better utilize other lower cost, highly qualified health care providers and services. The Canadian Nurses Association advocates the further development of multidisciplinary community health centres and home care services, with nurses and other health care providers serving as a first contact with the system for assessment, referral and care (CNA, 1983b, p. 4).

The representation was vigourous and prolonged. Members of the CNA Board lobbied members of Parliament on several occasions in 1983 and 1984; reports and analyses of individual meetings were published in bulletins and distributed to the membership. The CNA Executive and Staff held meetings with key members of the federal government and members of the civil service with responsibility for developing legislation. In a letter to members of the CNA Board, President Helen Glass (1983) urged:

> It's our responsibility to make nursing's voice heard—and soon. Even if you have already contacted your minister of health, we strongly urge you to keep up your lobbying efforts. Health department officials, leaders of opposition parties, opposition health critics and members of standing committees on health will be key targets (p. 1).

The Honourable Monique Bégin, Minister of National Health and Welfare, faced the difficult task of drafting the legislation and shepherding it through committees of the Cabinet and House of Commons before it could be introduced as a bill to be debated and acted on in the House of Commons. In her opening statement to the Conference of Federal and Provincial Ministers of Health in Ottawa in 1982, Bégin said:

> The health care system for which we are responsible is one of Canada's greatest social policy achievements. For Canadians it is the single most popular government program. To outside observers it is a source of great envy . . . However, our commitment to health care insurance in Canada is no easy task. Our governments are faced with major problems of financing in tough economic times . . . It is clear that Canadians today are particularly concerned about the future of their health care system (pp. 1-4).

The pressure to implement more directly and carefully the five basic principles identified, but loosely applied, in initial health insurance legislation was intense:

> The militancy of our associations of health care professionals has never been higher. Recurrent confrontations with doctors, nurses and hospital workers have troubled our system. Concern about the phenomena of opting out and extra-billing, about user fees and about the level of services provided in our hospitals is high. Most Canadians still have adequate access to health care, but many of them fear for the future of the health care system. I feel certain that most of us here today share these concerns. It is clearly up to us to act and act quickly (Bégin, 1982, p. 4).

The new legislation was passed in early April of 1984, amid intense publicity. Bégin became a high-profile figure, and the media focused on confrontations with health ministers in a number of provinces where elected officials considered the Canada Health Act an intrusion into the constitutional rights and powers of the provinces for health care. The CNA lobbied hard and was rewarded for its efforts with legislation that effectively ended the practices of extrabilling and user fees and with the introduction of a statement that provided federal funding for services provided by "health practitioners." The door was thus open for the inclusion in provincial health plans of specialized nursing services that were eligible for reimbursement for the first time. The wording of the legislation could also apply to services provided by other health-care professionals. Clearly, this was the first step in achieving the stated CNA goals: better utilization of nurses and more cost-effective health care. The Canadian Medical Association (CMA) lobbied equally hard against the legislation, but due to the popularity of national health insurance, the unpopularity of extrabilling and user fees, and strong political support for the legislation, it was unable to prevent the passage of the Canada Health Act.

■ ■ ■ ■

PRIVATIZATION OF HEALTH CARE

Recession has led not only to a general shortage of resources and retrenchment in the health-care system, but also to discussions of privatization of health care. The percentage of the gross domestic product that Canadians spend on health care is substantially lower at 9.9% than the 13.3% spent in the United States in 1991 (Health Canada, 1994). In the United States, some 35 million people are not even covered by public health-care financing arrangements, which exist only for those over 65 years of age. In that country the private sector is permitted to operate hospitals at a profit, even though their hospital costs are considerably higher (3.48% of Gross Domestic Product) compared to those in Canada which were 4.18% of Gross Domestic Product (Evans et al, 1989). At least two provinces have conducted experiments in privatization contracting with private organizations to run hospitals. However, the results of these experiments have not been made public by the governments providing the financing. Many were opposed to these ventures as they appeared to violate, at least in spirit, one of the five basic principles on which health legislation in Canada was founded (i.e., public administration).

However, arguments in favour of allowing market forces to prevail in health care are not easily dismissed, as they are continually raised by supporters. Rachlis and Kushner (1994) have countered:

> Explaining the basic economic principles affecting health care financing and delivery leads to conclusions that seem counter-intuitive: public health insurance is more efficient than private insurance; the knowledge gap between caregivers and patients almost eliminates price as an effective signal in the market (p. 187).

It is nevertheless likely that considerable opposition would surface if anything more than token experiments in privatization were undertaken. Despite its problems, most Canadians value their health-care system, and most would not want the system of public financing to be significantly altered.

■ ■ ■ ■

PHILOSOPHICAL BASIS OF HEALTH-CARE FINANCING LEGISLATION

The combined effect of the provisions of the 1948 federal legislation supporting hospital construction and the 1957 hospital insurance legislation set in motion a system in which "hospital-based patterns of practice were solidified" (Vayda, Evans, and Mindell, 1979). The number of hospital beds increased at twice the rate of population increase between 1961 and 1971, and occupancy rates were around 80%. Since outpatient care was not eligible for federal cost sharing, there was an incentive for choosing more costly hospital care over outpatient or home care. Community health services were also excluded from federal financing, and provinces were required to finance the operation of such services without assistance.

Another point that pertains to nursing and the services offered by other health-care professionals is that medical care insurance legislation provided federal cost sharing only for physicians' services. This was intended to constrain the development of the health-care system by providing a financial incentive for the proliferation of physicians' services. Since these were the most costly services of all of the health professions, this decision had serious financial repercussions for the health-care system.

One of the factors associated with the volume of health care services is the number of physicians. More surgeons are correlated with higher discretionary surgical rates and more physicians with an increased volume of medical services, just as more hospital beds are associated with greater bed use (Vayda, Evans, and Mindell, 1979, p. 220).

Projections of the number of physicians needed to care for the Canadian population were grossly overestimated in the 1960s. The Royal Commission on Health Services Report of 1964 assumed there would be a shortage, based on its projections of 1961 patterns of health-services utilization, and failed to account for "changes in technology and productivity" (Vayda, Evans, and Mindell, 1979, p. 219). The ratio of physicians to population rose dramatically, from 1:850 in 1961 to 1:600 by 1973. The financial repercussions for a physician-driven system in which the skills of other health professionals are not effectively employed are obvious. As Vayda, Evans, and Mindell (1979) have pointed out, "There are dangers inherent in health care decisions that are predicated solely on financial considerations; yet now governments not only know what the total health care bill is, they also have to pay that bill and deal with the issues (p. 230)."

■ ■ ■ ■

RESTRUCTURING THE HEALTH-CARE SYSTEM

There is ample evidence that, "although universal hospital insurance in Canada provided payment to hospitals, it did not mandate an organizational framework to deal with problems of efficiency or duplication of services" (Vayda, Evans, and Mindell, 1979, p. 219). When insurance for medical services was imposed on the existing structure of services, the environment for care was clearly the hospital. When new funding arrangements were implemented in the legislation of 1977, the federal government attempted to stop open-ended health-care financing by placing limits on the total amount of federal spending. Thus it sought to constrain its own financial commitment in a more predictable way, one that would encourage the provinces to manage their programs more efficiently (by removing any illusion that they are spending 50-cent dollars). The outcome has been a loss of federal control over health insurance programs. In retrospect it appears that the federal government was somewhat naive in believing that the nature of Medicare and hospital insurance would make them immune to provincial government encroachment (Brown, 1980, p. 525). It is not difficult to understand why restructuring and reorganizing the health-care system were not included in federal legislative proposals for funding provincial health-care services. The need for change had been recognized for some time; the Royal Commission on Health Services had recommended reorganization of health services in its 1964 report. Political considerations, the fierce determination of the provinces to retain their constitutional prerogatives for health care, and the opposition of powerful lobbyists were all factors that deterred needed change in the system. In the process of enacting new health-care financing legislation, such as the Canada Health Act of 1984, the federal government encountered difficulty implementing even a few changes; they were opposed by physicians and provinces. The need for a new approach to health care remains and is more urgent than ever, but the agenda for legislative change is a political minefield. The federal government that next addresses the need for action in health care will require a firm commitment to change and the courage of its convictions in the presence of strong political opposition.

Canada cannot afford to continue to support a system in which the physician is the "gatekeeper" to virtually all health-care services. Research indicates that using the services of nurses and other health professionals is a sensible and cost-effective approach to the provision of health-care services. A study of nurses providing primary care in rural Newfoundland demonstrated that acute-care hospital services decreased by 5%, while in the control area there was a 39% increase in a physician-based, acute care-centred system. The cost of providing services to the population in the experimental group was substantially lower (24%) than in the control group (Chambers et al, 1977, p. 971). An investigation in Manitoba demonstrated that physicians were less successful than nurse practitioners in helping comparable groups of patients control blood pressure and lose weight (Ramsay, McKenzie, and Fish, 1982). In a controlled trial, nurses were more successful in vaccinating elderly patients for influenza than were physicians—nurses immunizing 35% of clients compared with 2% by physicians (Hoey, McCallum, and LePage, 1982, p. 27). Until recently Canada has been one of few countries in the world where nurse midwives were not legally permitted to practise. Legislation legalizing midwifery came into force in Ontario on January 1, 1994, and Alberta passed such legislation in 1992, although it had not been proclaimed by the autumn of 1994. In Ontario a new university-level program in midwifery has been initiated, while in Alberta work is ongoing on the regulations for the midwifery legislation that has not yet been proclaimed. Several other provinces are currently studying this matter, and it is likely that the practice of midwifery will be eventually permitted in most provinces.

Because physicians have in the past opposed efforts to include services provided by nurses among those eligible for direct reimbursement in provincial health-care plans, it will not be easy to change existing provisions. Nevertheless, nurses provide a viable and cost-effective alternative in delivering certain kinds of health-care services, particularly those involving health promotion, health maintenance, and counseling activities in relation to health. In the presence of an environment characterized by fiscal restraint that has been accompanied by extensive layoffs of professional nurses and widespread salary reductions for health professionals and public sector workers, the entire system is open to question. Health-care legislation has imposed financial constraints on nursing roles and functions since nursing's inception in Canada. This has meant that change that might have occurred naturally in a free and open health-care environment has not occurred. To date, powerful physician-dominated lobby groups have successfully prevented major departures from the physician-centred health system maintained through the force of health-care financing legislation. Nurses are learning to develop effective lobby groups of their own to ensure that politicians understand the contribution nurses can make to the health-care system. Governments will be forced to consider alternatives, despite the pressure to resist change, as the limits of the public purse and the demand for improved health are recognized.

REFERENCES

Agnew, G.H. (1974). *Canadian hospitals, 1920 to 1970: A dramatic half century.* Toronto: University of Toronto Press.

Bégin, M. (1982). Opening statement to Conference of Federal and Provincial Ministers of Health. Ottawa.

Brown, M.C. (1980). The implications of established program finance for national health insurance. *Canadian Public Policy. 3,* 521-532.

Canadian Nurses Association. (1983a). The Canada Health Act: Where we stand. *Canada Health Act Bulletin IV.* Ottawa: The Association.

Canadian Nurses Association. (1983b). The Canada Health Act: Where we stand. *Canada Health Act Bulletin.* Ottawa: The Association.

Chambers, L.W. et al. (1977). A controlled trial of the impact of the family practice nurse on volume, quality, and cost of rural health services. *Medical Care, 15*(12), 971-981.

Evans, R.G., Lomas, J., Barer, M.L., Labelle, R.J., Fooks, C., Stoddart, G.L., Anderson, G.M., Feeny, D., Gafni, A., Torrance, G.W., and Tholl, W.G. (1989). Controlling health expenditures - the Canadian reality. *New England Journal of Medicine, 320,* 571-577.

Glass, H.P. (1983). Letter to Dr. Janet Kerr. *Provincial health insurance plans: Extra-billing/user charges by hospitals.* Ottawa: Health and Welfare Canada.

Health Canada. (1994). Preliminary estimates of health expenditures in Canada. *Provincial-Territorial Summary Report, 1987-1991.* Ottawa: Health Information Division, Policy and Consultation Branch, Health Canada.

Hoey, J.R., McCallum, H.P., and LePage, E.M. (1982). Expanding the nurse's role to improve preventive service in an outpatient clinic. *Canad Med Assoc J, 127* (1), 27-28.

LeClair, M. (1975). The Canadian health care system. In S. Andrepoulos (Ed.). *National health insurance: Can we learn from Canada?* (pp. 11-96). New York: John Wiley & Sons.

Rachlis, M., and Kushner, C. (1994). *Strong medicine: How to save Canada's health care system.* Toronto: Harper Collins Publishers Ltd.

Ramsay, J.A., McKenzie, J.K., and Fish, D.G. (1982). Physicians and nurse practitioners: Do they provide equivalent health care? *American Journal of Public Health, 72*(1), 55-57.

Taylor, M.G. (1978). *Health insurance and Canadian public policy: The seven decisions that created the Canadian health insurance system and their outcomes.* Montreal: McGill-Queen's University Press.

Vayda, E., Evans, R., and Mindell, W.R. (1979). Universal health insurance in Canada: History, problems, trends. *Journal of Community Health, 4*(3), 217-231.

Wallace, E. (1980). The origin of the social welfare state in Canada, 1867-1900. In C.A. Meilicke and J.L. Storch (Eds.). *Perspectives on Canadian health and social services policy: History and emerging trends* (pp. 25-37). Ann Arbor: Health Administration Press.

CHAPTER EIGHTEEN

Organizing for Nursing Care: Primary Nursing, Traditional Approaches, or Both?

JANNETTA MacPHAIL

I dentifying the ideal system for organizing staff to provide nursing care has been a goal of nursing service administrators for at least 4 decades. Because many factors influence assignment patterns, and are influenced by them, identifying the ideal system offers a challenge to administrators and their staffs. The administrator is concerned not only about quality and costs of care, but also about the satisfaction of nursing staff and the patients in their care. A historical review of the major organizational modes used since the early part of the century will provide a perspective of this continual challenge to administrators and nursing staffs.

■ ■ ■ ■

TYPES OF ORGANIZATIONAL MODES

Four major types of organizational modes can be identified from the literature and from accounts of nurses who have practised since the 1920s: functional assignment, case assignment, team nursing, and primary nursing. In the functional assignment mode, care is assigned by task or function; the primary considerations are efficiency and cost control. This mode was based on the work of Frederick W. Taylor (1912), the "father of scientific management," whose work dates back to the 1880s. Taylor's management concepts were first published in 1912. Drucker (1974) states: "Taylor was the first man in the known history of mankind who did not take work for granted, but looked at it and studied it" (p. 24). Unfortunately, his focus was on the individual task, not the end product, which he always took for granted (Drucker, 1974). The premises of his theory of management were that managers "are capable of thinking and planning" and that "the worker is viewed as needing close supervision and constant direction" (Beswetherick, 1979, p. 18).

The functional system is task-oriented and highly structured, with the charge nurse reigning supreme and operating according to the rules, regulations, and procedures. Tasks are assigned according to the ability and status of the various members of the nursing staff. Until World War II, and in some cases after that time, the staff consisted primarily of nursing students, and assignments were made according to their level of progression in the hospital diploma programs. Decisions were made by the charge nurse, to whom all reported and by whom all were evaluated. The charge nurse was the main communicator; thus the charge nurse, usually a registered nurse on days and a senior nursing student on nights, was in a position of power and control. This arrangement could be either beneficial or detrimental to patients and staff, depending on the charge nurse's knowledge base, decision-making ability, and leadership style. The advantages of the functional system were efficiency and cost. For example, if the ratio of staff to patients was low, it conserved both costs and energy. This system is still used, particularly when staff is limited. Three disadvantages of functional assignment are fragmented care, with the patients attended by many persons who have responsibility for only one or two aspects of care; limited responsibility on the part of the nursing staff; and limited opportunity to learn about decision making.

The case assignment method developed as a result of recognizing the limitations of the functional method and the need to provide continuity of care, a concern that was intensified by the change from 12- to 8-hour shifts, which occurred in the 1940s and 1950s. Case assignment was recognized by nurse educators as a way to teach total-patient care, which became increasingly important after the middle of the century. It was also the method of assignment used by private-duty nurses, who were prevalent in the first half of the century, practising in the home and hospital. In the case assignment system, the nursing student or staff nurse was assigned a certain number of patients for their total hospital stay; a new patient was assigned when one was discharged. Assignment was based on the severity of illness of patients and the abilities of the staff. Although it was still task-oriented to a great extent, the staff member provided total care. The charge nurse remained the central control figure and the main communicator in this system; she made all assignments and all staff reported to her. The advantages of case assignment include greater continuity of care and a more consistent view of the patient as a whole. The disadvantages are that control is still centralized and opportunities to learn decision making and responsibility are still limited, though greater than under the functional system. Another disadvantage of the system is that experienced staff with well-rounded abilities are needed to make this system work, and in many situations staff do not meet these requirements. In the 1950s changes began to occur in the way nurses viewed nursing. They began to identify nursing problems and realize that nursing was not merely a collection of tasks to be performed.

The third method of organizing nursing staff is team nursing. This mode was influenced by the shortage of nurses that occurred during World War II, when many nurses enlisted and the number of nursing students left to staff hospitals was not sufficient. As a result, assistants to nurses, usually nursing aides and nursing assistants or practical nurses, were recruited. The focus of this mode is the work group or team, which includes professional nurses and nonprofessional staff. The team is headed by a team leader, to whom members of the team report; the team leader reports to the head nurse and is responsible for the care of all patients assigned to the team and for the supervision of team members. The number of teams on a nursing unit depends on the size of the unit and the number of staff available. An advantage of this mode, as noted by proponents of team nursing (Lambertsen, 1953; Brooks, 1961; Williams, 1964; Kron, 1966; Douglass and Bevis, 1970) is that it improves patient care by using the diverse skills of team members to their full potential under the guidance of registered nurses. Other advantages are the ability to function with more nonprofessionals on the unit; an increase in opportunities for learning clinical decision making, particularly by the team leader; opportunities for the team leader to learn leadership and group skills; availability of a nurse's judgement to a larger number of patients; decreased number of staff needed to care for a patient; increased opportunity to share responsibility; and better use of individual abilities. Disadvantages of the team system are fragmentation of care; a tendency to place blame on others and not assume responsibility; possible resistance by nonprofessionals to direction by the team leader, which affects new graduates particularly; an insufficient number of team leaders who have the skills needed to direct staff; time devoted to supervising others instead of assessing care; and a tendency for staff dissatisfaction.

To address the disadvantages of team nursing and increase nurse and patient satisfaction, a fourth system of organization—primary nursing—was created in the 1970s. Hegyvary (1982) perceives primary nursing as "both a philosophy of care and an organizational design . . . not simply a way of assigning nurses to patients, but rather a view of nursing as professional, patient-centred practice" (p. 3). Although there are many definitions of primary nursing in the literature and in practice, it means essentially:

> . . . the nursing care of a specific patient is under the continuous guidance of one nurse from admission through discharge. One nurse on each shift provides total care for the same group of patients day after day. Round-the-clock care is coordinated for each patient by the nurse designated as the primary nurse for that patient (Hegyvary, 1982, p. 3).

Four essential elements of the primary nursing model, identified by Hegyvary, are: 1) accountability to the patient, family, professional colleagues, and institution; 2) autonomy, in that the nurse decides and acts on decisions about nursing care; 3) coordination of care, which promotes consistency and harmony; and 4) comprehensive care, or total patient care.

Several authors indicate that in this mode of organization the registered nurse's activities are changed from manager of care and organizer of personnel to care manager/care implementer (Ciske, 1974; Manthey, 1973; Manthey and Kramer, 1970; Manthey et al, 1971; Marram, 1976; Williams, 1975). Munson and Clinton (1979) also note that in this system, nurse's aide activities focus on equipment and supplies rather than on direct contact with patients, as in team nursing.

Many advantages of primary nursing are explicated in the literature. They include continuity of care, increased accountability, total patient care, highly individualized care, opportunity to implement the total process of nursing care and evaluate outcomes, increased autonomy and authority, and comprehensive and better coordinated care. Some have also claimed that there is improved quality of care (Felton, 1975; Leonard, 1975; Marram, 1976); faster recuperation for certain patients, with a corresponding decrease in length of stay and in cost per patient day (Brown, 1976; Henderson, 1982; Jones, 1975); increased patient satisfaction (Isler, 1976; Nenner, Curtis, and Eckhoff, 1977); increased nurse satisfaction, with a corresponding reduction in turnover rates and absenteeism (Ciske, 1974; Isler, 1976; Knecht, Schlegel, and Marram, 1973); reduction in errors of commission and omission; and improved relationships between nurses and physicians (Cicatiello, Zimmer, and Christman, 1977). Although not identified as disadvantages, some of the problems in implementing primary nursing are: 1) difficulties in maintaining a well-qualified staff because of turnover or poor staffing, and 2) changes required in hospital philosophy, structure, and process to accommodate the primary nurses' increased independence and autonomy that are essential to the system.

Munson and Clinton (1979) note that it is impossible to generalize the findings of various reports on primary nursing because of conflict among them, even though the findings may have been valid and relevant for the particular setting in which the research or activities occurred. In addition, finding a clear and definitive model of one of the modes consistently in operation is unlikely in most settings. Rather, there may be many combinations of the four modes, which makes comparison difficult and generalization of findings unreliable.

■ ■ ■ ■
COMPARISON OF ORGANIZATIONAL MODES

The four major organizational modes can be compared from many perspectives, although Munson and Clinton (1979) could not define them clearly enough to make rigourous comparisons. The key comparison factors identified by Giovanetti (1986) are major focus, accountability, lines of authority, communication patterns, basis of personnel assignment, and patient-care planning. The major focus in functional assignment is on tasks, in case assignment on patients and tasks, in team nursing on patients and managing team members, and in primary nursing on patients. Accountability is to the charge nurse in the functional assignment and case assignment modes, to the team leader in team nursing, and to the patient in primary nursing. Lines of authority are as follows: The charge nurse is in complete control in the functional and case assignment modes; the team leader reports to the charge nurse in team nursing; and the primary nurse is in charge in primary nursing.

Communication is channelled through the charge nurse in the functional and case assignment modes and through the team leader to the charge nurse in team nursing; in primary nursing all communication is directed to the primary nurse. Personnel assignment in both functional and case methods is based on tasks and the level of preparation of the worker. In team nursing, personnel are assigned according to the severity of illness of patients and the level of preparation of team members. In primary nursing, personnel are assigned according to patient needs. Involvement in patient-care planning and clinical decision making is centred in the charge nurse in functional and case assignment methods, in the team leader in team nursing, and in the primary nurse in primary nursing.

■■ ■■ ■■ ■■

ASSESSMENT OF PRIMARY NURSING

Primary nursing, introduced in the early 1970s, became very popular in the 1980s. It was advocated as the solution to many problems in organizing nursing staff to give quality care and increasing job satisfaction for nurses and patient satisfaction with care (Corpuz, 1977; Dawson and Wilson, 1983). A great many articles, reports, and books have been devoted to primary nursing, particularly in the nursing literature. Young, Giovannetti, Lewison, and Thoms (1981) identified more than 150 articles and reports on primary nursing, nearly 80% of which were not research based and overwhelmingly supported the concept. Giovannetti (1986) states that "the remaining research literature, consisting of evaluative studies and explorative non-comparative studies, also concluded with strong support for primary nursing, but in-depth analysis revealed serious methodological flaws leading the reviewers to question the largely positive results" (p. 127).

Giovannetti (1986) conducted a comprehensive survey of published and unpublished works pertaining to primary nursing between 1970 and 1984 to identify studies that met these criteria: "(1) be an evaluative study citing primary nursing as an independent variable; (2) be systematic; (3) include information on the methods and procedures for data collection; (4) present findings; and (5) be written and translated into English," (p. 128). Only 29 studies met these criteria. Several hundred articles, reports, and comparative studies were excluded. A major problem identified was the lack of an operational definition of primary nursing or of any other organizational mode studied. Although many investigators recognized this as a limitation and few stated that their findings could be generalized, Giovannetti identified this lack as a major problem. Moreover, although investigators did not suggest that their results could be generalized, many nurses in practice and in administration tend to do so.

Giovannetti (1986) completed an insightful critique of these 29 studies and identified basic problems with the research. She states:

> Although many methodological issues could be identified in research on primary nursing, instrumentation and research design are of particular importance. With few exceptions, the instruments used to measure the criterion variables lacked adequate reliability and validity assessment. In many instances, no reference was made to the psychometric attributes of the measurements. In the instances where standardized

measures were used, many investigators appeared to assume that previously established reliability and validity estimates were transferable. The inadequacies associated with instrumentation, coupled with the problems related to the operationalization of the independent variable, are not inconsequential. If it is not known what is going to be measured, and it is not known whether the instruments really measure what is to be measured, intelligible interpretations of the research effort cannot be made (pp. 130-131).

Several other investigators have noted similar inadequacies with the research of primary nursing. Steckel (1980) states, "There are insufficient data to demonstrate that primary nursing improves the quality of care, increases nurse or patient satisfaction, or is cost-effective" (p. 77). Prescott and Sorenson (1978) identified flaws in research design or outcome measures used in evaluations of primary nursing. Betz (1981) criticizes the wide variations in time periods used to compute turnover rates and failure to fully discuss the sample and methods used in reporting studies. Betz also states, "The claims in other reports are made so easily and with such cavalier disregard for the methods by which their data are measured, obtained, and computed that one does not know how seriously to read, let alone generalize, the findings" (p. 151).

Despite the lack of research evidence available to determine whether implementation of primary nursing will achieve all that it is purported to accomplish, the use of primary nursing became widespread in the 1980s. There are few negative reports in the literature, and those that are negative are not research based (Hylands and Sarnavka, 1984; Chavigny and Lewis, 1984). Because research evidence could not be found in the literature to support a change from team nursing to primary nursing in a Veteran's Administration (VA) Hospital, Chavigny and Lewis (1984) conducted an epidemiologic cohort design study to determine if there were differences between the two organizational modes in relation to patient health status, quality of care, costs, and job satisfaction. The only significant difference noted was in direct care time: Team nursing resulted in more contact with patients than did primary nursing, which supports the findings of Giovannetti (1981) and Shukla (1982a). The survey of nurses' job satisfaction indicated that the nursing staff perceived primary nursing as difficult and stressful; 73% of the registered nurses in the VA Hospital thought this method should not be used. Their decision to reject primary nursing was based on opinion, not on comparative data.

In an effort to find a sound scientific base for choosing primary nursing over team nursing, Shukla (1982a, 1982b, 1983) undertook extensive research to evaluate the cost benefits of the two modes. He controlled for the quality and quantity of registered nurses in the models compared, which had not been done in other studies. Shukla (1982b) concluded that individual factors, such as nurse competency, affect quality to a greater extent than the structural differences between team nursing and primary nursing. He states: "While the structure for primary nursing is generally found to be a better system for organizing care, its effectiveness is obviously not uniform for all types of nurses, patients, hospitals, and even nursing units within a single hospital" (p. 12). He identified two critical factors that should influence the choice of organizational mode: the efficiency of nursing support systems and the patients' degree of independence. The support systems include transportation systems, distribution systems, communication systems, and the unit management system. The more efficient these systems, the less time nurses have to spend on indirect care activities and the more time they can devote to direct patient care. This has been the basis for development and improvement of support systems in hospitals over the past four decades. In spite of the improvement, one of the chief complaints of nurses today, as indicated by surveys and study commissions in both Canada and the United States, is their frustration from having insufficient time to devote to direct care because of the time required for indirect care, due to inefficiencies or inadequacies in the nursing support systems. Efficient support systems for nurses, such as the Friesen Concept, were designed more than 20 years ago. Some aspects of the concept existed more than 40 years ago when the designer, Gordon Friesen, was a visionary and creative hospital administrator. Why then, do efficient support systems still not exist in all hospitals today? Cost is often cited as the reason. Would the cost not be offset by the reduction in costs of rapid nurse turnover, inefficiencies, dissatisfaction, and nurses leaving nursing?

Another factor to consider in selecting an organizational mode is nurses' satisfaction with the various delivery models. Betz and O'Connell (1987) conducted two studies to compare job satisfaction of nurses on primary nursing units and nurses on team nursing units. Like other investigators, they found no significant difference in satisfaction from the quantitative data collected (Alexander, Weisman, and Chase, 1981). Some researchers have speculated abstractly about their results, whereas others have searched further. Betz and O'Connell (1987) collected qualitative data as well and found that nurses practising in the primary nursing mode were enthusiastic about their increased autonomy, increased involvement in and responsibility for direct patient care, better nurse/patient ratios, and increased knowledge about their patients with which to make clinical decisions; dissatisfaction arose from insufficient help with low-level tasks and too much paperwork. The investigators suggest that the move to primary nursing contributes to two types of role strain: role overload and role ambiguity. Role overload is the result of increased responsibility and inadequate support systems for managing the increased responsibilities. Role ambiguity is a part of any role change, but it may be increased in cases where preparation for the change was insufficient, as has been reported by registered nurse students who had been involved in changes from team nursing to primary nursing in their work settings. Other research indicates that increased autonomy may not lead to increased satisfaction unless autonomy leads to control over pace and conditions of work (Karasek, 1976). The primary nurses who are responsible for low-level tasks that should be performed by efficient support systems do not have this control.

Nursing costs have been increasingly important to hospitals since the advent of diagnostic-related group-based (DRG) payment systems in the early 1980s, and are even more critical with the shortage of nurses. Studies of the costs of primary nursing have indicated inconsistencies: Some results show primary nursing to be less costly than team nursing (Marram, 1976); some show it to be more costly (Shukla, 1982a); and some show no significant difference in costs (Chavigny and Lewis, 1984). Wolf, Lesic, and Leak (1986) compared direct nursing care costs within specific DRGs between a primary nursing unit and a team nursing unit in a 474-bed acute-care community hospital. They endeavored to control for patient acuity but found the acuity level 28% higher on the primary nursing unit. This, however, was probably due to a factor that was previously unknown to the investigators: Physicians were asking the hospital admitting department to admit their more acute patients to the primary nursing unit because of the reputation it had earned for providing quality care. The findings showed that "the primary nursing unit's average daily cost per patient per DRG was $1.30 less than on the team unit" (Wolf, Lesic, and Leak, 1986, p. 11). Researchers speculate that the primary nursing structure may allow nurses to care for patients more efficiently, but they emphasize the need for additional study of the cost of primary nursing within the prospective payment system.

Glandon, Colbert, and Thomasma (1989) completed an extensive analysis of the cost of nursing in 392 nursing units in 62 U.S. hospitals that are part of the Medicus Systems Corporation. They compared nursing costs among four organizational modes: primary nursing, team nursing, modular nursing, and total patient care. Modular nursing is defined as "a geographic assignment of patients that encourages continuity of care by organizing a group of staff to work with a group of patients. The fixed geographic areas typically represent 10-12 patients per module" (Hegyvary, 1977, p. 189). It is a pragmatic mixture of team and primary nursing. Total patient care is "a case method for organizing nursing care where nurses are responsible for total care of a patient but only for the hours that a specific nurse is present" (Hegyvary, 1977, p. 190). The findings of the Glandon, Colbert, and Thomasma analysis revealed that small, primary nursing units using a high mix of registered nurses are the most costly per patient day, even after controlling for the patients' average nursing care needs. The investigators note that the nursing care delivery model used, size of nursing unit, and extent to which registered nurses are used all have significant effects on nursing costs. Moreover, they note that the delivery model and use of registered nurses are closely interrelated; they plan to use regression analysis to separate possible confounding influences. Glandon et al. (1989) emphasize that their analysis did not account for differences in quality of care and that decisions cannot be made solely on the basis of cost; the quality of care must also be considered. They conclude that, "in the current health care environment, there does not appear to be one best method to deliver care in a cost effective manner," and that, "more research is needed on the relationship of nursing care delivery to the quality of care and nurse satisfaction" (p. 33).

In response to criticisms of the sampling and time frames used for comparative studies of primary nursing and team nursing, a longitudinal study involving eight medical units in a tertiary-care teaching hospital was conducted over a 5-year period with external funding. Gardner (1991) and Gardner and Tilbury (1991) reported that the quality of care was higher, retention of nurses was better, and costs were less with primary nursing than with team nursing. Primary nursing produced a 6.5% cost reduction below the team nursing costs, which was attributed to lower unit-specific costs, higher nurse productivity, and lower use of agency nurses. The latter two factors were related to a much higher retention rate for primary nurses than team nurses (Gardner and Tilbury, 1991.) Retention rate was also found to be related to educational preparation, as reflected in 40% of nurses with a baccalaureate or higher degree being retained on primary nursing units after 2 years, while only 8% of nurses with this level of education were retained on team nursing units. The retention rate for nurses educated at the diploma level was 23% on primary nursing units in comparison to 42% on team nursing units, which also used more agency nurses (Gardner, 1991). While these findings are very persuasive, the investigators caution against generalizaing the findings because primary nursing models may not be comparable across settings.

Based on their research comparing the two organizational modes, McPhail, Pikula, Roberts, Browne, and Harper (1990) concluded that neither primary nursing nor team nursing was superior to the other on important clinical and administrative variables and hence, did not warrant implementing primary nursing in their setting. The variables examined were patient satisfaction, quality of care as perceived by physicians and allied health professionals, absenteeism and nurses' perception of their work environment. The setting was a 35-bed medical/surgical unit in a tertiary-care, teaching hospital. The study design was "a randomized crossover trial, where one-half of the nurses would carry out the present system of team nursing while the other half would employ primary nursing; then after five months, the primary nurses would cross over to team nursing and the former team nurses would practice primary nursing" (McPhail et al., 1990, p. 191). In critiquing their research, O'Connor (1990) considered it premature to reach this conclusion based on two trials and urged further replications using sensitive process and outcome measures and larger sample sizes. She encouraged investigating the conditions under which primary nursing is better than team nursing and beginning with "a conceptual analysis of: (a) the different needs that are met by the two systems (e.g., security versus autonomy); (b) the underlying mechanisms that explain the relationship between the nursing system and the quality of care, patient satisfaction, and nurse satisfaction; and (c) the conditions that may enhance or inhibit the relationship between the nursing system and selected outcomes" (O'Connor, 1990, p. 198).

■ ■ ■ ■

CASE MANAGEMENT AND MANAGED CARE

While the debates over primary nursing versus team nursing continue, case management and managed care have become the focus of much attention in the literature and at conferences. They are designed to control costs while endeavouring to achieve optimal outcomes in health-care delivery. The concepts are defined and developed quite differently in Canada and the United States because of the vast differences in the organization and financing of the health-care delivery systems in the two countries. Nonetheless, the ultimate goals are the same: to deliver quality care at less cost. Managed care in the United States refers to "a cost-containment process in which healthcare benefits are carefully controlled in terms of types, levels, and frequency of treatments; in terms of access to care; and in terms of the amount of reimbursement paid for healthcare services" (Brent,

1991, p. 8). It is most often associated with health maintenance organizations (HMOs) that try to provide services within cost-effective systems.

Case management is an integral part of such a system and is also becoming an integral part of health-care organizations in Canada as they endeavour to deliver better care at lower cost. King (1992) defines case management, "as a clinical system of health care delivery that organizes and sequences care at the patient-provider level to achieve cost control and optimal outcomes. The underlying aim is patient-centered, outcome-focused care within a fiscally responsible length of stay" (p. 15). The case management system developed at The Toronto Hospital was an innovation adapted from the New England Medical Center Model but is different from American models in that it is multidisciplinary, expecting and requiring the collective efforts of all providers and departments to contain costs, provide quality care and improve practice patterns. Basic assumptions underlying this model are:

> (1) Health care resources are finite; (2) Health care should proceed from a structured, multi-disciplinary plan; (3) Collaborative team efforts, with activities coordinated around defined, patient-centered outcomes, result in quality, cost-effective care; (4) Patients and families are empowered through informed and participatory decision making; (5) Accountability for optimal patient care and responsible use of resources is a health care imperative for institutions, professions and providers; and (6) Job and career satisfaction are enhanced in a work environment that enables one to practise in accordance with professional ideals and standards (King, 1992, p. 15).

Evaluation of the case management system in this setting revealed improvement in patients outcomes, reduced length of stay for certain patient categories, improved attraction and retention of nurses, and enhanced interdisciplinary relationships and partnerships.

Case management is not an organizational mode; rather it is superimposed on a mode and has been found to be very compatible with primary nursing (Zander, 1988; Olivas, Del Togno-Armanasco, Erickson, and Harter, 1989a, 1989b). It has also been adapted in the community (Parker et al., 1992; Sinnen and Schifalacqua, 1991; Holzemer, 1992). The case manager role is viewed as ideal for the clinical nurse specialist (Sparacino, 1991; Papenhausen, 1990), and as requiring a baccalaureate degree in nursing as minimal preparation (American Nurses Association, 1988). Case management is a concept that can be expected to be implemented widely in these times of budgetary constraints and limited resources.

■ ■ ■ ■

THE FUTURE IN ORGANIZATIONAL MODES

Identifying the best methods of organizing nursing staff to provide quality nursing care remains a challenge to all nurses. Because nurses are dissatisfied with existing systems, they seek other approaches and are strongly influenced by the proponents of new methods presented in the literature and at conferences. They are asked to demonstrate cost-benefit ratios before implementing a new approach, although this is not usually required of other health professionals with new ideas. In many settings, primary nursing, or the application of some attributes of primary nursing, seems to be achieving the desired outcomes in nurse satisfaction and patient satisfaction. Although it is not unusual that nurses wish to share their ideas with others, it is important that scientifically sound research be completed to evaluate the outcomes of different approaches before they are used so that false claims are not made. It is important that the research be designed with expert consultation to ensure its quality and ability to be replicated. Replication of research is needed to provide nursing with a sound base for proceeding in new directions.

Giovannetti (1986) suggests that, if primary nursing is partially a philosophy of care (as many have suggested [Hegyvary, 1982; Marram, Schlegel and Bevis, 1974]), we should proceed with philosophic rather than scientific inquiry. Attempts to use scientific means alone to measure the effects of primary nursing are premature; without philosophic inquiry the measurements will continue to be ineffective. Philosophic questions are not answerable through the scientific method. Whatever the source of these problems, they must be addressed; to ignore them is to assure that research in nursing does not provide a sound basis for making decisions about improving nursing care (Giovanetti, 1986).

The major factors that influence nursing assignment patterns are patient characteristics, nursing resources, and organizational support. The method of combining these factors will influence the degree of continuity and integration and the type of coordination that can be achieved. The challenge for the future is to consider all factors and support sound scientific and philosophical inquiry that will help identify the best methods for organizing nursing care at an affordable cost. There may not be a "best" mode, due to the variability of patient characteristics and nursing resources that exist in the various health-care settings that constitute Canada's health-care system. The goal in all settings is to promote, facilitate, and support professional nursing practice in a cost-effective manner.

REFERENCES

Alexander, C.S., Weisman, C.S., and Chase, G.A. (1981). Evaluating primary nursing in hospitals: Examination of effects on nursing staff. *Medical Care, 19*(1), 80-89.

American Nurses Association. (1988). *Nursing Case Management*. Kansas City, MO: Author.

Beswetherick, M. (1979). A review of past and current systems of nursing care delivery. *The Canadian Nurse, 75*(5), 18-22.

Betz, M. (1981). Some hidden costs of primary nursing. *Nursing and Health Care 2*(3), 150-154.

Betz, M., and O'Connell, L. (1987). Primary nursing: Panacea or problem? *Nursing and Health Care, 8*(8), 457-460.

Brent, N.J. (1991). Managed care: Legal and ethical implications. *Home Healthcare Nurse, 9*(3), 8-10.

Brooks, E.A. (1961). Team nursing: 1961. *American Journal of Nursing, 61*(4), 87-91.

Brown, B. (1976). The autonomous nurse and primary nursing. *Nursing Administration Quarterly, 1*(3), 31-36.

Chavigny, K., and Lewis, A. (1984). Team or primary nursing care? *Nursing Outlook, 32*(6), 322-327.

Cicatiello, J., Zimmer, M.J., and Christman, L. (1977). NAQ forum: Primary nursing—why not? *Nursing Administration Quarterly, 1*(2), 82-83.

Ciske, K.L. (1974). Primary nursing: An organization that promoted professional practice. *Journal of Nursing Administration, 4*(1), 28-31.

Corpuz, T. (1977). Primary nursing meets needs, expectations of patient and staff. *Hospitals, 51*(6), 95-96.

Dawson, P., and Wilson, N.M. (1983). What nurses say about primary nursing. *The Canadian Nurse, 79*(6), 37-41.

Douglass, L.M., and Bevis, E.D. (1970). *Team leadership in action: Principles and application to staff nursing situations.* St. Louis: The CV Mosby Co.

Drucker, P.F. (1974). *Management: Tasks, responsibilities, practices.* New York: Harper & Row.

Felton, G. (1975). Increasing the quality of nursing care by introducing the concept of primary nursing: A model project. *Nursing Research, 24*(1), 27-32.

Gardner, K. (1991). A summary of findings of a five-year comparison study of primary and team nursing. *Nursing Research, 40*(2), 113-117.

Gardner, K., and Tilbury, M. (1991). A longitudinal cost analysis of primary and team nursing. *Nursing Economics, 9*(2), 97-104.

Giovannetti, P. (1981). *A comparative study of team and primary nursing care.* Unpublished doctoral dissertation. Johns Hopkins University, Baltimore.

Giovannetti, P. (1986). Evaluation of primary nursing. In H. Werley, J. Fitzpatrick, and R.L. Taunton (Eds.). *Annual Review of Nursing Research* (Vol. 4) (pp. 127-151). New York: Springer.

Glandon, G.L., Colbert, K.W., and Thomasma, M. (1989). Nursing delivery models and RN mix: Cost implications. *Nursing Management, 20*(5), 30-33.

Hegyvary, S.T. (1977). Foundations of primary nursing. *Nursing Clinics of North America, 12*(6), 187-196.

Hegyvary, S.T. (1982). *The change to primary nursing: A cross-cultural view of professional nursing practice.* St. Louis: The CV Mosby Co.

Henderson, C. (1982). Can nursing care hasten recovery? *American Journal of Nursing, 64*(6), 80-83.

Holzemer, W.L. (1992). Linking primary health care and self-care through case management. *International Nursing Review, 39*(3), 83-89.

Hylands, J., and Sarnavka, A. (1984). Primary nursing or total patient care? *Dimensions, 61*(9), 36-38.

Isler, C. (1976). Rx for a sick hospital: Primary nursing care. *RN, 39*(2), 60-65.

Jones, K. (1975). Study documents effect of primary nursing on renal transplant patients. *Hospitals, 49*(24), 85-89.

Karasek, R. (1976). *Impact of work environment on life outside the job.* Unpublished doctoral dissertation, Massachusetts Institute of Technology, Boston.

King, M.L. (1992). Case management. *The Canadian Nurse, 88*(4), 15-17.

Knecht, A.A., Schlegel, M.W., and Marram, G.D. (1973). Innovation on Four Tower West (3 Parts). *American Journal of Nursing, 73*(5), 808-816.

Kron, T. (1966). *Nursing Team Leadership* (2nd ed). Philadelphia: WB Saunders.

Lambertsen, E.C. (1953). *Nursing team organization and functioning.* New York: Bureau of Publications, Teachers College, Columbia University.

Leonard, M. (1975). Health issues and primary nursing in nephrology care. *Nursing Clinics of North America, 10*(3), 413-420.

Manthey, C., et al. (1971). Primary nursing: A return to the concept of "my nurse" and "my patient." *Nursing Forum, 9*(1), 65-83.

Manthey, M., and Kramer, M. (1970). A dialogue on primary nursing. *Nursing Forum, 9*(4), 356-379.

Manthey, M. (1973). Primary nursing is alive and well in the hospital. *American Journal of Nursing, 73*(1), 83-87.

Marram, G.D. (1976). The comparative costs of operating a team and primary nursing unit. *Journal of Nursing Administration, 3*(4), 21-24.

Marram, G.D., Schlegel, M.W., and Bevis, E.O. (1974). *Primary Nursing: A model for individualized care.* St. Louis: The CV Mosby Co.

McPhail, A., Pikula, H., Roberts, J., Browne, G., and Harper, D. (1990). Primary nursing: A randomized crossover trial. *Western Journal of Nursing Research, 12*(2), 188-197.

Munson, F.C., and Clinton, J. (1979). Defining nursing assignment patterns. *Nursing Research, 28*(4), 243-249.

Nenner, V.C., Curtis, E.M., and Eckhoff, C.M. (1977). Primary nursing. *Supervisor Nurse, 8*(5), 14-16.

O'Connor, A.M. (1990). Commentary on McPhail et al. study of primary nursing: A randomized crossover trial. *Western Journal of Nursing Research, 12*(2), 197-198.

Olivas, G.S., Del Togno-Armanasco, V., Erickson, J.R., and Harter, S. (1989a). Case management: A bottom-line care delivery model, Part I: The concept. *Journal of Nursing Administration, 19*(11), 16-20.

Olivas, G.S., Del Togno-Armanasco, V., Erickson, J.R., and Harter, S. (1989b). Case management: A bottom-line care delivery model, Part II: Adaptation of the model. *Journal of Nursing Administration, 19*(12), 12-17.

Papenhausen, J.L. (1990). Case management: A model of advanced practice? *Clinical Nurse Specialist, 4*(4), 169-170.

Parker, M., Quinn, J., Viehl, M., McKinley, A., Polich, C., Detzner, D., Hartwell, S., and Korn, K. (1992). Case management in rural areas. *Journal of Nursing Administration, 22*(2), 54-59.

Prescott, P., and Sorenson, J. (1978). Cost effectiveness analysis: An approach to evaluating nursing programs. *Nursing Administration Quarterly, 3*(3), 17-39.

Shukla, R.K. (1982a). Nursing care structures and productivity. *Hospital and Health Services Administration, 27*(16), 45-58.

Shukla, R.K. (1982b). Primary or team nursing? Two conditions determine the choice. *Journal of Nursing Administration, 12*(11), 12-15.

Shukla, R.K. (1983). All-RN model of nursing care delivery: A cost-benefit evaluation. *Inquiry, 20*(2), 173-184.

Sinnen, M.T., and Schifalacqua, M.M. (1991). Coordinated care in a community hospital. *Nursing Management, 22*(3), 38-42.

Sparacino, P.S. (1991). The CNS-case manager relationship. *Clinical Nurse Specialist, 5*(4), 180-181.

Steckel, S. (1980). Introduction to the study of primary nursing. *Nursing Dimensions, 7*(4), 74-77.

Taylor, F.W. (1912). *The principles of scientific management.* New York: Harper & Row.

Williams, L.B. (1975). Evaluation of nursing care: A primary nursing project. Report of the controlled study. *Supervisor Nurse, 6*(1), 32, 35-36, 38-39.

Williams, M.A. (1964). The myths and assumptions about team nursing. *Nursing Forum, 3*(4), 61-73.

Wolf, G.A., Lesic, L.K., and Leak, A.G. (1986). Primary nursing: The impact on nursing costs within DRGs. *Journal of Nursing Administration, 16*(3), 9-11.

Young, J.P., Giovanetti, P., Lewison, D., and Thoms, M.L. (1981). *Factors affecting nurse staffing in acute care hospitals: A review and critique of the literature (DHEW Publication No. HRP 0501801).* Hyattsville, MD: Department of Health, Education and Welfare.

Zander, K. (1988). Nursing case management: Strategic management of cost and quality outcomes. *Journal of Nursing Administration, 18*(5), 23-30.

CHAPTER NINETEEN

The Practising Nurse and the Law

JANET ROSS KERR

L egal challenges to nursing activities were once rare and posed little concern in the nursing profession. There were also very few legal disputes involving medical practice in Canada. This situation, however, is changing. The consumer movement, the extension of the nurse's scope of practice, substantial improvements in salaries and working conditions for nurses, and a greater propensity for the public to seek damages for professional negligence are all reasons for nurses to be aware of their responsibilities and the law to avoid civil suits and criminal prosecutions.

This chapter provides an overview of the law and the principal areas of nurses' involvement in the legal system. This information is not intended as a comprehensive treatment of the subject, but rather as a cursory review to emphasize areas of concern, stimulate thinking about issues, and encourage additional research. The potential benefit of understanding rights and responsibilities under the law, particularly as they apply to the health-care field, is easily identified when one considers the close and continuing contact between clients and nurses in health-care environments. Nurses' responsibilities traditionally have been thought of as falling largely in the area of comfort and less in the area of treatment procedures. However, the continuous transfer of functions from medicine to nursing and the exponential increase in knowledge and technology relating to health have had a far-reaching impact upon nursing and nurses' roles. The expanded scope of practice in nursing has been such that nurses have taken on performing procedures that have considerable risk attached to them, a situation that was not the case in the past.

■ ■ ■ ■

AN OVERVIEW OF THE LAW

Canadian law was derived from Roman civil law and English common law. Roman law can be traced from the Twelve Tables of Rome (450 B.C.), through codification by Justinian in 533, and development of the French Code of

Napoleon in 1804 (Merryman, 1969). English common law has a more recent history, beginning with the Norman conquest of 1066 (Plucknett, 1956). In Canada, English common law forms the basis of the legal system in all provinces except Quebec, where Roman civil law is the dominant influence. As Dais (1973) has noted,"The two traditions have much in common in terms of the legal rules they apply. Their essential difference has to do with culturally conditioned attitudes about the relation of law to society, the limits on government in using law, and the techniques and intellectual skills for making, interpreting, applying and teaching law" (p. 4).

Although the law refers to a clearly defined system of rules for the conduct of human activities and sanctions for violations of these, in practical terms the law is viewed in a wider sense and is,

> ... seen as a set of institutions, roles and procedures for ordering human behaviour in accordance with social values and political policies. . . It punishes deviance from basic social values (criminal law). It remedies harms intentionally, negligently or accidentally inflicted (tort law). It allocates scarce resources for satisfying human needs (property law). It facilitates productive enterprises (contract law) (Dais, 1973, p. 4).

In our society the institutions that serve the law are the legislatures of the provinces and the Parliament of Canada by making laws, the police by enforcing laws, the courts by judging disputes, and the prisons by applying punishments.

Case law and enacted law are the two primary types of law. In the Roman tradition, enacted law assumes greater importance because less freedom for judicial interpretation is allowed; under English common law, however, case law is dominant. The judicial process begins when there is disagreement about whether a matter meets the terms of the law. The courts are often thought of as the principal component of the judicial system; however, other important components include the legal profession and the adversary system. It should be noted that jury trials are rare in civil cases in Canada because of the expense involved; jury trials are primarily conducted in criminal cases.

It is helpful to know the distinctions between the various types of law. Civil law, also known as private law, comprises contract law, tort law, and property law, while public law is concerned with constitutional law, administrative law, and criminal law. International law may be considered private or public law, depending on whether the dispute is between individuals or between governments (Dais, 1973).

■ ■ ■ ■

RESPONSIBILITIES OF NURSES UNDER THE LAW

In a professional field such as nursing, legal obligations to the public are particularly important. Nurses are entrusted with the lives and health of other people throughout the course of their duties. The law has become increasingly complex, and it is important for all citizens to be aware of the laws that govern everyday life. On a daily basis, nurses are at great risk of violating the legal rights of others. The public expects nurses to practise competently and to do no harm to those who entrust nurses with their care. The concept of the provision of a reasonable standard of nursing care has been upheld by the courts in case law. Thus it is essential that nurses be knowledgeable and competent in the practice of their profession as well as being aware of and respecting the legal rights of their clients.

■■ ■■ ■■ ■■

RIGHTS OF THE HEALTH-CARE CONSUMER

As Storch (1982) has pointed out, rights are the product of social history and are based in law and ethics. As a self-governing profession, nursing has a statutory responsibility to protect the public interest in the course of providing the service at the basis of its practice. Reference to a code of ethics or ethical principles is embodied in provincial statutes regulating nursing. A code of ethics, one of the hallmarks of a profession, represents an attempt to document appropriate conduct.

It was not until after World War II that codes of ethics were developed and accepted by nursing organizations. Unacceptable experimentation on and treatment of human beings by the Nazis during the war led to the Declaration of Universal Human Rights in 1948, and the health-care professions focused attention on the necessity of protecting individuals from unscrupulous, unethical, and incompetent practitioners. The Code of Ethics developed by the International Council of Nurses in 1953 was used as the standard for measuring nurses' conduct for many years. The Canadian Nurses Association's (CNA) first code of ethics, developed in 1980, was replaced by a new version in 1985. The latter was succeeded by another revision in 1991. Today, most provincial nursing associations use the CNA code as the standard.

As important as codes of ethics may be, they are not a panacea for all the ethical concerns and dilemmas that arise in nursing practice. The difficulties have been noted by Storch (1982): "Health-care codes ... may not include all issues of concern to the patient . . . codes are limited because moral dilemmas in health care and nursing do not generally occur as a series of problems and questions to be solved with a series of guidelines. Rather, moral dilemmas are situations of complexity and conflict" (p. 20). Codes of ethics may be used by the profession to promote function in an ethical manner, but nurses must also have good intent, understand the facts of a situation that has ethical dimensions, exhibit clear thinking in weighing a situation, and be able to use basic ethical principles or theory in decision making (Storch, 1982).

Consumer rights in health care, as proclaimed by the Consumers' Association of Canada, include:

> . . . the right to be informed, the right to be respected as the individual with the major responsibility for his own health care, the right to participate in decision-making affecting his health, and the right to equal access to health care regardless of the individual's economic status, sex, age, creed, ethnic origin and location (Storch, 1982, p. 186).

The right of individuals to be informed about their health care is protected legally in tort law, which requires informed consent, and ethically in the principles of autonomy, veracity, and beneficence. The client's right to read and examine health-care records about personal health is an issue that arises in discussing this right. The right to be respected as an individual is a more elusive concern, raising ethical questions of autonomy, nonmaleficence, and beneficence. From a legal standpoint, the client's right to confidentiality and to refuse treatment is associated with the right to be respected and the right to privacy. The right to participate in decision making about health care is primarily ethical in nature; the principles of autonomy and responsibility are at issue. The right to equal access to health care finds its origin in the principle of justice (Storch, 1982).

■■■■

CONSENT TO NURSING CARE

A fundamental human right, historically respected in law, is the right to be free from interference. The tort of battery involves intentional touching of another person; there need not be any injury for the charge to be upheld by the courts. Because nursing practice involves a great deal of touching clients, it is important that client consent be obtained for any nursing procedures that involve touching. In most cases, clients will not initiate legal proceedings unless serious harm has resulted from the touching, but nurses must be aware of the importance of client consent. Nurses are taught the importance of explaining to a client, before beginning a nursing procedure, what is involved and why it is necessary. The importance of communicating effectively and ascertaining client consent to nursing care cannot be overstated.

Nurses often encounter problems in obtaining informed consent. The consent is legally valid only if a number of conditions are met, including the requirement that the client be properly informed about the procedure and clearly understand its nature and risks. Age, health, and mental status of clients, and circumstances surrounding the situation often make it difficult for nurses to obtain informed consent. Nurses usually rely on the client's verbal expression of consent to nursing-care activities. In the past the majority of these activities have been considered low risk; however, with the steady expansion of the scope of nursing practice and the increase in independent nursing functions, many current nursing-care procedures are considered high risk. Consent to care may be expressed, implied, or inferred. Philpott (1985) asserted that health-care workers who rely on implied consent in the absence of emergency or for high-risk procedures are exposing clients to unauthorized invasion and themselves to possible liability (p. 55).

Philpott (1985) identified six elements that must be present in legal consent:

1. The consent must be genuine and voluntary.
2. The procedure must not be an illegal procedure.
3. The consent must authorize the particular performer of the treatment or care.
4. The consenter must have legal capacity to consent.
5. The consenter must have the necessary mental competency to consent.
6. The consenter must be informed (p. 57).

■ ■ ■ ■

TELEPHONE ORDERS

A related concern is the problem inherent in nurses' acceptance of telephone orders from physicians for treatment. Many health-care agencies accept telephone orders only in emergency situations. If telephone orders are considered acceptable by an agency, the nurse may be liable in the event of later disagreement about the orders. If telephone orders are deemed acceptable by the agency, provision should be made for validation of the order, such as taping the conversation or having a second person confirm the orders with the physician. The complexity of health care and the potential for problems with modern drugs and treatments increase legal risks for nurses. If there is disagreement between physician and nurse on what transpired, external validation of the orders would strengthen the nurse's legal position. The decreased potential for error benefits the client as well.

■ ■ ■ ■

NEGLIGENCE

Complaints of negligence are the basis of most lawsuits against health-care professionals. Negligence is commonly defined as that which a reasonable and prudent nurse would or would not do in particular health-care circumstances. Philpott (1985) has noted that certain conditions must be present for a defendant to be liable in actions involving negligence and for damages to be awarded by the court:

1. The presence of a duty of care by the defendant to the plaintiff.
2. The defendant's conduct must constitute a breach of that duty of care, i.e., must have failed to comply with the required standard of care.
3. The plaintiff must have suffered a material injury.
4. The negligent conduct must have been the proximate cause of the injury.
5. There must not have been contributory negligence on the part of the plaintiff and he must not have voluntarily assumed the risk (p. 25).

The standard of care a reasonable and prudent nurse would use in a particular situation is established by the courts in a number of ways: articles and books by nursing authors that document the acceptability of certain practices, nursing practice standards developed by national and provincial professional nursing associations, curriculum content in schools of nursing, and testimony by expert witnesses who are nurses. The individual nurse's practice, educational background, and experience will be scrutinized by the court. The professional activities of a nurse whose practice is being questioned may also be considered relevant. In one important case, a nurse was found negligent after the court learned that the nurse, who had worked in a physician's office in Alberta for 22 years, had failed to take any continuing education courses since the year after she had graduated, 40 years before (Dowey v. Rothwell, 1974).

Krever (1973) states that the term *malpractice* is commonly used as a synonym for negligence. He points out that, although malpractice is a popular term that has even found its way into writings of the Supreme Court of Canada, it is a term that "tends to cause confusion, because of its very imprecision" (p. 109). As Krever notes, not only does the term malpractice refer to negligent practice by someone authorized to practise a profession, it also includes the practice of a profession by an unauthorized person. The latter situation would fall under the category of battery.

Although health-care professionals, including nurses, tend to view actions involving negligence as negative to reputation and integrity, Krever (1973) points out that "moral blamelessness is not involved" (p. 109). The purpose of the law pertaining to torts is to compensate the party who is injured through the actions of another. The issue here is not punishment; it is compensating the plaintiff for injury by moving responsibility for loss from the plaintiff to the defendant. Noting that any citizen can be sued for negligence, Krever (1973) states that a higher standard of care is expected of the professional. The question of foresee-ability of outcome of nursing-care activity or lack of activity is important in cases involving negligence. Krever (1973) states, "A person must take reasonable care to avoid acts or omissions which he can reasonably foresee would be likely to injure other persons so closely and directly affected by his act that he ought reasonably to have them in contemplation as being so affected when he is directing his mind to the acts or omission in question" (p. 110). Commenting on a determination of negligence when burns resulted from a diathermy treatment that was improperly performed, Krever (1973) points out that, "it was clearly foreseeable that burns would result from a failure to use that degree of care which objectively could be expected from a reasonable person with the nurse's training" (p. 112). The client had placed his trust in the nurse and had a right to expect the best possible care based on a reasonable standard of skill and knowledge.

■ ■ ■ ■

NURSING DOCUMENTATION

Nurses' records of the care and progress of clients in their care are important documents. In 1970 nurses' notes were declared admissible as evidence by the Supreme Court of Canada.

> Hospital records, including nurses notes made contemporaneously by someone having a personal knowledge of the matters then being recorded and under a duty to make the entry or record should be received in evidence as *prima facie* proof of the facts stated therein. This should in no way preclude a party wishing to challenge the accuracy of the records or entries from doing so (Ares v. Venner, 1970, p. 608).

Before this decision, nurses' notes were considered hearsay evidence and were not admissible in court. As Grady (1973) has observed, the legal system has gained a great deal from this decision, for:

> . . . if the nurse is (1) dead; or (2) for any sufficient reason unavailable to give evidence . . . or (3) unable to testify with regard to the accuracy of the facts stated in nurses' notes (for example, because of the many patients attended and the time lapse since the notes were taken), these notes may be introduced as evidence and proof of the facts stated therein. Such facts could be used to support a case, either for or against a nurse, doctor, or hospital (p. 128).

There are differences, however, among provinces as to whether various kinds of nursing records that form a part of the hospital record are admissible as evidence in court. Philpott (1985) notes that the Canada Evidence Act and the majority of provincial laws concerning evidence accept those parts of the record that are considered business records. However, there are variations in nursing records from agency to agency, and whether any part or all of a record is consistent with the definition of business records is decided by the province involved.

Ross (1973) emphasizes the importance of ". . . the virtues of accuracy, legibility, . . . brevity practised faithfully by the nurse" (p. 102) in recording descriptions of care or progress. Ross (1973) also refers to descriptions of unusual occurrences involving clients. These "unusual occurrence" or "incident" records are most often written by nurses, who may or may not have been present when the events took place. The desired characteristics of nursing notes, as previously mentioned, could include the need for contemporaneous recording by the nurse who had firsthand knowledge of what was described in the record and who was responsible for the record. The importance of a "cool, dispassionate, and thoughtful" approach to preparing a "factual, concise and totally objective" record of the event is reinforced by the fact that the record could be introduced as legal evidence to support or defend a damage claim (Ross, 1973, pp. 102-103).

In many cases, problems with nursing notes introduced as evidence in court have engendered criticism in court records of the proceedings. Frequent criticisms include failure to record events contemporaneously, gaps in recording, and recording of care by someone other than the nurse who provided the care. In general, it is difficult to verify that any care not recorded was actually provided. Cases often come to trial long after the events in question occurred. In these circumstances it is difficult for principals to remember details of what happened. Thus clear, accurate,and complete recording of events is essential. Nevertheless, many believe that there is a good deal of unnecessary charting in which nurses are required to spend a great deal of time recording routine care. This is wasteful both in terms of the highly skilled professional and in terms of storage and retrieval processes. Thus charting by exception is being used in many centres. This is a method by which unusual occurrences and reactions only are recorded, and if it were to become the norm, this method would allow the efforts of nurses to be directed more toward caring for the needs of clients.

There have also been cases of falsification and destruction of nursing records by nurses. These occurrences are sad commentaries on the trust and confidence placed in nurses by a public that expects honesty and integrity in all aspects of care. Nurses may be considered negligent in these cases simply because the court must assume that important facts were hidden and the person or persons responsible for the act were acting in self-interest. It is evident that dishonesty in matters pertaining to care will usually be discerned in court proceedings and will not reflect positively on the character, conduct, or professionalism of the nurse or nurses involved.

Computerization in hospitals is another development that is changing the way hospital records are developed and maintained. Programs written to support computerized nursing records are designed to facilitate nurses' recording of notes. Typewritten entries eliminate legibility problems, but the issues associated with the nature and quality of the recording remain. Computer programs can also be designed to note the correct time on all entries and to eliminate interlineations. Although signatures are not possible, a unique identification code can be assigned to each user to attribute entries to the correct individuals. Issues of client confidentiality are important and the parameters of maintaining confidentiality do not change with computerization. However, the fact that it is possible for many people to access computerized records underscores the need to ensure that systems are put in place that allow only those with the right to access the client's records to do so. The storage of hospital records in computer files will allow for a highly efficient means of maintaining, storing, and retrieving client records.

■— ■— ■— ■—

CONFIDENTIALITY

Statutes of the provinces that include laws addressing the client's right to confidentiality in health records are usually included in hospital acts, although acts that regulate nursing also contain provisions that reiterate the nurse's professional responsibility to maintain client confidentiality. To fail in this responsibility is to be subject to allegations of professional misconduct. Other areas of law where client confidentiality is protected include contractual and common law. Four provinces protect the right of privacy by statutory means: Quebec, British Columbia, Manitoba, and Saskatchewan. It has been noted that "where statutory rights to privacy are recognized, the client's right to consent and withdraw consent to privacy is valued and enforceable" (Philpott, 1985, p. 134). However, such is not the case in other provinces, where the only references to privacy are in hospital acts, which do not provide the same protection. There is an area of the law that as yet remains unexplored in relation to the provisions of section 7 of *The Charter of Rights and Freedoms* (Government of Canada, 1992). This provides that "Everyone has the right to life, liberty and security of the person and the right not to be deprived thereof except in accordance with the principles of fundamental justice" (p. 11). Challenges by clients to this section of the *Charter* may well be forthcoming with the passage of time.

Exceptions to the responsibility for maintaining confidentiality include: (1) client consent for disclosure of personal information to persons other than those named in the hospital act of the province, (2) statutory provisions for reporting certain diseases and child abuse to appropriate health and social services personnel, and (3) court orders, which are often used to obtain health records for the use of plaintiffs or defendants in trials.

In the past the client's right to view personal records has been a controversial issue. Historically lawyers acting for clients in suits against a hospital or its employees have had to gain access to the records by court order. Health-care agencies have traditionally been reluctant to release client records. However, there has been recognition that clients have the right to see their records, and the development of new legislation dealing with confidentiality should allow clients easier access to their own records.

▬ ▬ ▬ ▬

UNDERSTANDING LEGAL ASPECTS OF NURSING

It is evident that the professional nurse must have some knowledge of the law, legal processes, the judicial system, and client rights. The increasing complexity of professional practice has been associated with increased risks in nursing procedures, and higher risk procedures increase the potential for legal action. There have been many changes in the nurse's role over time, and the pace of development has accelerated in recent years. The effort to establish the baccalaureate standard for entry to practice in the profession is likely to result in even more change in the direction of augmented responsibility and increased risks for the nurse. There is no substitute for maintaining a high level of competence in nursing practice, excellent communication with clients, and awareness of the risks involved in performing various procedures.

The Canadian Nurses Protective Society (CNPS) was established by the CNA in 1988 at the request of the provincial/territorial professional associations in nursing as a result of escalating costs for professional liability insurance. It is a nonprofit organization that offers liability insurance purchased by 10 of the 12 provincial/territorial associations on behalf of their members. It also offers advice about professional liability to nurses from 0845 to 1630 hours, Monday through Friday, EST. Nurses may call CNPS if they have had personal involvement or knowledge of any situation in which there are ethical/legal implications of concern by calling a toll-free number: 1-800-267-3390 outside Ottawa or 237-2133 in Ottawa. CNPS offers the opportunity to speak with a nurse-lawyer who will give advice immediately and provide assistance with the steps to be taken in documenting an unusual occurrence, in understanding legal processes that might be applicable, and in referring nurses to experienced legal counsel.

The assumption is that the knowledgeable nurse will have a good understanding of the legal aspects of the relationship with the client, but few schools of nursing devote courses or units within courses to legal issues in nursing practice. Likewise, there are few continuing education programs that offer topics on legal issues for staff nurses who wish to enhance their understanding of the law as it relates to professional practice. Indeed, the in-service education departments of acute-care agencies deal with this subject only rarely in the programs they offer, perhaps because those who are responsible for teaching and programming have not had formal instruction in the legal aspects of nursing and may not consider this area an essential component in the curriculum or in-service education programs. They may also be unaware of the increasing legal risks for nurses in practice. However, as the 21st century approaches, new educational standards will be needed for the professional environment. The nurse of the future will need extensive knowledge and skills for competent and ethically based practice. Nursing practice will require a fundamental understanding of the law and the legal aspects of nursing.

REFERENCES

Ares v Venner (1970). S.C.R., 14, D.L.R. (3d) 4 (S.C.C.), p. 608.

Dais, E.E. (1973). Canadian law: an overview. In S.R. Good and J.C. Kerr (Eds.), *Contemporary issues in Canadian law for nurses* (pp. 3-14). Toronto: Holt, Rinehart & Winston.

Dowey v Rothwell (1974). 5 W.W.R. 311.

Government of Canada. (1992). *The charter of rights and freedoms: A guide for Canadians.* Ottawa: Minister of Supply and Services Canada.

Grady, P.E. (1973). The law and nurses' notes. In S.R. Good and J.C. Kerr (Eds.), *Contemporary issues in Canadian law for nurses* (pp. 127-129). Toronto: Holt, Rinehart & Winston.

Krever, H. (1973). Liability for negligence. In S.R. Good and J.C. Kerr (Eds.), *Contemporary issues*

in Canadian law for nurses (pp. 107-116). Toronto: Holt, Rinehart & Winston.

Merryman, J.H. (1969). *The civil law tradition.* Palo Alto, Calif: Stanford University Press.

Philpott, M. (1985). *Legal liability and the nursing process.* Toronto: W.B. Saunders.

Plucknett, T.F.T. (1956). *A concise history of the common law.* Boston: Little, Brown & Co.

Ross, M.W. (1973). The nurse as an employee. In S.R. Good and J.C. Kerr (Eds.), *Contemporary issues in Canadian law for nurses* (pp. 95-106). Toronto: Holt, Rinehart & Winston.

Storch, J. (1982). *Patients' rights: Ethical and legal issues in health care and nursing.* Toronto: McGraw-Hill Ryerson Ltd.

CHAPTER TWENTY

Ethical Issues and Dilemmas in Nursing Practice

JANNETTA MacPHAIL

C losely related to the issues pertaining to legal aspects of nursing practice are issues and dilemmas concerning professional ethics. Health professionals have always been faced with ethical dilemmas and have had to make ethical decisions; however, the dilemmas are more complex today. Factors contributing to this complexity are the rapidly expanding body of medical knowledge and the development of new technologies to save or prolong human life. At the same time, changes in societal values have increased recognition of individual rights and freedoms and responsibility for protecting those rights. Another influential factor is the availability of education, resulting in a better-informed public who are more questioning and expect to be more involved in decisions about their own lives and health. Because of the eradication of many diseases, increasing control over other diseases, and improved living standards, people are also living longer, which creates new ethical questions in terms of making decisions about prolonging life. The finite amount of resources available is another factor that raises questions about priorities in the health-care system; when there are insufficient resources to meet all needs, complex decisions must be made about who will receive care and how funds will be spent.

Because of these interacting factors, health professionals face many dilemmas. Who decides what is right for the individual or family involved? Is there always a right answer? Curtin (1982) defines ethics as "a discipline in which we attempt to identify, organize, analyze, and justify human acts by applying certain principles to determine the right thing to do in a given situation" (p. 1). Thus ethics is concerned with judgment of actions, not judgment of human beings.

■ ■ ■ ■

CODES OF ETHICS

A code of ethics is one of the characteristics of a profession. It is defined by the profession through the professional association and serves to inform members of that profession and society about the profession's expectations in ethical matters. For many years physicians, upon graduating from medical school, have taken the Hippocratic Oath, which was derived from the time of Hippocrates. Although it provides some ethical direction, it also commits the physician to saving and prolonging life at any cost, which is one of the factors leading to difficulties between physicians and nurses today. For example, there is often a difference of opinion between these two professions about prolonging life. This difference has led to stressful interprofessional relationships in terms of who should make the decision. Many physicians believe it is their responsibility, whereas many nurses believe the individual or family should be involved in making a decision that affects their lives.

Although some nurses have taken the Florence Nightingale pledge (which did not originate with Florence Nightingale but with Harper Hospital School of Nursing in Detroit), this pledge does not provide ethical direction for the issues and dilemmas encountered in practice. In 1955 the Canadian Nurses Association (CNA) adopted the code of ethics developed in 1953 by the International Council of Nurses (ICN) and replaced in 1973 by *The ICN Code for Nurses—Ethical Concepts Applied to Nursing*, which guided members in ethical decision making until the 1970s. At its 1978 annual meeting, the CNA made the development of a new national code a priority. A new code was approved in 1980, but revisions were deemed necessary soon after. An ad hoc committee appointed to make the revisions sought input from nurses across Canada and after lengthy deliberations published *Code of Ethics for Nursing* in 1985 (CNA, 1985). Within a few years it became apparent that this Code needed further study and assessment based on nurses' experience in using it in practice. The outcome was a revised *Code of Ethics for Nursing* published in November 1991 and distributed to all CNA members.

> This Code expresses and seeks to clarify the obligations of nurses to use their knowledge and skills for the benefit of others, to minimize harm, to respect client autonomy and to provide fair and just care for their clients. For those entering the profession, this Code identifies the basic moral commitments of nursing and may serve as a source of education and reflection. For those within the profession, the Code also serves as a basis for self-evaluation and for peer review. For those outside the profession, this Code may serve to establish expectations for the ethical conduct of nurses (CNA, 1991, p. ii).

The Code presents values—or broad ideals—and obligations arising from each value that provide direction in particular circumstances. Some values pertain to clients or patients; other values are concerned with nursing roles and relationships. An example of a value and the obligations deriving therefrom is shown in the box on page 253.

A tentative code of ethics for nurses in the United States, adopted by the American Nurses Association (ANA) in 1926, was revised a number of times

---

VALUE IV . . .

Dignity of Clients

VALUE

The nurse is guided by consideration for the dignity of clients.

OBLIGATIONS

1. Nursing care must be done with consideration for the personal modesty of clients.
2. A nurse's conduct at all times should acknowledge the client as a person. For example, discussion of care in the presence of the client should actively involve or include that client.
3. Nurses have a responsibility to intervene when other participants in the health care delivery system fail to respect any aspect of client dignity.
4. As ways of dealing with death and the dying process change, nursing is challenged to find new ways to preserve human values, autonomy and dignity. In assisting the dying client, measures must be taken to afford the clients as much comfort, dignity and freedom from anxiety and pain as possible. Special consideration must be given to the need of the client's family or significant others to cope with their loss.

Source: Canadian Nurses Association. (1991). *Code of ethics for nursing*. Ottawa: Author, p. 7.

---

over the years. The ANA code of ethics for professional nurses, adopted in 1950, was revised in 1960 to become the *Code for Professional Nurses*. After additional revision in 1976, the ANA adopted the *Code for Nurses with Interpretive Statements* (ANA, 1976; Flanagan, 1976). Earlier codes of ethics, prescriptive in nature, were essentially rules to govern the personal and professional conduct of members of a profession; recent codes are more similar to guidelines for practice that provide a framework for nurses to make ethical decisions and fulfil their responsibilities to the public and the profession. Although codes of ethics may or may not be part of statutory regulations, in most provinces there is a statutory requirement within the Act governing the nursing profession that mandates that nurses uphold ethical standards as defined by the nursing profession. This means that not only are individual nurses expected to uphold the precepts contained in codes of ethics, but are also to hold colleagues accountable for adhering to them.

Because of the complexity of the ethical dilemmas nurses confront today, they need more than a code of ethics. Storch (1982) believes that at least four conditions are necessary for ethical decision making: (1) desire and commitment to do what is right and good; (2) knowledge of relevant facts of the particular situation; (3) clarity of thought, rather than emotionalism, in dealing with the facts; and (4) some understanding of basic principles or concepts of ethics. In recent years nurses and other health-care professionals have recognized the importance of examining and clarifying values that may influence their actions and the importance of becoming more sensitive to the values of their patients or clients.

Rather than prescribing a set of values for nurses and nursing students as in the past, values clarification strategies are being used increasingly in both nursing education programs and continuing education programs for practising nurses.

■ ■ ■ ■

PRINCIPLES AND CONCEPTS OF ETHICS

A prerequisite to applying ethics in nursing is having a theoretical base in ethics, just as basic knowledge in the biologic and behavioral sciences is requisite to the application of principles and concepts from those sciences to nursing. Without a theoretical base, discussion of ethical issues may be merely sharing of opinions. Two basic theoretical approaches are: (1) teleological, which is goal-directed or consequence-oriented, and (2) deontological, which is duty-oriented or focused on rules. Kluge (1992) identifies the difference between the two approaches "in the sorts of considerations they find relevant in reaching their conclusions" (p. 17). The teleological approach focuses on the anticipated outcome of actions, whereas "the deontological approach concentrates on balancing rights and duties . . . and considers them independently of outcome considerations" (Kluge, 1992, p. 17).

Although it is not feasible to provide a theoretical base for ethical decision making in this context, basic concepts of ethics can be identified. They include: (1) personhood, of which self-awareness is a basic quality (Storch, 1982); (2) autonomy, which implies not only freedom to decide and to act, but also to acknowledge and respect the dignity and autonomy of others (Francoeur, 1983); (3) veracity, which includes obligation to tell the truth and to use good judgment in determining what the patient wants to know or can withstand; (4) paternalism, which refers to restricting the liberty of an individual without his or her consent with the justification of trying to do good, such as not telling a person about his or her diagnosis and condition because of a poor prognosis; (5) confidentiality, which must be maintained but balanced against the rights of others, including society (Francoeur, 1983); (6) beneficence, or doing what is best for an individual while balancing the risks and benefits in a given situation; (7) nonmaleficence, or not inflicting intentional harm or risk of harm and preventing evil or harm whenever possible; and (8) justice, which pertains to ensuring that individuals get what they deserve according to individual need, worth, and merit and also involves enforcing the concept of distributive justice, which "has to do with the distribution of good and evil, of burdens and benefits in any society when resources are limited" (Davis and Aroskar, 1983, p. 45).

The question of justice presents an ethical dilemma frequently described in the literature today because of inadequate staffing due to cutbacks in funding causing nurses to make difficult decisions about apportioning care when all needs cannot be met. A thorough knowledge of basic ethical concepts is necessary for nurses to be able to address the increasingly complex issues encountered daily in practice settings. Although there is a tendency to consider only the dilemmas faced in acute-care settings, the issues are different but equally complex for practitioners in long-term care and home and community settings due to increased longevity, early discharge from hospitals, and the use of technologies in the home that were previously limited to acute-care settings. Robillard et al. (1989) point out that there has been little research on the ethical issues in primary care, although most health care is provided in primary care settings. Their study revealed that the issues are most frequently pragmatic, not dramatic, and are concerned with "patient self-determination, adequacy of care and professional responsibility, and distribution of resources" (p. 9). Thus nurses practising in all types of health-care settings need a knowledge base in ethical concepts and principles, as well as support and expert resources to assist them in ensuring that basic human rights are recognized and respected.

■ ■ ■ ■

BASIC HUMAN RIGHTS ABOUT HEALTH AND HEALTH CARE

Basic human rights in health care, which are increasingly recognized today, are the right to be informed, the right to be respected, and the right to self-determination. Each has great implications for ethical decision making and the responsibility of health professionals to protect these rights. These rights also cause debate over some ethical issues and are the bases for confrontation between nurses and physicians. For example, there may be differences of opinion between nurses and physicians about the meaning of being informed and whose responsibility it is to inform the individual or family. A confrontation may occur when information is withheld by a physician who believes it is in the best interest of the patient and the nurse believes that the patient should be informed and is asked directly for such information. The right to be informed has increased the need for obtaining informed consent before medical interventions are instituted and before patients or clients are asked to participate in research. Until the 1970s there was no expectation or requirement for obtaining informed consent for participation in research, and people were sometimes exploited. For example, in an experiment at the Allen Memorial Institute in Montreal in the late 1940s, patients were given mind-altering drugs, such as lysergic acid diethylamide (LSD), which had far-reaching effects; recompense was sought in the mid-1980s.

The right to be respected has great implications in approaches to patients and is interrelated with the right to be informed. Providing an interpretation of care and explaining medical conditions are two methods of showing respect for patients. Respect also has implications for confidentiality, which has been a problem in terms of information shared among health professionals. Although nurses and physicians may respect confidentiality to the point of not sharing information with persons outside the health professions, there has been a tendency to share information openly in discussion where it can be overheard. Confidentiality also requires that written records be carefully protected, which, with the development of computers, has great implications for the protection of rights.

The right to self-determination implies that individuals or families have the right to make decisions about matters that affect their health and their lives.

Ensuring that this right is protected is complex; for example, it involves deciding if an individual is capable of making decisions and if not, who should be involved in the decision making. Making decisions about matters that affect a patient's health and life involves giving people the opportunity to decide not to have treatment recommended by a physician. This is a difficult situation for health professionals because they are faced with an individual refusing treatment that they believe is best for the individual. There may be circumstances in which not consenting to certain treatment is logical in terms of an individual's prognosis and desire not to undergo possible adverse side effects. For example, cancer therapy might be refused by a patient when the disease has progressed beyond redemption. On the other hand, some individuals choose to have treatment almost to the end, even if there is no hope of cure or remission.

Self-determination is not limited to life and death matters, but also involves making decisions about life-style. For example, individuals make decisions to continue with life-styles and behaviour patterns that are known to be detrimental to their health and well-being, such as smoking, overeating, excessive drinking, refusing to wear seat belts, and engaging in sexual relations with people likely to be carriers of the human immunodeficiency virus (HIV), which causes AIDS. Although efforts to educate the public about the hazards of such habits are meeting with some success, many persons still choose to do things that are harmful to their health.

■ ■ ■ ■

THE RIGHT TO MAKE CHOICES IN RELATION TO DEATH

Dying and death give rise to many ethical issues and dilemmas. Davis and Aroskar (1983) identify three issues: (1) possible interventions by health professionals, such as resuscitation and passive euthanasia; (2) possible interventions by the family or significant others, such as helping a terminally ill person to hasten death and end suffering; and (3) possible interventions by the afflicted person, such as suicide, use of a living will, and claiming "a right to die."

> The ethical, legal, medical, social, cultural, psychologic, and economic factors to be considered in types of intervention will vary with the individual and family involved. Decisions about types of intervention are extremely complex for everyone involved because of the numbers and kinds of factors intersecting in each individual situation. There are significant implications from the decisions made in individual situations for individuals and the community in terms of the moral principles of respect for the person, doing no harm, and justice (Davis and Aroskar, 1983, pp. 136-137).

The word *euthanasia* is derived from Greek and means good or pleasant death. Is death ever preferable to life? That question is difficult to answer; it must consider the specific situation and distinguish this from the interests and values of the care provider and the institution. Some believe that euthanasia should be considered only for those who can ask to die, which would eliminate newborns, infants, and individuals who are kept alive by machines and are unable to speak for themselves. Others believe that in certain circumstances some severely deformed newborns should be allowed to die by withdrawing or withholding treatment, and that the decision should be made by the parents and their professional advisors, who are usually physicians (Duff and Campbell, 1973; McCormick, 1974; Shaw, 1973).

Passive euthanasia, or "letting someone die," may be done by not initiating treatment or by stopping treatment, with or without the consent of the individual. These measures, although used in some hospitals, are still morally controversial. Active euthanasia means providing an individual with the means to end life or directly bringing about the individual's death with or without consent (Brody, 1976). How does the concept of protecting human rights fit into euthanasia? Does a person ever have the right to die? Can one refuse life-saving treatment? Is lack of clear-cut policies and guidelines to help health professionals in addressing such complex questions a reflection of there being no right or wrong answer? Some believe that death should never be hastened; others believe that a person whose death is imminent should be allowed to die to relieve pain and suffering, and that the right to refuse treatment should be respected. Some fear that if euthanasia as a kindly act—beneficent euthanasia—can be morally justified, euthanasia for other purposes may also be justified and practised (Dyck, 1975).

■ ■ ■ ■

DO NOT RESUSCITATE ORDERS

In recent years more has been written about the ethical dilemmas faced by nurses in relation to "do not resuscitate (DNR)" or "no code" orders (Campbell and Field, 1991; Honan et al, 1991; Ott and Nieswiadomy, 1991; Slomka, 1992; and Toth, 1991). If there are no written DNR orders and a patient arrests, is the nurse expected to "code" the patient? Who is or should be involved in making such a decision? Are there or should there be a difference in DNR policy in long-term care institutions versus acute-care settings? The development of guidelines for resuscitation has been encouraged through a joint effort of the Canadian Medical Association (CMA), Canadian Nurses Association (CNA), Canadian Hospital Association (CHA), and Canadian Bar Association (CBA), which resulted in a "Joint Statement on Terminal Illness" published in *The Canadian Nurse* (CNA, 1984). The guidelines have been used in formulating institutional policy and procedure; however, they address only patients who are terminally ill and do not address such issues as chronic illness and age. Toth (1991) states unequivocally that CPR should not be performed "on a patient for whom such an intervention would prolong the dying process rather than extend life," and that "strong consideration should be given to a policy that would make CPR the exception rather than the rule in long-term care institutions" (p. 5). The University of Alberta Hospitals' policy for a "No Cardiopulmonary Resuscitation Order" (see box p. 258) reflects some of Toth's thinking, and addresses the issue of CPR in long-term care settings in Item 2.3 in terms of the frequency of reviewing a "no CPR" order.

University of Alberta Hospitals Policy 4.1.1.6
No Cardiopulmonary Resuscitation Order (No CPR Order)
Issued 12 August 1991

1. RATIONALE

1.1 Cardiopulmonary resuscitation (CPR) should *not* be attempted in cases in which such an intervention is not in the best interests of the patient. CPR performed for inappropriate indications may prolong the dying process rather than extend life and may lead to futile suffering of patients.

1.2 Physicians and other health care professionals have a duty to inform themselves of the results of studies of outcomes following attempted CPR in different age groups and disease states so that decisions concerning the appropriate indications for CPR are scientifically based.

1.3 Patients have the right to accept or refuse beneficial treatment; however, the physician is not obligated to provide treatment which is not in the best interest of the patient.

2. IMPLEMENTATION

2.1 Physicians shall leave clear written orders that CPR should not be attempted when
   a) the patient has a condition which is irreversible and/or has caused irreparable damage and for whom CPR would not be in the best interests of the patient; or
   b) the patient or the legal guardian requests that such an order be written. The patient, or legal guardian(s) of the patient (if the patient is not competent), or family member(s) (if there is no legal guardian and if there is a "family" which appears to be interested in the welfare of the patient) should be informed that CPR will not be performed.

2.2 Discussion of the "no CPR" order with the patient, guardian and family should be documented in the progress notes. These discussions should include the irreversible and/or irreparable condition of the patient, the patient's life expectancy, and the consequences of the order.

2.3 A "no CPR" order shall be written and signed by the attending physician covering each hospital admission of a patient. The attending physician shall review the order every seven days or sooner as clinically appropriate. In patients in the long term care areas (Station 82, 95 and 97) a "no CPR" order shall be reviewed every three months or sooner as clinically appropriate.

2.4 In urgent circumstances, a "no CPR" order may be given by the attending physician over the telephone. Such an order must be countersigned within 24 hours.

2.5 A second opinion shall be obtained from another physician if there is doubt about the decision. Such a consultant shall record his/her opinions as a consultant's note. The attending physician and/or the second staff physician may consult with the Ethics Consultation Service. Further details may be obtained from the Vice-President, Medical Affairs (6822).

2.6 If the clinical criteria leading to the decision to write a "no CPR" order appear to have changed or become invalid, another physician or nurse may rescind the order until the situation can be reassessed. The patient, guardian or involved family should be notified.

2.7 A "no CPR" order in no way limits the implementation of any other medically indicated interventions. All other measures to assure the mental and physical comfort of the patient shall be enacted.

Source: University of Alberta Division of Bioethics. (September 1991). *The Bioethics Bulletin*, 3(3), 6.

Although it is the physician's responsibility to write a DNR order and also convey the meaning of it to the nursing staff, there should be opportunity for nursing input into the development of such guidelines. Davis and Aroskar (1983) point out that "nurses are in a key position to notify the physician if the patient's condition changes, which change would indicate that the orders may need reassessment" (p. 149). This reinforces the need for careful nursing assessment and clear communication with physicians and the need for flexibility and wise judgment in applying orders based on changes in the patient's condition.

The policy indicates the importance of discussing the DNR order with the patient, guardian, and family and also recording this in the progress notes; however, the literature raises questions about the extent to which patients are involved in such decisions. In a study of older adults in an acute-care and a long-term care setting, Godkin (1992) found that most of the patients had limited knowledge of CPR and its possible outcomes, and that it was gained primarily through television in which most of the attempts to resuscitate were successful. The question of CPR had not been discussed by a physician with the majority, and most had not discussed their wishes regarding care with anyone. Nonetheless, if given an opportunity, 85% would have chosen to be involved in deciding whether to have CPR, and 75% "hoped that their physician would inform them if they thought that CPR would be of no benefit to them" (Godkin, 1992, p. 114). Most of the patients favoured a collaborative approach to decisions about CPR, involving physicians, themselves, nurses, and family members. Most DNR policies in hospitals pertain to terminally ill patients only. Godkin (1992) suggests that such policies be made known so that every individual understands that current policy requires that CPR be performed on other patients unless a DNR order is recorded on the chart. This would require that the issue be addressed, which could reduce the dilemmas faced by families and staff regarding CPR, could reduce costs of administering CPR that was not desired by the patient, and could prevent the situation of the patient being unable to participate in the decision by the time any discussion is initiated.

Although autonomous decision making by the patient is highly valued by both nurses and physicians, recent research shows that frequently the patient is not involved in the decision where participation is possible (Bedell and Delbanco, 1984; Bedell, Pelle, Maher, and Cleary, 1986; Evans and Brody, 1985; Savage, Cullen, Kirchhoff, Pugh, and Foreman, 1987). Bedell and Delbanco (1984) surveyed 154 physicians whose patients had been resuscitated and found that only 19% of the patients had discussed resuscitation with the physician before cardiac arrest occurred. They found also that 33% of the families were consulted about resuscitation before the arrest, but patient competency to be involved in the decision was not addressed. Youngner (1987) identifies some possible reasons physicians may not discuss resuscitation with their patients: lack of awareness; pressure of time; feeling uncomfortable about discussing such matters; and/or the paternalistic attitude of doing what the physician feels is best for the patient. Such reactions fail to support the patient's right to self-determination and autonomy.

In a study of the influences for DNR policies and end-of-life decisions in acute-care and long-term care settings in Alberta, Wilson (1993) found that 73%

of 135 accredited health-care facilities had a written DNR policy. Most had been developed in the 1990s to optimize decision making and involve the patient in the process; however, these purposes had not been achieved in general. In-depth surveys of four of the facilities indicated that DNR policies were not commonly followed and that in almost one-third of all instances they were not implemented at all. Problems generally arose from late decision making that excluded the patient from end-of-life decisions. Hence DNR policies seemed to have limited effect on practice. Wilson (1993) identifies the need for internal assessment to determine the extent to which nurses and physicians are knowledgeable about the DNR policy. Further, she believes that if the policy is retained, adherence should be emphasized because "lack of adherence to organizational policy places health care facilities in legal and ethical jeopardy" (p. 127). She suggests implementing additional education about the policies and perhaps designing a separate DNR chart to improve recording and to help guide decision making about DNR.

Wilson (1993) also found that no-CPR decisions were usually made late and therefore did not create an ethical or legal dilemma for health-care professionals or family members "as everything possible appeared to have been done to restore health and prevent death" (p. 129). She noted that it was common practice for health-care professionals to use at least one life-sustaining technology, such as oxygen or intravenous fluids, to promote comfort during the end-stage dying process. Questioning whether comfort was always the outcome, Wilson (1993) identifies the need for research to substantiate or refute whether such measures promote comfort or just extend the dying process.

Yarling and McElmurry (1983) propose authorizing both the responsible physician and the responsible nurse to write DNR orders, depending on the situation. Although this may seem like an onerous responsibility for the nurse, is it any greater than having to perform CPR when the nurse knows that the patient does not want it? While it seems unlikely that nurses will be granted such a privilege, it is important that nurses and physicians have mechanisms to discuss such questions and differences of opinion. Also, it is important that patients have opportunity to participate in making such profound decisions in advance of the critical occurrence, such as provided by advance directives.

■■ ■■ ■■ ■■

ADVANCE DIRECTIVES

In recent years much attention has been given to developing directives in advance to serve as guidelines for health-care practitioners and family members when an individual is no longer capable of making decisions. A report, *Advance Directives and Substitute Decision-Making in Personal Care*, recommends that:

> legislation be introduced to enable individuals to execute a healthcare directive, in which they can (1) appoint someone as their healthcare agent, who will have authority to make healthcare decisions on their behalf in the event of their becoming incapable of making those decisions personally; (2) identify anyone whom they do not wish to act as their healthcare proxy; and (3) provide instructions and information concerning future healthcare decisions (Alberta Law Reform Institute, March 1993, p. 94).

Similar legal developments have taken place or are in process in Manitoba, Ontario, Newfoundland, British Columbia, and Saskatchewan. In an unpublished 1991 study, Storch and Dosseter found overwhelming support for the concept of advance health-care directives in a survey of Edmonton residents. Similarly, strong support was found by Hughes and Singer (1992) in their survey of 1000 family physicians in Ontario; however, their findings also revealed that most respondents rarely discuss the idea with their patients.

Advance health-care directives may be prepared in the form of a living will that enables individuals to indicate in advance whether they want "heroic or extraordinary measures" in the event they are unable to make known their wishes. This approach was rejected by the Alberta Law Reform Institute and Health Law Institute because of problems of interpretation with the use of such vague terms as "heroic" and "extraordinary" measures. For example, do they refer to CPR only, or do they include tube feeding and other measures designed to prolong life? They also rejected the "endurable power of attorney" approach which "enables an individual, while mentally competent, to appoint someone who will have the authority to make health-care decisions on the donor's behalf once the donor becomes mentally incapable of making these decisions" (Alberta Law Reform Institute, 1993, p. 7). Their approach, instead, is to legalize the concept of health-care directives so individuals can have control over who will make decisions on their behalf when they become unable to do so and can also have some control over the content of decisions by including specific instruction in the directive, if desired.

Wilson (1993) emphasizes that, if the advance treatment directives are enacted by the Alberta legislature, health-care facilities will need to review, and perhaps revise, their DNR policy to change the method in which life support preferences are determined and used in decision making about care. Wilson's findings indicate a need for action to enhance patient self-determination even if advance treatment legislation is not enacted.

Flarey (1991) identified three major advantages of the use of advance directives: (1) ensures that one's predetermined wishes are followed; (2) helps family members in making complex decisions; and (3) provides guidance to health professionals regarding the individual's wishes in such circumstances. As found by Wilson (1993), the attainment of these goals will depend on the extent to which health-care agencies develop and implement such policies and inquire of patients whether they have developed an advance directive. Nurses can play an important role in ensuring that these goals are attained in their work settings by gaining representation on ethics committees and policy-making bodies on advance directives and by educating colleagues and the public about individual rights to self-determination.

■ ■ ■ ■

THE RIGHT TO LIVE AS PERSONS, AND RESPONSIBILITIES FOR CHANGING BEHAVIOUR

Many complex ethical questions derive from efforts to effect a change in deviant behaviour. Bandman and Bandman (1978) state:

Once a set of persons occupies a place within the circle of life, the problem of the right to live as persons arises. The limits to this right are found in the right a person has to be free to live well, without unjustified interferences of his or her freedom. Conversely, being free—and one can only be free if unmolested and free from unjustified harm, injury or threat of violence—is the presence of rules and norms for changing undesirable behavior. To induce changed behavior, reward and punishment are commonly used (p. 4).

Although few people would argue about the need to control violence against others, what constitutes deviant behaviour is worthy of discussion. What establishes norms of standard behaviour? What authorizes persons to try to change behaviour that does not meet these norms and under what conditions? Specific groups in society, such as prisoners, children, older persons, and the mentally ill, are particularly vulnerable to having their rights disregarded when professionals use behaviour modification methods.

Peplau (1978) identified a major problem in defining mental illness with the contradictory views of professionals. She believes that "the difficulties of the `mentally ill' are conceptualized in different ways by health professionals, and each viewpoint gives rise to a different form of treatment" (p. 208). She also notes that problems with self-identity, relationships, and function within social systems do not fit easily into the cause-effect, disease-oriented medical model. How do we ensure protection of the human rights of the "mentally ill" who have long been considered incompetent and unable to judge the necessity of treatment? They are not given the opportunity to refuse treatment. Moreover, many of the therapies used for these patients have been designed to change behaviour in the direction of obedience, compliance, and conformity. Coercion has been used to force patients to accept treatment. Whittington (1975) believes it would be best to admit we often do not know what is best for an individual or group and give them more choices.

Another concern about allowing the mentally ill to refuse treatment is that, if untreated, their conditions will become chronic and they will become an economic burden on society. Peplau (1978) believes that releasing these patients into the community, which has been done in Canada and the United States for almost two decades, is not as much a matter of their being a danger to society as their being a burden on others. In addition, they are in danger of being exploited by others ready to take advantage of the already disadvantaged. It is probably more appropriate to give them the opportunity to choose from available treatments or grant them the right to refuse treatment after participating in "sessions designed to investigate conceptions of treatment offered and reasons for refusing" (Peplau, 1978, p. 212).

■— ■— ■— ■—

ETHICAL DILEMMAS RELATED TO CHILDBEARING

The major ethical issue pertaining to childbearing is abortion. The issue is "the status of the fetus as a member of the human species when the existence of the fetus poses a threat to physical, psychological or social well-being of a pregnant woman and/or other family members" (Curtin, 1982, p. 240). Anti-abortionists claim that the personhood of the fetus is being denied, wheras pro-abortionists maintain that the woman's right to self-determination cannot be denied. They emphasize the burden imposed on society by an unwanted pregnancy and the possible outcomes for the welfare of the child in the future. Between the two extremes are those who favour abortions depending on circumstances surrounding the pregnancy, such as rape and incest.

The Supreme Court of Canada's decision, made in 1988, endorses women's rights to self-determination in relation to abortion. This has been challenged many times, but the challenges have not been supported. For example, Bill C43, passed in 1990 by the House of Commons, would permit abortion only if a continued pregnancy would jeopardize the woman's physical or mental health, as diagnosed by one physician only. Physicians adamantly opposed this change because of the possibility of criminal charges against them, and because they would be required to provide pre-abortion and post-abortion counseling. Bill C43 was struck down and hence the Supreme Court's decision still prevails.

The question of abortion may present problems for the individual nurse who is expected to participate in abortions within a health-care agency. It is important that the nurse know the agency's policies about such participation before accepting a position. Health-care agencies must have clearly defined policies that can be communicated to potential employees and referred to when situations arise that present an ethical dilemma to staff members. The nurse is responsible, legally and morally, for ensuring that patients' needs are met and that patients are not neglected because of differing values (Curtin, 1982).

■ ■ ■ ■

ALLOCATION OF HEALTH-CARE RESOURCES

Ethical issues pertaining to allocation of health-care resources may be encountered at several levels. At the government level, public policies are established that determine what type of health care can be provided. Nurses and other health professionals have a responsibility to exercise their prerogatives and communicate with legislators to influence these policies. For example, as a result of a government's decision not to require seat belt use by law, a considerable portion of the health-care dollar is spent on persons involved in automobile accidents.

Policies that influence the use of health-care resources are also established at the institutional level. Too often nurses have little influence on such policies and they need to take action to affect decision making and priority setting. Decisions to develop programs are often made without adequate consideration of the implications for nursing practice; new medical programs, such as heart transplants and hip replacements, have enormous impact on the need for nursing care and could affect nurses' ability to respond to the demands placed on them. At the unit level, nurses have to delineate problems that result from new programs and provide data that will facilitate a reasoned decision, although values and emotions often enter into these decisions. Fortunately, nurses have become more vocal in expressing their concerns and in providing facts that can influence decision making, rather than merely responding to the decisions made by physicians and hospital administrators.

Is it ethically and morally right to support activities that may jeopardize the patient or result in unequal or unfair distribution of resources among different programs within a health-care institution? Who decides the priorities in allocating resources, and what facts are considered?

With the increasing proportion of older persons in Canada and other developed countries, the question of age may influence decisions. For example, a 99-year-old man had surgery for removal of an esophageal pouch that was making adequate nutrition impossible. He had been advised 17 years earlier not to have surgery because of his age, but the predictors of his life expectancy were inaccurate. Although he survived the surgery, it might have been easier at age 82. Many disadvantaged groups such as the physically handicapped, the cognitively impaired, the poor, and ethnic minorities, are also exploited by such decisions and their rights are neglected.

Other factors that influence allocation of resources in health-care legislation include consumer unrest and the patients' rights movement. Davis and Aroskar (1983) believe that "health care policy cannot be the monopoly of providers any more than scientists should have the only say on biomedical research" (p. 206). Reasons for such a position are: 1) possible conflicts of interest; 2) large amounts of taxes are used to provide health care; 3) nonmedical dimensions of health problems may be critical aspects; and 4) "individual liberty and autonomy extend not only into the political arena but also into health care" (Davis and Aroskar, 1983, p. 206). Although nurses, individually and collectively, have become more involved in influencing public policy through lobbying and working effectively with consumers and providers of care, their involvement needs to be increased. In addition to responding to particular issues, the professional organizations are working diligently to influence public policy about the allocation of health-care resources.

■ ■ ■ ■

STRATEGIES FOR ADDRESSING ETHICAL DILEMMAS IN PRACTICE

The number and variety of ethical dilemmas that nurses encounter in practice have increased because of advancements in scientific knowledge and the development of technologies. Nurses and physicians often become embroiled in ethical dilemmas in which opinions differ, leading to decreased communication and failure to work together in the interests of patients. These results can be detrimental to patient care and to the mental health and well-being of nursing staff, particularly in intensive care units, where nurses and physicians may disagree on life and death decisions, on approaches to care, and on setting priorities.

Some health-care agencies address these dilemmas through an ethics committee, which is called on an *ad hoc* basis to address dilemmas presented by nurses or physicians. In some large teaching hospitals an ethicist is employed to provide expert assistance and guidance. At Montreal General Hospital, Dr. David Roy, an internationally recognized physician-ethicist, has been helping nursing and medical staff address complex issues for many years.

Institutional ethics committees are not a new venture in Canadian hospitals. The Canadian Hospital Association (CHA) issued a policy statement recommending them in 1986 (CHA, 1986). In 1984 Avard, Griener, and Langstaff (1985) conducted a survey to determine the extent to which ethics committees exist, as well as their composition and modus operandi. Their findings revealed a great deal of variability in size, composition, and functions and showed that they were primarily advisory. A second survey conducted by Storch, Griener, Marshall, and Olineck in 1989 (cited in Storch and Griener, 1990) was designed to try to determine the effectiveness of committees in addressing the ethical problem of self-determination. The data revealed that the status of ethics committees in Canadian hospitals in 1989 was very similar to that in 1984. The most evident change was an increase from 18% to 58.3% of the hospitals having an ethics committee. Most respondents indicated that the committees serve primarily in an advisory capacity; however, it is not known whether such advice must be followed. To seek an answer to this question and others regarding the effectiveness of committees, a second phase of the study was undertaken through site visits to five selected hospitals for in-depth review, but the findings have not been reported to date (Storch and Greiner, 1990).

A preventive strategy is to improve the teaching of ethics in nursing education by ensuring that ethics is an official part of nursing curricula on the undergraduate and graduate levels and is taught by experts, not left to "chance" to be integrated into all teaching. Thompson and Thompson (1989) are advocates of this approach. They identify the goals of teaching ethics to professional students and professionals as: "to stimulate the moral imagination; recognize ethical issues; elicit a sense of moral obligation; develop analytical skills; and tolerate and reduce disagreements and ambiguity" (p. 86). They recommend using case studies, as do many textbooks on ethics; however, expert guidance should be provided during the process of analyzing the ethical issues and dilemmas presented.

Since many practising nurses who face ethical dilemmas every day have not had the benefit of this education, discussion of ethics should be included in in-service education and continuing education. After nurses have learned the theoretical foundation of ethics, ongoing Bioethics Rounds can be organized for nurses and physicians. Bioethics Rounds are not intended to address ethical issues encountered in the care of a specific patient, but to provide opportunities for open discussion of ethical issues when the professionals involved can consider various viewpoints and are not facing a specific ethical issue requiring an immediate decision.

This approach has been developed through a Joint-Faculties Bioethics Project undertaken in 1987 by the University of Alberta, the University of Alberta Hospitals, and the Cross Cancer Institute. The project, a result of a collaborative effort to address ethical dilemmas, has equal representation from medicine, nursing, and philosophy through directors who plan and conduct Bioethics Rounds and are responsible for joint teaching in ethics for nursing and medical students. Such a collaborative approach facilitates addressing issues involving both professions so they are deliberated together, and collaborative decisions are reached that are in the best interests of the patients and the health-care providers. This approach is based on the belief that collaboration in the delivery of health care is required to address complex ethical dilemmas; there are no right or wrong answers, but decisions must be made that will meet the needs of the consumers of health care.

■ ■ ■ ■
CONCLUSION

This chapter has highlighted a few ethical issues and dilemmas; many more are addressed in books and journals for health professionals. The amount of literature on ethics has increased at a phenomenal rate in the past two decades, helping health professionals determine what action to take ethically in situations encountered in practice. Although there are no easy answers to ethical questions, health professionals must have resources available, in the literature and through ethicists, and they must use these resources in dealing with complex issues and dilemmas.

REFERENCES

Alberta Law Reform Institute. (March 1993). *Advance directives and substitute decision-making in personal health care (Report No. 64).* Edmonton, Alberta: Alberta Law Reform Institute and the Health Law Institute.

American Nurses Association (1976). *Code for nurses with interpretive statements.* Kansas City, MO: American Nurses Association.

Avard, D., Griener, G., and Langstaff, J. (1985). Hospital ethics committees: Survey reveals characteristics. *Dimensions, 62*(2), 24-26.

Bandman, E.L., and Bandman, B. (1978). *Bioethics and human rights.* Boston: Little, Brown & Company.

Bedell, S., and Delbanco, T. (1984). Choices about cardiopulmonary resuscitation in the hospital. *New England Journal of Medicine, 300,* 310-317.

Bedell, S., Pelle, D., Maher, L., and Cleary, P. (1986). Do not resuscitate orders of critically ill patients in the hospital. *Journal of the American Medical Association, 256,* 12.

Brody, H. (1976). *Ethical decisions in medicine.* Boston: Little, Brown & Company.

Campbell, D. (1984). Surrogate mothers—controversy continues. *Nursing Mirror, 158*(5), 5.

Campbell, M., and Field, B. (1991). Management of the patient with do not resuscitate status: Compassion and cost containment. *Heart and Lung, 20*(4), 345-348.

Canadian Hospital Association. (1986). *Institutional ethics committees: Recomendations for action.* Ottawa: Author.

Canadian Nurses Association. (1985). *Code of ethics for nursing.* Ottawa: Author.

Canadian Nurses Association. (1991). *Code of ethics for nursing.* Ottawa: Author.

Canadian Nurses Association, Canadian Medical Association, and Canadian Hospital Association. (1984). Joint statement on terminal illness: A protocol for health professionals regarding resuscitative intervention for the terminally ill. *The Canadian Nurse, 80*(4), 24.

Curtin, L.L. (1982). Case study v: Abortion, privacy and conscience. In L. Curtin and M.J. Flaherty, *Nursing ethics: Theories and pragmatics* (pp. 239-254). Bowie, MD: Robert J. Brady Company.

Curtin, L.L. (1985). Developing a professional ethic. *AARN Newsletter, 41*(10), 1, 3-6.

Davis, A.J., and Aroskar, M.A. (1983). *Ethical dilemmas and nursing practice* (2nd ed). Norwalk, CT: Appleton-Century-Crofts.

Duff, R.S., and Campbell, A.G.M. (1973). Moral and ethical dilemmas in the special-care nursery. *New England Journal of Medicine, 289,* 890-894.

Dyck, A.J. (1975). Beneficent euthanasia and benemortasia: Alternative view of mercy. In M. Kohl (Ed.), *Beneficent euthanasia* (pp. 120-126). Buffalo, NY: Prometheus.

Evans, A., and Brody, B. (1985). The do not resuscitate order in teaching hospitals. *Journal of the American Medical Association, 253,* 15.

Flanagan, L. (1976). *One strong voice: The story of the American Nurses Association.* Kansas City, MO: American Nurses Association.

Flarey, D. (1991). Advanced directives: In search of self-determination. *Journal of Nursing Administration, 21*(11), 16-22.

Francoeur, R.T. (1983). *Biomedical ethics: A guide to decision making.* Toronto: John Wiley & Sons.

Godkin, M.D. (1992). *Cardiopulmonary resuscitation: Knowledge, attitudes and opinions of older adults in acute care and long-term care settings.* Unpublished master's thesis, University of Alberta Faculty of Nursing, Edmonton.

Honan, S., Helseth, C., Bakke, J., Karpuik, K., Krsnak, G., and Torkelson, R. (1991). Perception on "no code" and the role of the nurse. *Journal of Continuing Education in Nursing, 22*(2), 54-61.

Hughes, D.L., and Singer, P.A. (1992). Family physicians' attitudes toward advance directives. *Canadian Medical Association Journal, 146*(11), 1937-1944.

International Council of Nurses. (1973). *ICN code for nurses—Ethical concepts applied to nursing*, Geneva: International Council of Nurses.

Kluge, E.W. (1992). *Biomedical ethics in a Canadian context*. Toronto: Prentice-Hall Canada, Inc.

McCormick, R.A. (1974). To save or let live: The dilemma of modern medicine. *Journal of the American Medical Association, 229*, 172-176.

Ott, B., and Nieswiadomy, R. (1991). Support of patient autonomy in the do not resuscitate decision. *Heart and Lung, 20*(1), 66-74.

Peplau, H.E. (1978). The right to change behaviour: Rights of the mentally ill. In E.L. Bandman, and B. Bandman (Eds.), *Bioethics and human rights* (pp. 207-212). Boston: Little, Brown & Company.

Robillard, H.M., High, D.M., Sebastian, J.G., Pisaneschi, J.I., Perritt, L.J., and Mahler, D.M. (1989). Ethical issues in primary care: A survey of practitioners' perceptions. *Journal of Community Health, 14*(1), 9-17.

Savage, T., Cullen, D., Kirchhoff, K., Pugh, E. and Foreman, M. (1987). Nurses' response to do not resuscitate orders in the neonatal intensive care unit. *Nursing Research, 36*, 6.

Shaw, A. (1973). Dilemmas of "informed consent" in children. *New England Journal of Medicine, 289*, 885-890.

Slomka, J. (1992). The negotiation of death: Clinical decision making at the end of life. *Social Science Medicine. 35*(3), 251-259.

Storch, J.L. (1982). *Patients' rights: Ethical and legal issues in health care and nursing*. Toronto: McGraw-Hill Ryerson.

Storch, J., and Griener, G. (June 1990). Ethics committees in Canadian hospitals: Report on 1989 survey. *The Bioethics Bulletin, 2*(2), 1-3. (Available from University of Alberta Division of Bioethics, Edmonton, Alberta).

Thompson, J.E., and Thompson, H.O. (1989). Teaching ethics to nursing students. *Nursing Outlook, 37*(2), 84-88.

Toth, E. (1991). Commentary on the national guidelines for no resuscitation orders. *The Bioethics Bulletin, 3*(3), 4-5. (Available from University of Alberta Division of Bioethics, Edmonton, Alberta).

Whittington, H.G. (1975). A case for private enterprise in mental health. *Administration in Mental Health, 25*(1), 23-27.

Wilson, D.M. (1993). *The influences for do-not-resuscitate policies and end-of-life treatment or non-treatment decision*. Unpublished doctoral dissertation, University of Alberta, Edmonton.

Yarling, R.R., and McElmurry, B.J. (1983). Rethinking the nurse's role in "Do not resuscitate" orders: A clinical policy. *Advances in Nursing Science, 5*(4), 1-12.

Youngner, S.J. (1987). DNR orders: No longer secret, but still a problem. *Hastings Center Report, 17*(1), 24-33.

CHAPTER TWENTY ONE

Emergence of Nursing Unions as a Social Force in Canada

JANET ROSS KERR

A prediction made 25 years ago about the direction and management of determining nurses' salaries would make interesting reading today. Whether the rise of powerful and independent nursing unions was foreseen is not known, but it is probable that this development would have seemed unlikely. One wonders how the health-care system and the public in general would have reacted if nurses had used the ultimate union weapon, the strike, a quarter of a century ago (Muyskens, 1982). Because striking employees in the public sector are viewed negatively by a certain proportion of the public, the image of nurses on picket lines would probably have seemed far-fetched, if not impossible (Rotkovich, 1980). The power of unions in general, however, has been challenged by some provincial governments, and as the 1990s unfold, it would appear that unions, including nursing unions, have felt the impact of these threats to their hard-earned power base.

The approach of the 21st century has brought with it many changes that once seemed improbable. Nurses in Canada today are at the helms of organizations that promote their social and economic welfare by influencing and participating in the collective bargaining process. When collective bargaining activity began in nursing, nurses made an effort to become knowledgeable about labour relations, anticipating control of salaries and wages through mastery of the process (Ponak, 1981). Although there is considerable variation among provinces in approach and achievement, the thrust in nursing unions has been increasingly directed to consolidating membership, withstanding the threats to structural integrity and maintaining the right to negotiate collective agreements on behalf of members of unions. The impact of a worldwide climate of economic uncertainty has raised the tenor of the debate on health-care reform. Widespread public sector salary reductions in a number of provinces, including Ontario and Alberta, have created an environment in which all unions are struggling to preserve their mandate.

■ ■ ■ ■

THE RISE OF NURSING UNIONS

In Canada, as well as in other countries, professional nursing associations have played key roles in the development of nursing unions. However, since 1973 events in Canada can be differentiated from those in other countries because of the decision made in a Saskatchewan case that was appealed to the Supreme Court of Canada. The issue was a dispute between the Service Employees International Union and the Saskatchewan Registered Nurses Association (SRNA) over the SRNA's application for certification as a bargaining agent. The union charged that the SRNA should not be permitted to act as a trade union because its Board of Directors included nursing managers. The decision, which ruled in favour of the union, radically altered labour relations in nursing in Canada in little more than a decade. Because the rules governing the structure of the SRNA allowed for the election of nursing managers to its governing body, the association was presumed to have an inherent bias or conflict of interest that precluded participation in collective bargaining. Thus the way was paved for establishing new organizations across the country. The new unions took over the collective bargaining functions that had been performed exclusively by the professional associations.

Both the Canadian Nurses Association (CNA) and the American Nurses Association (ANA) approved the principle of collective bargaining for nurses in the 1940s, and, at that time, both organizations affirmed that the bargaining agent at the provincial/state level should be the professional association. The passage of the Labour Relations Act at the national level in 1944, which gave federal employees collective bargaining rights, was probably instrumental in the 1944 CNA decision to support collective bargaining among its member associations. The CNA and the ANA were also on record as supporting a no-strike policy. This stand, however, became controversial 2 decades later and was repealed by both organizations in the 1960s.

Rowsell (1982) notes that nurses were concerned about possible management domination from the boards of directors of provincial associations after the 1944 decision. Because there was no formal collective bargaining at that time, the provincial associations struggled with the issues inherent in being at the forefront of the process. Shortly after that, having studied the issues, member organizations informed the CNA that it was not legally possible for them to act as bargaining agents. The first breakthrough in provincial labour legislation appeared in 1946, when the Registered Nurses Association of British Columbia (RNABC) became the first provincial association to apply successfully for certification as a bargaining agent under a labour relations act, beginning a movement that would eventually involve all provinces.

Although they were not permitted to be formally involved in collective bargaining, the other nine provincial associations became engaged in promoting the social and economic welfare of their memberships in a less formal and proactive manner. It became customary in most provinces to publish annual personnel policies that included recommendations about salaries and working conditions. The associations then discussed the recommendations with employers or hospital associations. Although the recommendations in the document resulted from agreement between employers and employees, they were not binding and often not implemented, which led to progressive disillusionment with the process and its results. The recognition of failure to make any progress using the personnel policy approach led to a search on the part of the associations for a more effective method of involvement influencing salary and wage decisions.

During the expansionist decade of the 1960s, the majority of the provincial associations began to become more assertive in applying for the right to bargain collectively for the large groups of nurses employed in provincial health-care agencies. A number of factors were important in setting the stage for this new phase of development in nursing organizations. With the economy finally booming after gradual recovery through the postwar period, workers were making gains in financial status because the country could finally afford it. There were new opportunities for students as an egalitarian mood swept the postsecondary education system, and ability and willingness to work diligently became the new entrance standards. Wealth and social status were no longer required as competitive scholarships became available to the most academically qualified students. The Royal Commission on the Status of Women drew attention to the need for equal opportunity for women in society and for removing inequities in a system that inadequately remunerated women. The new optimism in society brought what in the past had seemed impossible into the realm of the possible.

Because provincial nursing associations in all provinces except British Columbia could not be certified under provincial labour laws in the early 1960s, the associations established an important role for themselves by teaching staff nurses in hospitals and community health agencies about collective bargaining and helping them organize staff nurses' associations at the agency level. These organizations became the bargaining units that were eventually certified under the various labour acts. The exception to this process was Prince Edward Island where collective bargaining rights were written into the Prince Edward Island Nurses' Act (PEI Nurses' Act).

The provincial associations laid the groundwork for involvement in the collective bargaining process. By the time the Supreme Court decision was made that led to the separation of professional associations and unions, nurses had gained some experience and expertise in collective bargaining, and the transition from a single organization to two was facilitated. There were difficulties in moving from one structure to another in some provinces, but by 1981 the process was complete and the dual structure was in place in all provinces. The last to complete the process was Prince Edward Island.

There were many advantages to the new organizational structure. Professional associations became more credible. Because they were not responsible for collective bargaining, they were no longer protecting their economic interests in public statements on health-care issues, particularly those that involved financing health care. Annual membership fees to professional associations no longer supported collective bargaining. Because collective bargaining is a labour-intensive process that involves extensive time commitments from a bargaining team and the involvement of labour relations consultants, lawyers, and others, it is an expensive process. Management involvement in professional associations and the fact that members' fees supported collective bargaining had always been sensitive issues. Complaints about the associations' strong thrust in the bargaining arena came from those not affected by the bargaining process. Creating two organizations from one addressed these complaints. Also, the removal of responsibility for collective bargaining enabled the professional association to focus on serving the public interest through self-regulatory functions, improving standards of nursing education and practice, promoting nursing research, and interacting with government and other health-care professions as the official voice of the profession (Beletz, 1980; Eldridge and Levi, 1982; Hopping, 1976; Jacox, 1980).

Many were disappointed when the alternatives narrowed as a result of the Supreme Court decision, and the inevitability of separating professional associations and unions across the country became clear. It was difficult for nurses to think about separating and maintaining distinct and autonomous organizations (Cleland, 1978). It was also difficult for many nurses to understand that the professional association now stood truly apart from the bargaining function and could no longer intervene at difficult times to support a union stance in the face of a strike action.

This did not keep some provinces from developing excellent working relationships between the professional association and the union (Conroy and Hibberd, 1983). In Ontario there was a good working relationship between the organizations until 1988. In 1961 self-regulatory functions had been transferred to the College of Nurses. The Registered Nurses Association of Ontario (RNAO) performed all other professional functions, including bargaining. After the Ontario Nurses Association (ONA), the major nursing union, was created in 1975, there were three organizations, and each was concerned with a different area of professional activity. When the RNAO began losing members at a rapid pace in the late 1970s and early 1980s, it established an agreement with the ONA. The terms of the agreement, which became effective in 1983, enabled the union to purchase a block membership in the RNAO. The agreement also provided for a reduced RNAO membership fee for union members, with no reduction in services. Although there was some concern that the terms of the agreement might compromise the RNAO's autonomy and freedom to address health-care issues, this was an excellent example of cooperation and collaboration between the two organizations. A change in union leadership in 1987 destroyed the collaborative relationship and block membership was terminated.

■ ■ ■ ■

ESTABLISHMENT OF THE NATIONAL FEDERATION OF NURSES' UNIONS

Parallel to the development of provincial nursing unions as separate bargaining units, efforts were being directed at establishing a national voice for unionized nurses. By the late 1960s, provincial labour relations staff began meeting through the Committee on Socio-Economic Welfare of CNA. With the controversial implementation of wage and price controls and a code of ethics by the CNA, unionized nurses were convinced of their need for a more formal national structure. In 1977 a labour relations service department was established under the auspices of the

CNA to disseminate information on collective bargaining and to provide educational assistance to members. In 1981 the National Federation of Nurses' Unions (NFNU) was formalized to represent unionized Canadian nurses in both watchdog and lobbying activities. By 1984 NFNU member unions included British Columbia, Alberta (Staff Nurses' Association), Manitoba, New Brunswick, Prince Edward Island, and Newfoundland/Labrador (Connors, personal communication, 1994).

■ ■ ■ ■

THE ORGANIZATIONS: ESTABLISHMENT AND CONSOLIDATION

The development of separate and unique organizations for collective bargaining occurred within a relatively short time after the Supreme Court decision in 1973. Only 8 years elapsed between the inception of the first such organization, the Saskatchewan Union of Nurses, and the conclusion of the process with the establishment of the last, the PEI Nurses Union, in 1981.

British Columbia

As previously noted, the organization that first acquired formal authority, in that it was legally recognized as the official bargaining agent for nurses in the province, was the RNABC. In the early years it operated on the basis of personnel policies approved each year at the annual meeting; the bargaining that took place between the RNABC and the hospital boards was based on these approved recommendations. This process was similar to that used in other provinces. The difference was the legal recognition of the RNABC's role as bargaining agent. In British Columbia and other provinces, dissatisfaction arose with the personnel policies route by 1959. Many disputes went to conciliation and strike votes were taken in a number of health-care agencies. It was evident that a different approach was needed.

The new approach was the process of collective bargaining in the sense that it is used today where the agencies and the nursing groups each have a primary bargaining agent who bargains on behalf of all that wish to be a part of the process. This proved to be a reasonably successful approach over the next decade and a half. The bargaining structure within the association remained stable until 1974, when the RNABC disassociated the collective bargaining program from other association activity. This initial response to the Supreme Court decision may have been an attempt to determine if anything other than total separation was possible and to obviate the need for developing a totally separate organization for collective bargaining.

In 1974 the British Columbia government approved legislation that gave government employees the right to bargain collectively and the right to strike. However, a decade later, new legislation revoked the right to strike for those designated as essential employees, which included some nurses. Although there was a good deal of protest, the government stood firm in its decision. A nurses' strike in May and June 1989 provided an interesting example of the lack of solidarity between the union and its leadership because the membership repudiated the memorandum of agreement approved by union leaders. An agreement was reached eventually, but the startling anger of the membership with their union leaders was evident.

In late 1989 under new leadership, structural changes resulted in much greater cohesiveness in the membership. Subsequently the BC Nurses' Union and the remaining two provincial unions representing health-care workers—the Hospital Employees Union representing support staff, and the Health Sciences Association representing other professional groups such as laboratory and x-ray technicians and others—negotiated a landmark employment security agreement. This tripartite agreement between the union, employer, and government, in effect until March 31, 1996, ensures that should their present positions be abolished, nurses belonging to the union will be reemployed in a similar position in an appropriate locale. This agreement, now the envy of many other provinces, also included retraining arrangements and early retirement packages. It represented the successful amalgamation of independent unions in the pursuit of common goals. In September 1993, unionized nurses moved to a 36-hour work week retaining the same salary agreements. While this applies to nurses employed in hospitals only, discussions are presently under negotiation to have community health nurses included in this contract.

Alberta

Nurses in Alberta became concerned about their social and economic status in the early 1960s, and organizational meetings were held to decide what should be done. The Alberta Association of Registered Nurses (AARN) led this movement and worked to help nurses in hospitals develop staff nurses' associations for bargaining. Amendments made to the Registered Nurses' Act in 1965 allowed the AARN to act as bargaining agent for the nurses. The AARN, like the RNABC, made bylaw changes in 1974 to create a unit for collective bargaining that would function separately from the rest of the Association. However, nurses in Alberta made the decision that a separate and autonomous structure for collective bargaining was really what they wanted, and in 1977 the United Nurses of Alberta was selected to act in this capacity. Shortly thereafter the first nurses' strike occurred. Seven hospitals and 2000 nurses participated. Government intervened and ordered the nurses back to work, appointing a tribunal to rule on the items in dispute. Subsequently, two nurses' strikes occurred in Alberta, one in 1980 and another in 1982. In 1983 the Alberta government enacted legislation that made it illegal for hospital nurses to strike. However, in January, 1988, Alberta nurses defied the Labour Act and went out on an 18-day illegal strike.

As in many other provinces, Alberta nurses have become much more politically astute and assertive. Between the time of the 1988 nurses' strike and 1994, two contracts have been negotiated, each resulting in much less friction than in previous negotiations. The strong stand that nursing has taken has resulted in greater respect for nurses at the bargaining table.

Saskatchewan

In Saskatchewan the SRNA became involved in collective bargaining before 1973, primarily in response to a demand from members employed in non-governmental positions. Government-employed nurses who were represented by unions achieved significant improvement in salaries throughout the 1960s, whereas SRNA members who had had no bargaining agent before 1968 did not. By 1972 collective agreements between the SRNA and the Saskatchewan Hospital Association encompassed about half of Saskatchewan hospitals (Botterill-Conroy,

1980). As previously noted, the amendment to the Trade Union Act that resulted from the question of the legality of the SRNA's role as bargaining agent for the nurses was ratified by the Supreme Court's 1973 decision. The Saskatchewan Union of Nurses (SUN), created after the decision was made, has continued its efforts to improve the social and economic welfare of nurses.

Health-care reform translated into the implementation of a process of regionalization in Saskatchewan with the appointment of regional health boards and the closing of a number of small acute-care hospitals. The SUN has refocused its efforts to argue for a "wellness model" consistent with the changes. Since many nurses have had to relocate, the union has directed its attention to ensuring labour adjustment strategies were in place to protect nurses from the impact of the sweeping changes in the health-care system. Two strikes occurred in Saskatchewan, one in 1988 and the other in 1991. The last strike focused on professional issues and resulted in the inclusion of a professional responsibility clause giving nurses a mechanism to deal with concerns involving patient care. A panel of nursing experts has since been used successfully to adjudicate on issues that remained unresolved in the workplace.

Manitoba

Although nurses in Manitoba asked the Manitoba Association of Registered Nurses (MARN) to represent them in collective bargaining as early as 1953, the MARN did not become formally involved in this activity until 1969. Because the MARN had not begun to participate actively in bargaining, the Winnipeg Civic Registered Nurses' Association was organized in 1965 to serve as an alternative to the provincial employee union, the Federation of Civil Employees. Even after 1969, when the MARN became involved in bargaining, some ambivalence about that involvement continued within the Association because the Labour Relations Act clearly specified that unions must operate separately from management. As a result, the MARN followed the precedents set in Alberta and British Columbia where the collective bargaining sector of the organization was segregated to function at arm's length from the rest of the Association. As in the other provinces, this was a short-term solution to the problem, and in 1975 the Manitoba Organization of Nurses Association (MONA) was established (Botterill-Conroy, 1980). This union later became the Manitoba Nurses' Union (MNU), and, as in Nova Scotia and Saskatchewan, included licensed practical nurses and registered psychiatric nurses in its membership. As a result of a month long strike in 1991, MONA emerged more cohesive than previously and members were satisfied with an agreement that included joint trusteeship of pension plans, a responsibility clause, and differential salary increases for RNs and LPNs. The union has continued to make strides in the political arena, particularly in relation to health-care reform in Manitoba.

Ontario

As previously discussed, events took a different course in Ontario, beginning with the creation in 1961 of a quasi-governmental body, the College of Nurses of Ontario. Collective bargaining rights were not secured easily in Ontario, and nurses tried unsuccessfully from 1958 until 1965 to gain legal recognition of bargaining for nurses. Even so, after 1965 bargaining had to be done individually, agency by agency. Not until 1973 did the Ontario Hospital Association approve centralized bargaining, on monetary issues only, for nurses (Botterill-Conroy, 1980). Although the RNAO had assumed the bargaining function for many years, a decision to form a nurses union was made at an annual RNAO meeting, and the Ontario Nurses' Association (ONA) was established. The ONA separated from the RNAO in 1975, following the trend that by now was well established in the rest of the country, but bargaining at the provincial level did not begin until 1979. Legislation passed in 1965 had prevented nurses in hospitals and nursing homes from striking since that time. However, community health nurses continue to maintain that right.

The ONA has a very active legislative committee, which lobbies provincial members of the legislature on health-care issues. This political action has no doubt been instrumental in obtaining an amendment to the Public Hospital Act which now must include an elected staff nurse on the Fiscal Advisory Committee. In 1991 the ONA successfully negotiated a contractual agreement that included 10 incremental steps. For the nurse with a lengthy service record, expert clinical skills and mentorship functions were formally recognized, giving these individuals an annual income of more than $50,000 per annum.

Quebec

In Quebec, nurses were given legislative approval for collective bargaining in 1946 under the Quebec Nurses' Act. However, the Association of Nurses of the Province of Quebec did not develop a bargaining program. The reasons for this are unclear. However, after the enactment of the omnibus legislation, which applied to a number of professional groups, and the development of the Professional Code in Chapter 43 of the legislation applying to nursing, registration in the province became mandatory. The Order of Nurses of the Province of Quebec (ONQ/OIIQ) was disqualified as bargaining agent, not because of management domination but because the right of free association guaranteed by the Quebec Labour Code was precluded by the mandatory membership provisions of the Act. Therefore nurses sought other representation in the socioeconomic domain. Several unions were formed—l'Alliance des Infirmières et Infirmiers du Québec, la Fédération des Syndicats Professionels d'Infirmières du Québec (FSPIIQ), and in 1967, the United Nurses of Montreal (UNM). L'Alliance and FSPIIQ bargained separately for staff nurses and management nurses whereas the UNM represented all nurses, including management nurses. This changed in 1970 when the UNM split into separate staff and management organizations— United Nurses' Inc. (UNInc.) and United Management Nurses' Inc (UMNInc.).

In 1972 many public services were affected by a strike of the Quebec Federation of Labour that involved nurses who were members of l'Alliance. These nurses were ordered to return to work when the Quebec National Assembly passed legislation to end the interruption in public services. In 1975 UNInc. joined the Corps des Organismes Professionels de la Santé (COPS) for the purpose of bargaining. Representing the vast majority of unionized nurses in

Quebec, the organization also included among its members the FSPIIQ and many other groups in the health professions (Botterill-Conroy, 1980). A number of strikes have occurred in Quebec since the one in 1972. However, because of the number of organizations that serve as bargaining agents in Quebec, the strikes have usually involved only certain sectors of the nursing population and other health workers.

Three nursing unions merged in December, 1987, to form the Federation of Nurses of Quebec, resulting in greater union strength in bargaining for salary increases for nurses in Quebec, traditionally among the lowest paid nurses in Canada. The illegal walkout of members of the new organization and the subsequent standoff between the nurses and the Premier and his government in the midst of an election campaign unified nurses and gained them considerable public support for their cause. Their gains in this confrontation were impressive, and their public image improved. The merger has been very successful in creating the umbrella under which nurses are affiliated and able to speak with a more unified and therefore stronger voice. The Federation has an unusually large but highly effective board of 500 nurses who have been very successful in putting forward issues of concern to their members. As a result, there is legislation that addresses employee concerns, namely occupational health and safety issues, and issues pertaining to pregnancy and breast feeding of infants. This achievement has been the envy of other nursing unions.

Over the years Quebec has seen a substantial change in the way health care is being delivered. The Centres Locaux de Services Communautaires (CLSC), community health centres, has been a widely accepted and much envied concept for the delivery of health and social services based in the community. Attributable to the efforts of the Federation, collective bargaining rights have automatically been extended to these areas as nurses formerly based in hospitals move out to these centres.

New Brunswick

In the 1960s nurses in New Brunswick became concerned about their socioeconomic status and disenchanted with the procedure for determining salaries. Originally the New Brunswick Association of Registered Nurses (NBARN) provided recommendations on salaries and working conditions to the government on an annual basis. The first step in the process that would accord nurses more power was the NBARN's Social and Economic Welfare Committee's acquisition of standing committee status in 1967. After acquiring this status, the committee began helping nurses in health care agencies to organize staff associations throughout the province. In 1968 the NBARN Provincial Collective Bargaining Council was established as a separate entity from the NBARN.

The first serious collective bargaining in New Brunswick began in 1969, when employers agreed to negotiate with the NBARN Provincial Collective Bargaining Council. When a stalemate occurred in the negotiations, the majority of New Brunswick nurses resigned. These resignations were withdrawn when the employer group agreed to go back to the bargaining table to negotiate in a fair and equitable manner. An agreement was signed by both parties soon after. In the same year, provisions of the Public Service Labour Relations Act gave nurses in the public sector the right to bargain collectively. The right was extended to the private sector 2 years later through the Industrial Relations Act. The NBARN Provincial Collective Bargaining Council disassociated itself from the NBARN by becoming the New Brunswick Nurses' Provincial Collective Bargaining Council, although it had been a distinct and separate organization from its inception. Due to the legislative division between public and private sector bargaining provisions, another organization was formed: the New Brunswick Civil Service Nurses' Provincial Collective Bargaining Council. The two organizations merged in 1978 and became the New Brunswick Nurses Union (NBNU) (Botterill-Conroy, 1980).

In 1991 the provincial government rescinded a previously agreed to salary adjustment, and the NBNU threatened to strike. Although a strike did not materialize, nurses found that issues they subsequently raised were being heard and government was increasingly involving nurses in health-care policy discussions. However, the increases that were negotiated did not go into effect until 1993 (Madeleine Steves, NBNU, personal communication, January 11, 1995).

Nova Scotia

In 1966 the Registered Nurses Association of Nova Scotia (RNANS) organized a Committee on Social and Economic Welfare as a tangible means of increasing their influence on salaries and working conditions. In 1968 members decided that the RNANS should act as a bargaining agent for nurses employed in agencies, but professional nursing legislation made no provision for collective bargaining. The RNANS helped nurses in health-care agencies to seek certification as bargaining agents through the Trade Union Act. The first certifications were granted in 1969, and nurses began to consider the possibility of bargaining collectively. The staff associations first worked as a committee under the RNANS, but in keeping with the national trend, organized the Staff Nurses' Association of Nova Scotia. This organization was the forerunner of the Nova Scotia Nurses Union (NSNU), which was organized 3 years later in 1976.

In 1971 a brief strike at Amherst Hospital resulted in an agreement. Longer strikes took place at two institutions in 1972, and in 1975 nurses in 15 institutions withdrew their services because of a bargaining impasse. At that time, bargaining was still primarily at the local level, but nurses realized that greater gains could be made by working together. The first joint bargaining session took place in 1978. By 1979 most agencies were involved in the process (Botterill-Conroy, 1980). In the past few years, the NSNU has been included in health-policy discussions and has been a part of how health care will be provided in Nova Scotia in the future. Nurses have successfully lobbied members of Parliament and felt that their voices were being heard.

Prince Edward Island

As previously noted, collective bargaining rights for nurses were included in the PEI Nurses' Act when it was amended in 1972. The reason for that amendment was that nurses were specifically excluded from the PEI Labour Act. This legislation made the Provincial Collective Bargaining Committee, an arm of the Association of Nurses of Prince Edward Island (ANPEI), legally responsible for collective bargaining for nurses in the province. Although the Act was amended in 1972, the first collective agreement was not produced until 1974 because the government and the ANPEI did not agree on the regulations to implement the Act. Although nurses in PEI did not have the right to strike, a "showdown" between the nurses and the government was resolved when the government agreed to a compromise after most of the nurses threatened to resign. For a time it seemed that Prince Edward Island might be the only province that would not establish a separate organization for collective bargaining, but in 1981 the PEI Nurses' Act was amended to remove responsibility for collective bargaining from the ANPEI and the Labour Act was amended to ensure that nurses would not be excluded from its provisions.

As a result of major initiatives taken in health-care reform, efforts have been directed toward establishing one large union that would represent all health-care workers, including nurses. This move toward consolidation, as in other provinces, would provide a more broadly based and more powerful group from which to argue for common issues of concern. Nevertheless, because of the broad range of interests that would be represented, it threatens to dilute profession-specific concerns.

Newfoundland

The Association of Registered Nurses of Newfoundland (ARNN) annually prepared recommendations for nurses' salaries and submitted them as part of a brief to the Cabinet until 1970, when the process was discontinued because the nurses did not see positive action being taken. The nurses then voted to establish the ARNN as their bargaining agent for nurses in the civil service to engage in collective bargaining with government, and the Newfoundland Hospital Association for those employed by nongovernmental agencies. The process occurred on a voluntary basis at the outset, and the first collective agreement was concluded in 1970. The passage of the Public Service Act in 1972 provided legal recognition of collective bargaining rights for nurses and other health workers. This legislation reflected the spirit and intent of the 1973 Supreme Court decision. Therefore the ARNN was precluded from involvement in collective bargaining. The Newfoundland Nurses' Union was established in 1974 to take responsibility for the socioeconomic welfare of nurses.

The Newfoundland economy has been severely affected by the recession. From 1991 to 1994 nurses have been subject to a wage freeze and have seen government withdraw its share of contributions to the pension plan. Nurses believe the quality and safety of health care in their province has dimished. An information campaign has been launched to sensitize the public to nurses' perceptions of what is happening to the health-care system in Newfoundland.

■■ ■■ ■■ ■■

UNION OR MANAGEMENT: WHERE TO DRAW THE LINE

It is difficult to describe the bargaining unit because of uncertainty about the appropriate classification of some supervisory positions. The dilemma is most prevalent at the level of first-line managers, and there are differences of opinion among the provinces as to whether certain employees can be included in the bargaining unit. In some areas the "hiring and firing" standard has been used. Managers who perform these functions are disqualified. In some instances management has redefined functions to ensure that first-line managers are not included in the bargaining unit. This redefinition has often occurred in provinces where the union has the right to strike. Management may perceive the need for expert assistance on the front lines in the event of strike.

Many nurses do not wish to be removed from the bargaining unit because they will no longer have the security of a contract. However, it must be noted that by 1994 the "contract" clearly did not carry the same assurances and security as in the past. There is little protection for management nurses in comparison to that provided by the collective agreement. Only the province of Quebec has a union for nurse managers that actively represents them. Nurses who hold administrative positions are thus at the mercy of their employers as far as salaries and benefits are concerned. Perhaps more important, they are also vulnerable in terms of job tenure, particularly in the 1990s where all middle-management positions are endangered as organizations strive for the greater financial efficiency of "flat" structures. Employers are aware of the potential power of the nursing department, the largest and most costly sector of activity in any hospital. In some instances administrators have been so threatened by strong nursing leaders that they have dismissed them and replaced them with a new individual, or a new arrangement, that appeared to be less threatening.

▬ ▬ ▬ ▬

PROFESSIONAL RESPONSIBILITY CLAUSES

In recent years one of the trends in negotiations across the country has been to focus on the climate of the setting in which nurses are expected to function. The advent of professional responsibility clauses as part of collective agreements is tangible evidence of this trend. Emphasis is shifting away from concern with salaries and wages as the first priority. Nurses are deeply concerned about the quality and safety of the care they can provide in certain settings. Structuring the collective agreement to allow nurses to negotiate with the employer about certain resources that may be necessary to provide safe care is attractive to many unions. Examples of difficulty in providing adequate care—as documented in waivers, or disclaimer of responsibility forms, and diaries—have been used to provide data to support concerns discussed at meetings with management on professional responsibility committees.

▬ ▬ ▬ ▬

IMPACT OF LOSS OF THE RIGHT TO STRIKE

The denial of the right of a particular professional group to strike is unusual and represents legislative interference with freedom to engage in the usual processes associated with collective bargaining (Anderson and Anderson, 1982). Ontario nurses lost the right to strike when the Hospital Disputes Arbitration Act of 1965 was passed (Botterill-Conroy, 1980). The right to strike was denied to nurses employed in hospitals in Alberta in 1983 after a period of acrimonious labour relations among Alberta nurses, the provincial government, and the Alberta Hospital Association. Three legal nurses' strikes between 1977 and 1982 motivated the Alberta government to enact legislation that denied hospital nurses (and some other workers) the right to strike because their services were essential. This legislation imposed severe penalties on those who defied the law. Penalties under this legislation were imposed as a result of an illegal strike in 1988. It is possible that events in Alberta convinced the government of British Columbia that legislation to prevent nurses' strikes was necessary. A question that is often asked is whether the presence or absence of freedom to strike compromises a union's position at the bargaining table (Amundsen, 1975). In Ontario, nurses in hospitals and nursing homes have not had the right to strike for 2 decades, but salary levels appear to be comparable with those in other provinces. Until Alberta nurses asserted themselves in the wake of a booming economy in the late 1970s and early 1980s, Ontario nurses had the highest salaries in Canada.

■ ■ ■ ■

PUBLIC IMPACT OF COLLECTIVE BARGAINING IN NURSING

It is difficult to determine the effect of the collective bargaining movement in nursing on public perceptions of nurses (McClelland, 1983). Stereotypic images of nurses as passive and unassertive have been undermined, particularly in provinces where nursing unions have been militant, and relations with employer groups and governments have been acrimonious (Baumgart, 1983; Kalisch, Kalisch, and Young 1983; Kluge, 1982). Public response to nurses' strikes has varied. In Alberta in 1977, public sympathy was against the nurses. However, in 1979 there was a virtual outpouring of sympathy for the bargaining position of the nurses, and the public as well as members of other unions joined the picket lines, resulting in a large salary settlement. When Alberta's nurses went on strike again in 1982, there was little public support. In 1988 the Alberta public was reasonably supportive of the nurses during their illegal strike. Except for the fines levied against the union, few repercussions against nurses resulted from this illegal walkout.

There have been some notable and successful efforts by provincial governments in Alberta and British Columbia to restrict the activities and processes that unions can use to exert pressure on their employers in the collective bargaining process. The fact that public protest did not persuade either government to reconsider its decision about passing the legislation and in fact exerted pressure to stimulate the development of the legislation suggests a lack of public support for the unions and their activities. The fact that both provinces were entering periods of recession when this legislation was enacted indicates that the factors and pressures that influenced its development were economic.

Nurses represent the largest group of health professionals in the labour force, and even small increases in nurses' salaries affect the total budget of a health-care agency significantly. Thus employers may often attempt to keep nurses' salaries at a minimum level to effect cost savings and to balance budgets. Although collective bargaining rights for nurses did not appear to change the goals of employer negotiating groups, it gave the process of negotiation a higher profile and gave nurses more power (Luttman, 1982; Zimmerman, 1985). Having fought hard for and achieved the right to bargain collectively with their employers, it is unlikely that nurses will ever again be remunerated so inadequately for their services (Stern, 1982; Numerof and Abrams, 1984). Financing of nursing services has acquired new dimensions since nurses' salaries showed higher proportionate increases to other comparably prepared professionals. The severe impact of the worldwide economic recession in the 1990s on publicly funded health and social services has left governments at federal and provincial levels hard pressed to find short- and long-term solutions to using decreasing tax revenues to benefit the consumer. Although nurses are likely to be reasonable in an economic downturn when public sector wages are being frozen and even reduced, they are nevertheless unlikely to give up the salaries and benefits and indeed, the respect for which they have had to fight so persistently over such a long period of time.

REFERENCES

Amundsen, N. (1975). Alternatives to strike in collective bargaining. *Journal of Nursing Administration* 5(1), 11-12.

Anderson, J., and Anderson, M. (Eds.). (1982). *Union-management relations in Canada.* Don Mills, Ontario: Addison-Wesley.

Baumgart, A. (1983). The conflicting demands of professionalism and unionism. *AARN Newsletter* 39(6), 2-7.

Beletz, E. (1980). Organized nurses view their collective bargaining agent. *Supervisor Nurse* 11(9), 39-46.

Botterill-Conroy, M.D. (1980). *Labour relations, collective bargaining and nursing.* Unpublished manuscript, The University of Alberta, Division of Health Services Administration and Community Medicine, Edmonton.

Cleland, V.S. (1978). Shared governance in a professional model of collective bargaining. *Journal of Nursing Administration* 8(5), 39-43.

Conroy, M.D., and Hibberd, J. (1983). Areas for cooperation and conflict between nursing associations and negotiating bodies. In S. Quinn (Ed.), *Cooperation and conflict: Caring for the carers.* Geneva: International Council of Nurses.

Eldridge, I., and Levi, M. (1982). Collective bargaining as a power resolution for professional goals. *Nursing Administration Quarterly* 6(2), 29-40

Hopping, B. (1976). Professionalism and unionism: Conflicting ideologies. *Nursing Forum* 15(4), 372-383.

Jacox, A. (1980). Collective action: The basis for professionalism. *Supervisor Nurse* 9(9), 22-24.

Kalisch, B., Kalisch, P., and Young, R. (1983). Television news coverage of nurses' strikes: A resource management perspective. *Nursing Research* 33(3), 175-180.

Kluge, E.W. (1982). The profession of nursing and the right to strike. *Westminster Institute Review,* 2(1), 3-6.

Luttman, P.A. (1982). Collective bargaining and professionalism: Incompatible ideologies. *Nursing Administration Quarterly* 6(2), 21-28.

McClelland, J. (1983). Professionalism and collective bargaining: A new reality for nurses and managers. *Journal of Nursing Administration* 13(11), 36-38.

Muyskens, J.L. (1982). Nurses' collective responsibility and the strike weapon. *Journal of Medical Philosophy* 7(1), 101-112.

Numerof, R.E., and Abrams, M.N. (1984). Collective bargaining among nurses: Current issues and future prospects. *Health Care Management Review* 9(2), 61-67.

Ponak, A.M. (1981). Unionized professionals and scope of bargaining: A study of nurses. *Industrial and Labor Relations Review* 34(3), 396-407.

Rotkovich, R. (1980). Do labor union actions decrease professionalism? *Supervisor Nurse* 9(9), 16-18.

Rowsell, G. (1982). Bargaining: A means of conflict resolution. *International Nursing Review* 29(5), 141-145.

Stern, E.M. (1982). Bargaining: A means of conflict resolution. *Nursing Administration Quarterly* 6(2), 9-21.

Zimmerman, A. (1985). Collective bargaining in the hospital: The nurse's right, the professional association's responsibility. In J. McCloskey and H. Grace (Eds.), *Current issues in nursing.* Boston: Blackwell Scientific Publications.

CHAPTER TWENTY TWO

Unionism and Professionalism: Conflicting or Compatible Processes?

JANET ROSS KERR

The establishment of independent nursing unions, leading to at least two powerful organizations representing nurses in each province, has brought to the fore, issues of relationships between professional organizations and unions. Historically the collective bargaining function in each of Canada's 10 provinces was assigned to a branch of the professional association, and it gradually became an important part of the association mandate. The situation changed markedly after the 1973 Supreme Court decision, *Service Employees International Union v. Saskatchewan Registered Nurses Association* (SRNA). The Court agreed with the union's contention that the SRNA could not legally represent staff nurses in Saskatchewan because of management domination. This decision led to separation of professional associations and unions across the country (Rowsell, 1982).

Because the core membership and the professional and socioeconomic welfare interests of both organizations are the same, their relationships are strong. In most provinces the professional nursing association is the largest professional organization and, although nursing unions are usually smaller than the professional organizations, their memberships are substantial. Because health-care services are publicly financed, and because nursing services constitute a significant portion of health-care budgets, activities of nursing unions engender considerable public interest and media comment.

▬ ▬ ▬ ▬

CHARACTERISTICS OF PROFESSIONAL ASSOCIATIONS AND UNIONS

Professional associations and unions have many common goals, including promoting the welfare of members and improving their working conditions.

Since professional associations include many who are not members of nursing unions and whose economic interests are not served directly by unions, they continue to play an important role in advising and assisting. Most nurses in management are included in this group. Professional associations are also interested in ensuring that salaries and benefits for staff nurses are maintained at sufficiently high levels to maintain the status of the profession and to encourage prospective candidates to enter nursing. All professions have an interest in seeing that members are appropriately remunerated, because the value that society places on services is reflected, at least in part, by the level of remuneration.

Professional associations and unions in nursing also share a concern for professional ethics, although it is the provincial association that is responsible for ensuring that the standard of professional conduct reflected in the code of ethics is practised. Professional maturity has been observed during the past decade in the attention given to developing and approving a code of ethics at the national level. Before the Canadian Nurses Association (CNA) Code of Ethics was approved and published in 1981, most provincial professional associations accepted the standard established by the International Council of Nurses (ICN) Code published in 1953. Subsequent revisions to the CNA Code of Ethics in 1985 and 1991 have ensured that its provisions are current (CNA, 1991).

Although they do have common interests, professional organizations and unions are also different in many ways. The service ideal that is deeply embedded in the professional consciousness is reflected in legislation that regulates discipline of their members. This is true in every province except Ontario, where the College of Nurses of Ontario, a separate, quasi-autonomous body, partially funded by government, is responsible for regulatory functions. Thus the focus of professional associations on the health and safety of recipients of nursing services is in the public interest. Standards of practice that support the public right to safe and competent care are of paramount importance. Unions are not legally bound to protect the public interest. They focus almost exclusively on the socioeconomic needs of members.

Unions are concerned with the development of legally binding agreements that regulate staff nurses' salaries, working conditions, and other negotiable benefits. Professional associations, although concerned that salaries remain at appropriate levels and that good working conditions be maintained, are not responsible for developing these agreements and therefore are not active in this area. In fact, professional associations must avoid involvement in the collective bargaining process because any interference may be viewed negatively by sectors of the membership and result in controversy and conflict. In times of labour unrest, many professional associations have been pressured by both union members and management nurses to take a position on issues on the negotiating table. These situations are difficult for professional associations, and any action must be based on maintaining appropriate standards of nursing care and serving the public interest.

The mandate of professional associations is also aimed at improving and maintaining standards of nursing education. In most provinces the professional association is legally authorized to monitor standards in programs of basic nursing education. However, in Alberta this responsibility is delegated to the Universities Coordinating Council through the provisions of the Nursing Profession Act. In Ontario the responsibility belongs to the Ministry of Colleges and Universities of the Government of Ontario under the Health Disciplines Act. In Quebec, where nursing programs are governed by the Ministry of Higher Education and Science, a mechanism for approval of diploma nursing programs has been developed with the advice of the Ordre des Infirmières et Infirmiers du Québec (OIIQ), and university nursing programs are subject to the approval process of all educational programs in their respective universities. Since the mid-1950s there has been a drive to establish master's programs in nursing and to ensure their availability in various regions of the country. More recently, professional associations have focused their efforts on promoting doctoral education in nursing in Canada. The first fully funded doctoral program in nursing in Canada was established at the University of Alberta on January 1, 1991, although several universities had special case arrangements for students to study at the PhD level in nursing prior to that time, including McGill University and the University of Alberta. The second program was established later in 1991 at the University of British Columbia and accepted the first students in September of that year. Programs followed at McGill University and the University of Montreal (joint program) and the University of Toronto in the fall of 1993. Approval of a program at McMaster University led to the registration of the first students in the program in the fall of 1994. Thus within the short space of three and a half years, five doctoral programs in nursing were initiated.

Efforts to ensure opportunities for graduate study have coincided with a movement toward baccalaureate education in nursing as a requirement for entry to practice. The CNA and all member associations support the requirement of baccalaureate status for entry to practice by the year 2000. Although there has been union support for educational standards and improvements in programs, unions tend to be less concerned with education and educational standards even for advancement in the profession. The principle of seniority is normally the basis for unions' approaches to advancement and other workforce decisions. Competence, skill, and educational background are not usually the primary considerations when unions choose staff members for positions. Opportunity is based on seniority in the health-care agency.

Finally, professional associations tend to value autonomy and independent action on the basis of individual evaluation and judgement. An individual approach to solving problems is contradictory to the approach taken by unions to achieve goals in collective bargaining. Individual needs are supplanted by those of the majority when pressing for contract demands, and the egalitarian view prevails: What is good for the average member is good for all members. Professional associations attempt to respond to the needs of various sectors of the membership and take public stands that will enhance standards of care and address needs of different categories of members. Unions must negotiate agreements that incorporate all the items agreed to by unions and management; therefore the needs of the "average" member prevail.

■ ■ ■ ■

FACTORS INFLUENCING COOPERATION AND CONFLICT

There is considerable controversy about whether it is possible for professional associations and unions to coexist in areas in which their objectives are sufficiently dissimilar to engender conflict. Conroy and Hibberd (1983) have postulated two propositions to address the question: "Where collective bargaining is controlled by nurses and where professional values predominate, the greater the likelihood of cooperation between the professional body and the negotiating body" and "Where collective bargaining is controlled by nurses and where union values predominate, the greater the likelihood of conflict between the professional body and the negotiating body" (p. 84). The underlying principle is that predominantly professional values are believed to encourage good relationships and cooperation, whereas the reverse may lead to conflict between the organizations.

In Quebec, where there are many large nurses' unions, the Order of Nurses of the Province of Quebec (OIIQ, 1982) took an unusual step in 1982 when it issued a public statement that the professional association would not endorse the use of strike tactics if patient care was jeopardized:

> Governed by its mandate to ensure the protection of the public, the Bureau of the Ordre declares it is against withdrawal of services in the health field. This is the position it has taken following its study, having considered the different components of the context of the organization of health services, those of labour relations and the harm suffered by the population (p. 14).

At the same time, the OIIQ suggested to the Commission Permanente du Travail et de la Main-d'Oeuvre de l'Assemblé Nationale du Québec that a new approach to collective bargaining was needed, recommending compulsory arbitration that would require participation by professionals and consumers. Very few professional associations in nursing or in other professions have taken a similar stand, undoubtedly because of the likelihood of a negative interpretation by a large section of the membership. The willingness of the OIIQ to take this stand is impressive, possibly due in part to the fact that union membership in Quebec is scattered across several organizations and in part to the strength of Quebec legislation for nursing to incorporate mandatory registration empowering the OIIQ to vigorously monitor standards of nursing practice in the province.

Unions, a new genre of nursing organization since 1973, have introduced a range of new interorganizational and intraorganizational challenges. The development of leadership and of organizational culture and norms takes time, as both are evolutionary processes. Nurses have had to learn about the collective bargaining process and how to use collective power to advantage. Professional nursing associations, dating formally from 1910 and informally for many years before that, have had a much longer history than nursing unions. The maturity that characterizes the relationship between professional associations and unions is extremely important, as it will define the nature of the interactions between them. The initial growth period of unions has been characterized by positive and negative relationships between these organizations. Because unions were organizational newcomers in a relative sense, the independence and determined challenges from them may have come as a surprise to professional associations who had not expected to be at odds over issues with their sister groups.

The potential or actual use of the strike as a weapon may also be a source of conflict between professional organizations and unions. Historically, nurses have been ambivalent about the use of strike. The no-strike policy of the CNA was not eliminated until the 1960s, when collective bargaining was becoming important to nurses across the country. Although it may have been difficult for many of them, nurses were prepared to go on strike if labour negotiations did not produce the necessary outcomes. Kluge (1982) has examined the arguments about whether it is ethical for the nurse to withdraw services: "It is by no means a foregone conclusion that depriving individuals within society, no matter how strategically placed they may be, of their fundamental rights as persons will advance the public good" (p. 6). However, Kluge (1982) did conclude that such a right exists "because of the nature of contracts and the fact that the nurse herself is an autonomous moral agent with the usual corresponding rights; qualified because she is a member of a monopolistic service group" (p. 6). Nevertheless, the right is deemed to be "severely limited" by the public welfare concern.

Initially, nurses had the right to strike in all provinces except Prince Edward Island. However, as some of the provincial governments realized the tremendous effect of nurses' strikes, they attempted to eliminate the strike option. The right to strike was eliminated in Ontario in 1973 and in Alberta in 1983. In New Brunswick and Newfoundland the right to strike still exists, but there is legislation that requires designated employees to remain on the job to maintain essential services in the event of a strike. In British Columbia it is now illegal for nurses and other public sector workers to strike, and although Newfoundland has been reviewing its legislation with a view to eliminating public sector employees' right to strike, nurses continued to have the right to strike at the outset of 1995. In Quebec the right to strike still exists, but legislation passed in 1981 and modified in 1986 requires nurses to maintain 90% staffing in health-care agencies. Therefore, the effect of strike action is considerably limited. In Manitoba the right to strike still exists, but there is an agreement between labour and management to maintain essential services in the event of a strike (K. Connors, personal communication, June 22, 1987). Although elimination of the right to strike is believed to hamper bargaining power, nurses' salaries in Ontario have been among the highest in the country during the decade and a half since the right to strike was denied. The legislation introduced by the Alberta government to deny essential workers, including nurses, the right to strike involved imposing severe penalties for violations, indicating that there was concern within government ranks that nurses might engage in illegal walkouts. The 19-day illegal strike of Alberta nurses in 1988 substantiated this concern, and it resulted in heavy fines for the union and the appointment of a government commission to study the issues. In Quebec an illegal walkout of nurses in 1989 resulted in a confrontation between the striking nurses, the Premier, and other government officials. The nurses emerged from the bitter confrontation relatively unscathed and their salary demands were met. Although striking nurses were subject to lose their seniority in health-care agencies, most agencies failed to implement this punitive measure.

■■ ■■ ■■ ■■

RELATIONSHIPS BETWEEN PROFESSIONAL ASSOCIATIONS AND UNIONS

The history of collective bargaining in Canada indicates that the development of nursing unions was influenced by professional associations. In some cases there have been "growing pains" as fledgling unions separated from the professional associations. A few of the provincial nurses unions have joined the trade union movement and severed their connections with the more professionally directed organizations, perhaps reflecting a process of maturation as the new organization searches for its own identity. This association with the trade union movement, however, could adversely affect some members and the professional association. Because trade unions were originally founded by factory workers and employees in the unskilled labour category, the processes, language, and strategies used are not those of professionals. The image of nurses adopting the language and actions of general trade unionists may be abhorrent to many professional nurses, the professional nursing association, and other professional associations.

Although trade union alliances for nursing unions may result in fewer beneficial outcomes due to lack of member support for a less professional image, solidarity between groups in the trade union movement could benefit the union membership as a whole. The sharing of resources, strategies, financial assistance, and moral support may benefit a nursing union. The professional association cannot provide support during periods of labour unrest because of its statutory mandate to serve the public interest before the professional interest. Nevertheless, the price of closer ties may require members to march with locals of other unions on strike. Media coverage that might ensue may not be pleasing to all members of the professional organization and may engender a less professional public image.

The development of a professional model of collective bargaining has been proposed by Cleland (1978). In essence, this model would promote stronger professional ties for the nursing unions. Although the Cleland model was developed for the United States, where professional nurses' associations are often involved in bargaining, it includes some important perspectives on professional unionism that apply to the Canadian situation. New developments in unionism have resulted in the formation of more professional unions from highly educated professional groups, such as professors. Although most physicians are self-employed, the advent of medicare since 1957 has meant that payment for services comes primarily from the public purse. Economic decline, the accumulation of large federal deficits, and the need to control public sector spending have led to controls on reimbursement of medical services under provincial health-care plans. Physicians' strikes have been infrequent, the two most notable being in Saskatchewan in 1962 and in Ontario in 1986. The increasing size of the professional sector of the union movement allows for the development of alliances, whereas nursing unions previously had little alternative but to form alliances with the trade union sector.

The American Nurses Association's (ANA) Commission on Nursing Services developed a statement designed to encourage good relationships between professional and negotiating bodies entitled the *Characteristics of a Professional Climate of Administration and Practice in a Nursing Department* (1979). The characteristics listed include: 1) a system of shared governance; 2) planning for quality of nursing staff as well as optimal staffing levels to meet patient needs; 3) encouraging continuing education for staff; 4) recognizing educational background, professional experience, and level of clinical competence; 5) appointing administrators with educational and experiential background appropriate for their positions; 6) emphasizing nursing research in the practice setting; and 7) establishing a joint practice committee to promote collegial relations between nurses and physicians.

Professional associations and nursing unions in most jurisdictions in Canada will probably establish relationships that allow each to perform its functions to the best advantage. Intolerance of the unique mandate of the negotiating body and the professional body may have clouded perceptions of the appropriateness of the other's actions in the past. With time may come understanding and acceptance of the role and functions of each type of organization. Many agencies, alliances, and relationships may be needed to help the profession accomplish its goals in the diverse areas noted. Communicating with the large membership complement of the profession to increase understanding on the part of its members presents challenges that are difficult but not insurmountable. No doubt, compromise will characterize relationships between groups and affect the development of positive relationships. As Zimmerman (1983) has noted, "The history of organized nursing has been the history of a profession seeking to assert itself, to define and control its own body of knowledge and practice, to win recognition, respect and just reward for its contributions" (p. 603).

REFERENCES

American Nurses Association. (1979). *Characteristics of a professional climate of administration and practice in a nursing department.* Kansas City, MO: The Association.

Canadian Nurses Association. (1985). *Code of Ethics.* Ottawa: The Association.

Canadian Nurses Association. (1991). *Code of ethics.* Ottawa: The Association.

Cleland, V.S. (1978). Shared governance in a professional model of collective bargaining. *Journal of Nursing Administration, 8*(6), 39-43.

Conroy, M.D. and Hibberd, J.M. (1983). Areas for cooperation and conflict between nursing associations and negotiating bodies. In Quinn, S. (Ed.), *Cooperation and conflict: caring for the carers.* Geneva: International Council of Nurses.

Kluge, E.W. (1982). The profession of nursing and the right to strike. *Westminster Institute Review,* pp. 3-6.

Order of Nurses of the Province of Quebec. (1982). *Labour relations and withdrawal of services within the health sector.* Brief presented at the meeting of the Comité Permanante du Travail et de la Main-d'Oeuvre de l'Assemblé Nationale du Québec. Quebec: The Association.

Rowsell, G. (1982). Changing trends in labour relations: effects on collective bargaining for nurses. *International Nursing Review, 29*(5), 141-145.

Zimmerman, A. (1983). Collective bargaining in the hospital: The nurse's right, the professional association's responsibility. In McCloskey, J. and Grace, H. (Eds.), *Current issues in nursing.* Boston: Blackwell Scientific Publications.

PART IV

Educating Nurses for the Future

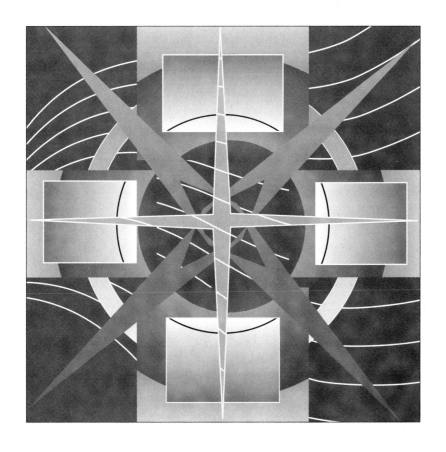

The Origins of Nursing Education in Canada: An Overview of the Emergence and Growth of Diploma Programs: 1874 to 1974

JANET ROSS KERR

H igher education in formal settings outside the home was not available to women at the beginning of the 19th century. Just before the turn of the century at the time when a crusade to allow women to gain entry into institutions of higher education began, Mary Wollstonecraft presented an articulate case for the schooling of women (1786, 1792). However, it was not until the middle of the century that the struggle to open the universities and professions to women began to gain momentum. Teaching was among the first professions to accept women, and in the western United States, seminaries and normal schools for women were founded,

> . . . where from the 1830s onward women teachers were churned out by the thousands for the numerous but very elementary schools of the expanding American republic. When universities opened in the new mid-western and western states in the 1860s and 70s, for example in Michigan, Wisconsin, Iowa and Utah, the need for fees fully as much as frontier egalitarianism dictated that these state-funded land-grant institutions would be coeducational from the outset (Jackel, 1985 p. 3).

The more tradition-bound eastern states did not move as quickly. As a substitute for the full admission of women to existing institutions, such as Harvard and Yale, a number of universities, such as Radcliffe, Smith, Vassar, Bryn Mawr, and Wellesley, were formed expressly for women. In Great Britain the outcome of the debate about the education of women was affected by the fact that women great-ly outnumbered men: at mid-century by 650,000 and in 1900 by 1.5 million. Jackel (1982) notes:

> "Distressed gentlewomen," as impoverished middle-class women were called, was no mere phrase, therefore; the privations of these women when male breadwinners died or lost their incomes were very real, and they were not only material, but psycho-logical and emotional as well. Consequently the plight of the single educated woman without means became one of the most widely debated social issues of nineteenth-cen-tury Britain (pp. xvi-xvii).

The situation was particularly acute for middle-class women because social norms dictated that an unmarried woman should depend on her male relatives for financial and social support; however, the surplus of women supported the argument to allow women to become educated and use their skills in gainful employment so that they would not be dependent on male family members. Many women became active in the movement for higher education for women, including Florence Nightingale (1929), who eloquently put the question as, "Why have women passion, intellect and moral activity—these three—and a place in society where no one of the three can be exercised" (p. 396)?

EARLY PREPARATION FOR NURSING PRACTICE

Although nurses had some preparation for practice in the early days of the profession, it was largely informal. Observation, passing knowledge from one person to another, and on-the-job training were the principal forms of educational preparation for nurses in the 17th, 18th, and 19th centuries. The three Augustinian nuns, who arrived in 1639 and who share the distinction of being the first trained nurses practising in Canada, received their preparation within their order, which had dedicated itself to the care of the sick. For several centuries women who joined religious orders were taught the skills of nursing by experi-enced members of the sisterhood. Jeanne Mance, the first lay nurse with prepara-tion, designed her own course of study, travelling to several centres in France to learn care methods before emigrating to Canada to take up her vocation.

THE NIGHTINGALE MODEL

The setting in which education for the practice of nursing was born and nur-tured was the hospital. The founding of the first school of nursing, by Florence Nightingale in 1860 in conjunction with St. Thomas' Hospital in London, was evi-dently a development that was needed in western society, for the idea swept the world and many hospital training schools were established throughout Europe and America. The term "historical accident," coined by Esther Lucile Brown (1948) referred to the failure to apply the fundamental philosophy of the Nightingale model in the majority of the new schools (p. 164). In many of the new schools, the concept of autonomy was lost in the financial administration of the enterprise. Such schools became completely dependent on the financial stability of the hospital with which they were associated, and their policies were dictated by a board of trustees. The educational orientation was forgotten as the new schools-cum-service ministered to the needs of the sick. As a result, little attention was given to opportunities for instruction in the classroom or during clinical experience, and educational preparation was considered secondary to the needs of the hospital nursing service.

Certain principles of the first Nightingale school were present in new schools: women who were as well prepared in nursing as possible were placed in charge of the schools, courses were spread over a period of 2 or 3 years, and incidental instruction was accompanied by extended periods of practice. It was an apprenticeship system that lacked a master craftsman. In North America, students who did not have responsibilities for patient care on the nursing units attended one or two hours of lectures that were given each week by a physician or the superintendent of nurses. Those who could attend related the information to those who could not.

One of the first schools in North America to advocate the principles of Florence Nightingale was the Bellevue Training School for Nurses; it was established in New York in 1873 by Sister Helen Bowden, an Anglican sister who had been educated at University College Hospital in England. Many Canadian women went to the United States to study during this period, and some, including Isabel Hampton Robb, Mary Adelaide Nutting, and Isabel Maitland Stewart, later became leaders in American nursing. Close contact was maintained between nurses in Canada and the United States through professional nursing organizations.

■■ ■■ ■■ ■■

THE FIRST CANADIAN NURSING SCHOOLS

The first hospital diploma school in Canada, the St. Catharine's Training School, was initiated on June 10, 1874 by Dr. Theophilus Mack, an Irish-born physician who was convinced that "the prejudice held by many sick people against going into public hospitals could best be overcome by building up a profession of trained lay nurses" (Gibbon and Mathewson, 1947, p. 144). Healey (1990) notes that the date of the inception of the school "so closely parallels the start of Bellevue that in later years there will be those who seek to prove it was the first on the Continent to incorporate Nightingale's ideas" (pp. 31-32). Healey (1990) also indicates that "Dr. Mack is credited with having the idea [for the establishment of the school] as early as 1864" (p. 43). Constraints were again imposed, as "nursing was considered an undesirable vocation for a refined lady, the only acceptable profession being teaching" (Healey, 1990, p. 44).

Admission standards were "plain English education, good character, and Christian motives" (St. Catharines Annual Report [cited in Healey, 1990]). The philosophy of the school is reflected in a statement concerning instruction (Healey, 1990, p. 45):

> Every possible opportunity is seized to impart instruction of a practical nature in the art of nursing, while teachings will be given in Chemistry, Sanitary Science, Popular Physiology and Anatomy, hygiene and all such branches of the healing art as a nurse ought to be familiar with . . . . The vocation of nursing goes hand in hand with

that of physician and surgeon, and are absolutely indispensable one to the other. Incompetency on the part of a nurse renders nugatory the best effects of the doctor in the critical moments and has frequently resulted in loss of life. All the most brilliant achievements of modern surgery are dependent to a great extent upon careful and intelligent nursing . . . The skilled nurse, by minutely watching the temperature, conditions of skin, pulse, respirations, the various functions of all the organs and reporting faithfully to the attending physician, must increase the chances of recovery twofold" (Healey, 1990, pp. 45-46).

The School for Nurses associated with the Toronto General Hospital was established in 1881; 17 students enrolled, but 8 resigned or were dismissed (Gibbon and Mathewson, 1947). When Mary Agnes Snively was appointed Superintendent of the school in 1884, there were no systems for work or study, no written orders, no history records, and no systems for obtaining ward supplies. The living conditions were distressing. The school was gradually reorganized and the modern plan developed (Gibbon and Mathewson, 1947). In 1894 53 candidates for the program were selected from 647 applications. Also in 1894, 21 graduands and 4 graduate nurses held staff positions. The program's size made it the largest nursing education program in Canada (Gibbon and Mathewson 1947). Miss Snively worked hard to improve the educational component of the program as it developed. In 1896 a 3-year course was introduced that included "84 hours of practical nursing and 119 hours of instruction by the medical staff" (Gibbon and Mathewson, 1947, p. 154).

Miss Snively's involvement with the International Council of Nurses (ICN) began in 1899, the year the council was founded. She became the first honourary treasurer of the organization, and her efforts in establishing the Canadian National Association of Trained Nurses (later the Canadian Nurses Association [CNA])and in serving as its first president are an indication of the stature she achieved (Canadian Nurses Association [CNA], 1968). Written records of CNA meetings indicate that Miss Snively supported changes designed to improve nursing education programs. Commenting on the recently introduced plan to devote the first part of the training period to a preliminary course at a meeting, she stated:

> They are also taught anatomy, physiology and simple lessons in nursing and practical demonstrations during the three-months period. We have a room fitted up with bedding and linen and all the necessaries, there the nurses are taught to do practically all the work that will be required of them after they enter the school as nurses. At the end of three months, probationers pass an examination in all they have been taught theoretically, and also in practical work (Gibbon and Mathewson, 1947, p. 155).

At the Montreal General Hospital, which was founded in 1822, early interest in establishing a school of nursing led to the Committee of Management's correspondence in 1874 to secure assistance in developing "a system of trained hospital nurses such as approved of in England" (MacDermot, 1940, p. 17). Communication may have been initiated by Miss Maria Machin, a native of Quebec who was engaged in nursing in London at the Nightingale Home (Baly, 1986, p. 143). Baly (1986) notes that: "It is unlikely that Miss Nightingale would have selected Miss Machin, for her loss as Home Sister to the Nightingale Home would be irreparable for she had not long been installed and was regarded as the one person who could keep the peace with Mrs. Wardroper" (p. 144).

Correspondence that ensued with Florence Nightingale and her brother-in-law Henry Bonham Carter, the President of the Fund, dealt primarily with plans for the new hospital building that had been promised by the Committee of Management. Miss Machin set out for Montreal with four Nightingale nurses, but the mission failed. The difficulties that arose during Miss Machin's tenure at the hospital included a high staff turnover rate, and "there is reason to believe there was 'a lack of adaptability on the part of Miss Machin whose uncompromising purpose was to apply Nightingale principles of nursing care at whatever cost and without much thought for diplomacy' (Redpath [cited in Baly, 1986, p. 146]). The problems she encountered and her failure to accomplish her initial objective, establishing a training school for nurses, led to her perception of failure in her mission and she returned to England in 1878. Baly (1986) notes that the Council of the Nightingale Fund did not make much of their efforts in Montreal or elsewhere because Cook (Nightingale's biographer) had only given Montreal a passing reference, and Carter clearly thought that the entire issue should be forgotten. Baly (1986) has taken issue with "nursing historians" who "have claimed that Nightingale missioners took reformed nursing to both Canada and Australia and have made much out of little evidence" (p. 147).

The School for Nurses at the Montreal General Hospital was finally initiated in 1890, under the direction of Nora Livingston, who was born the daughter of English parents in Sault Ste. Marie, Michigan, raised in Como, Quebec, and educated at the New York Hospital's Training School for Nurses. When she arrived in Montreal, "Conditions at the General were deplorable . . . and within a year of her entrance she had so revolutionized the organization of the hospital as to make it almost unrecognizable compared with conditions of the previous year" (*Famous nurses in history*, undated).

The popularity of the school increased rapidly. Miss Livingston reported 169 applications in the first year, 80 of which were accepted on probation. Of the 80 that were accepted, 42 of them proved satisfactory, 4 resigned, and 2 were dismissed (Gibbon and Mathewson, 1947). Recollections of Miss Livingston's abilities are positive:

> . . . what an extraordinary amount of tact and gumption this remarkable woman possessed. Not only had she to change the incredible conditions of nursing but above all she had to change the attitudes of the administrators, men animated by good intentions but more accustomed to conducting the affairs of business than those of a hospital (Desjardins, 1971, p. 103).

The nursing education program gradually took shape; one of the early graduates recalls: "Thinking of those days so long ago, I think I hear Miss Livingston say—'Nurse—the patient—always the patient first!' I think that spirit still lives within these old walls" (Gibbon and Mathewson, 1947, p. 149).

The move to establish hospital schools of nursing swept the country. The Winnipeg General Hospital initiated the first Training School for Nurses in the west in 1887, which served all of the west in its early years. Gibbon and Mathewson (1947) note that 134 graduates of that school served as matrons and nursing sisters in World War I. In the maritime provinces, the Saint John General Hospital in Fredericton and the Victoria Public Hospital in Saint John opened training schools for nurses in 1887, and the Victoria General in Halifax and the Prince Edward Island Hospital in Charlottetown followed suit in 1890. In Vancouver the General Hospital began an educational program in 1891, and in Alberta a school was initiated at Medicine Hat in 1894. By 1930 there were approximately 330 schools of nursing in Canada (Canadian Nurses Association, 1968).

■ ■ ■ ■

RECOGNIZING THE NEED FOR IMPROVEMENT IN STANDARDS

Because hospitals were staffed primarily by students in the late 19th and early 20th centuries, there were few opportunities for securing a staff position after graduation. Graduates who practised their profession usually did so as private duty nurses in the homes of the sick. Therefore one of nurses' first struggles after the hospital-based system of nursing education was established involved replacing students with graduate nurses as the primary providers of nursing care. Mabel Holt (1936) writes of an "experiment" in a Montreal hospital in which a nursing unit was totally staffed with graduate nurses and justified the endeavour as follows:

> There are, however, other and even more important benefits, affecting the nursing profession as a whole, which have come about as a direct result of this new policy. Instead of adding to the output of graduate nurses during these difficult years by increasing the enrolment of our school of nursing, we have created employment for those who otherwise would have been obliged to enter an overcrowded and highly competitive field. I also consider it to be a great factor in the education of the public concerning its responsibility to nurses and nursing that a Board of Directors should be willing to try out the difficult experiment of staffing a complete unit with graduate nurses (p. 10).

In view of the firm establishment and acceptance of the hospital-based educational system, the difficulty that the university-based system encountered in establishing its credibility in the eyes of patients, the public, and even nurses is easily understood. Bonin (1976) commented: "So deeply time-honoured became this system of nursing education that it became difficult to imagine nursing, like other professions, as belonging to a university setting for the education of its practitioners" (pp. xii-xiii).

Increased awareness of deficiencies resulted in a number of surveys of nursing education in Canada and the United States. In 1923 the Goldmark Report, commissioned by the Rockefeller Foundation to investigate conditions in schools of nursing in the United States, described appalling conditions. The report advocated more attention for the educational preparation of nurses, more stringent admission requirements for nursing schools, and provision of federal grants to assist schools in raising their educational standards. In Burgess (1928) and the Committee on the Grading of Nursing Schools (1934), reports of a joint committee of several professional nursing associations and professional organizations of related health fields on the grading of schools of nursing restated the shortcomings of the system. It was concluded that:

1. No hospital should be expected to bear the cost of nursing education out of funds collected for the care of the sick. The education of nurses is as much a public responsibility as the education of physicians, public school teachers, librarians, ministers, lawyers, and other students planning to engage in professional public service, and the cost of such education should come, not out of the hospital budget, but from private or public funds.
2. The fact that a hospital is faced with serious financial difficulties should have no bearing upon whether or not it will conduct a school of nursing. The need of a hospital for cheap labour should not be considered a legitimate argument for maintaining such a school (Burgess, 1928, p. 447).

Regarding the institutions that conduct schools of nursing: "The Grading Committee reports showed clearly that the system of hospital-owned and operated schools of nursing was still practically universal. The proportion of university schools was so small in 1932 that they scarcely figured numerically, however important their influence might be individually" (Stewart, 1947, p. 213).

The significance of the 1910 Flexner Report on medical education and its impact on nursing education have been noted by Allemang (1974). Funded by the Carnegie Foundation, the Flexner Report was commissioned because of concern for the quality of medical practice and medical education and the concomitant inability of the American Medical Association and the Council on Medical Education to achieve reforms. As a result of the Flexner Report, the character of medical education changed quickly; the proprietary schools that operated for profit were closed, and standards in medical education began to rise as the universities assumed major responsibility for the support and direction of the enterprise. According to Allemang (1974): "The Flexner report on medical education provided a model for the new approach to nursing reforms" (pp. 115-116). Thus the call for improved standards of nursing education became more intense as the 20th century began.

In Canada, unrest similar to that in the United States surfaced a few years later over conditions in schools and hospitals. In 1927 a joint committee of the Canadian Medical Association (CMA) and the CNA was organized to study the problems. The Committee appointed Dr. George Weir, of the Department of Education at the University of British Columbia, to conduct a survey to address these matters. The study documented the problems and drew attention to the changes needed to improve standards of education and service. The fact that small hospitals had established schools of nursing led to a presumption that the size of a hospital was important because there could be a lack of variety in clinical experience in small institutions. The survey indicated that this presumption was educationally unsound, but it also indicated that schools associated with hospitals with fewer than 75 beds were more concerned with the financial needs of the hospital than with the educational needs of nursing students in operating programs (CNA, 1968; Gibbon and Mathewson, 1947; Weir, 1932). This suspicion about the general motives of hospitals in offering educational programs led to the recommendation that authority and responsibility for schools of nursing be vested within the general provincial system of education. "The development of training schools for nurses primarily as educational institutions functioning as an integral part of the general educational system of the province and financed on the same principle as are normal schools, should be made an immediate objective" (Weir, 1932, p. 116).

This recommendation was repeated many times in the years before the basic diploma nursing education program began to move within the purview of the general postsecondary system of education. After the Weir Report was tabled, nurses turned their attention to developing strategies to improve the quality of education in schools of nursing.

> Moved by the recommendations in the Weir Report indicating the need for immediate correction of defects in administrative and teaching policies of hospital schools of nursing, in 1932, the Canadian Nurses' Association . . . organized a National Curriculum Committee with the responsibility of constructing a curriculum guide (Letourneau, 1975, p. 6).

The curriculum guide, published in 1936, was intended to serve as an interim measure that would help schools of nursing during their transfer to provincial educational systems (CNA, 1936).

The Demonstration School

The minimal progress through the next decade led the CNA to secure Red Cross funding for a demonstration school that would ascertain the feasibility of preparing a nurse in less than 3 years. The school, known simply as the Demonstration School, was established in 1948 in conjunction with the Metropolitan Hospital in Windsor, Ontario. Red Cross funding enabled the Demonstration School to be financially independent from the hospital. The experiment continued until 1952, when the Demonstration School reverted to its former status of financial dependence on the hospital. An extensive evaluation, conducted by a joint committee (chaired by A.R. Lord) of the CNA and the Canadian Education Association (CEA), indicated that the venture was a success; it was possible to prepare a nurse for practice in 2 years.

> The conclusion is inescapable. When the school has complete control of students, nurses can be trained at least as satisfactorily in two years as in three, and under better conditions, but the training must be paid for in money instead of in services. Few students can afford substantial fees nor can the hospital pass on such additional costs to the "paying patient." Some new source of revenue is the only solution (Lord, 1952, p. 54).

The Centralized Teaching Program

In Saskatchewan there was increasing consternation about the lack of foundational courses in basic sciences for nursing students in diploma programs and the general shortage of suitably qualified faculty. The Saskatchewan Registered Nurses Association (SRNA) sought and secured financial support from the W.K. Kellogg Foundation to centralize teaching of basic sciences for all schools of nursing in the Saskatoon and Regina areas. The program provided for:

... a duly authorized sixteen weeks' program of instruction in the basic sciences for nursing students. It is an integral part of the curriculum plan of the hospital school of nursing provided apart from the hospital school at a designated centre permitting centralization of effort and resources not immediately available in the local setting of the participating schools (Schmitt, 1957, p. 6).

Although considerable effort was directed to organizing this effort and it was declared a success, it was not considered a panacea for the ills of basic nursing education. Although many areas of the country decided not to offer basic science instruction on a regional basis, this endeavour provided a solution to some problems and issues in basic diploma nursing education.

Accreditation

The CNA next directed attention to the quality of instruction in schools of nursing. A pilot project under the direction of Executive Director Helen Mussallem was designed to determine whether schools were ready for a national voluntary accreditation program. The findings were somewhat disappointing; only 16% of schools met the criteria for accreditation. It was also determined that little progress had been made in improving the quality of schools since Dr. Weir had made his report public some 30 years before. Dr. Mussallem thus recommended that the CNA not embark on an accreditation program, but rather a school improvement program that would lead to accreditation in the future (Mussallem, 1960). The CNA implemented Dr. Mussallem's recommendation, and accreditation was not seriously discussed again until the late 1970s. At that time, because of the costs associated, accreditation was not considered for diploma schools in the absence of an organization willing to provide the necessary funds.

The Royal Commission on Health Services

A trend gradually became evident in the majority of the 2-year schools that were established. In the brief presented to the Royal Commission on Health Services, the CNA favoured "introducing diploma schools of nursing into the post-high school system of the country" (Mussallem, 1964, p. 137). The Royal Commission on Health Services, or the Hall Commission, surveyed the entire range of health services (including nursing) that were provided and reported in 1964. Nursing education programs that took fewer than 3 years and functioned independently from the hospital were recommended.

> The Commission believes this to be the right approach. The educational system for nursing should be organized and financed like other forms of professional education. An additional reason for the change in nursing education is not only that we shall obtain equally, if not better, qualified personnel in shorter time, but that a substantial part of hospitalized patient-care will no longer depend, as it does now, upon apprentices (Government of Canada, 1964, pp. 64-69).

A certain momentum created by the increased pace of change after the release of the Hall Commission Report may have led to the CNA's plan for the development of nursing education programs within the general educational system. Mussallem (1964) declares that:

Whether nursing education should be placed within the general educational system can no longer be considered a point of debate. It is possible and it can be done . . . The Canadian Nurses' Association, in cooperation with its provincial counterparts, should take steps to implement the plan present in the study . . . leading to the inclusion of all nursing education within the general educational system of each province (pp. 183-185).

■■ ■■ ■■ ■■

THE MOVEMENT TO ESTABLISH 2-YEAR SCHOOLS

Saskatchewan

Saskatchewan was the first province to consider implementing 2-year diploma nursing schools. The Regina Grey Nuns Hospital School of Nursing requested and received permission from the Saskatchewan Registered Nurses Association (SRNA) to develop a 2-year diploma program in nursing on an experimental basis. This led to the establishment of 2-year diploma programs in the two major cities of the province in 1967. Letourneau (1975) cites the difficulties that occurred because "Saskatchewan had forged ahead in legislating change without having an educational system fully established to absorb programs" (p. 25). To avoid the development of isolated institutions that would be for nursing only, the SRNA (1966) insisted "that diploma nursing for nurses be established in post-secondary institutions for higher education" (p. 1). In Saskatchewan "the trend was not for hospital schools of nursing to transmute to an educational institution, but rather to gradually phase out by ceasing to admit students" (Letourneau, 1975, p. 27). The two new 2-year programs in Saskatchewan were developed at the Kelsey Institute in Saskatoon and at Wascana Institute in Regina.

Quebec

In Quebec, the Royal Commission of Inquiry on Education, also known as the Parent Commission, reported its findings in 1966, recommending not starting one or two 2-year schools as suggested by the Association of Nurses of the Province of Quebec (ANPQ), but a total transfer of programs to the general system of education. The contention of this report was that the entire education system was examined by the Commission, and the nursing recommendations were totally consistent with findings in other fields. Campbell (1971) has commented about the impact of the Parent Commission's report. "It would be difficult to name any royal commission in the history of Canadian education whose judgements more profoundly altered the structure and process of the entire educational system of a province and with greater speed" (p. 54).

In 1967 three programs were selected for transfer to the Collèges d'Enseignement Général et Professionnel (CEGEP) to serve as pilot projects; 17 were selected in 1968, and others after that. "In 1972, the last Schools of Nursing attached to hospitals closed, ending three-quarters of a century of history. Now a network of 40 nursing options exist throughout "la belle province"' (ANPQ, 1972, p. 1), and with the two English-language CEGEPs that have diploma programs, the number of programs was 42. Also, "A distinctively unique characteristic of education offered in a CEGEP is that it is tuition free for all full-time students"

(Letourneau, 1975, p. 77). Thus as nursing schools became part of the community college system in Quebec, nursing students began receiving the same educational benefits as students studying in other professions and vocations.

Ontario

Elsewhere in Canada, models for 2-year programs emerged as independent, freestanding institutions. The Nightingale School of Nursing in Toronto, established in 1960, was financed by the Ontario Hospital Services Commission. Situated in close proximity to New Mount Sinai Hospital where nursing clinical experience was obtained, the school was administered by an independent board of directors. The Quo Vadis School of Nursing was established in 1964 under the auspices of the Catholic Hospital Conference of Ontario. Again, financial support was provided by the Ontario Hospital Services Commission and the school was administered by an independent board of directors. This school had a mandate to structure its educational program to attract mature students (McLean, 1964).

The School of Nursing established at Ryerson Polytechnical Institute in Toronto in 1964 had the distinction of being the first nursing diploma program in Canada to be initiated in an educational institution (Letourneau, 1975). The efforts of the Registered Nurses Association of Ontario (RNAO) were influential in instigating this effort; Ryerson's administration and board reviewed the RNAO's proposal carefully, decided to establish the school, and accepted the first class in 1964. Similar programs were developed in colleges across the country. Although Ryerson's program was initially structured as a 3-year program, it was later converted to a 2-year program. Dr. Moyra Allen of McGill University and Professor Mary Reidy of the University of Montreal evaluated the Ryerson program after 5 years and confirmed the soundness of the program. The findings "point to the potential value of preparing a nurse in a college-level institution within the general system of education" (Allen and Reidy, 1971, p. 262).

In 1967, 20 colleges of applied arts and technology (CAAT) were created in the province by order of the Ontario government. In 1969 Humber College was the first of these institutions to develop a nursing program. Ontario moved ahead on another front before it began to develop schools of nursing within the CAAT system on a large scale; freestanding schools of nursing called regional schools were developed apart from the general education system. There were no regional schools in 1965, but "by the end of 1967 there were eight, and ten more . . . expected within the next five years" (Murray, 1970, p. 132). The government also decided, in spite of the reservations expressed by the College of Nurses of Ontario, to move to "two plus one" programs, initially in a "ten-year plan leading to a gradual shortening and regionalization of schools of nursing" (Letourneau, 1975, p. 144). This change occurred rapidly, but it was a passing phenomenon; the move to establish 2-year schools under the aegis of the CAATs was overwhelming, and "in 1972, policies with regard to free room and board were altered; the year of internship was discontinued, and nursing students were required to pay tuition fees" (Letourneau, 1975, p. 145). Thus by 1973, 56 schools had been absorbed by 23 CAATs.

British Columbia

In British Columbia, the first diploma nursing program to be established within the general educational system was a jointly planned venture of the British Columbia Institute of Technology (BCIT) and the Registered Nurses Association of British Columbia (RNABC) in 1967. The RNABC's (1967) position was well known:

> Nursing can no longer be taught by apprenticeship methods; yet the students are part of the hospital service personnel . . . We believe that the method of financing nursing education partly through hospital operating costs and partly through service rendered by students is no longer an adequate or desirable one (p. 20).

Funding for this program was obtained through an agreement between the federal and provincial governments for vocational-technical education. During the development of the program the RNABC successfully lobbied for changes in existing legislation to allow for development of new and innovative models of diploma nursing programs. Thus community colleges throughout the province were able to develop nursing programs, and in 1965 Vancouver City College in Langara and Selkirk College in Castlegar initiated programs. By 1974 four programs had been developed, and several others were in the planning stages, although four hospital diploma programs still remained in operation.

Alberta

In Alberta the transfer of diploma programs to the community colleges also was incomplete by 1974. Mount Royal College in Calgary was the first college in the province to develop a diploma nursing program in 1967. Others included Red Deer College and College St. Jean (merged with Grant MacEwan Community College in 1972) in 1968, Lethbridge Community College in 1969, Medicine Hat College in 1970, and Grant MacEwan Community College in 1972. Although seven hospitals had phased out their schools, six were still in operation in the province in 1974 (Letourneau, 1975). A report prepared by Dr. G. R. Fast in 1971 recommended the transfer of remaining diploma programs to the Alberta college system; however, the recommendation was not well received by all stakeholder groups, reportedly because of a lack of consultation and discussion preceding the release of the report.

Manitoba

The transfer of diploma nursing programs to the colleges in Manitoba was also incomplete by 1974, with five hospital-based programs continuing to operate. The first and only college diploma program was established at Red River Community College in 1970, the result of "action on the part of the Departments of Health and Education and the adjoining cooperative efforts of the MARN" (Letourneau, 1975, p. 253). The Manitoba Association of Registered Nurses (MARN) was influential in establishing the program because it supported the inclusion of diploma nursing programs in the general system of education and shortening their duration to 2 years (Manitoba Association of Registered Nurses [MARN], 1968).

The Atlantic Provinces

By the end of 1974 there had been some activity in the Atlantic provinces in relation to the movement that was sweeping other parts of the country, but activity was limited. A study conducted by Katherine MacLaggan of nursing education in New Brunswick resulted in a recommendation that the general educational system be vested with responsibility for diploma nursing education (MacLaggan, 1965). According to Letourneau (1975): "conflicting forces have rendered impossible the actual transfer of hospital programs to the system of education" (p. 275) In 1971 the Abbis Report recommended that four independent schools be established similar to a pilot program at the Saint John School of Nursing, which had been converted to a 2-year program, but financed through health dollars from the Department of Health (Study Committee on Nursing Education, 1971). Because the document contained controversial recommendations about registration and standards in addition to recommendations about diploma nursing education that were not entirely satisfactory, the New Brunswick Association of Registered Nurses (NBARN) (1971) indicated that it was "gravely alarmed at the import of these recommendations and quite surprised that they appear in the Report . . . earnestly recommend that they be rejected" (p. 23)

Because there was no authority for establishing community colleges in New Brunswick until 1974, transfer of diploma nursing programs to the system of general education across the province was not possible. Thus four independent schools and one hospital school were established in Bathurst, Edmunston, Moncton, and Saint John (Letourneau, 1975). These programs were autonomous in all respects except finance. However, as Letourneau (1975) observed: "Trends point to an eventual orderly transfer of independent programs to the provincial system of education, but first the community college system must develop sufficiently to absorb these programs" (p. 290).

The Registered Nurses Association of Nova Scotia (RNANS) had a leading role in pressing for changes in the system of nursing education in that province. The RNANS' appointment of a curriculum council to determine each school's plan for change may have hastened and facilitated self-study by the schools so that: "Seven hospital schools of nursing were authorized, in the period extending from 1969 to 1970, to begin a two-year program or to effect a change in this direction" (Letourneau, 1975, p. 293). As with nurses across the country, in 1969 nurses in Nova Scotia had to stop an attempt to remove the regulatory powers vested in their association. Nova Scotia also faced the problem of having a community college system that needed to "develop sufficiently to absorb these programs" (Letourneau, 1975, p. 290).

The Association of Nurses of Prince Edward Island (ANPEI) requested that the three existing hospital schools of nursing in its province be phased out and replaced by one program to make the best use of staff and facilities and to provide the best possible education for students (Letourneau, 1975). The organization also sponsored a study to assess the climate and readiness for change in the diploma nursing education system; this study indicated that it was not the right time right for major change (Rowe, 1967). In 1968 the ANPEI again pressed for change in the system, and this time the government responded by providing authority for developing one independent "two plus one" program for the province, replacing the three hospital schools (Letourneau, 1975). Efforts in 1974 to link the school with the community college, Holland College, were unsuccessful.

Letourneau (1975) stated: "The transfer of hospital schools of nursing to the system of education is, as in other Atlantic provinces, non-existent in Newfoundland" (p. 308). Four hospital schools of nursing continued to exist there, although the Association of Registered Nurses of Newfoundland (ARNN) tried to encourage change. Arpin (1972), a consultant hired by the ARNN to help formulate goals, recommended that "the three schools of nursing in St. John's develop their curriculum plans so that the theory and experience essential for meeting the school objectives is included in the first two years of the program" (p. 1). By 1973 the three schools in St. John's had established "two plus one" programs and the Corner Brook program had reduced its length to 2 years.

■ ■ ■ ■

CONCLUSION

In 1974, 100 years after the inception of the Mack Training School for Nurses in St. Catharine's, the system of diploma nursing education had undergone a transformation. In 1874, despite the wide recognition of Florence Nightingale's work around the world and despite the historic work of the nursing sisterhoods in Canada dating from the 17th century, it was still not socially acceptable for a woman to do nursing in a hospital or leave home to enter a school to acquire knowledge and skills for that work. In 1974, 109 basic diploma schools of nursing (Letourneau, 1975) operated across the country, and widespread debate continued about the quality of instruction and the expectations for nursing students in comparison to those for other students in the system of postsecondary education. Issues change over time; the comparison of diploma nursing education to that provided at the university level as the most appropriate level for beginning practice is a current issue of concern in the profession that is discussed in more detail in Chapters 24 and 25. Nevertheless, one can see both a progression and transition of nurses' ideas about their educational system. It is evident that there is a fundamental concern for standards of education and practice in view of the responsibility for safe patient care. With the development of the discipline and the expansion of the knowledge base, the appropriateness of the environment in which learning takes place is at issue. The fact that nursing is one of the last sex-segregated professions has led to attention to the potential for differential treatment, with improvement in the status of women as they gradually gained fundamental rights and privileges previously accorded only to men. Although it is difficult to say what the next 100 years will mean to nursing and nursing education, it is likely that nurses will continue to work to improve standards of education and practice.

REFERENCES

Allemang, M.M. (1974). *Nursing education in the United States and Canada, 1873-1950: Leading figures, forces, views on education.* Doctoral dissertation, University of Washington, Seattle.

Allen, M., and Reidy, M. (1971). *Learning to nurse: The first five years of the Ryerson nursing program.* Ontario: Registered Nurses Association of Ontario.

Arpin, K. (1972). *Report of visit to the Association of Registered Nurses of Newfoundland.* St. John's: AARN.

Association of Nurses of the Province of Quebec.

(1972) *CEGEP nursing education after five years*. Montreal: Author.

Baly, M. (1986). *Florence Nightingale and the nursing legacy*. London: Croom Helm.

Bonin, M.A. (1976). *Trends in integrated basic degree nursing programs in Canada: 1942-1972*. Doctoral dissertation, University of Ottawa, Ottawa.

Brown, E.L. (1948). *Nursing for the future*. New York: Russell Sage Foundation.

Burgess, M.A. (1928). *Nurses, patients and pocketbooks*. New York: Committee on the Grading of Nursing Schools.

Campbell, Gordon. (1971). *Community colleges in Canada*. Toronto: McGraw-Hill.

Canadian Nurses Association. (1936). *A proposed curriculum for schools of nursing in Canada*. Montreal: Author.

Canadian Nurses Association. (1968). *The leaf and the lamp*. Ottawa: Author.

Committee on the Grading of Nursing Schools. (1934). *Nursing schools today and tomorrow*. New York: Author.

Desjardins, E. (1971). *Heritage: History of the nursing profession in the province of Quebec*. Quebec: Association of Nurses of the Province of Quebec.

Famous nurses in history. undated. "Gertrude Elizabeth Livingston." Guelph: The Sterling Rubber Company Ltd.

Gibbon, J.M., and Mathewson, M.S. (1947). *Three centuries of Canadian nursing*. Toronto: Macmillan.

Government of Canada. (1964). *Royal Commission on health services* (Vol. I) (Emmett M. Hall, Chairman). Ottawa: Queen's Printer.

Healey, P. (1990). *The Mack training school for nurses*. Unpublished doctoral dissertation, University of Texas, Austin, TX.

Healey, P. (1989). *The Mack training school for nurses*. Unpublished manuscript.

Holt, M. (1936). Staffing with graduate nurses. *The Canadian Nurse*, 32(1), 5-10.

Jackel, S. (1985). *Women in Canadian universities: A historical overview*. Keynote address to the Conference and Annual Meeting, Western Region, Canadian Association of University Schools of Nursing, University of Alberta, Edmonton, Alberta.

Jackel, S. (Ed.). (1982). *A flannel shirt & liberty*. Vancouver: University of British Columbia Press.

Letourneau, M. (1975). *Trends in basic diploma nursing programs within the provincial systems of education in Canada 1964-1974*. Doctoral dissertation, University of Ottawa, Ottawa.

Lord, A.R. (1952). *Report of the evaluation of the Metropolitan School of Nursing, Windsor, Ontario*. Ottawa: Canadian Nurses Association.

MacDermot, H.E. (1940). *History of the School of Nursing of the Montreal General Hospital*. Montreal: The Alumnae Association.

MacLaggan, K. (1965). *Portrait of nursing: A plan for the education of nurses in the province of New Brunswick*. Fredericton: New Brunswick Association of Registered Nurses.

Manitoba Association of Registered Nurses. (1968). *A position paper on nursing in Manitoba*. Winnipeg: Author.

McLean, C.D. (1964). *A report on the establishment of the Quo Vadis School of Nursing and the selection of the first class of students*. Toronto: Quo Vadis School of Nursing.

Murray, V.V. (1970). *Nursing in Ontario: A study for the committee on the healing arts*. Toronto: Queen's Printer.

Mussallem, H.K. (1964). *A path to quality: A plan for the development of nursing education programs within the general educational system of Canada*. Ottawa: Canadian Nurses Association.

Mussallem, H.K. (1960). *Spotlight on nursing education: The report of the pilot project of the evaluation of schools of nursing in Canada*. Ottawa: Canadian Nurses Association.

New Brunswick Association of Registered Nurses. (1971). *Position paper*. Fredericton: Author.

Nightingale, F. (1929). *Cassandra: An essay*. Old Westbury, NY: Feminist Press.

Registered Nurses' Association of British Columbia. (1967). *A proposed plan for the orderly development of nursing education in British Columbia: Part One—Basic nursing education*. Vancouver: RNABC.

Rowe, H.R. (1967). *A study of transition in nursing education in Prince Edward Island*. Charlottetown: ANPEI.

Saskatchewan Registered Nurses' Association. (1966). *Brief presented to the joint committee on higher education*. Regina: Author.

Schmitt, L.M. (1957). *Basic nursing education study: Report of the status of basic nursing education programs in Saskatchewan*. Regina: Saskatchewan Registered Nurses Association.

Stewart, I.M. (1947). *The education of nurses*. New York: Macmillan.

Study Committee on Nursing Education. (1971). *A study committee on nursing education*. New Brunswick: Department of Health.

Weir, G.M. (1932). *Survey of nursing education in Canada*. Toronto: University of Toronto Press.

Wollstonecraft, M. (1787). *Thoughts on the education of daughters*. Clifton, NJ: A.M. Kelley.

Wollstonecraft, M. (1792). *A vindication of the rights of woman*. London: J. Johnson.

CHAPTER TWENTY FOUR

A Historical Approach to the Evolution of University Nursing Education in Canada: 1919 to 1974

JANET ROSS KERR

T he history of nursing education in Canada parallels that of the country, as it is intimately related to social and economic developments. The health-care system has tended to expand and move ahead in times of prosperity. This has included building more hospitals and health-care facilities, all of which require nursing staff. As the recruitment of nurses has direct implications for nursing education, developments in schools of nursing have been conditioned by society. Standards of education in schools of nursing have been an important concern of the profession over the years and therefore have been subjected to considerable scrutiny and discussion. This chapter focuses on some of the major forces that have shaped the nature and form of the current system of nursing education at the university level in Canada. The focus is on undergraduate nursing education; graduate education is dealt with in some detail in Chapter 32.

■ ■ ■ ■

EMERGENCE OF UNIVERSITY SCHOOLS OF NURSING

University education for nurses was the subject of an address by Dr. Malcolm T. MacEachern to the British Columbia Hospitals Association in July 1919, after the May 26 Board of Governors' decision to approve the Senate's recommendation that a department of nursing be established at the University of British Columbia (Street, 1973). The founding of the department, a precedent in the history of Canadian nursing, occurred 4 years after the 1915 establishment of the university, largely through the efforts of Dr. MacEachern, the progressive medical superintendent of the Vancouver General Hospital. Universities were founded in the west as early as the second decade of the 20th century, when agricultural and technical education were receiving attention from the federal government. The utilitarian, philosophic orientation of the new western universities rationalizes the location of the first school of nursing in the West—in British Columbia.

When the decision was made to establish the University of British Columbia's Department of Nursing, the source of funding for the school was reviewed:

> The Board was advised that the Department would not involve any additional expense to the University. The minutes of this meeting do not add a fact of which the Board was aware: that the Vancouver General Hospital would pay the full salary of its director of nursing, who would also take charge of the University's Department of Nursing (Street, 1973, pp. 118-119).

In subsequent communication to the Senate to inform members of the disposition of the recommendation, it was ``emphasized that the action was taken on the understanding that the establishment of this Department would not involve any additional expense to the University" (Street, 1973, pp. 118-119). Under the terms of such a favourable arrangement, where the operating costs of the new department were to be borne by the hospital, the university was undoubtedly more easily persuaded by the persistent Dr. MacEachern that the entry of nursing to the academic world of the university was both possible and desirable.

The appointment of Ethel Johns as Director of the new department was fortuitous; she was energetic, articulate, and of independent spirit. These qualities would be an asset, because in the beginning the way would not be easy for the first university school of nursing in the country. Street (1973) alludes to the "precarious early years" (p. 115) of the new program. In an address to a joint session of the British Columbia Hospitals Association and the Canadian Public Health Association in Vancouver in June 1920, Miss Johns had an opportunity to appeal for positive attitudes, which had prevailed among physicians, toward the new development in nursing education:

> To those who are in opposition or are in doubt, one last word, if there are any of such here: Will you not listen to the appeal of those upon whose shoulders you yourselves lay such heavy burdens? You see so many faults, so many blunders in our nursing service. So do we; they are not hidden from us. You cannot imagine why things should not run more smoothly, but we can; we know it is because of insufficient teaching and supervision. You do not realize how complex your own profession has become. How can we expect you to realize how difficult it is for us, with few of your educational advantages, to keep up with the advance shown in medicine? (Street, 1973, p. 132).

The degree program thus established was based on the prevailing American model and "became the Canadian prototype of the pattern which came to be known as the non-integrated degree nursing course, or the 2+2+1 or 1+3+1 course, in which the university assumed no responsibility for the 2 or 3 years of nursing preparation in a hospital school of nursing" (Bonin, 1976, p. 7). The new program gradually became established. After the program was approved for its 5th year there was a request from the Library Committee:

> ... for a grant of two hundred fifty dollars with which to purchase books for the Department of Nursing. But the Board had a long memory. After some discussion, it was decided to direct the attention of the Library Committee to the undertaking of the Hospital authorities that the University would not be asked to assume any financial responsibility in respect to the Department of Nursing. It was decided that a sum not to exceed one hundred dollars should be granted for books (Street, 1973, p. 127).

■■ ■■ ■■ ■■

THE IMPACT OF RED CROSS FUNDING

After World War I the Canadian Red Cross Society participated in the formation of the League of Red Cross Societies and the planning of an international program for peacetime activity in public health. "It was decided that there should be a great worldwide public health organization to help bring up the standards of physical and mental fitness of the world . . . the promotion of health, the prevention of disease and the mitigation of suffering throughout the world" (Gibbon and Mathewson, 1947, p. 342).

In Canada the Red Cross Society first directed its efforts to providing funds for the provision of facilities for postgraduate instruction in public health nursing "by subsidizing special courses for three years at the Universities of Toronto, McGill, British Columbia, Alberta, and Dalhousie" (Gibbon and Mathewson, 1947, p. 342). The financial incentive provided by these grants contributed to the creation of departments for the study of nursing at four of the institutions and encouraged the extension of what had been initiated the previous year at the University of British Columbia:

> In April 1920 the University of British Columbia accepted a proposal from the Provincial branch of the Canadian Red Cross Society to the effect that a Red Cross Chair of Public Health be established. For a period of three years from date of acceptance by the University, the Red Cross Society would pay five thousand dollars toward the salary of the professor. The expectation was that "the cause of Public Health, which everywhere is being regarded as of great importance, will be materially advanced throughout British Columbia." The Senate approved the proposal (Street, 1973, p. 128).

The Red Cross funds must have seemed like a windfall to the young institution, which had been founded during wartime and had received little tangible support from the liberal government that was in power in the province at the time.

In addition to providing funds to the institutions to stimulate the creation of new programs in public health nursing, the Canadian Red Cross Society provided financial aid to students who wanted to attend programs initiated under their sponsorship (King, 1970, p. 70). These actions were met with enthusiasm, and continued increases in enrolment ensured the survival of most of the universities after the 3-year period of institutional grants had ended. Not surprisingly, these certificate courses became the first in a series of such courses that were offered by the universities and also led to the development of degree programs in most of the institutions. However, these developments in 1920 were preceded by years of effort on the part of nurses to secure advanced preparation. King (1970) notes that:

> The first documentation concerning efforts to establish a university nursing program in Canada appeared in 1905 when a memorandum was submitted by the Graduate Nurses' Association of Ontario to the University of Toronto requesting the university "to offer a course of training and education of nurses" (p. 70).

In 1918 Dr. Helen MacMurchy, a physician and the first editor of *The Canadian Nurse,* wrote to the presidents of the universities to urge them to encourage establishment of nursing programs at their institutions (MacMurchy, 1918). Although the influence of such communication remains a matter of speculation, it is reasonable to assume that it at least made administrators of higher education more aware of the needs and issues in nursing education. As one author concluded: "One of the most significant developments during the period from 1910 to 1930 was the growth of positive attitudes toward university education for nurses" (Allemang, 1974, p. 137).

The one exception to the lasting success of the stimulus provided by the Red Cross for establishment of university nursing education was the public health nursing certificate program begun at Dalhousie University, which was also the first of its kind to be initiated (Tunis, 1966). The program at Dalhousie was short-lived and, for financial and perhaps other reasons, did not survive after 1922. It is noteworthy here that, although Dalhousie's program was the first to be initiated through Red Cross funds, the nature of the support differed; it consisted of direct funding of students rather than institutional grants. Thus the assistance provided to Dalhousie was far less substantial than that given to other universities during those same years.

■ ■ ■ ■

CRISIS AT McGILL

The year 1929 spelled the end of a decade in which university nursing education in Canada improved by leaps and bounds. According to Allemang (1974), the stock market crash in the fall of 1929 "and the economic depression that followed brought unemployment and hardship to nurses" (p. 172). Nurses had experienced difficulties in securing employment before 1929, and because of the worldwide economic depression, the situation rapidly worsened. Patients could no longer afford to employ private-duty nurses, and private duty had been the most promising area of employment for graduate nurses (Gunn, 1933, p. 141).

For universities in general, the Depression meant a period of significant adjustment, which included reduced revenues, staff layoffs, and difficult working conditions. However, despite this adverse environment, enrolments continued to show generally slow but steady growth throughout the decade; perhaps because no employment was available for people who had completed their high school educations, many chose to remain in school. The impact of the Depression on an institution in Canada was determined to a large extent by the amount of external support it received from government and private sources.

The Depression was hard on McGill University. McGill received only token funding from its provincial government from the earliest times. As a private institution, its mandate was to raise funds from private sources to operate its programs or reduce the size of its enterprise. This mandate made financing difficult enough during prosperous times; during the lean years of the Depression, it became an onerous task. The School for Graduate Nurses at McGill was subjected to the impact of the financial crunch for more than a decade.

Helen Reid, a member of the first class to graduate from McGill, was a strong proponent of the establishment of a school of nursing at McGill because she felt this would give women another means of entering the university. Although she had originally envisioned a 2-year degree course at McGill, in 1920 advice from Isabel M. Stewart, the Canadian-born professor of nursing at Teacher's College, Columbia University, suggested that "to attempt at present in any way to arrange for two-year courses would be a real injury to the undertaking" (Tunis, 1966, p. 22). The final announcement of the course reflected the intent to begin a degree program "in the near future" (Tunis, 1966, p. 22). The issue was raised again after the death of the Director of the School for Graduate Nurses, Flora Madeline Shaw, in 1927, and the matter was referred to committee (Tunis, 1966, p. 22). After Canadian-born nurse educator, author, and administrator from Yale, Bertha Harmer, was appointed Director of the School in 1928, the Committee recommended "that a six-year undergraduate course leading to a degree be established at the School for Graduate Nurses" (Tunis, 1966, p. 42). It is reported that the attitude of the Principal and Vice-Chancellor was encouraging, as exemplified in his promise to Miss Reid: "When we establish the degree course we can promise that Miss Harmer's rank will be that of professor" (Tunis, 1966, p. 42).

Because there was reason for optimism, work went forward under Miss Harmer's direction to develop a framework for the curriculum that would facilitate the transition to the degree program when it was established. Students could select from five new areas of focus, each of which could lead to a university diploma rather than a certificate after 2 years of study. To implement the new programs, four new faculty members were appointed for the 1929-30 academic year. Despite the optimism, however, the financial uncertainty under which the school operated after the termination of Red Cross funding in 1923 was a threat to its viability. To the new director this uncertainty must have been a continuing source of anxiety, which can be detected in her query to the Acting Principal:

> I have just returned to the office after a repeated attack of illness and had hoped to find a favourable decision of the Finance Committee awaiting me. At the risk of seeming to trouble you unduly I am writing to ask the decision of the Finance Committee in regard to our budget. I should not trouble you if it were not that so many important matters are depending on it (Harmer, 6 May 1929).

The undercurrent of suspicion toward nursing's place in the university environment surfaced again: "There are so many professors in the University who most cordially disapprove of schools of this kind. Their antagonism becomes more marked because of the necessity of reducing their salaries" (Currie, 27 June 1932).

A crisis was imminent and the facts were given to Miss Harmer by Sir Arthur Currie, the Acting Principal:

> I quite agree with you that the School has had an increasing attendance, that it has done excellent work, and that the influence of its graduates on nursing and nursing education and administration has been most valuable. But there is the eternal question of finance. How are we to get the money to continue this School? (Currie, 27 June 1932).

In the face of the university's economic difficulties because of the Depression, the school would not be permitted to continue to drain McGill's financial resources. It was given only one alternative to closure; it would have the opportunity to raise an endowment of $40,000 to provide for the annual operating expenses of $8000, "which would keep it going for the next five years, in the hope that by that time financial conditions would be such that the expense of the School could be more readily provided for" (Currie, 27 June 1932).

The Alumnae Association and the Advisory Committee convened in joint session to consider the crisis that had beset the school and offered support for a national fund-raising effort (Tunis, 1966). An appeal was sent to the presidents of all provincial nursing associations to assist with the campaign. In Miss Harmer's (1932) words:

> The nursing profession has many interested and grateful friends who appreciate the service which it renders, and it is quite right and just that they, in addition to the provincial and city government boards, and boards of hospitals and public health and welfare associations, should now be asked as individuals to contribute to the support of nursing education (1 December 1932).

Support was also to be solicited from foundations, businesses, and corporations; however, the appeals to these organizations failed and the response was a great disappointment. "All was not lost, however, for the appeal to Canadian nurses did not go unheard and 'miraculously the money poured in. Within two months, more than $5,000 in cash was on hand and over $12,000 pledged'" (Tunis, 1966, p. 56).

The role of alumnae groups all over the country in ensuring the survival of the McGill School for Graduate Nurses was the critical factor in the resolution of the financial crisis that spanned more than a decade. In the process, the stature of nurses and nursing was raised, as nurses demonstrated a single-minded commitment to continuing the good work that had been started at McGill. The documents that pertain to the crisis also indicate an element of surprise on the part of McGill administrators that nurse alumnae members and others would have sufficient interest or strength of purpose to donate funds so generously. Although the total amount raised never reached the goal of $40,000, about $20,000 was raised, which was applied directly to the operating costs of the school on an annual basis.

The fact that $20,000 was sufficient to see the school through 10 difficult years was attributed to strict control over spending by school administrators (Tunis, 1966). An example of the nature of the commitment and dedication to the school is found in Miss Harmer's report (1933) to the principal on the results of the first, and possibly the most important, phase of the campaign:

> I am enclosing a statement showing results of the efforts of nurses to raise $40,000 to endow the School for the next five years. As it seemed hopeless, however, under present conditions, to raise this sum, efforts were concentrated on raising $8,000 in the hope that better times would enable us to raise an endowment later. Deducting my salary, (my services were offered at the end of the year when it seemed the only hope of saving the School) left $5,000 as the objective. As the enclosed statement shows we have pledges for $5,597 for the next year, and $6,355.52 toward the next four years.

In addition, many special lecturers who gave series of lectures in courses in the program accepted reduced fees for their services or waived them altogether. Operating costs were lowered further when faculty members bought books for the library and supplies out of their own pockets (Tunis, 1966). Sir Arthur Currie's announcement (1933) that sufficient funds had been received in the first five months of the fund-raising campaign to continue the school for one more year was a cause for rejoicing among faculty, alumnae, and friends of the school:

> On the understanding that the Budget for the next year does not exceed the year just closing, and relying on the pledges outlined in your letter of May first, 1933, I shall recommend to the Board of Governors that the School for Graduate Nurses be continued for another year, that is, until June 30, 1934. (Currie, 12 May 1933).

The struggle was to be long, however, and neither Miss Harmer nor Sir Arthur Currie would live to see its conclusion. After Miss Harmer's resignation and death in 1934, the continuing struggle for existence was carried on under the direction of Marion Lindeburgh as Acting Director until 1939 and as Director thereafter. The stringent economies that were practised required that fewer courses be taught and that the 2-year diploma programs initiated by Miss Harmer be dropped in favour of the 1-year certificate programs (Tunis, 1966). The degree program had to be postponed until much later because, for many years, program development priorities had to focus on retaining the programs that remained operational.

■ ■ ■ ■

THE DEVELOPMENT OF AN EXPERIMENTAL SCHOOL OF NURSING AT TORONTO

It is ironic that at the very moment that the McGill School for Graduate Nurses was served with notice of intent to terminate its programs by its administration, the University of Toronto School of Nursing received financial and philosophic encouragement to continue the innovative experimentation with basic curriculum design that had begun in 1926, a program that was the vision of Edith Kathleen Russell. However, this event had been preceded by many years of groundwork by Kathleen Russell, and the grant was not the first the school had been awarded by the Rockefeller Foundation for the development of its program. The program established in 1926 and the improved one begun in 1933 were diploma rather than degree programs. Their importance for Canadian nursing was that they were radical departures from existing philosophy in university education for nurses. These events took place at a time when the content and form of university nursing programs and courses were somewhat fluid and undefined, and when nurses in many other university centres were constantly trying to justify their existence to skeptical and budget-minded administrators.

Miss Russell, who came to the university very early in the national development of higher education in nursing, was blessed with good health, a sound mind, and rare qualities of leadership. She had time to establish herself at the university and to think critically, thus developing her ideas about the pursuit of knowledge and truth as applied to nursing in the university setting. The credibility of the work at the university School of Nursing and Kathleen Russell's unique capabilities for leadership were remarkable. Ultimately, these factors augured well for the University of Toronto because, as Carpenter (1970) has indicated, "In the 30-year period ending in 1953, the Foundation supported the development of nursing education in 48 countries. The University of Toronto was the only Canadian university to receive this support" (p. 94).

The proposal for the 1933 program, which also established the School of Nursing as an autonomous unit within the administrative framework of the university and provided it with a status that would allow it to participate fully in university governance, was first submitted to the Rockefeller Foundation in 1929. The Foundation agreed to support the project if support was also obtained from the university and the Ontario government; those guarantees were subsequently provided. The major feature of this 39-month program, which was unique from a developmental standpoint and made this curriculum model stand apart from the nonintegrated curriculum pattern, was the principle that the faculty of the school would assume total responsibility for the education of the student. Because the school was administratively independent from the hospital, new value was placed on clinical teaching. Student learning needs would no longer be put aside in favour of pressing hospital nursing service demands because students were not utilized in "staff" positions. They were viewed as learners, with the rights and responsibilities that accompany that role; the role of the faculty member in the clinical setting was one that was critical in facilitating the integration of theory and practice and fostering creative thinking and a questioning attitude (Carpenter, 1982). The function of the university school, as conceived by Miss Russell (1956), was as follows:

> The intention of the University School of Nursing is to prepare professional women who, through studies in the humanities and social sciences, will grow in understanding and wisdom; with this education in the realm of human values they may approach with some degree of safety the work which is awaiting them (p. 35).

■ ■ ■ ■

UNIVERSITY SCHOOLS IN THE DEPRESSION YEARS

The 1930s were extremely difficult years for Canadian universities, and the annual reports of presidents of the major institutions of higher education through these years are replete with accounts of the impact of the economic situation, which produced conditions that were unfamiliar to the universities. The 1920s had been productive years, during which adequate financial support had been available to support programs and expansion into new fields. During this period nursing had entered the university scene in Canada with the development of programs in six universities. However, growth and expansion in these institutions after 1929 was limited because of the general lack of economic resources. There are frequent references to salary cuts that professors accepted rather than see colleagues lose their positions because of financial constraints. Evidence of the lack of growth in the decade after the stock market collapse was observed in all institutions, but particularly those in western Canada.

During the 1920s, several new 5-year, non-integrated degree programs were initiated at Canadian universities, similar to the 1919 degree program established at the University of British Columbia. The second degree program was established at the University of Western Ontario in 1924, followed in 1925 by one at the University of Alberta and in 1926 by a program at l'Institut Marguerite d'Youville. The University of Toronto experimented throughout the 1920s and 1930s with a new model of a diploma program that would evolve into the integrated degree program, while McGill was involved in a difficult struggle to maintain its certificate programs in the 1930s.

The religious order associated with the University of Ottawa initiated what was essentially a hospital diploma program in 1933. Only three degree programs were initiated during that decade, and then only during the later years. The University of Saskatchewan and the University of Ottawa introduced degree programs in 1938; St. Francis Xavier University began a program in 1939. Thus by the end of the 3rd decade in the history of university nursing education in Canada, five degree programs were operational and two other universities offered diploma or certificate programs.

■■ ■■ ■■ ■■

NEW INITIATIVES AND INCENTIVES IN UNIVERSITY NURSING EDUCATION BETWEEN 1940 AND 1955

In 1940, as Canada became involved in World War II, the sluggish national economy improved because of the need for manufactured goods. The war also affected higher education. Education in the health sciences became a priority; the nation quickly recognized the need for health professionals to care for military personnel and the civilian population and placed a new value on services provided by practitioners in these professions.

In the nursing profession pressures arose from the conditions of returning prosperity in 1940; as these mounted, the balance between supply and demand reversed abruptly from what it had been during the 1930s. Where there had been oversupply, there was now a distinct shortage. With increasing prosperity, the return of the demand for private duty nurses in both hospitals and homes was partially responsible for this turn of events, which placed the profession and health services in general in a tight squeeze. The economic conditions of the 1930s had forced many small hospitals to close their schools of nursing and hire from the large pool of unemployed nurses who would work for very low wages.

By the end of the decade, general staff nursing in hospitals had become a major form of employment among nurses (Allemang, 1974). This contrasted sharply with the previous decade, in which there were few staff nurse positions in hospitals and graduate nurses generally sought employment as independent practitioners whose services were retained by families to care for ill family members in hospitals and homes.

Other factors that contributed to the development of the shortage included the wartime demands on a profession with a contribution to make:

> Nursing administrators, supervisors, head nurses, teachers and public health nurses left their civilian positions for those of military service. These were key people in providing quality in nursing services and nursing education. Since bedside nursing care accompanied by supervision and ward teaching was considered the core of the curriculum, their loss was deeply felt (Allemang, 1974, p. 211).

Nurses were also needed in wartime industries, which generally offered better salaries and working conditions. For the most part, the shortages were most acute in rural areas for hospital and public health positions, as well as in special areas, such as tuberculosis sanatoria, isolation hospitals, and psychiatric institutions, where nurses were badly needed. In fact, the needs became so great and the possibilities for meeting them were so limited that a new category of health worker was created to fill the gap—the certified or registered nursing assistant or licensed practical nurse. Although some consideration was given to shortening nursing programs in Canada to meet specific needs related to war, this development never occurred because enough nurses volunteered for the armed services (Lindeburgh, 1942).

University schools of nursing soon began to reap benefits from federal interest in higher education, both from subsidizing the operations of the institutions and from its considerable response to the assistance requested by the professional organizations. Federal funds for nursing education, distributed through the Canadian Nurses Association (CNA) to the schools, amounted to $150,000 in 1942 and $250,000 each in 1943 and 1944. The program was maintained until the end of the war. Funds were then awarded through the provincial nurses' associations to the diploma and university schools of the provinces. In addition, the W.K. Kellogg Foundation initiated a program of fellowships in nursing and, between 1941 and 1959, granted $11,680 to institutions and agencies to be awarded to Canadian nurses for additional study. The university schools of nursing received the greater part of these funds so that they could upgrade the academic qualifications of their faculties. The fellowships were tenable in the United States and, during that period, there were no master's programs for nurses in Canada. The new funds, most of which were provided between 1941 and 1945, provided a stimulus to nursing education at a time when it was needed.

The W.K. Kellogg Foundation also made scholarship and loan funds available for students in programs at five universities between 1942 and 1944. Under this program, McGill University, l'Université de Montréal, the University of Toronto, and the University of Western Ontario each received $4000, and Laval University received $6000. For students seeking certificate or baccalaureate preparation, the Victorian Order of Nurses, a national agency that needed nurses with specific preparation in public health nursing, reactivated the bursary program initiated during the 1920s and discontinued in 1933. The Canadian Red Cross Society also made scholarships in public health nursing available (Tunis, 1966).

An awakened interest in nursing and nursing education in the post-war period, evidenced by the availability of extra university funding, appears to have been a prime factor not only in consolidation and growth of existing schools but also in the founding of new programs in nursing in several universities. Queens University (1941) and McMaster University (1941) initiated programs early in the decade, the University of Manitoba in 1943, Mount St. Vincent University in 1947, and Dalhousie University in 1949. Clearly, federal funds made available for schools and fellowship and bursary programs under the auspices of private foundations and agencies played an important role in the new developments that occurred. As in 1920, universities became aware of potential benefits to their institutions from the sponsorship of nursing programs.

At McGill the influx of additional funds was considerable and continuous. The courage and perseverance of those faculty, alumnae, and friends who had held out for the retention of the school through the long Depression and war years were rewarded; their steadfast conviction that the school had a significant and critical function to fulfil at McGill was vindicated. The funds provided to the McGill School from the federal grant program administered by the CNA included: "$2,100 [in 1942] an amount that was increased to $6,000 in 1943, and which by 1945 totalled $27,750" (Tunis, 1966, p. 73). The impact on programs has been described as follows:

> Conditions at the Schools were affected with startling rapidity. For the first time since the crisis of 1932, a programme of expansion could be considered. Two 4-month courses were undertaken in 1942, one in administration and supervision in public health nursing, the other in clinical supervision, in an effort to meet war-time demands for trained personnel. These courses, which were offered annually until the autumn of 1945, could be used as credits toward the 1-year certificate course (Tunis, 1966, p. 73).

Nursing faculty at McGill were again able to entertain the idea of a degree program. Preparations began in 1941 for a 5-year nonintegrated degree course, the proposal for which was subsequently approved; the first students were accepted in 1944. In 1945 the alumnae of the school disbanded their Special Finance Committee, which had served the school so well during the Depression and war years, but simultaneously revitalized earlier efforts to establish a Flora Madeline Shaw Endowment Fund to establish a chair in nursing (Tunis, 1966).

■ ■ ■ ■

DIPLOMA TO DEGREE: THE INCEPTION OF THE BASIC DEGREE PROGRAM AT THE UNIVERSITY OF TORONTO

The development of curricula in baccalaureate education for nursing has not been without difficulties. These difficulties have centred largely around contractual agreements between the university schools of nursing and hospitals and other agencies used for clinical experience. In her postwar report on the state of nursing education, Esther Lucile Brown (1948) defined the responsibility of the university school:

> One general principle, however, must be kept clearly in mind. The university school should enter into relations with other institutions exclusively to obtain necessary clinical laboratories, not to help provide nursing service for patients. Regrettably some university schools find themselves in the same situations as most hospital schools, where students are expected to supply nursing care at the expense of the educational process (p. 157).

Brown (1948) cited two reasons to explain why these issues arose as major problems: the traditional outlook of the hospital viewing nursing education as service, and the meagre financial resources of many university schools and students.

Probably the most influential event in the history of Canadian degree programs was the introduction of the basic degree program at the University of Toronto in 1942. This was not an isolated event, but one step in a process that began some 16 years earlier. It provided an alternative to the existing pattern of baccalaureate nursing education. In this integrated program, studies in the arts and sciences were combined with the nursing component. Courses were carefully planned and sequenced so that individual student development would be enhanced. The departure from the previously established pattern was striking:

> It is of particular interest that for the first time in a nursing undergraduate degree programme full authority and responsibility for the teaching of nursing rested in the university. The nursing courses were planned, taught, and evaluated by full-time university teaching staff. This simple fact, nonetheless, was a radical departure from existing degree programmes, the roots of which, by this time had been firmly established in both Canada and the United States (King, 1970, p. 72).

It is always difficult to break with tradition, and in nursing, the nonintegrated degree pattern had established its stepladder approach to nursing education well over 20 years before. In addition, the hospital programs on which this approach leaned had been entrenched for an even greater number of years. Effecting a change that made the basic degree program stand apart from its nonintegrated counterpart required a great leader and, as previously noted, Edith Kathleen Russell was such an individual. In instituting this change, she exerted a profound influence on the thinking of her colleagues in nursing, and she was able to enlist the moral support of the Faculty of Medicine and the President of the University of Toronto, as well as the financial support of the Rockefeller Foundation. In regard to her influence, Emory (1964) notes: "It has been said that greatness is attained through changing the course of events and changing them for always. If this be true, then in retrospect there can be detected in Edith Kathleen Russell's professional life and work an element of true greatness" (p. 7).

■ ■ ■ ■

A SECOND BASIC DEGREE PROGRAM BEGINS

Bonin (1976), who studied basic degree programs in Canada, said: "The most salient driving forces which spurred the establishment of basic degree programs are key persons, especially Kathleen Russell and Gladys Sharpe, in two pioneering universities" (p. 178). Four years after the introduction of the University of Toronto basic degree program, a second basic degree program was developed at McMaster University under the direction of Gladys Sharpe, who was largely responsible for phasing out the early degree and diploma program called *Arts and Nursing*, which had begun in 1941 at McMaster, and introducing a new basic degree program. At McMaster the initiative of the Hamilton General Hospital had been important in developing the earlier affiliation between the hospital and the university, and the hospital continued to support the new program and its director. Support from an associated hospital, while not always forthcoming, occurred in 1919 with the establishment of the University of British Columbia School of Nursing. It was also evident that there was an extremely close working relationship between the Toronto General Hospital and the School of Nursing at the University of Toronto. In the early 1930s, consideration was given to combining the Toronto General nursing program with that of the University of Toronto (Carpenter, 1970).

■ ■ ■ ■

SURVEYS OF NURSING EDUCATION

In the history of Canadian nursing education, periodic surveys have been undertaken by professional organizations and government to assess the prevailing situation and aid in making improvements in areas where weaknesses were demonstrated. Kathleen Russell carried out a survey in New Brunswick that addressed the whole gamut of issues in nursing education in that province and had considerable impact on the thinking of nursing educators. The establishment of the School of Nursing at the University of New Brunswick in 1959 was a direct result of her conclusions and recommendations about higher education in nursing in New Brunswick (Russell, 1956). Soon afterward the CNA, under the direction of Dr. Helen K. Mussallem, launched the Pilot Project for Evaluation of Schools of Nursing. This study, designed to determine the feasibility of and issues associated with a system of accreditation of schools of nursing in Canada, was published in 1960.

One of the recommendations from the Mussallem (1960) study was: "1. That a re-examination and study of the whole field of nursing education be undertaken" (p. vii). This recommendation was implemented within a very short time; a Royal Commission was appointed by the federal government to investigate the problems and issues related to all aspects of the delivery of health services in Canada. The report of that commission recommended that 10 more university nursing programs, under administratively autonomous schools of nursing, be established in Canada as soon as possible (Royal Commission on Health Services, 1964). It also recommended elimination of nonintegrated basic programs at a time when admissions were 22% higher than admissions to integrated programs. The impact of this report was impressive; only 4 years later "admissions to integrated pro-grammes constituted ninety-seven percent of all admissions to baccalaureate programmes" (King, 1970, pp. 178-79). In addition, the number of candidates seeking postbasic degrees after graduation from hospital or college programs doubled during the same period. Because there is normally a limitation on enrolment in schools of nursing due to the constraints imposed by available clinical facilities, schools of nursing began to make concerted efforts to increase their maximum enrolment levels in response to the Royal Commission recommendation:

> It is of the utmost importance that these schools be expanded in number to enable them to prepare approximately one-fourth of the total recruits to the nursing force. It is from this pool that the instructors, supervisors, administrators and other leaders in the profession must come (Royal Commission on Health Services, 1964, p. 67).

Since 1965 the ratio of diploma- to baccalaureate-prepared nurses has increased to approximately 1 in 10 nationally. In addition, all of the 10 new university schools recommended by the Royal Commission were established. However, enrolments in university schools are still very low in comparison with those in diploma programs. In Chapter 25, questions pertaining to entry to practice are considered.

■ ■ ■ ■

CONCLUSION

This chapter has identified and documented events and trends of major sig-nificance to university nursing education. The enterprise began with informal and on-the-job training. Hospital schools of nursing began to develop after 1874 and university schools after 1919. Community college nursing education pro-grams, which began to appear in the 1960s, also offered diploma preparation. Today in Canada, nursing education is offered under the auspices of the three types of schools. However, the profession's entry to practice position has led to a drive for expansion of university programs at both the basic and post-RN levels. Contemporary approaches to educational issues of importance are discussed in other chapters.

REFERENCES

Allemang, M.M. (1974). *Nursing education in the United States and Canada, 1873-1950: Leading figures, forces, views on education.* Unpublish-ed doctoral dissertation, University of Washington, Seattle.

Bonin, M.A. (1976). *Trends in integrated basic degree nursing programs in Canada: 1942-1972.* Unpublished doctoral dissertation, University of Ottawa, Ottawa.

Brown, E.L. (1948). *Nursing for the future.* New York: Russell Sage Foundation.

Canadian Nurses Association. (1968). *The leaf and the lamp.* Ottawa: Author.

Carpenter, H.M. (1970). The University of Toronto School of Nursing: An agent of change.

In M.Q. Innis (Ed.), *Nursing education in a changing society* (pp. 86-108). Toronto: University of Toronto Press.

Carpenter, H.M. (1982). *Divine discontent: Edith Kathleen Russell—Reforming educator.* Toronto: Faculty of Nursing, The University of Toronto.

Currie, Sir Arthur W. Letter to Bertha Harmer, 12 May 1933. *Financial crisis: 1933 to 1943* (Acc. 2432, File). Montreal, Quebec, McGill University Archive.

Currie, Sir Arthur W. Letter to Dr. Helen R.Y. Reid, 27 June 1932. *Financial crisis: 1933 to 1943* (Acc. 2432, File). Montreal, Quebec, McGill University Archive.

Emory, F. (1964). *Edith Kathleen Russell: An appreciation of her professional life and work.* 6 March. (Acc. A-73011, mimeographed). Faculty of Nursing, University of Toronto.

Gibbon, J.M., and Mathewson, M.S. (1947). *Three centuries of Canadian nursing.* Toronto: Macmillan.

Gunn, J.I. (1933). Educational adjustments recommended by the survey. *The Canadian Nurse,* 29(3), 139-145.

Harmer, B. Letter to Dr. C.F. Martin, 6 May 1929. *Financial crisis: 1933 to 1943* (Acc. 2432, File). Montreal, Quebec, McGill University Archive.

Harmer, B. Letter to presidents of provincial nursing associations, 1 December 1932. *Financial crisis: 1933 to 1943* (Acc. 2432, File). Montreal, Quebec, McGill University Archive.

Harmer, B. Letter to Sir Arthur W. Currie, 1 May 1933. *Financial crisis: 1933 to 1943* (Acc. 2432, File). Montreal, Quebec, McGill University Archive.

King, M.K. (1970). The development of university nursing education. In M.Q. Innis (Ed.), *Nursing education in a changing society* (pp. 67-85). Toronto: University of Toronto Press.

Lindeburgh, M. (1942). Important emergency measures. *The Canadian Nurse,* 38(12), 925-926.

MacMurchy, H. (1918). University training for the nursing profession. *The Canadian Nurse,* 14(9), 1284-1285.

Mussallem, H.K. (1960). *Spotlight on nursing education: The report of a pilot project for the evaluation of schools of nursing in Canada.* Ottawa: The Canadian Nurses Association.

Royal Commission on Health Services. (1964). Vol. I. Ottawa: Queens Printer.

Russell, E.K. (1956). *The report of the study of nursing education in New Brunswick.* Fredericton: Government of the province of New Brunswick.

Street, M. (1973). *Watch-fires on the mountains: The life and writings of Ethel Johns.* Toronto: University of Toronto Press.

Tunis, B.L. (1966). *In caps and gowns.* Montreal: McGill University Press.

CHAPTER TWENTY FIVE

Entry to Practice: Striving for the Baccalaureate Standard

JANET ROSS KERR

The baccalaureate degree as the minimum educational qualification for entry to the practice of nursing has been a highly controversial and hotly debated issue in the nursing profession (Besharah, 1981). Strong emotions have been generated in the entry to practice debate, because comprehensive restructuring of the educational system in nursing has been both perplexing and threatening to many. However, the discussion and debate stage of the "pros" and "cons" of the entry to practice position would appear to be almost a thing of the past as the movement to implement the baccalaureate standard has taken hold across the country. The steps that have been taken in the various provinces are outlined in this chapter.

Underscoring the movement to implement the entry to practice position, it should be noted that nurses' contributions to the promotion, maintenance, and restoration of health have made the nursing profession one that is held in public esteem. Their contributions have also moved nursing to the threshold of the university because of the complexity of knowledge and skills required, and the fact that it is through the educational process that nursing students acquire the essential foundation for practice. It is thus necessary and important to understand and appreciate nursing as a complex, multifaceted process embracing many roles and functions.

■ ■ ■ ■

ENTRY TO PRACTICE: THE POSITION, ITS DEVELOPMENT AND RATIONALE

The entry to practice position is often misunderstood. It refers to all those graduating from schools of nursing and entering the practice of nursing in the year 2000. The graduates in the year 2000 and those in subsequent years would require a baccalaureate degree in nursing in order to practise. Those who will graduate from diploma nursing programs in the year 1999 or before would not be required to have the baccalaureate credential. This approach, often termed "grandparenting," means that the new standard is phased in gradually, allowing ample time to make changes and adjustments in systems and resources. The right to practise nursing would not be jeopardized for those who qualified for practice prior to the year 2000.

Some 2 decades have passed since the first statement of the entry to practice position by the Alberta Task Force on Nursing Education (Government of Alberta, 1975). Since then a fundamental shift has occurred in the approach taken to the entry to practice position as endorsed by the Canadian Nurses Association (CNA) and the provincial nursing associations. Strategies to facilitate implementation of the policy commonly called EP2000 have been developed at provincial and national levels by professional associations over the past decade and a half. There has also been a concomitant increase in the demand for post-RN baccalaureate education by members of the profession qualified at the diploma level. Many of these nurses recognize a personal need for additional preparation, and there is also the inescapable fact that additional study may improve one's competitive position in applying for positions, particularly those at a leadership level.

When discussing educational opportunities for registered nurse students, it is important to remember that the entry to practice position does not refer to RNs who have already qualified to practise nursing, however important it may be to make baccalaureate preparation available to those in this group who desire it. It is a position that applies to new nursing graduates entering the profession in the year 2000 and thereafter. The achievement of such a goal is itself a monumental undertaking because of the number of students who will need to receive their education under the auspices of the university.

The voice of the profession on this matter has become an increasingly united one, as one provincial nursing association after another has espoused commitment to the position that all new nurses entering the profession should be qualified at the baccalaureate level by the year 2000. Initial leadership came, however, neither from the profession nor from university faculties of nursing, but from a government-appointed committee established to study needs in relation to nursing education in the province of Alberta, the Alberta Task Force on Nursing Education. Although the Alberta government subsequently issued a denunciation of its committee's recommendation, stating that it did "not agree with making the baccalaureate degree a mandatory requirement for practice," the profession did not allow the matter to rest there (Government of Alberta, 1977, p. 6).

Discussion of the controversial document ensued among all interested parties immediately after its publication. The Alberta Association of Registered Nurses (AARN) issued an endorsement of the Task Force recommendations shortly thereafter (AARN, 1976). The year 2000 was subsequently suggested by the AARN as a more realistic target date for implementation of the entry to practice position than the 1995 goal suggested by the Task Force (AARN, 1978, 1979). In Vancouver at the 1980 Biennial Convention of the Canadian Nurses Association, delegates found themselves debating a resolution to develop a statement on the minimum educational qualification needed to enter the profession. Following approval, the resolution became a priority for the 1980-82 biennium. Momentum began to grow with the establishment of a committee to study the issue, and articles appeared in *The Canadian Nurse* debating both sides of the question (Kerr, 1982; Rajabally, 1982). The decision to endorse the baccalaureate standard was taken by the CNA Board of Directors in February 1982 when the Report of the Committee was presented. Support was high and the motion was carried unanimously. Delegates to the 1982 Biennial Convention, in Newfoundland, added further strength to the position by adopting a motion of support.

Support for the position became strong within the profession as the issues were debated in provinces that had not already adopted a position on the matter. Gradually, province by province, positions in support of EP2000 have been taken. The enthusiasm and eagerness to reach the goal by the year 2000 is evident as nurses from one end of the country to the other identify and develop mechanisms to ensure that logical, well-articulated, reasonable plans are made for its achievement. If they are to be successful, such plans must result in public policy commitments to the baccalaureate standard as additional years of university-level nursing education for students require commitments to redistribute existing resources.

The question of why EP2000 was supported so strongly by the nursing profession is often asked. The reason is to be found in the changing nature of practice and the knowledge necessary to engage in practice. Attempting to raise professional status through higher educational standards does not constitute good and sufficient reason for implementing the baccalaureate standard for entry to practice. Two or three decades ago, there were five or six distinct areas of hospital and community-based practice. Today there are upwards of 30 or 40, if not more, different clinical nursing areas, each requiring mastery of a unique and specialized knowledge base. The era of specialization in nursing arrived some time ago. No longer is it possible, if in fact it ever was, to graduate "a finished product." It is now accepted that the new nursing graduate is a beginning practitioner just as new graduates in other fields are considered to be. Further, like other professionals, registered nurses must be lifelong learners. There is no way one can be master of all knowledge in nursing, either within the context of a program of basic nursing education or after graduation when concentrating on a field of practice. The rapid rate with which care based on new knowledge is integrated into practice makes continuing education an individual, organizational, and professional responsibility to ensure that practitioners remain abreast of new developments in their areas of practice.

Advances in the health sciences have meant that today's programs of basic nursing education are hard-pressed to offer curricula that address the depth and breadth of theoretical content and related clinical experience for safe and effective practice. The impact of technology and changing roles requires the acquisition of appropriate knowledge and the development of new skills. The expansion of the knowledge required for competent practice and the range of responsibilities expected of the nurse at all levels provide substantial rationale for an increase in the length of the basic nursing program and for the standard of educational preparation offered at a baccalaureate level. The movement of nursing education to the university level is also seen as a women's issue, for educational preparation at the level of complexity seen in nursing in male-dominated disciplines has long been the responsibility of the university.

■■ ■■ ■■ ■■

STANDARDS OF NURSING EDUCATION: A HISTORICAL PERSPECTIVE

Florence Nightingale founded the first modern school of nursing in 1860 in conjunction with St. Thomas' Hospital in London. The idea was novel and soon became the model for the establishment of hospital training schools throughout Europe and America. However, in the translation of the model to North America, the idea of financial independence of the school of nursing was lost, and the new schools became dependent upon hospitals to sustain them. The Nightingale school was an independent school supported by the Nightingale Fund, a substantial endowment resulting from gifts to support the success of her mission of caring for British soldiers during the Crimean War. Nightingale's reputation from her service in the Crimea was such that her idea for a school of nursing was taken up readily and the nurses she prepared in her school were widely sought to lead new developments elsewhere.

Standards of education have historically been a primary concern of the nursing profession. There is considerable evidence that the quality of nursing education was one of the early issues addressed by professional organizations. During the 1920s and 1930s, after the successful resolution of the struggle to achieve nursing registration in each province, the profession became concerned with achieving higher educational standards through the development and adoption of a standard curriculum for schools of nursing. Undoubtedly these efforts, which were spearheaded by the CNA, did much to raise educational standards in schools of nursing (Weir, 1932). Although today the idea of a national standard curriculum may seem somewhat strange and rather prescriptive, undoubtedly there was a need for this kind of guidance because educational standards at the time were described as deplorable by many observers.

With the initiation of the first university degree program in Canada for nurses at the University of British Columbia in 1919 under the direction of Ethel Johns, a new era in nursing education began. Red Cross funding to six Canadian universities after World War I encouraged the establishment and development of a variety of nursing programs in these institutions. They included the University of British Columbia, University of Alberta, University of Western Ontario, University of Toronto, McGill University, and Dalhousie University. Most began as certificate programs, and all eventually developed into degree programs. The first degree programs were based on the prevailing American model and were termed nonintegrated programs. In such programs, the principle of university control over university courses and hospital control over the clinical nursing part of the program became firmly entrenched (Kerr, 1978).

In 1926, dissatisfied with the prevailing pattern of university degree programs in nursing, which she termed "an ill-arranged program of studies" (Russell, 1932, p. 87), E. Kathleen Russell, Director of the Department of Public Health Nursing at the University of Toronto, set out to demonstrate that a nurse could be prepared in a much more effective and educationally sound manner by establishing the principle of university direction and control over all courses in the program. Although close cooperation with health-care agencies was maintained, faculty who were responsible for clinical nursing education were employed by the university. A substantial Rockefeller Foundation grant was obtained to fund this innovative experiment in basic degree nursing education resulting in the first integrated program in Canada at the University of Toronto in 1942. With its initiative to develop a basic integrated baccalaureate degree program in nursing in 1946, McMaster University became the second university in the country to do so.

In the formative years between 1940 and 1955, university schools of nursing became firmly established and began to accommodate ever increasing numbers of students and administer increasingly large budgets. It is interesting that until 1965, no additional integrated degree programs besides those at Toronto and McMaster were established in any Canadian university. However, the *Report* of the Royal Commission on Health Services (1964) was to change university nursing education dramatically and rapidly with recommendations that were highly critical of the existing system. Among the recommendations were those that proposed that 10 more university nursing programs under administratively autonomous schools of nursing be established in Canada as soon as possible, and that nonintegrated basic degree programs in universities be eliminated. This came at a time when admissions to nonintegrated programs were 22% higher than admissions to integrated programs. The impact of this report was impressive. Only 4 years following its publication "admissions to integrated programmes constituted ninety-seven percent of all admissions to baccalaureate programs" (King, 1970, pp. 78-79). The Royal Commission (1964) also recommended that baccalaureate programs "be expanded in number to enable them to prepare approximately one-fourth of the total recruits to the nursing force" (p. 67).

■■ ■■ ■■ ■■

MOVING TOWARD THE YEAR 2000

Although we have been dealing with questions involving standards of education in nursing since the profession became formally established in this country, the issues of today are quite different. Everything has changed—the settings, conditions of practice, health needs and problems, beliefs about individual responsibility in health care, and performance expectations for nurses in all settings. This is not surprising because change is, after all, the inexorable reality of our existence. Choices for the profession and its practitioners involve ways of influencing the direction of change in the manner most appropriate for the service rendered. Indeed, we have moved from questions of "why" and "what" to those of "how" and "when" in relation to the baccalaureate standard for initial entry to practice. The educational and service sectors are preparing for the changes that are occurring. The process of developing collaborative partnerships between diploma and degree programs to produce a baccalaureate-level practitioner is well underway across the country, but there is some distance to go before one could even say that the end is in sight. Creative new nursing education program models are being developed to facilitate the implementation of the baccalaureate standard. Hospitals and other health agencies, colleges, and universities are increasingly recognizing that they must become partners in planning and promoting an integrated system of nursing education that will benefit the health-care consumers of the next century.

The respective roles of the provincial and national nursing associations in the process of encouraging the implementation of baccalaureate entry to practice will undoubtedly continue to be critical factors in influencing opinion and action among health professionals and the general public. After adoption of the entry to practice resolution by the Board of Directors in 1982, the CNA quickly moved to adopt a proactive stance on the issue. Committees were appointed to develop long-term goals and plans, discussion papers and annotated bibliographies on the subject, and strategies to achieve goals. CNA efforts were directed at encouraging member associations to develop specific plans for their provinces. A 5-year National Plan for Entry to Practice was adopted by the Canadian Nurses Association in March 1989. Professional nursing associations in all provinces except Ontario are charged with legislative authority for the registration and discipline of nurses (see Chapter 27). In Ontario the College of Nurses carries out regulatory functions for the profession. Except in Alberta, Ontario, and Quebec, the provincial nursing associations also have statutory responsibilities for nursing education (see Chapter 27). All are committed to improving standards of nursing education. The grassroots campaign to implement the baccalaureate standard for entry to practice has taken place at the provincial level because that is where authority for health and education rests. Since the provincial ministries of education and health are charged with the responsibility for allocating resources for postsecondary education and for health personnel, the question of implementation of the entry to practice position is of vital concern at the provincial level.

Because of the complexity of determining costs of student education, conclusions based on inadequate information or comparisons have, in the past, led some to assume that exorbitant costs are associated with implementation of the baccalaureate standard, a conclusion the CNA has termed "unclear, unfounded, unwise and unwarranted" (CNA, 1984, p. 1). It was concluded that there were no well-designed studies of the cost of nursing education in Canada and that "institutional costs per 'student year' or per 'student credit hour' or per 'student years of future graduates' might well have been lower in universities than in other institutions" (CNA, 1984, p. 1). The CNA made it clear that the conclusion that a baccalaureate nursing program was more expensive than other types of nursing programs had no basis in fact, and that the actual situation might have been quite the reverse.

Nursing faculty in universities were articulate proponents of the baccalaureate standard for entry to nursing practice from the outset. The fact that academic units in nursing in universities were likely to sustain extensive change as a result of the tremendous impact of implementation did not deter faculty members from being proactive about EP2000. It was clear also that all sectors of the nursing education enterprise would be dramatically affected by adoption of the entry to practice position. Issues of concern continue to include those of the availability of qualified faculty. Many university faculties of nursing have devoted considerable effort to assisting faculty without doctoral degrees to achieve that level of preparation and indeed to go on to postdoctoral work. Recruitment of qualified faculty will continue to be a difficult issue for university schools as collaborative efforts take shape, for universities will be offering courses to a greater number of undergraduate students and the need for a larger number of qualified faculty members in order to do this will be pressing.

It is thus evident that the preparation of faculty is a critical issue in relation to achieving EP2000. Therefore graduate programs strong in clinical and research preparation are key elements in expanding the ranks of well-prepared nursing faculty in universities. The development and expansion of university programs in nursing at the baccalaureate level cannot be accomplished without the infusion of considerable numbers of faculty prepared at the master's and doctoral levels. Master's programs have been established in most regions of the country. However, whether or not there is sufficient capacity in existing master's programs is a matter that is open to debate. The CNA (Winter 1992-93, p. 2) has pointed out in its newsletter on nursing education that "the rate of growth in admissions [to master's programs in nursing] has not kept pace with the growth in applications." While applications to master's programs went up 50% between 1987 and 1991, admissions only rose 24% in the same period of time. It has further been observed that while there were 12 master's programs for 262,288 registered nurses in Canada employed in nursing in 1991, there were 16 master's programs in social work for 48,591 social workers (CNA, Winter 1992-93, p. 2).

Although the development of doctoral programs in nursing was slow to get started, development and expansion of programs has occurred relatively rapidly since the establishment on January 1, 1991 of the first fully funded program at the University of Alberta. Other programs followed in rapid succession at the University of British Columbia (September, 1991), a joint program between McGill University and the University of Montreal (Fall, 1993), the University of Toronto (Fall, 1993) and McMaster University (Fall, 1994). Although admission quotas are still relatively small, enrolment in doctoral programs in nursing is growing steadily. Whether or not there is sufficient capacity for student positions in the doctoral programs remains a concern because of the increasing role of the university in nursing education. Strong and productive graduate programs will be essential in all approaches to implementing the entry to practice position.

The effect of program expansion on health-care agencies will be considerable. A key factor will be partnership in the planning and development processes. Health-care reform initiatives across the country have already meant dramatic changes in care environments including roles of nurses. It will be essential for universities to ensure that there is meaningful participation by health-care agencies in the plans for development of new goals, program changes, and in the teaching and learning process. There are many ways in which working together can be fostered, including the use of joint appointments, secondment arrangements, shared projects, and organizational structural changes to foster partnership for mutual benefit. Many university schools and faculties of nursing are working collaboratively with health-care agencies in these kinds of activities as well as in others.

There is evidence that students are enroling in existing baccalaureate programs at increased rates. From 1985 to 1988, admissions to basic baccalaureate programs climbed 31%. In the same period, full-time enrolment in post-RN baccalaureate programs decreased by 0.6%, while part-time enrolment rose by 24.4% (CNA, 1989). In 1993 CNA statistics reported that university enrolments in baccalaureate programs in nursing were relatively constant at a figure between 5000 and 6000 students in the years from 1987 to 1991 (CNA, Spring 1993, p. 3). Expansion and development in baccalaureate programs in universities will take place gradually with the number of baccalaureate students rising steadily as degree programs become available to students across the country. Students in basic and post-RN baccalaureate programs comprised 29.3% of all nursing students enroled in Canada in 1991, while the comparable figure for 1981 was 26.3% (CNA, Spring 1993, p. 3). Although this may seem like very slow progress toward achieving the entry to practice position, it must be recognized that there are large and populous regions of the country that are not served well by opportunities for students to pursue baccalaureate education in nursing. It will take time for all regions of the country to develop collaborative models and other arrangements to offer new and expanded baccalaureate programs in nursing. In the meantime, the movement to implement the entry to practice position is gaining momentum.

■ ■ ■ ■

PROVINCIAL DEVELOPMENTS
The First Steps

The transition of the Vancouver General Hospital School of Nursing from diploma nursing education to baccalaureate nursing education through a collaborative effort with the University of British Columbia, and the enrolment of the first class in the newly structured program in September 1989 were the first of many such joint ventures at the discussion and approval stages to be implemented (CNA Connection, 1989a). Planning for this merger began in 1988 and plans were translated into action quickly to allow the program offered by the University of British Columbia School of Nursing to be extended to the Vancouver General Hospital School of Nursing site, with all subsequent students being admitted to the 4-year program (CNA, June 1991, p. 3).

Planning began in 1985 in Alberta for an innovative arrangement between the University of Alberta Faculty of Nursing and Red Deer College that resulted in the implementation of a collaborative model for a 4-year baccalaureate program in nursing. This collaboration between a community college and a university to award a degree was the first such model of its kind in the country when the first students enrolled in the program in September 1990. In this unique arrangement all courses throughout the 4-year program were offered on the Red Deer site. This collaborative model was extended to include the diploma schools of nursing at the University of Alberta Hospitals, Grant MacEwan College, the Misericordia Hospital, and the Royal Alexandra Hospital, and students at those sites were enrolled in the program in September 1991. This effort was unique in that all diploma schools in Edmonton including the hospital schools and the college program were integral partners in the collaboration from the outset.

Collaboration Between Diploma and Degree Programs Increases

In Calgary, government approval of the conjoint program between the University of Calgary Faculty of Nursing and the two diploma schools of nursing at Mount Royal College and the School of Nursing at Foothills Hospital allowed for implementation of the program in September, 1993 (CNA, Summer 1993, p. 1). The government of Alberta announced early in 1994 that all hospital diploma schools of nursing in Alberta would be closed and their programs transferred to the general education system. Although this involved a 50% cutback in the resources of the hospital diploma schools in Edmonton and Calgary, it meant that there was a transition of student places to the University of Alberta and Grant MacEwan College in Edmonton and to the University of Calgary and Mount Royal College in Calgary. The fact that collaborative programs had been operating for 2½ years in Edmonton and for 1 year in Calgary meant continued smooth operation of courses and continuation of programs.

Further developments in British Columbia led to the development of a collaborative program between the University of Victoria and several colleges—Camosun, Cariboo, Malaspina and Okanagan College. As it was anticipated from the outset that degree granting power would be eventually granted to Okanagan and Cariboo University Colleges, a different arrangement was developed between these institutions and the University of Victoria where the University worked with college faculty offering the courses throughout the 4 years. Although Malaspina College is also a university college, their participation initially took the form of offering some post-RN courses. As there is now a proposal for Malaspina to offer the full program to both post-RN and continuing students, it seems likely that they will move into the same arrangement as the University has with Okanagan and Cariboo University Colleges. The University of Victoria has also taken on some additional partners—Langara College, North Island College (first students admitted September, 1993), and Selkirk College (first students admitted September, 1994). Two additional colleges, Douglas College and Kwantlen College in Vancouver, have asked to join the partnership and will admit their first students in September, 1996 (Molzahn, personal communication, September 2, 1994). The collaborative initiatives at the basic baccalaureate integrated program level were the logical extension of the University of Victoria's initial development of its post-RN program on the campuses of Okanagan and Cariboo colleges further to the 1987 provincial government resolution to increase access to post secondary education (CNA, March 1992, p. 3). Still newer developments in British Columbia have taken place at the University of Northern British Columbia. This is a newly established institution with a nursing program that has collaborated with several colleges—Northern Lights Community College, and the College of New Caledonia. A third college, Northwest College, had initially been a partner in this consortium, but did not admit students in September, 1994 as originally planned. A collaborative, 4-year curriculum was developed in a relatively short period of time because of the fact that the three colleges already had a common curriculum and there was considerable support from the colleges for moving to a baccalaureate curriculum. The program had yet to receive government funding approval at the outset of 1995. Although a 6-month diploma exit formed a part of the proposal, it was reported that it was unknown whether or not the provincial government would fund this part of the proposal (Dana Edge, personal communication, January 4, 1995).

In Saskatchewan, a Nursing Education Coalition between the College of Nursing at the University of Saskatchewan and the diploma programs at Kelsey (Saskatoon) and Wascana (Regina) Institutes were working to develop a new nursing degree program in the spring of 1994 and planned to have a program proposal to send to the University, the Saskatchewan Institute of Applied Arts and Technology (SIAST), and the Saskatchewan Registered Nurses Association (SNRA) for approval by the fall of 1995. The program was envisioned as being 4 years in length with a diploma exit at the end of the 3rd year. In the meantime, diploma programs at Kelsey and Wascana Institutes would continue to operate (SNRA, 1994, p. 10).

The initial collaborative initiative that was implemented in Manitoba in 1991 developed into a consolidated effort by 1994. The 4-year baccalaureate degree program in nursing that was developed was offered at the University of Manitoba and, beginning in 1991, at the Manitoba Health Sciences Centre. At the latter site and at the St. Boniface site, which joined the collaboration in 1992, 1 year of the program was added per year until all 4 years were operational. As the initiative was implemented and in view of the changing health-care context and health-care reform, a consolidated arrangement was developed so that blended teaching teams at the various sites were being used to avoid duplication of effort (Bramadat, September 2, 1994). At the University of Brandon where a 2-year, post-RN degree program had been offered, a collaborative arrangement with the Brandon General Hospital and the Grace Hospital in Winnipeg has led to the development of a 4-year degree program in nursing offered at these sites.

In the provinces of Ontario, Quebec, and Saskatchewan in the 1970s, all hospital-based diploma schools of nursing had been transferred to the colleges as a result of provincial government decisions. In Ontario there are 9 university nursing programs and 23 diploma programs in the colleges, and planning for baccalaureate entry to practice is perhaps more complex than in some of the other provinces. However two proposals for restructuring basic nursing education to ensure students will have the opportunity to earn a baccalaureate degree in initial programs of nursing education were funded by the Ontario government (CNA, Winter 1992-93a). The first project involves two universities and two community colleges. In the collaborative effort being undertaken between Laurentian University and Cambrian College, implementation of the new collaborative program, which is four years in length, is planned for the fall of 1996. It is not known whether or not a diploma exit will be part of the program (Vanderlee, personal communication, January 4, 1995). Collaboration between the University of Western Ontario and Fanshawe College has led to the development of a collaborative program that still requires approval by the senate of the University. Here, a 4-year program with a common curriculum at both sites is planned. However, a decision has not been taken on a diploma exit (Bramwell, personal communication, September 1, 1994). At the outset of the development of the joint working groups at the Ontario institutions, the Ministry of Health "decreed that a consortium be formed to formulate 'a coherent and consistent province-wide approach', which provides for 'accessibility and equity' without threat to the diploma exit" (CNA, Winter 1992-93b, p. 1).

In the other project funded by the Ontario government, Queen's University is collaborating with four college nursing programs—St. Lawrence College-St. Laurent in Kingston, Brockville and Cornwall, and Loyalist College in Belleville. In this project, which is still at an early stage, a committee with representation from the five institutions is meeting and working on a collaborative curriculum as well as on transfer of credits. Although a model has not yet been selected, it is envisaged that the program that results will have a common curriculum, be 4 years in length, and offer a diploma exit (Estabrook, personal communication, August 31, 1994).

In Quebec, the Collèges d'Enseignement et Professionel (CEGEP) system of preparation allows for 2 years of preparation in the college system followed by 3 years at the university level leading to a degree in nursing. The colleges also offer diploma programs in nursing that those not planning to take a degree in nursing may select. To date there is no word on collaborative initiatives between the CEGEP nursing programs and the universities. Because Quebec is the province with the largest number of nurses in the country, the development and implementation of collaborative initiatives would be an important step forward in the movement to achieve the entry to practice position.

The announcement in 1988 of the decision by the government of Prince Edward Island to "phase out diploma education in favour of a degree program" (CNA Connection, 1989b) was the culmination of many years of effort on the part of nurses in Prince Edward Island to secure a baccalaureate program of nursing in their province. It is obviously more complex to envision implementing the baccalaureate degree as the basis for entry to practice in a large populous province with many schools of nursing than it is in a small one, such as Prince Edward Island. However, the model established by the province of Prince Edward Island was an important one for the nation.

Plans are underway in Newfoundland, Nova Scotia, and New Brunswick to develop collaborative baccalaureate programs. Working under the auspices of the New Brunswick Association of Registered Nurses (NBARN), the Nurse Educators Interest Group has taken leadership in discussions relative to collaboration between the five diploma and two university programs in nursing. There has been no official announcement on closure of the diploma schools of nursing as of the time of writing (Wiggins, personal communciation, September 1, 1994). Collaborative initiatives in Nova Scotia have resulted in collaboration between Dalhousie University and two diploma programs in that province (CNA, September, 1992). A program involving the three institutions is to commence in the fall of 1995 when the two diploma programs (Victoria General Hospital - Camp Hill Medical Complex and Yarmouth Regional Hospital School of Nursing) will close. There will be one curriculum that was developed collaboratively for the three sites with no diploma exit, and all nursing students will be registered at Dalhousie University (W. Dundas, personal communication, September 1, 1994). Memorial University of Newfoundland and four diploma schools of nursing have planned a degree program in nursing in which there is no diploma exit. The diploma schools included the General Hospital, the Salvation Army Grace General Hospital, St. Clare's Mercy Hospital, and Western Memorial Regional Hospital (CNA, Winter 1992-93c).

The tasks ahead are difficult and challenging. However, a cursory glance through the pages of nursing history confirms that the road has never been easy, and nursing is at this educational crossroads today because there have been leaders with vision and courage who developed and found support for wise initiatives. Unity of purpose and action have characterized what the nursing profession has accomplished in moving towards successful achievement of its educational goals. The rationale for implementation of the baccalaureate standard for entry to practice can only be understood and accepted on the basis of the nature and range of knowledge and skills required to practise nursing and the right of the health-care consumer to receive care from a well-prepared professional nurse. In the end it is likely that the success of the transition to the baccalaureate entry-level standard will be achieved through the efforts of nurses at all levels and in all settings who were convinced of the importance of the issues involved and who worked tirelessly to make it happen.

REFERENCES

Alberta Association of Registered Nurses. (1976). *The response of the Alberta Association of Registered Nurses to the Government of Alberta's Position Paper on Nursing Education.* Edmonton: Author.

Alberta Association of Registered Nurses (1978). *Postition paper on nursing.* Edmonton: Author.

Alberta Association of Registered Nurses (1979), *Postition paper on nursing.* Edmonton: Author.

Alberta Task Force on Nursing Education. (1977). *Position paper on nursing education: Principles and issues.* Edmonton: Author.

Besharah, A. (1981). When will the shouting start? *The Canadian Nurse, 77*(3), 6.

CNA Staff. (1984). *Entry to practice bulletin.* Ottawa: Author.

CNA Staff. (1989). *Entry to practice newsletter,* 5(3), 1-3.

CNA Staff. (June 1991). VGH/UBC Prepare for third year of collaboration. *Edufacts,* 1-4.

CNA Staff. (September 1991). Manitoba phasing out two programs: Joint program begins. *Edufacts,* 1-4.

CNA Staff. (March 1992). University-College Collaboration in BC. *Edufacts, 2*(1), 1-4.

CNA Staff. (Winter 1992-93a). Do we have enough master of nursing programs? *Edufacts,* 1-4.

CNA Staff. (Winter 1992-93b). Ontario edging closer to entry to practice? *Edufacts, 2*(4), 1-4.

CNA Staff. (Spring 1993). Tracking enrolments. *Edufacts,* 1-4.

CNA Staff. (September, 1992). New BN education—Nova Scotia style. *Edufacts, 2*(3), 1.

CNA Staff. (Winter, 1992-93). Joint funding for Newfoundland collaboration. *Edufacts, 2* (4), 4.

CNA Staff. (Summer 1993). Calgary Conjoint Nursing Program. *Edufacts,* 1-4.

CNA Connection. (1989a). VGH School joins UBC. *The Canadian Nurse, 85*(2), 12.

CNA Connection. (1989b). Baccalaureate education comes to PEI. *The Canadian Nurse, 85* (3), 10.

Government of Alberta. (1975). *Report of the Alberta Task Force on Nursing Education.* Edmonton: Author.

Government of Alberta. (1977). *Position paper on nursing education: Principles and issues.* Edmonton: Author.

Kerr, J.C. (1978). *Financing university nursing education in Canada from 1919 to 1976.* Unpublished doctoral dissertation, The University of Michigan, Ann Arbor, MI.

Kerr, J.C. (1982). The shouting starts. *The Canadian Nurse, 78*(2), 42-43.

King, M.K. (1970). The development of university nursing education. In M.Q. Innis (Ed.). *Nursing education in a changing society,* (pp. 67-85). Toronto: University of Toronto Press.

Rajabally, M. (1982). We have seen the enemy. *The Canadian Nurse, 78*(2), 40-42.

Royal Commission on Health Services. *Report.* (1964). Ottawa: Queen's Printer.

Russell, E.K. (1932). The teaching of public health nursing in the University of Toronto. In *Methods and problems of medical education,* (pp. 82-88). New York: The Rockefeller Foundation.

Saskatchewan Registered Nurses Association. (August 1994). *ConceRN.* Regina: Author.

Weir, G.M. (1932). *Survey of nursing education in Canada.* Toronto: University of Toronto Press.

CHAPTER TWENTY SIX

Collaboration Between Nursing Education and Nursing Practice for Quality Nursing Care, Education, and Research

JANNETTA MacPHAIL

I nadequacies in relationships between nursing education and nursing service have been recognized increasingly as a major issue in Canada and the United States, particularly in the 1970s and 1980s. The risks and benefits pertaining to this issue have been identified in the literature and at national and international conferences by proponents of unifying nursing education and nursing practice through a number of mechanisms and strategies. The benefits pertain to the recipients of care and the nursing staff in health-care agencies, as well as to the students and faculty involved in education, practice, and research.

■ ■ ■ ■

HISTORICAL INFLUENCES ON SEPARATION BETWEEN EDUCATION AND SERVICE

Historically, nursing education was developed within hospital training schools in Canada and the United States. Training schools were developed to staff the hospitals regardless of a hospital's size. Until the late 1930s and even into the 1940s in some hospitals, nursing care was provided primarily by nursing students; the only registered nurses held such positions as superintendent of nurses, supervisor, and perhaps head nurse. Thus the hospitals were dependent on students to staff them around the clock, throughout the year. One of the unfortunate consequences of this arrangement was that the need for students to provide care or meet service needs usually took precedence over students' educational or learning needs. Until the middle of this century, students were exploited to meet service needs, without regard for learning needs (Schlotfeldt and MacPhail, 1969a). Although nurse writers may not have identified this problem directly, the history of hospitals in both countries records this method of staffing. Moreover, many retired and older nurses, educated before the middle of the century, can attest to the fact. One of the consequences of this situation was that nurse educators became increasingly frustrated because of their lack of control over the learning opportunities provided to students and the planning of students' time. The solution of the educators was to separate the school of nursing from the hospital nursing service, although both were under the same administration, board, and budget.

Another factor that influenced the separation between service and education was the development of nursing programs in universities and later in community colleges that had no clear delineation of relationship to service. Although the first university school of nursing was established in Canada in 1919 at the University of British Columbia, the early university programs did not promote separation because they were not designed as separate entities. The first university nursing programs were 5 years in length, with students enroling for 1 year in liberal arts courses, then entering a hospital school of nursing for 3 years, and returning to the university for the 5th year, in which they specialized in either teaching and supervision in nursing, or public health nursing. Programs of this design have been referred to as *"sandwich"* baccalaureate programs because the nursing component, which was not under the control of the university, was *"sandwiched"* between 2 years in the university. Such programs continued in many parts of Canada into the 1960s. In 1933 Kathleen Russell, a visionary and effective leader, developed the first integrated baccalaureate program, with nursing courses and liberal arts courses integrated throughout, at the University of Toronto. This program was also 5 years in length. Although this type of program was much more sound educationally, it resulted in a clear separation between education and service, as did the nursing programs that were developed later in colleges. Faculty in such programs became "guests" in the clinical agencies where the faculty placed students for practice and supervised them in practice. Faculty did not have, and in most cases still do not have, any control over the practice environment and the role models involved in practice. Their modus operandi became one of persuasion and compromise, which was sometimes to the detriment of learning opportunities provided to students.

Another factor influencing the separation between education and service was the tendency of nursing instructors in educational institutions to separate themselves from practice. This was evidenced by their withdrawal from the practice setting except to supervise students. In some cases, instructors chose to wear a lab coat instead of a uniform to differentiate themselves from the nursing staff. This served as an additional impediment in relationships between nursing educators and nursing staff, since attire has always tended to be a status symbol and an important means of identifying people in hospital settings. In some cases, nursing instructors were perceived by nursing staff as having chosen teaching to escape from practice. In fact, the instructors were allowed limited involvement in practice by the nursing education administrators. One consequence was that there were often negative attitudes toward the nursing faculty and students.

In many cases, learning opportunities were inadequate because of lack of staff support and interest in facilitating students' learning. Another outcome was the tendency to "label" each other, with the result that a lack of respect and trust developed between nursing educators and nursing service personnel. This further resulted in limited communication between the two groups and sometimes open conflict and negative controls.

Clearly, the organization and structure of nursing school/faculties had no relationship to the organization and structure of health-care agencies, even in academic health centres. Chater (1983) states "University-owned and university-affiliated hospitals became part of academic health centers so that medical schools could have control over the environments for patient care and guaranteed access to the mix of patients required for the clinical programs" (p. 59). Have nursing schools/faculties obtained similar control of care and patient access as the medical schools/faculties in Canada and the United States?

Theoretical Framework

Organizational theorists have identified factors that contribute to separation between organizations and factors that promote interaction (Blau, 1975; Stinchcombe, 1968; Ullrich and Wieland, 1980). Batey (1983) applies this theoretical knowledge to nursing, showing how structure influences interaction between persons in an organization. She defines structure as: "A network of relationships among social positions that effects differences in role relations and social integration" (p. 3). One would expect more interaction among members of like groups than among members of different groups. It is also known that status differences influence interaction. One of the outcomes of interaction within an organization is for members to develop shared values. If interaction is limited, there is less opportunity to develop shared values; there may even be conflicts among different groups (Batey, 1983).

To what extent have such outcomes occurred in nursing? One need only reflect on some of the differences in values that can be found between education and service, such as the importance of research; conceptualizations of practice; priorities for care; and theoretical foundations of practice. Given the differences between faculty and nursing staff in health-care agencies on such variables as education, work setting, autonomy, and status, clearly "the structured forces against integration are stronger than the forces for it" (Batey, 1983, p. 5). Although it is important to recognize differences, it is equally important to take steps to reduce them and increase interaction in order to strengthen values and to work together to overcome deterrents to the common goals of nursing: quality care, quality education, and quality research.

Means of Overcoming Deterrents

One means of overcoming deterrents to interaction is to develop a collaboration or unification model, such as those developed at a few universities in the United States and Canada. The first such model was developed in 1959 at the University of Florida by Dorothy Smith, then Dean of the College of Nursing (Smith, 1959; Smith, 1965). Although this model did not survive, it made an important contribution to the promotion of collaboration. Smith later acknowledged that her model had not been based on organizational theory, nor had it used role theory; she perceived that these factors contributed to its demise. Such theories were considered carefully and used in the development of subsequent models. The next application of an interorganizational model was at Case Western Reserve University and University Hospitals of Cleveland in the 1960s under the direction of Schlotfeldt and MacPhail (MacPhail, 1972, 1975, 1980, 1983; Schlotfeldt, 1980; Schlotfeldt and MacPhail, 1969a, 1969b, 1969c). Other examples are the application of a unification model, beginning in 1972 at the University of Rochester and Rush University in Chicago. Subsequently, a "contractual agreement approach" was developed at Rutgers University (Joel, 1985); a "partnership plan" was developed at the University of Pennsylvania (Fagin, 1985); and a "partnership model" was designed and tested at the University of South Carolina (Baker, Boyd, Stasiowski, Simons, 1989a; Baker et al, 1989b). Although all were designed to promote and facilitate interinstitutional collaboration, each was a different model, on a different scale, designed to fit a particular situation. This is an important concept to consider when making an effort to foster collaboration. Despite these efforts, most university nursing schools in the United States are still separated organizationally and structurally from the health care agencies in which students practise and faculty and graduate students conduct research.

In an effort to promote more collaboration between education and practice, the American Association of Colleges of Nursing (AACN) membership approved almost unanimousluy that "AACN establish the goal that all member schools of nursing develop collaborative relationships with practice settings to advance the goals of nursing practice, education and research" (Hegyvary, 1991, p. 148). By establishing this goal, AACN communicates an expectation for more schools to develop interinstitutional arrangements that will promote collaboration. "Collaborative relationships were defined as substantive interchange of human and/or material resources for the purpose of advancing common goals in practice, education, and research" (Hegyvary, 1991, p. 148). Even though AACN, which is similar to the Canadian Association of University Schools of Nursing (CAUSN), has no means of enforcing such changes, their programming could help to facilitate them through education and recognition of successful interinstitutional models. CAUSN could also encourage the development and evaluation of such models through their programming and recognition of changes in structure and roles that strengthen the relationships between education and practice settings, such as the 1993 Western Region CAUSN Conference which focused on "Collaboration: A Time to Evaluate *(CAUSN Newsletter,* June 1993). CAUSN could also consider recognizing successful collaborative relationships and efforts to develop joint appointments through their accreditation program.

■ ■ ■ ■

INTERINSTITUTIONAL LINKAGES TO PROMOTE COLLABORATION

The two types of interinsitutional models that are most widely known are the unification model, such as implemented and evaluated at the University of Rochester and Rush University beginning in 1972; and the collaboration model, such as developed and assessed at Case Western Reserve University in the late 1960s and early 1970s. Because the unification model requires a university and hospital under one administration and one chief executive officer for nursing that encompasses the positions of dean of nursing in the university and director of nursing of the major university hospital (Ford, 1980a; Ford, 1980b; Sovie 1981a; Sovie 1981b), it has not been regarded as a feasible approach for most faculties/schools of nursing. The collaboration model, as developed at Case Western Reserve University and the University Hospitals of Cleveland beginning in 1966, has been considered more feasible because it involves two independent organizations, each with a head of nursing who has a secondary appointment in the other organization. The heads of nursing delegate responsibility for practice, education, and research to clinical directors who also serve as chairs of the faculty groups. To facilitate and promote interaction and opportunities to develop shared values, three types of joint appointments were developed: shared cost, clinical, and associate. Cost-sharing may be on different percentage bases (50% to 50%; 75% to 25%; or 80% to 20%), depending on the needs of the two organizations. Clinical appointees are nurses with at least master's preparation who hold leadership positions in the hospital or other health-care agency and a clinical appointment in the school of nursing. Associate appointees are faculty members who hold an associate in nursing appointment in a hospital or other health-care agency. There is no cost-sharing for these two types of appointments, but there is sharing of time and talents to contribute and fulfill responsibilities to the other organization.

Although the collaboration and unification models differ in specific structures, roles, and titles, all models contain an organizational structure that facilitates and ensures interaction and communication between education and service, and opportunities to develop shared values. All models have the same goals: (1) improving the quality of nursing care through research and strong clinical leadership; (2) enhancing the learning climate and learning opportunities for nursing students and nursing staff; (3) promoting nursing research and the application of valid and reliable research findings in practice and education; (4) fostering interprofessional collaboration, particularly between nurses and physicians; and (5) using human and material resources cost-effectively.

Theoretical Bases and Outcomes of the Models

The development of organizational structures that are based on these models has required major changes in the organizations involved and in the relationships between the organizations. The structures were based on organizational theories and theories of planned change. Changes in roles and relations were based on role theory, emphasizing the importance of the five factors known to influence role development: education; experience to reinforce the education; reference group identification or role modeling; the status system in the organization; and the incentive system of the organization. All of the models have involved decentralization of authority and responsibility within nursing service; restructuring within each organization and between organizations; redefining roles and role relations; changing expectations for role incumbents by those with whom they interact, including nurses, physicians, and patients; developing strong leadership in nursing; and increasing the involvement of faculty in practice.

Outcomes of these models have been development of strong leadership within the educational institution and the health-care agency; attraction of faculty and clinical specialists to the settings; increased attraction and retention of nursing staff in the health-care agencies; and increased resources and expertise available to both organizations, with sharing of resources between service and education. A major consequence experienced by all involved in those settings has been increased interaction between the incumbents of roles in both education and service, with the opportunity to develop mutual trust and respect, and shared values.

Criticism of Collaboration and Unification Models

There has been criticism that collaboration and unification models increase workloads and contribute to burnout (Blazek, Selckman, Timpe, Wolfe, 1982; Ford, 1980b; Powers, 1976; Sovie, 1981b; and Spero, 1980). These problems have occurred in some settings; however, one can learn from the mistakes of others and try to avoid such pitfalls. The administrators who develop the model must set reasonable expectations and provide guidance and flexibility to joint appointees to try to prevent them from attempting to assume two full-time jobs. This hazard applies particularly to persons in shared-cost appointments.

The models have also been criticized for decreasing research productivity and publication; however, most models have facilitated and ultimately increased scholarly endeavours. Problems tend to arise if the nurse administrator in each institution is not familiar with the expectations held for the joint appointees in the other institution and if guidance and incentives are not provided for role incumbents to meet all expectations to a reasonable degree. For example, one cannot expect a joint appointee in a 50% to 50% position to maintain the same teaching responsibilities in the school of nursing or to have the same involvement in agency programs as the person who does not hold such an appointment.

All collaboration and unification models have contributed to enhancing the learning environment for students by virtue of the improved quality of care, exemplary role models, and the supportive learning climate provided by staff. The old "we-they" concept no longer exists, because everyone involved collaborates in developing shared values and pursuing common goals. Rather than being ignored, head nurses and staff nurses are helped to see their importance in students' learning and are used to advantage, thus minimizing negative attitudes.

Faculty Practice

Over the past two decades, increasing attention has been given to faculty practice, particularly as an integral part of collaboration and unification models. Unfortunately, the schism between nursing education and nursing practice resulted in many nursing faculty members failing to maintain involvement in practice and not being perceived as role models by either nursing students or nursing staff. Much of the impetus for the focus on faculty practice was derived from the publication, "Statement of Belief Regarding Faculty Practice" (1979), which was written by 13 nursing leaders in the United States who were highly committed to collaboration and keenly aware of the difficulty many faculty members were experiencing in incorporating practice into their roles. The statement called for legitimizing nursing practice as an integral part of the faculty role; developing incentives to promote and reward practice as a means of enhancing practice, education, and research; and adapting organizational structures and policies to facilitate faculty practice. The American Academy of Nursing sponsored four annual symposia from 1983 to 1986, the first three of which were partially funded by the Robert Wood Johnson Foundation, a philanthropic organization that is strongly committed to promoting faculty practice to improve patient care (Barnard, 1983; Barnard and Smith, 1985).

Several definitions of faculty practice can be found in the literature. Ford and Kitzman (1983) defines it as activities related to the care of patients that must meet two criteria: (1) "be scholarly in orientation with associated scholarship outcomes;" and (2) "have the care of patients or clients as the central focus" (pp. 13-14). Faculty practice may involve any roles that faculty members play in service agencies that meet the criteria. These roles include activities in the direct and indirect care of patients and participation in programs, such as staff development, quality assurance, clinical advancement, and administrative and committee assignments (Ford and Kitzman, 1983). Other definitions exclude indirect care activities and limit faculty practice to direct care of patients (Algase, 1986; Anderson and Pierson, 1983). Faculty practice is perceived as quality care through which clinical judgement is enhanced. It has the potential for enriching teaching; generating credibility in students, nursing staff, and colleagues in other disciplines; influencing the selection of research problems to be investigated and the methods of inquiry used; promoting application of research findings in practice; sensitizing nurse educators to nursing service issues and problems; increasing the testing of theory in practice; and enhancing the quality of care provided to patients and the education of students.

Faculty practice is and integral part of collaboration and unification models and of partnership models developed by Fagin (1985) and Baker et al (1989a and 1989b). Fagin believes that any pattern adopted to promote partnership "must be flexible enough to fit the vast variety of circumstances and settings in which nursing education and nursing practice occur" (1986, p. 144). Moreover, she thinks collaborative models should have "potential for uniting people rather than organizations" and that "faculty practice designs that do not reflect the research agenda are doomed from the start" (Fagin, 1986, p. 144).

Deterrents to Collaboration Between Service and Education

If collaboration between service and education, of which faculty practice is an integral part, is possible and can accomplish the objectives stated previously, one may ask why more such models are not developed. Some of the factors identified to date are lack of interest by either faculty or nursing service personnel; skepticism by faculty members or nursing leaders who seem to have difficulty believing that the system can work; fear of heavy work load, leading to burnout; faculty role strain and role conflict (Barger and Bridges, 1987); limited access to practice sites due to inflexible policies that permit practice on a limited basis (Millonig, 1986); failure to adapt criteria for promotion and tenure to recognize and reward faculty practice; and lack of organizational support through formalized practice policies, expectations, or remuneration mechanisms to promote and facilitate faculty practice (Lambert and Lambert, 1988). Additional factors include insufficient clinical expertise of faculty who are threatened by the expectations required in the clinical settings, and an inadequate number of risk-takers in nursing. Other possible deterrents to promoting collaboration are insufficient communication and interaction between nurses in education and service to develop shared values and common goals; fears of faculty members that research productivity will be decreased because of additional commitment to practice; and obvious differences in values, status, and education between the stakeholders in nursing education and those in nursing service.

Joint Appointments as Facilitators of Interaction

A collaboration or unification model is not feasible in all settings. Another means of facilitating collaboration and achieving at least some of the goals of collaboration is to develop a system of joint appointments between nursing education and the health-care agencies, in which students practise and in which research is conducted by faculty members and students. Joint appointments are designed to increase interaction; nurture shared values; and promote a sense of joint accountability for quality nursing practice, quality education, and quality research.

The development of joint appointments is the approach used to facilitate interaction and collaboration in 11 of the 23 Canadian university faculties/schools of nursing, based on responses from 19 of the deans/directors to and inquiry sent by the author. McMaster University has had a system of joint appointments for the greatest number of years, beginning in 1968 when the first joint appointment as a Clinical Associate in the School of Nursing was negotiated by Alma Reid, Director, for the Director of the Nurse Practitioner Programme based in the Family Practice Unit of the School of Medicine (Royle, 1984). During the early 1970s when planning for the opening of McMaster's Health Sciences Centre, a committee of nursing faculty members and the head of nursing in the Medical Centre were appointed to explore "the nature of the interrelationships to be established between the University Hospital and the School of Nursing" (Royle, 1984, p. 5). Existing models of joint appointments were examined and two committee members attended the 1971 *Final Report on the Nursing Demonstration Project,* directed by the author, through which the collaboration model was developed at Case Western Reserve University and the University Hospitals of Cleveland with the aid of a 5-year grant from the W.K. Kellogg Foundation (MacPhail, 1972). Subsequently, a system of joint appointments, similar to this model, was developed at McMaster University under the leadership of Dorothy Kergin, Associate Dean, Nursing. By 1981 nine such appontments had been made, of which two were hospital staff with appointment to the University; seven were nursing faculty given an appointment to a hospital or the Victorian Order of Nurses (VON). Eight of the nine were cost-shared appointments (Royle, 1984). In concluding her *Report on Joint University/Hospital/Health Care Agency Appointments in Nursing,* Royle (1984) stated: "McMaster University

School of Nursing and the Hamilton hospitals and community agencies have achieved an effective system of shared appointments in nursing" (p. 18). The system of joint appointments was reported to be operational in 1994, with 13 of 47 faculty members jointly appointed with cost-sharing, and 86 nurses in clinical settings holding clinical faculty appointments.

Eight of the 19 universities from which a response was received (Alberta; British Columbia; Calgary; Dalhousie; McMaster; Ottawa; Toronto; and Victoria) have three types of joint appointments, which may be described generically as: agency/faculty; faculty/agency; and shared-cost, although the latter type may not be filled continuously. The two categories of appointees that most frequently have a shared-cost appointment are clinical nurse specialists and researchers. Since salary and fringe benefits can be received from only one source, the role incumbent must choose the organization in which to have the primary appointment. Varied titles are selected for the two types of joint appointments that do not involve cost-sharing, such as "Clinical Associate" for those whose primary appointment is in a health-care agency, and "Faculty Associate" for faculty with an appointment in a health-care agency. There is no consistency among institutions, which makes it difficult to interpret titles on curricula vita. Responses from three universities (McGill, Queen's, and Saskatchewan) indicate that they offer adjunct appointments in the faculty to selected health-care agency personnel, but do not have appointments for faculty in health-care agencies. Most of the eight respondents who do not have a system for joint appointments indicated interest in them. In fact, l'Université de Montréal was reported to be in the process of developing a collaboration model. Information could be shared to facilitate the development of collaborative endeavours and perhaps achieve more consistency in titles, role expectations, and incentives pertaining to joint appointments.

The system of joint appointments at the University of Alberta was designed in the 1982-1983 academic year through a group effort involving representatives from four health-care agencies and three representatives from the university's Faculty of Nursing. Two types of joint appointments exist: *faculty-agency*, with the primary appointment in the faculty; and *agency-faculty*, with the primary appointment in the health-care agency. There may or may not be sharing of costs in these two types of appointments; however, most do not involve cost-sharing. In a shared-cost appointment, the incumbent must hold a primary appointment in either the educational institution or the health-care agency, and the other institution is billed for its share of salary and fringe benefits, as mutually agreed. The privileges and responsibilities entailed in the two types of appointments have been specified; they serve as a guide for incumbents of the joint appointments and provide a basis for writing an annual report on an individual's participation in the other organization. It is vitally important to have reasonable expectations in both organizations and to have flexibility in evolvement of the role. Some shared-cost appointments involve faculty members who serve as clinical nurse researchers for a portion of their time in a health-care agency, which may be on a 50% to 50%, 30% to 70%, or 20% to 80% basis. Others are clinical nurse specialists in a health-care agency with an appointment in the university's Faculty of Nursing or a unit supervisor with master's preparation (head nurse) who provides clinical supervision for students placed in the unit.

The privileges and responsibilities of the two types of joint appointments have been developed with careful attention to balance or equality in each of the items (Faculty of Nursing, University of Alberta, 1983). For example, an individual from a health-care agency who holds an associate faculty appointment is listed in the Faculty of Nursing Calendar, obtains a library card, and has opportunity to participate in faculty meetings with voice, but not with a vote. The person has access to faculty development programs and opportunity to gain knowledge of and contribute to the development of curricula. There may also be opportunities to serve as preceptor for students or teach in courses related to their expertise and to increase research competence through conducting research and using consultation resources.

In a similar vein, a faculty member who holds an Associate in Nursing appointment in a health-care agency may participate in administrative or clinical meetings and contribute to staff development programs in the agency. The person has opportunity to gain knowledge of and contribute to nursing practice and program development in the agency. There are opportunities to practise or conduct research in the agency, although ethical clearance must be obtained to do research. Faculty members who hold such an appointment may use it to assist staff in research development and contribute to staff development. An individual may choose to contract to practise a certain proportion of time weekly, serve as consultant to staff, or be involved in several activities.

All privileges and responsibilities are negotiated with the person responsible for programs in the other organization. Negotiation is logical since persons in leadership positions have knowledge of the programs and know what would be appropriate and what areas need involvement. In addition, persons in leadership positions are the individuals ultimately responsible for evaluating the performance of the joint appointee and deciding whether the appointment will be continued.

Most of the deans/directors, responding to the author's inquiry, were very positive about joint appointments and shared clearly delineated role expectations and a system for evaluating performance and deciding about continuation of appointment. It was encouraging to find emphasis placed on research as an expected outcome and support for joint research endeavours by faculty and agency personnel. In most settings the number of agency/faculty appointments exceed the number of faculty/agency apppointments by three to four times, which may reflect a difference in the value placed on such and appointment, or fear of overload which has been identified in the literature as a possible outcome (Acorn, 1990; Blazek et al, 1982; Ford, 1980b; Powers, 1976; Sovie, 1981b; Spero, 1980). Another factor influencing the greater number of agency/faculty appointments, is the number of different health-care agencies needed to accommodate both students and faculty for practice and research.

Other Strategies to Promote Collaboration

Several of the dean/director respondents shared other strategies used to promote collaboration. Since 1986 the University of Toronto has established five clinical teaching units in health-care agencies. Each unit has a faculty member with expertise in the nursing specialty of that unit, who is assigned to it on a continuing basis. The head nurses and several staff nurses are given joint appointments as clinical assistants in the Faculty of Nursing, and may precept students if they are prepared at the baccalaureate level in nursing. Faculty and staff may engage in joint initiatives, such as the development and evaluation of a pain scale and reporting their findings at research conferences. A joint research project has been conducted to assess this role.

In 1992 the University of Toronto initiated another collaborative project that involves six teaching hospitals and two health units from which 40 preceptors prepared at the baccalaureate level are recruited and given a clinical assistant appointment. Twenty-four 4th-year students are involved, as are 2 faculty members. The 24 students have three major differences in their programs from those of classmates. Their fourth year is extended to 10 months and the 24 students commence their final year on June 1 following the third year. Each of the 24 students has a faculty member assigned for the full fourth year and a preceptor with whom they practise for extended periods, thus having more than one preceptor over the course of the year. They also have paid employment for 3 months during the summer while under the guidance of a preceptor, with a faculty member on call during July and August. A preceptor meets at least monthly with the faculty member assigned to her/his students. These 24 students meet the same objectives as the others, but their course content is organized differently and they have only one course with the rest of the class. To date, both faculty and the 24 students are very satisfied with this approach, and the students feel much more secure in the practice environment than do their counterparts.

Several universities reported favourable outcomes from having nurse researchers with doctoral preparation in shared-cost appointments (Alberta, British Columbia, Dalhousie, Montreal, and Ottawa). This approach has enhanced the research climate, increased research that has been undertaken, and promoted application of research findings in practice. Since 1991, the University of Toronto has gradually located six senior researchers in practice settings where the hospitals involved provide office and research space, some support services, and space for graduate students. This approach is making research more visible in the practice environment, helping to involve staff in research and application of findings, and making research more relevant as the questions arise from nursing practice. Currently, l'Université de Montréal has seven professors serving as members of research centres within four hospitals. One such appointment involves cost-sharing. Each of the centres has a clinical focus, such as care of the aged, AIDS, mental illness, cardiology, and all are funded by grants from le Fonds de recherche en sante du Quebec, which is a provincial health research council.

The University of Western Ontario reports involvement in a Nursing Research Consortium, which is a network among health-care agencies and faculty and graduate students, designed to help generate researchable problems from practice; facilitate communication among researchers, clinicians, and graduate students; facilitate cross-agency involvement in research; and foster interdisciplinary research. The University of Ottawa reported positive outcomes from organizing a nursing research committee that includes researchers from the faculty and practice settings who work together to facilitate collaborative research projects, present monthly research seminars, distribute a research newsletter, and sponsor nursing research events. In the past decade, there has been a notable increase in faculties/schools of nursing and health-care agencies that conjointly sponsor nursing research conferences on a local, regional, national, and even international basis, as reflected in the conferences advertised in *The Canadian Nurse, CAUSN Newsletter,* and provincial nurses' association newsletters. For example, in less than a decade, the University of Alberta involved faculty and clinical faculty in the organization and presentation of the following two major, international nursing research conferences: the Second International Nursing Research Conference in 1986, which attracted over 800 nurses from 38 countries; and the First International Community Health Nursing Research Conference in 1993, which was attended by over 900 nurses from 40 countries. The latter conference was sponsored jointly by the Faculty of Nursing and the Edmonton Board of Health.

Another type of collaborative endeavour undertaken by faculty and health-care agency colleagues is the development of certificate courses in specialty practice (Alberta and Manitoba). These courses have been successful in improving the quality of courses and care and also in enabling students to earn credit toward a baccalaureate degree, which often encourages them to enroll in a program and earn a baccalaureate degree. The University of New Brunswick is developing this approach in collaboration with Memorial University of Newfoundland to offer certificate course via distance education to nurses in the Atlantic region.

The most recent development in collaboration is the collaborative approaches designed by faculties/schools of nursing and diploma programs to prepare more nurses at the baccalaureate level and move toward the profession's goal of a baccalaureate degree for entry into nursing practice by the year 2000. These approaches are reported in Chapters 4 and 25.

■■ ■■ ■■ ■■

EVALUATION OF OUTCOMES

One criticism of the collaboration and unification models and of joint appointments has been insufficient effort to evaluate outcomes to demonstrate benefits. Admittedly, in the early collaboration models, much effort went into developing the models, with less attention devoted to evaluation of outcomes. In addition, some of the outcome measures used by proponents of the models to demonstrate results have involved inconclusive data because of the nature of the phenomena being evaluated.

A major objective of joint endeavours is to improve nursing practice. Such improvement is evident in the amount of research conducted and the extent to which research findings are applied in practice. Neither of these aspects has as yet been documented systematically, but they could be in future models or joint appointments. If one believes that research is necessary to improve practice and that it is through research that knowledge is advanced and practice improved, this would seem to be a logical means of evaluation.

Documenting the initiation of new programs of care by experts who have been attracted to leadership positions in these collaboration models is often used as evidence of improvement in care. To have such systematic documentation, it is necessary to obtain baseline data about the programs of care before a model is implemented, which in most cases has not been feasible. Nonetheless, one can reflect on the nature of programs of care at the outset and document progressive programs that have been implemented. Some examples in maternity nursing might include preparation for childbearing, support of parents who have had such preparation by staff, and father and sibling visitation programs. Examples in other areas of nursing would be parent participation in child care and educational programs pertaining to particular kinds of health problems for patients and families.

Patient satisfaction studies are another method of evaluating care. These have been used to some extent, although the validity and reliability of the instruments have presented problems in such studies over the years. Sovie (1981a) notes that care in the Rochester model was evaluated as excellent by patients and families, physicians, and staff. Similar outcomes are reported by MacPhail (1972) in relation to the Case Western Reserve University/University Hospitals of Cleveland model. Sovie (1981a) also identifies excellent patient and family teaching programs and materials as an outcome of the Rochester model. Another mechanism that verifies improvement of care is the accreditation report, through which written and verbal comments are received about the quality of nursing care and the extent to which standards are met and surpassed (Sovie, 1981a). Some nursing service leaders refer to the outcomes measured by quality assurance indicators; however, others are reluctant to use such indicators because of problems with the validity and reliability of some of the quality assurance indicators.

Another outcome is enhancement of the learning climate and learning opportunities for students and staff. This outcome may be evaluated by evidence of changes in access to patients by faculty, improvements in student learning, changes in attitude of staff toward learners, types of learning experiences made available to students through collaborative efforts and sharing of information, and improved role models for students. It is logical to expect a clinical setting in which students gain experience to be characterized by high quality of care. It has been clear to observers that this has been an outcome of collaborative efforts in all three models previously described due to joint decision-making at the clinical leadership level.

Another objective of collaboration pertains to the promotion and facilitation of research endeavours. This can be documented by collecting data about the number and nature of studies conducted over time and about efforts to apply research findings in practice. Data reflecting these efforts include conferences and research rounds to share research findings and assist staff nurses in applying the findings, as well as the actual application of findings in specific situations. Other indications of research endeavours include publications; presentation of papers, and active research promotion activities in both nursing education and nursing service, such as a research day or research week conducted as an annual activity in a health-care agency, and evidence of attention to research in internal nursing newsletters.

Another objective of joint endeavours is to enhance interprofessional collaboration. This can be documented by change in the number and nature of joint meetings and collaborative or interdisciplinary endeavours. Changes in joint planning on hospital units and joint educational efforts between and among educational programs would also indicate success in meeting this objective. Sovie (1981b) refers to collaboration between nursing and medicine by designing innovative approaches to the organization and delivery of ambulatory care. Other measures of success would be respect and recognition between the professions, and the position of influence and power obtained by nursing through such a joint endeavour. Reference has been made to these outcomes by Sovie (1981b) and MacPhail (1972).

Results of changes in the organizational structure to facilitate interaction and development of shared values can provide powerful and persuasive evidence of movement toward goals. Such evidence can be documented in terms of joint meetings, collaborative endeavours, new programs developed jointly, and the extent to which values are shared versus differences emphasized on a long-term basis.

■■ ■■ ■■ ■■

CONCLUSION

There are undoubtedly other ways to promote collaboration between nursing education and nursing service and to overcome barriers between them. The study of organizational theories and structures leads one to conclude that structures are required to promote and facilitate interaction and communication between education and service that is needed to develop shared values and goals. In addition, there is need for carefully designed strategies to promote and facilitate collaboration by using existing knowledge of planned change, role development, and other organizational concepts that enter into such a collaborative endeavour. Educators and practitioners need to respect and trust each other, not lay blame. The achievement of this goal requires good communication; interaction; openness; objectivity; readiness to examine beliefs, attitudes, and values; and willingness to recognize that compromises are needed to move toward the goal of collaboration and joint accountability for practice, education, and research. Together, educators and service leaders can develop the quality of nursing practice to which nurses in general aspire, as well as an exemplary learning environment for both nursing students and staff. Creating a supportive research environment will help improve the quality of practice through research and encourage the application of research findings for the benefit of both the consumers of nursing care and the nurses providing care.

REFERENCES

Acorn, S. (1990). Joint appointments: Perspectives of nurse executives. *Canadian Journal of Nursing Administration, 3*(4), 6-9.

Algase, D. (1986). Faculty practice: A means to advance the discipline of nursing. *Journal of Nursing Education, 25,* 74-76.

Anderson, E.R., and Pierson, P. (1983). An exploratory study of faculty practice: Views of those faculty engaged in practice who teach in an NLN-accredited baccalaureate program. *Western Journal of Nursing Research, 5,* 129-143.

Baker, C.M., Boyd, N.J., Stasiowski, S.A., and Simons, B.J. (1989a). Interinstitutional collaboration for nursing excellence: Part 1, Creating the partnership. *Journal of Nursing Administration, 19*(2), 8-12.

Baker, C.M. Boyd, N.J., Stasiowski, S.A., and Simons, B.J. (1989b). Interinstitutional collaboration for nursing excellence: Part II, Testing the model. *Journal of Nursing Administration, 19*(3), 8-13.

Barger, S.E., and Bridges, W.C. (1987). Nursing faculty practice: Institutional and individual facilitators and inhibitors. *Journal of Professional Nursing, 3*(6), 338-346.

Barnard, K. (1983). Preface. In K. Barnard (Ed.). *Structure to outcome: Making it work* (pp. v-vi). Kansas City, MO: American Academy of Nursing.

Barnard, K., and Smith, G. (Eds.). (1985). *Faculty practice in action.* Kansas City, MO: American Academy of Nursing.

Batey, M. (1983). Structural consideration for the social integration of nursing. In K. Barnard (Ed.), *Structure to outcome: Making it work* (pp. 1-11). Kansas City, MO: American Academy of Nursing.

Blau, P.M. (1975). *Parameters of social structure: Approaches to the study of social structure.* New York: Free Press.

Blazek, A.M., Selckman, J., Timpe, M., and Wolfe, Z.R. (1982). Unification: nursing education and practice. *Nursing and Health Care, 3*(1), 18-25.

Canadian Association of University Schools of Nursing. (June 1993). Collaboration: A time to evaluate, *CAUSN Newsletter, 4,* WRCAUSN annual meeting and conference.

Chater, S. (1983). Faculty practice considerations in academic health centers' schools of nursing. In K. Barnard (Ed.), *Structure to outcome: Making it work* (pp. 59-65). Kansas City, MO: American Academy of Nursing.

Faculty of Nursing University of Alberta. *Joint appointments: Terms of reference.* Unpublished statement of definition, policies and procedures, role expectations and privileges, University of Alberta, Edmonton.

Fagin, C. (1985). Institutionalizing practice: Historical and future perspectives. In K. Barnard and G. Smith (Eds.), *Faculty practice in action.* Kansas City, MO: American Academy of Nursing.

Fagin, C. (1986). Institutionalizing faculty practice. *Nursing Outlook, 34,* 140-144.

Ford, L.C. (1980). Unification of nursing practice, education and research. *International Nursing Review, 27*(6), 178-183, 192.

Ford, L.C. (1981). Creating a center for excellence in nursing. In L.H. Aiken (Ed.), *Health policy and nursing practice* (pp. 242-255). New York: McGraw-Hill.

Ford, L.C. and Kitzman, H.J. (1983). Organizational perspectives on faculty practice: Issues and challenges. In K. Barnard (Ed.), *Structure to outcome: Making it work* (pp. 13-29). Kansas City, MO: American Academy of Nursing.

Hegyvary, S.T. (1991). Collaborative relationships for education and practice. *Journal of Professional Nursing, 7*(3), 148.

Joel, L. (1985). The Rutgers experience: One perspective on service-education collaboration. *Nursing Outlook, 33*(5), 220-224.

Lambert, C.E., and Lambert, V.A. (1988). Faculty practice: Unifier of nursing education and nursing service? *Journal of Professional Nursing, 4*(5), 345-355.

MacPhail, J. (1972). *An experiment in nursing: Planning, implementing, and assessing planned change.* Cleveland: Case Western Reserve University.

MacPhail, J. (1975). Promoting collaboration between education and service. *The Canadian Nurse 71*(5), 32-34.

MacPhail, J. (1980). Implementation and evaluation of the Case Western Reserve University unification model. In L.H. Aiken (Ed.), *Health policy and nursing practice.* (pp. 229-241). New York: McGraw-Hill.

MacPhail, J. (1983). Collaboration/unification models for nursing education and nursing service. In N.L. Chaska (Ed.), *The nursing profession: A time to speak* (pp. 637-649). New York: McGraw-Hill.

Millonig, V. (1986). Faculty practice: A view of its development, current benefits, and barriers. *Journal of Professional Nursing, 2*(3), 166-172.

Powers, M. (1976). The unification model in nursing, *Nursing Outlook, 24*(8), 482-487.

Royle, J. (1984). *Joint university/hospital or community health care agency appointments in nursing: History, structure and function.* Unpublished munuscript, McMaster University School of Nursing, Hamilton, Ontario.

Schlotfeldt, R.M. (1980). The development of a model for unifying nursing practice and nursing education. In L.H. Aiken (Ed.), *Health policy and nursing practice.* (pp. 218-228). New York: McGraw-Hill.

Schlotfeldt, R.M., and MacPhail, J. (1969a). An experiment in nursing: Rationale and characteristics. *American Journal of Nursing, 69*(5), 1018-1023.

Schlotfeldt, R.M., and MacPhail, J. (1969b). An experiment in nursing: Introducing planned change. *American Journal of Nursing, 69*(6), 1247-1251.

Schlotfeldt, R.M., and MacPhail, J. (1969c). An experiment in nursing: Implementing planned change. *American Journal of Nursing, 69*(7), 1475-1480.

Smith, D.M. (1959). Practice: A part of teaching. *Nursing Outlook, 7(3),* 134-135.

Smith, D.M. (1965). Education and service under one administration. *Nursing Outlook, 13*(2), 54-56.

Sovie, M.D. (1981a). Unifying education and practice: One medical center's design. I. J*ournal of Nursing Administration, 11*(1), 41-49.

Sovie, M.D. (1981b). Unifying education and practice: One medical center's design. II. *Journal of Nurs ing Administration, 11*(2), 30-32.

Spero, J. (1980). Faculty practice as one component of the faculty role. New York: National League for Nursing.

U.S. Nursing leaders. (1979). Statement of belief regarding faculty practice. *Nursing Outlook, 27*(3), 158.

Stinchcombe, A.L. (1968). *Constructing social theories.* New York: Harcourt, Brace & World.

Ullrich, R.A., and Wieland, G.F. (1980). *Organization theory and design.* Homewood, Ill: Richard D. Irwin.

CHAPTER TWENTY SEVEN

Monitoring Standards in Nursing Education

JANNETTA MacPHAIL

N ursing education programs in Canada were originally developed in hospital schools of nursing, primarily for the purpose of staffing the hospitals. This was the standard means of staffing, regardless of the size of the hospital. Indeed, some hospitals admitted as few as 10 to 12 students per year even in the 1950s. The only registered nurses in the hospitals were the head nurses, supervisors, and the director of nursing. Nursing students received instruction from a few nurses, who taught such courses as anatomy and physiology and nursing arts (basic procedures) in the classroom, and from physicians, who taught courses about diseases and medical or surgical treatments. The only clinical supervision was provided by head nurses and supervisors.

Schools of this nature proliferated in the early part of the twentieth century and continued into the 1940s and early 1950s, despite the recommendation of the Weir Report in 1932 that nursing education be organized and administered separately from the hospitals. This independent pattern of organization was promoted by Florence Nightingale in the nineteenth century. Nursing leaders, such as Isabel Hampton Robb and Mary Adelaide Nutting, recognized the need for a system to monitor standards of education, and worked for nurses within the professional nursing organizations to assume the monitoring role. Their goal was to devise a system requiring approval for new nursing programs, standards for existing schools of nursing that were equal to the new schools, and regular inspection of all programs to ensure that standards continued to be met.

■ ■ ■ ■

NURSING EDUCATION STANDARDS

Standards in nursing education are delineated by knowledgeable nurse educators who have expertise in the practice of nursing and in methods of education. Standards range from minimal to ideal, depending on the purpose for which they are defined. There are two basic mechanisms for monitoring educational programs: approval and accreditation. Approval is a process used to designate an educational institution's competence to prepare practitioners for entry to nursing practice; that is, it gives permission to operate a nursing program (Committee on Credentialing, 1979). The standards set by the monitoring body are usually minimal, whereas the standards established for accreditation of programs are intended to promote quality. "Accreditation is a process whereby institutions or programs are assessed and measured using a set of predetermined criteria which, if met, connote a basic level of quality" (Committee on Credentialing, 1979, p. 33).

Approval is a mandatory process, and minimal standards are established by a body authorized by provincial legislation or regulations pursuant to that legislation. Accreditation, voluntary and national in scope, measures institutions against criteria established by the accrediting body to promote quality. Accreditation of educational programs exists in many professions, but approval and monitoring of programs are unique to nursing. No other profession is governed by legislation that regulates the conduct of educational programs; however, nursing is the only profession that does not require university-level preparation for entry to practice. Because diploma-level education continues to exist in nursing, there is a potential for wide variability in standards; hence, the monitoring mechanism of approval is considered essential.

The purpose of any credentialing mechanism is to protect the public and ensure accountability to consumers. In nursing education programs, the consumers are the students, and patients are the ultimate consumers of the services provided by nursing students and by graduates of nursing programs. Because any system of credentialing also benefits those who are credentialed, whether institutions or individuals, a system of checks and balances within the credentialing mechanism is necessary to ensure that the public is protected. In approval and accreditation, standards provide the checks and balances that ensure that the practitioners prepared in nursing education programs are competent to enter the practice of professional nursing.

Approval of Programs in Nursing Education

In Canada, constitutional responsibility for education and health care rests with the individual provinces. Consequently, policies and mechanisms for monitoring standards in nursing education are defined by each province. This responsibility is delineated in legislation that regulates the conduct of educational programs, whether the programs are conducted in universities, colleges, or hospital schools of nursing. In all provinces except Alberta, Ontario, and Quebec, the responsibility for defining and monitoring standards in nursing education is assumed by the provincial nursing association. Although specific mechanisms for defining standards and the process for approval of basic nursing programs may vary among provinces, the profession controls the educational standards for the admission of new practitioners to the profession. (See Chapter 3.)

In Alberta, responsibility for approval of nursing programs is delegated by the Universities' Coordinating Council (UCC), which, under the terms of the Universities' Act, has ultimate responsibility for defining and monitoring standards for all postsecondary education in the province. The responsibility for regulating and monitoring nursing education is delegated by UCC to a Committee on Nursing Education, which is responsible to UCC and includes five representatives, two of whom are from college programs, two from hospital nursing programs, and one from university nursing programs. This committee sets standards and approves functions for the seven diploma programs located in community colleges and the four hospital schools of nursing (Nursing Education Committee, 1982). Because the two basic baccalaureate degree programs (University of Alberta and University of Calgary) must meet the standards and obtain approval within each university as designated by UCC for all university programs, they are not monitored and approved by the Nursing Education Committee.

In Ontario, the Health Disciplines Act was enacted in 1974 to "govern nursing as well as dental, medical, optometric and pharmaceutical practitioners, a unique approach to nursing legislation in Canada" (Prowse, 1983 p. 20). The College of Nurses of Ontario (CNO), which is responsible to the Minister of Health, fulfills the registration and discipline functions for registered nurses and registered nursing assistants in that province. Monitoring and approval of nursing education programs for the 23 diploma programs in community colleges, is conducted by the CNO, which has a contractual arrangement with the Ministry of Colleges and Universities for this purpose. The standards of the CNO were originally delineated through the Provincial Advisory Council on Nursing Education, which was later dissolved. The responsibility for standards was transferred to the Council of Regents, advisory to the Minister of Colleges and Universities, and in 1989 to the Ministry of Colleges and Universities (J. Legg, personal communication, April 17, 1990). One exception to this approval mechanism is the diploma program at Ryerson Polytechnical Institute, where the Academic Council is authorized for the monitoring and approval functions. This exception may be explained by the fact that Ryerson has degree-granting privileges and grants a degree in nursing. Monitoring and approval of the nine basic baccalaureate degree programs in universities is one of the major responsibilities of the Ontario Region Chapter of the Canadian Association of University Schools of Nursing (ORCAUSN), as mandated by the CNO to establish standards and an approval process. "The Approval Committee has an arm's length relationship with ORCAUSN Council. . . .Schools/faculties are reviewed at least every five years. This process now articulates with the CAUSN accreditation process so that programs that choose accreditation rather than approval, are not subject to two review processes" (CAUSN Anniversary Report, 1992, p. 12).

In Quebec, all postsecondary education, including nursing programs, is governed by the Ministry of Higher Education and Science. There has been no mechanism for approval of nursing programs, but a mechanism for approval is being developed for the diploma programs of the Collèges d'Enseignement Generals et Professionnels (CEGEP). University nursing programs are subject to the approval process required of all educational programs in their respective universities. The Ministry of Higher Education and Science, which was established in 1985, studied nursing manpower needs and diploma programs and decided that an approval and monitoring system was needed to ensure that standards are maintained. An approval program was tested and implemented in

1988 as a five-year monitoring process. The standards were developed with advice from the Ordre des Infirmières et Infirmiers du Quebec (L. Michon, personal communication, July 23, 1987).

Thus primary responsibility for approval of nursing education programs is delegated to the provincial nursing association in all provinces except those previously mentioned. One can expect considerable differences in the systems for regulation and monitoring because of the variety and number of nursing education programs. All provinces now have at least one university nursing program. Prince Edward Island was an exception with only one diploma program; however, "On November 9, 1988, a provincial government decision to phase out diploma nursing education in favour of a degree program was announced . . . a move supported by the professional nursing association, nurses' unions, employers and educators alike" (CNA Connection, 1989, p. 10). With the official opening of the baccalaureate degree in September 1992, Prince Edward Island became the first province in Canada to achieve the goal of a baccalaureate degree as the minimal entry level into nursing.

Nursing education programs in colleges exist in all provinces except Newfoundland, New Brunswick, Nova Scotia, and Prince Edward Island. Hospital schools of nursing, which were initially the only type of nursing education program in all provinces, ceased to exist in Ontario, Quebec, and Saskatchewan in the 1970s. The governments in those three provinces phased out hospital schools of nursing and transferred the responsibility for diploma-level education to the college system. In 1989, the last remaining hospital school of nursing in British Columbia at Vancouver General Hospital was phased out when it was merged with the University of British Columbia School of Nursing. By 1994 there were in Canada 30 university baccalaureate degree programs holding membership in the CAUSN and 111 diploma programs, of which 19 are hospital schools of nursing; 80 are located in colleges; and 12 are collaborative programs with a baccalaureate degree program offering the option of a diploma exit. The collaborative programs developed to date are identified in Chapters 4 and 25.

The standards for nursing education programs in each province cover areas such as administration and general organization, philosophy and objectives; faculty; students; curriculum; educational resources and facilities, records, and reports; and evaluation. Approval must be obtained to establish a new program in nursing, and monitoring for continued approval occurs at 5-year intervals. Approval must also be obtained to eliminate a nursing program. The approval process involves submitting a report before a visit by persons designated by the authorized body to assume this responsibility. These individuals are normally qualified registered nurses who report their recommendations to the appropriate body. In most provinces, nursing education programs in universities are required to meet the standards defined by the university according to an Act governing the universities; it is not usually necessary for these programs to participate in the approval process defined for the diploma programs located in colleges and hospital schools of nursing.

Although the approval mechanism in all provinces is designed to ensure compliance with minimal standards, it is important that the standards and the process by which they are implemented ensure that nursing students are adequately prepared to enter practice. Delineating adequate preparation for entry is the subject of much debate and has always been a major issue in nursing education. In the days when almost all nursing students were prepared in hospital schools of nursing and each hospital recruited its own graduates, few questions were asked about the adequacy of preparation. The inbreeding that resulted from this system may have fostered obedience and strict adherence to the status quo. At that time, the emphasis was on procedures and technical preparation as opposed to the broader education that was encouraged after the initiation of university nursing programs. It has been difficult for some nurses in practice settings to accept the fact that graduating students are novices, not expert practitioners, as tended to be the perception regarding new graduates in the past. However, such an attitude was unrealistic because new graduates, even then, had much to learn. No other profession expects expert performance from newly graduated practitioners.

Another issue in the approval process pertains to the delineation of minimal standards. Who decides what constitutes minimal and what standards are considered more than minimal? It is important that standards be defined by well-prepared, competent nurses. Definition is possible within the professional associations and also in Alberta by the Committee on Nursing Education that is responsible to the UCC. In Alberta, when the Nursing Profession Act of 1984 was being formulated, the professional association's goal was to transfer responsibility for the approval process from the UCC to the professional association. Because the Alberta government demanded conditions the profession could not accept as the price for such a change, thus endangering the new act, responsibility for the approval process was left with the UCC. Although the responsibility for delineating standards and the approval mechanism remains with professional nurses, there is no doubt that the ideal in all provinces is to have the authority for this important regulatory mechanism remain with the professional associations. One exception may be Ontario, where the CNO, rather than the Registered Nurses Association of Ontario (RNAO), has the responsibility for registration and discipline.

The question of whether all programs should be under the same approval mechanism will continue as long as there is more than one type of program preparing students for entry to nursing practice. This will no longer be an issue when the goal of a required baccalaureate degree for entry to practice is attained. We hope this will be the case by the year 2000. Nurses in all provinces are working diligently to attain that goal even though they are fully aware of the barriers to be overcome and the resistance raised by nurses who feel threatened in spite of a grandparenting clause that would apply for those graduating before the year 2000. There is also some opposition to the position from outside the profession. Another problem that is prevalent in imposing regulatory mechanisms is avoiding rigidity in the standards and allowing for flexibility within the system. It is important that standards be defined broadly enough to allow for differences and creative approaches while maintaining basic accountability to the public and to the students, who are direct consumers of nursing education.

■ ■ ■ ■

ACCREDITATION OF NURSING EDUCATION PROGRAMS

No system for accreditation of nursing education programs was present in Canada until 1986, when the Canadian Association of University Schools of Nursing (CAUSN) approved the establishment of an accreditation program for university nursing programs after devoting 12 years to the development of an accreditation program. The major impetus for the program was that nursing was one of the few health sciences educational programs that did not have a system for accreditation (Joint Working Group, 1977). French states:

> In 1972 CAUSN was designated as the accrediting agency for university programs in nursing. In 1974 CAUSN established a committee on accreditation to develop a program of accreditation for university based programs in nursing. Recognizing the need for a method to stimulate the development of educational programs that are responsive to societal needs, and the dangers inherent in the accreditation process, CAUSN demanded a program that would support and promote change. The criteria on which the accreditation process was to be based had to reflect attributes of change and development. The major objective of the program of accreditation was to ensure that the educational programs were preparing the quality of practitioner required to deal effectively with existing and future health problems. Through the process of accreditation, institutions would be encouraged to engage in a process of self-evaluation, i.e., to study the goals of its educational program(s) and the means of attaining those goals (1982, p. 2).

From 1974 to 1984, the CAUSN Committee on Accreditation examined existing programs of accreditation, including the National League for Nursing (NLN) accreditation program in the United States, which had existed since 1952. The nursing accreditation program was conducted from 1939 to 1952 by the National League for Nursing Education, precursor of the NLN. Three major qualities were proposed by Allen (1977) and adopted by CAUSN as the criteria by which programs would be evaluated. These qualities were: (1) relevance to the trends in society that have an impact on the health needs of the community; (2) accountability, defined as the extent to which the program teaches students that the primary responsibility in nursing is to the client; and (3) relatedness or the extent to which parts of the program support and build on other parts, thereby promoting the achievement of goals. Subsequently, a fourth criterion, uniqueness, was adopted. It was defined as "the extent to which a program capitalizes on the resources within its particular setting" (CAUSN, 1978, p. 3).

The CAUSN Committee on Accreditation developed procedures for applying these criteria in the process of accreditation. A number of university nursing programs across Canada were involved as test sites in developing standards and instruments. Thus, the program of accreditation for university-based nursing programs evolved over 12 years before being accepted for general implementation by CAUSN Council in June, 1986. This accreditation program was launched in May of 1987 (Kirkwood and Bouchard, 1992).

CAUSN implements its accreditation function through a Board of Accreditation, which includes six members appointed by CAUSN Council who function within the policies and guidelines established by the Association. To provide an additional link between the CAUSN Executive Committee and the Board of Accreditation, and to facilitate future planning, the President Elect of CAUSN was assigned in 1994 specific responsibility for monitoring the accreditation program (Wood, 1994). By 1994, 12 of the university nursing programs that are members of CAUSN, were reviewed and accredited either for a 3- or 7-year period (McBride, 1994). Initially, most of the programs seeking accreditation were in Ontario, Quebec and Nova Scotia, the three provinces in which accreditation is an option to the program approval mechanism (J. Bouchard, personal communication, August 24, 1993; CAUSN Newsletter, December, 1991; CAUSN Newsletter, December, 1993). New baccalaureate degree programs have an option of being reviewed for candidacy while still in a developmental stage (CAUSN Newsletter, September 1989). To date two programs have been granted candidacy status. Ten programs have been scheduled for accreditation review over the next 5 years, 4 of which are reaccreditation reviews (McBride, 1994).

Within CAUSN's framework, "accreditation has two main purposes: (1) the support and improvement of standards of baccalaureate and graduate nursing programs in CAUSN member institutions; and (2) the recognition of programs that have been reviewed and have met specific standards" (CAUSN Newsletter, 1989, p. 1). CAUSN's policy is "that once a member unit has received notice from the Board of Accreditation concerning its accreditation status, and has had opportunity to respond, and if no appeal is pending, then it becomes public information and it will be published in the CAUSN Newsletter" (CAUSN Council, 1989). Thus accreditation status will become known to recipients of the CAUSN Newsletter, including all 30 member institutions and all individual members of the four regional chapters of CAUSN: Atlantic Region (ARCAUSN), Quebec Region (QRCAUSN), Ontario Region (ORCAUSN), and Western Region (WRCAUSN). The information published in CAUSN Newsletters to date identifies 12 universities that have been reviewed and accredited, but not whether for a 3-year or 7-year period (CAUSN Newsletter, Summer 1994). There is no indication of a denial of accreditation. To date there has been no stated means of providing information about the accreditation status of schools to prospective students, to guidance counsellors, or to nurses interested in earning a baccalaureate degree in nursing. However, the CAUSN Council decided that such information should be in the public domain, and steps are to be taken to make it known to the groups mentioned (J. Bouchard, personal communication, April 25, 1990).

In the United States, where the National League for Nursing (NLN) has been responsible for accreditation of all nursing programs since 1952, the listing of accredited programs appears regularly in the official journal of NLN and is published annually in booklet form. However, it includes only accredited programs and does not provide information as to whether programs not listed have failed to meet required standards or simply did not seek accreditation, which is a voluntary process. McCloskey (1985) and others question whether the concept of public accountability is actually fulfilled when accreditation bodies publicize only programs that have been accredited and do not release information about those that have not.

■ ■ ■ ■

FINANCING ACCREDITATION

Financing the accreditation program has been a major concern. In 1977, CAUSN submitted a proposal to the WK Kellogg Foundation for possible funding; however, support was not obtained. The foundation was approached again in 1979, but by 1980 there were strong indications that support would not be forthcoming. Consequently, CAUSN proceeded with plans for implementing the program, and a special annual fee, assessed to all university nursing programs, was kept in reserve to support the accreditation program. This fee, which was initially $1000 per school per year, was reduced to $500 in 1981. When the accreditation program was implemented in 1987, thus completing a review of the first nursing program to seek accreditation, a specific fee for the review had not been established. Therefore, a fee was charged based on the amount of involvement with each nursing program (J. Bouchard, [personal communication], April 25, 1990). However, it became obvious that additional funding was needed. In November of 1989, CAUSN Council approved a fee of $3000 to be instituted in the 1989-90 academic year and to be increased to $4500 for 1990-91 and 1991-92. CAUSN Council also stated that the accreditation program should become a cost-recovery program over the next 5 to 7 years (CAUSN Council, 1989).

The cost of the program includes fiscal costs and costs related to the development of graduate programs, including the development of doctoral programs in nursing which began as recently as January 1991; development of research in nursing to advance nursing knowledge and improve practice; and development of exemplary nursing practice in settings where students learn to nurse and faculty continue to practice and conduct research. The problem is the amount of time required for a faculty or school to conduct a self-study and for faculty participation in the visitation and review processes for programs other than their own. Time thus expended is not available to pursue other goals. French (1984) states:

> A program of accreditation had to facilitate, not impede the achievement of these goals. Accreditation was to be conducted with a minimum of effort, cost and time. It was to promote the interest of the educational consumers and the public. Educational primacy and the portability of educational qualification were identified as basic objectives of accreditation (p. 3).

Thomas, Arseneault, Bouchard, Cote, and Stanton (1992) reported that the schools that completed the evaluation tools designed to evaluate the accreditation process, indicated that "the self-study process was found to be very time-consuming . . . even though it increased awareness and stimulated discussion about the programme among faculty and students" (p. 41). Thomas and Arseneault (1992) concur that the self-study is time-consuming and increases faculty workload and stress, but is also rewarding because it fosters self-development and reinforces issues that have already been recognized.

The programs that have not yet sought accreditation will have to decide if they will do so, since it is a voluntary option and not a mandatory requirement such as approval. The $3000 accreditation fee for 1989-90 was increased to $4500 for 1990-91, and to $5,000 in 1993 (J. Bouchard, personal communication, August 24, 1993). Their decisions may be based on the availability of financial resources and time to do the self-study, or on other factors, such as the benefits of having accreditation status within the system of higher education. There is no doubt that an accreditation system encourages self-study and peer review by faculty and staff of an institution. Self-study and peer review can be achieved through internal review, which is a common practice in most universities across Canada. In fact, internal reviews may be conducted every 5 years; in these cases, thought must be given to the number of times the self-study process and the review procedure can be carried out within an academic unit.

The major issue pertaining to the CAUSN accreditation program is whether 30 university nursing education units in Canada can support such a program with only annual membership fees plus a special accreditation fee and still obtain services from CAUSN. In 1985, the basic annual membership fee was increased from $1000 to $1500, along with the established fee of $3.00 per full-time (FTE) student, which could amount to a total annual fee of $4000 for schools with large enrollments. In 1988, the basic annual fee was increased by 15% to $1750 plus the same per FTE student fee; however, this fee structure was still not adequate for CAUSN to fulfill its goals. Consequently, in November 1989, CAUSN Council voted in a new fee structure that was begun in the 1990-91 academic year. It is based on the number of FTE students enrolled in a faculty/school of nursing, using the FTE formula (3.5 part-time students = 1 FTE) used by Statistics Canada. The range of annual membership fees is as follows: $3000 for 1 to 99 FTE students, $3500 for 100 to 199, $4000 for 200 to 299, $4500 for 300 to 399, $5000 for 400 to 499, and $5500 for more than 500 (CAUSN Council, 1989). Whether the annual income generated by this fee structure, along with the $5000 accreditation fee paid by universities seeking accreditation and the $500 accreditation program fee assessed the universities not seeking accreditation annually, will be enough to support all CAUSN programs, has yet to be determined. Thomas et al indicated that: "It is difficult at this time to evaluate the long term financial feasibility of the accreditation programme, given the variability in the number of programmes requesting reviews, particularly during times of budgetary constraint in post-secondary institutions. Financial viability must be monitored. The potential for multiple three-year reviews could affect the feasibility of the existing program" (1992, p. 44). Nor is it known whether universities will be able to afford the time required for the actual process if they seek accreditation and if faculty choose to be involved in the peer review process of accreditation in other institutions.

■ ■ ■ ■

OTHER ISSUES REGARDING ACCREDITATION

Many issues other than cost are related to accreditation in general and to accreditation in nursing education. One benefit purported by supporters of accreditation is that it facilitates transfer of students from one institution to another. This may be true in the United States where there are thousands of colleges and universities, including private ones; but it may not be true in Canada. Knowledge of accredited programs may help a student select a transfer institution, but transferability of courses depends on the equivalence of courses in the institutions and the student's achievement in these courses. In Canada, the low number of private institutions and the geography of the country discourage frequent transfer.

McCloskey (1985) questions the extent to which accreditation helps prospective students decide which institution to attend. She notes that most students are unaware of accreditation status and that it is doubtful that guidance counsellors in high schools use this information. Whereas accreditation status may have relevance for prospective students in the United States, where there are approximately 500 accredited baccalaureate nursing programs from which to choose, it is questionable if this would apply in Canada, where there are 30 baccalaureate degree programs located in public universities that are required to give preference to residents from their own provinces. Substantial provincial support for higher education has been responsible for this preference although provisions of the Canadian Charter of Rights may soon eliminate such policies.

One of the stated goals of CAUSN's accreditation program is to raise the standards of nursing education in Canada. The question of whether accreditation promotes quality is difficult to answer because of problems in measuring quality. Young (1976) states, "Accreditation has never defined 'quality of education' except in terms of numbers of Ph.D.'s produced, books published, grants received, and the like; the validity of these criteria has never been demonstrated" (p. 622). The task of evaluating the accreditation process was delegated by CAUSN Council to the Committee on Accreditation. Criteria for evaluation were identified and defined, as were sources of data for each criterion and the data collection instruments. Thus, CAUSN is endeavoring to assess the validity of the four criteria selected for the accreditation process, as well as the validity and reliability of the instruments used to collect data. This process will continue as other programs seek accreditation.

An important question that is often raised is the effect of accreditation on research, which is important in university nursing programs. In the past, faculty members have tended to devote more attention to teaching and curriculum development than to research. Unless the criteria emphasize and require research, the process of accreditation may not help promote it, as evidenced by events in the United States for many years. In fact, U.S. participants in accreditation have reported that the time and effort devoted to accreditation impeded the progress of research. The difficulties lie in the amount of time required by the self-study and visitation processes, and the time required for faculty to serve as visitors and review board members. This time could have been devoted to research. What can accreditation programs do to promote research? If an accreditation program does not promote research and the application of research findings in teaching and practice, can one say that it is promoting quality in nursing education? Another question to be addressed is whether accreditation will help programs obtain what they need. This is considered a potential benefit by some proponents of accreditation who assume that if the accreditors note a deficiency and the recommended action to correct it requires infusion of resources, this will influence the administration to grant funding. Although this may occur in some cases, in times of financial constraint it may not.

With the development of collaborative programs between diploma programs and basic baccalaureate degree programs in universities, a new issue will have to be considered. Which approval mechanism will be used for the diploma programs that are collaborating with baccalaureate degree programs, particularly since most of the collaborative programs offer the option of a diploma exit? For example, the University of Alberta Faculty of Nursing has a collaborative program with five diploma programs at the following educational institutions: Grant MacEwan Community College, Health Sciences Division; Misericordia Hospital School of Nursing; Red Deer College, Department of Nursing; Royal Alexandra Hospital School of Nursing; and the University of Alberta Hospitals School of Nursing.

Whether the accreditation program will be or should be extended to involve graduate education in nursing, as well as baccalaureate education, is another issue to be addressed in Canada. Wood (1994) states: "The issue of accreditation of graduate programs will be brought to the [CAUSN] Council meeting (December 1994) for discussion. If Council agrees, a process will be started to develop the criteria and system for graduate program accreditation" (p. 6). In the United States, master's degree programs in nursing have been part of the accreditation process for many years; however nursing education administrators and nursing faculty involved in doctoral education have strongly resisted any extension of accreditation to the doctoral level. To date, their resistance has been effective in preventing movement in this direction. Will the same issue arise in Canada with the development of doctoral education in nursing?

■ ■ ■ ■

CONCLUSION

It is important to have standards for nursing education and a system to monitor the achievement of standards and promote quality in nursing education. The question in Canada is whether the 30 university nursing education units that comprise the membership of CAUSN can afford to support and be involved in several systems of monitoring, the approval process in provinces where university programs are monitored, intrainstitutional evaluation programs where they exist, and the accreditation process. To advance nursing knowledge, improve practice, and gain acceptance of nursing as an equal and legitimate participant in universities, research must be advanced and made an integral part of the faculty role for all faculty in tenured/tenurable appointments.

The goal of accreditation, to promote excellence, depends on the extent to which the process influences standards of education. One of the hazards, as identified in the Study of Credentialing in Nursing, is that "continual upgrading or revision of standards, however, can sometimes create unrealistic movement away from the concurrent goals of society, as can static standards impede progress and innovation" (Committee on Credentialing, 1979, p. 34). There is need to focus on student outcome criteria as a more valid index of educational quality because the criteria have tended to be structure-process oriented, dealing more with the teaching-learning environment than with the actual learning that takes place (Committee on Credentialing, 1979).

Accountability to the public is of vital importance in any credentialing mechanism. This involves the development and maintenance of programs that the public expects will prepare practitioners who can deliver a high level of care. In addition, accountability involves the credentialing body. This organization must be willing "to assure that the standards, criteria, and process through which credentials are conferred and retained are valid and reliable measures of the quality of expertise or service associated with the credential" (Committee on Credentialing, 1979, p. 45). If the public is to be served, there must be a means to maintain standards and to demonstrate and assess the accountability factor.

REFERENCES

Allen, M. (1977). *Evaluation of Educational Programmes In Nursing*. Geneva: World Health Organization.

American Nurses Association Committee on Credentialing. (1979). *The study of credentialing in nursing: A new approach: Vol. 1. The report of the committee*. Kansas City, MO: Author.

Canadian Association of University Schools of Nursing. (1978). *Development of a method to promote growth and change in university schools of nursing and nursing in general*. Ottawa: The Association.

Canadian Association of University Schools of Nursing Council. Minutes of meeting of November 17, 1989.

Staff. (1989, September). *CAUSN Newsletter*, p. 1-4.

Staff. (1990, June). *CAUSN Newsletter*, p. 1-4.

Staff. (1991, December). *CAUSN Newsletter*, p. 1-4.

Staff. (1993, December). *CAUSN Newsletter*, p. 1-4.

Canadian Association of University Schools of Nursing. (1992). *Anniversary report*. Ottawa: Author.

Canadian Nurses Association. (1993). *Diploma schools of nursing in Canada: Admissions, enrollment and graduations, 1992*. Ottawa: CNA Research Department.

CAUSN Newsletter/ACEUN-Bulletin d'Informacion. (September 1989). p. 1-4.

CAUSN Newsletter/ACEUN-Bulletin d'Informacion. (June 1990). p. 1-4.

CAUSN Newsletter/ACEUN-Bulletin d'Informacion. (December 1991). p. 1-4.

CAUSN Newsletter/ACEUN-Bulletin d'Informacion. (December 1993). p. 1-4.

CNA Connection. (1989). Baccalaureate education comes to PEI. *The Canadian Nurse, 85*(3), 10.

Canadian Nurses Association. (1993). *Enrollment in university schools of nursing by programs, sex and full-time/part-time, 1992*. Ottawa: CNA Research Department.

Committee on Accreditation. (1985). *Accreditation: Criteria and Process for Baccalaureate Program in Nursing: Book I*. Canadian Association of University Schools of Nursing.

French, S. (1982). Design for accreditation of educational programs in nursing. In M.S. Henderson (Ed.), *Recent advances in nursing no. 4: Nursing education* (pp. 81-102). London: Churchill Livingstone.

French, S. (1984). *The development of an accreditation program for university programs in nursing in Canada*. Document submitted to Canadian Association of University Schools of Nursing.

Joint Working Group of the Association of Universities and Colleges of Canada and the Association of Community Colleges in Canada. (1977). *Report on the joint working group on coordination of accreditation of health, sciences, educational programs*. Ottawa: The Association.

Kirkwood, R., and Bouchard, J. (1992). *"Take counsel with one another": A beginning history of the Canadian Association of University Schools of Nursing, 1942-1992*. Ottawa: Canadian Association of University Schools of Nursing.

McBride, W. (1994). Executive Director's message, CAUSN Newsletter, Summer 1994, 2-3.

McCloskey, J.C. (1985). Accreditation of nursing education: An overview and issues. In J.C.

McCloskey and H.K. Grace (Eds.). *Current Issues in Nursing* (2nd ed.) (pp. 507-524). London: Blackwell Scientific Publications.

Nursing Education Committee, Universities' Coordinating Council. (1982). *Regulations governing nursing education programs in the province of Alberta Leading to nursing registration.* Edmonton, Alberta: Author.

Prowse, J.A. (1983). *Nursing Legislation in Canada: An overview for health services administration.* Unpublished master's thesis, The University of Alberta, Edmonton, Alberta: Department of Health Services Administration.

Thomas, B. Arseneault, A., Bouchard, J., Coté, E., and Stanton S. (1992). Accreditation of university nursing programmes in Canada. *The Canadian Journal of Nursing Research,* 24(2), 33-48.

Thomas, B., and Arseneault, A. (1992). Organizing your school for accreditation. *The Canadian Journal of Nursing Research,* 24(2), 58-59.

Wood, M. (1994). President Elect's message, CAUSN Newsletter, Fall 1994, 5-6.

Young, K.E. (1976). Issues in accreditation. *Nursing Outlook,* 24(10), 622-624.

CHAPTER TWENTY EIGHT

Credentialing in Nursing

JANET ROSS KERR

T he study of credentialing in nursing is illuminating, for it draws attention to the growth and development of nursing as a profession. The relation of credentialing to professionalization can be seen in what has been referred to as "the natural history of professionalization" (Moloney, 1986, p. 23). Wilensky (1964) has asserted that this history is recognizable and sequential in nature:

> There is a typical process by which the established professions have arrived . . . [they] begin doing the work full time and stake out a jurisdiction; the early masters of the technique or adherents of the movement become concerned about standards of training and practice and set up a training school, which, if not lodged in universities at the start, makes academic connections within two or three decades; the teachers and activists then achieve success in promoting effective organization, first local, then national. . . . Toward the end, legal protection appears; at the end, a formal code of ethics is adopted (p. 144).

The presence of a specialized knowledge base is fundamental to the processes and mechanisms of credentialing in nursing. Goode (1960) noted that the perception of the defining characteristics of this knowledge determines identification and acceptance of a field as a profession. These may be briefly summarized as follows: 1) the knowledge and skills are abstract and consist of principles considered relevant to everyday situations; 2) there is a belief that the specialized knowledge will produce positive results when applied to real problems; 3) those in the profession are involved in developing and applying the knowledge base and in providing expert opinion in difficult cases; and 4) the knowledge and skills are complex, and only a few have the ability to acquire them. (Goode, 1960).

In a historical sense, Canadian nurses recognized early in this century that the knowledge and skills fundamental to the profession were important and that unqualified and unskilled practitioners could harm patients for whom they cared. They concluded that not only was it important to ensure that nurses were graduates of recognized schools of nursing, but also that professional standards were needed to regulate nursing education and practice.

363

Hospitals in Canada did not need to be encouraged to establish schools of nursing in the late nineteenth and early twentieth centuries. They all sought to emulate the successful Nightingale model in Britain and to ensure an adequate number of staff members as well as a qualified and inexpensive staff. However, this design was the antithesis of what Nightingale intended, as her school was supported by the Nightingale endowment and was financially and administratively independent.

Evidence of graduation from a school of nursing was the earliest form of credentialing. The period during which this occurred was also characterized by a concerted drive by nursing leaders to secure legislation for registration of nurses to ensure that the educated would be differentiated from the uneducated for the protection of the public.

In a general sense, credentialing issues are similar today, although the nature and extent of knowledge and skills that must be acquired to practise nursing have changed. The need for recognizing standards in programs, knowing the meaning of a certificate, securing qualified staff for many areas of specialization, establishing standards at the national level, and ensuring that practitioners update knowledge and maintain competence throughout their careers are important areas for discussion and study. However, questions pertaining to protection of the public from unscrupulous, unqualified, and unskilled practitioners are fundamental to credentialing processes and mechanisms.

■■ ■■ ■■ ■■

CREDENTIALING MECHANISMS

The Canadian Nurses Association (CNA) (1982) has described credentialing as "a term used to refer to all those processes by which individuals or institutions (or one or more of their programs) are designated as having met established standards at a specified point in time, by an agent recognized as qualified to do so" (p. 5), which means recognizing the individuals who have met the established standards in particular areas by awarding credentials. Thus, individuals who have knowledge and skills in a certain area are distinguished from those who do not have such skills. Describing credentialing as a system of checks and balances seems appropriate. Nursing has two main credentialing mechanisms: professional and educational. On the professional side, registration and licensure are awarded to individuals for practice of the profession.

■■ ■■ ■■ ■■

THE MOVEMENT TO SECURE LEGISLATION FOR REGISTRATION

The drive for registration of nurses occurred early in the development of the profession in Canada. This was the issue that brought nurses together in professional organizations. The formation of the first national and international organization for nurses in 1893, the American Society of Superintendents of Training Schools for Nursing of the United States and Canada, was followed by the foundation of the Associated Alumnae of the United States and Canada in 1896. The purpose of the latter organization was "to secure legislation to differentiate the trained from the untrained" (CNA, 1968, p. 35). Both organizations were initially headed by one of the most important nursing leaders of the time, Isabel Hampton Robb, a Canadian nurse from Ontario who was the first superintendent of nurses at The Johns Hopkins Hospital in Baltimore, Maryland. These groups stimulated the formation of many other professional nursing organizations at the local, regional, and national levels in the United States and Canada, all of which worked to complete the groundwork necessary for the passage of legislation to regulate nursing in the provinces. The publication of the *American Journal of Nursing* in 1900 and the *Canadian Nurse* in 1905 helped the cause.

The American and Canadian groups separated as activity intensified, and it was evident that the battle for passage of the legislation had to be fought regionally. In Canada, it was fought in the provinces because the British North America Act of 1867 provided that the legislatures of each province be given exclusive right to make laws in relation to health and education. The Canadian Society of Superintendents of Training Schools for Nurses emerged in 1907, followed by the Provisional Society of the Canadian Nurses Association of Trained Nurses in 1908. The first president of both groups was Mary Agnes Snively, a graduate of Bellevue Hospital in New York who had headed the School of Nursing at Toronto General Hospital since 1884 (CNA, 1968).

From the beginning, there have been valid reasons for requiring registration. Professional registration and licensure makes the benefits that accrue from the services of a highly skilled group available to society and protects society from those who are not highly skilled, as well as from those who might knowingly misuse their knowledge and skills to the disadvantage of the populace. In each province in Canada, local graduate nurse groups joined forces to become provincial nurses' associations and sought legislation for registration of nurses. These nurses believed that registration acts that set standards for training schools would also improve the quality of care.

Two powerful social forces influenced the drive for legislation for the registration of nurses. The first was the consciousness-raising regarding women's rights that was part of the movement for the enfranchisement of women. The second was that nurses' services were especially valued during World War I, when many nurses served with dedication and valour. The passage of legislation in every province over a 12-year period may have been facilitated by these factors and represented general recognition of the need for a system to ensure that nurses were qualified.

There was considerable activity for a number of years before legislation was first passed in 1910, when Nova Scotia passed an act that made registration voluntary and allowed nongraduate nurses to register. Succeeding acts in other provinces were more restrictive regarding the standards incorporated into the legislation. Minimum standards for admission and curricula in schools of nursing were set, as were rules governing registration and discipline of practising nurses. Ontario was the last province to approve legislation for nursing because of a lobby against the legislation led by hospitals whose administrators feared that educational standards for maintaining schools could not be met. Opposition also arose from nurses who felt they could not meet the qualifications. These objections were overcome or overruled, and legislation was passed in that province in 1922 (Sabin, Price, and Sellers, 1973).

In all provinces, the initial legislation gave the provincial nursing association the responsibility for administering the legislation. In Alberta, the Registered Nurses Act was passed in 1916, and uniform registration examinations were instituted in 1919. This statute was unusual because it placed nursing education under the aegis of the Senate of the University of Alberta. A chronology documenting the process of securing registration in each of the provinces is presented in Table 28.1.

■ ■ ■ ■

THE CASE FOR MANDATORY LICENSURE

Licensure laws were designed to protect the public from unethical and incompetent practitioners, not to protect the nursing profession from competition. The only justifiable reason for adopting legislation to guarantee professionals such a right is to protect the public from unqualified and incompetent practitioners. The legislation cannot and must not bestow a special benefit on people who have completed a certain educational program and demonstrated certain qualifications where there is no public protective component. In recent years, there has been public concern about self-rule by professional groups, the fear being that power may be exercised in the interest of the profession. The thrust of the consumer movement is to present challenges in areas in which the consumer interest may not be protected (International Council of Nurses, 1986). The health-care field is no exception in such efforts. This phenomenon and the fact that it is not easy to change existing legislation that governs professional groups explain why all provinces have not yet replaced their original permissive legislation with mandatory statutes. However, the provinces that have achieved mandatory licensure have done so by emphasising the need to assure the public that licensed nurses have met an appropriate standard of practice, as determined by the profession.

All Canadian nursing jurisdictions with the exception of Manitoba and Ontario have legislative provision for mandatory registration of nurses. The presence of a statutory definition of the scope of nursing practice is an important feature of legislature in jurisdictions with mandatory licensure. The permissive Manitoba statute also contains a definition of practice. However, the Manitoba legislation places the onus on the employer to hire only registered nurses to perform functions incorporated in the definition of nursing. Nurses' functions are delineated more explicitly when a definition of nursing practice is incorporated into the statute. The potential for overlap with functions performed by other health-care workers that exists in mandatory jurisdictions may be addressed through specific exemptions or by extending rights only to health-care workers practising by virtue of other statutes (Prowse, 1983). In 1994, Ontario enacted legislation affecting all health professions. This legislation, the Regulated Health Professions Act (RHPA), provides for the regulation of 23 professional groups under 21 individual professional acts. Each individual act describes a scope of practice and allows for restrictive use of title. To ensure public protection, however, the RHPA identifies 13 controlled acts that may be performed only by specific registered members as identified in the individual act. In this manner, it is the activity that is licensed, not the individual provider.

TABLE 28.1 Chronology of Legislation Regulating Nursing in Canadian Jurisdictions

Province	Date Legislation First Enacted	Current Status of Legislation	Date Mandatory Legislation First Enacted
British Columbia	1918	Mandatory	1988
Alberta	1916	Mandatory	1983
Saskatchewan	1917	Mandatory	1988
Manitoba	1913	Permissive	—
Ontario	1922	Permissive	—
Quebec	1920	Mandatory	1964
New Brunswick	1916	Mandatory	1984
Nova Scotia	1910	Mandatory	1985
Prince Edward Island	1922	Mandatory	1969
Newfoundland	1931	Mandatory	1953
Northwest Territories	1975	Mandatory	1975
Yukon Territory	1994	Mandatory	1994

Sources: Good and Kerr, 1973, p.189; Prowse, 1983, pp.10-28, 36-41; L. Dekker (personal communication, July 13, 1994).

Registration and licensure ensure a minimum level of safe practice at the time of initial registration. Those registered are eligible for re-registration annually if practice requirements are met and there is no evidence of unsafe practice. New knowledge is continually introduced to the field, and the individual must maintain and extend competence to meet the changing requirements. The nursing profession has wrestled with the problem of maintaining competence in an effort to demonstrate public accountability. As Prowse (1983) has noted, "As a peer review mechanism, the registration/licensure provisions of Canadian nursing statutes have . . . an explicit or implicit capacity for assuring the continued competence, capability and good conduct of nursing practitioners" (p. 65). The merits of mandatory versus permissive continuing education programs have been debated at length. In most provinces, mandatory continuing education has been rejected in favour of requiring a certain number of days of employment within a specified time period and a record of satisfactory practice as evidence of current knowledge and skills.

The move toward offering refresher courses for those who have been out of practice, upgrading programs, and providing opportunities for continuing education has become an integral and essential part of the nursing education system, as the practice of a profession must incorporate a commitment to lifelong learning. The nurse has a legal and ethical duty to maintain competence. In the event that a nurse's conduct is questioned by a client, the practitioner may be called upon in a hearing of peers or in a court of law to provide evidence that reasonable effort has been expended to attend continuing education seminars and workshops in order to maintain competence in practice.

▬ ▬ ▬ ▬

REGISTRATION AND LICENSURE

Registration allows the profession to maintain an official roster of member nurses. To be named on a register, a nurse must be a member in good standing of the organization incorporating the statutory responsibility for registration. In the provinces that still have permissive registration, the legislation protects only the title of the registered nurse; that is, a person may practise nursing without being registered but may not use the initials *RN*. In acts that provide for mandatory registration, the nature of the service provided by the profession is defined. This means that those who do not meet the requirements of the legislation may not practise the profession. Title is protected, as in permissive acts, but the definition of nursing and the restriction of practice as it applies to registered nurses are the critical features that differentiate the two forms of legislation.

Requirements for initial registration are similar in all provinces. An applicant must be a graduate of an approved school of nursing. Minimum standards for nursing education are established by an approval body. In all provinces except Alberta, Ontario, and Quebec, the approval body is the professional association. In Alberta, the Universities' Coordinating Council has been designated under the Nursing Profession Act as the approval body. In Ontario, the Health Disciplines Act and the Regulated Health Professions Act give authority for approval and monitoring of diploma programs to the Ministry of Education and Training (for college programs) and to the Canadian Association of University Schools of Nursing, the Council of Ontario University Programs in Nursing, and the university senate or governing council (for university programs). In Quebec, the Ministry of Higher Education and Science holds responsibility for monitoring diploma programs in the Collèges d'Enseignement Général et Professional (CEGEP).

The terms *registration* and *licensure* have different meanings, although they are used interchangeably in some situations. As previously noted, *registration* refers to the listing of a member in good standing of an organization on the roster of members. *Licensure* refers to the granting by a government body of the exclusive right to practise nursing to a member in good standing. In provinces where registration is mandatory, the same process may also be described as *licensure*. Practice of the profession by any person who has not been granted such a right is prohibited and punishable by law.

▬ ▬ ▬ ▬

SPECIALIZATION IN NURSING

The tremendous change in the nature and scope of nursing practice in Canada in this century has taken place almost imperceptibly, but it has been an evolution with a profound effect on health care and society. It has become increasingly difficult to master the knowledge required for practice in every area in which nurses function. The burgeoning increases in knowledge in the health-care field have led to specialization in nursing, which has raised questions about ensuring competence in those practising in specialized areas.

The medical profession itself is highly specialized. The movement toward specialization in medicine has been strong and, to a certain extent, has influenced nursing. Although there has been an attempt to place more value on the role of the general practitioner in medicine, more physicians are specializing. Given the tremendous increase in medical knowledge, this trend is not surprising. Nursing is influenced by many of the factors that have led to more specialization in medicine, and the outcome has been the development of discrete and increasingly complex nursing specialties.

Transfer of functions from medicine to nursing is also of interest. Many functions that were previously restricted exclusively to medical practice have been redefined as nursing responsibilities. Although this is primarily a task-oriented approach to practice in an area in which functions overlap, it is important because the changes in medical practice that produce the changes in nursing practice are immediately apparent. It is also important to recognize that (1) transfer of functions among the health professions is an ongoing process; and (2) there will always be overlap of functions among professions. With increases in knowledge, skills, and functions, the nurse is in a pivotal position in the delivery of health care. The nurse of today assumes roles and functions that were expected of the general medical practitioner of yesterday. In fact, the general practitioner of yesterday might be overwhelmed at the complexity of nursing roles of today!

The reasons for the trend toward specialization in the nursing profession are the increase in knowledge and the corresponding increase in skill needed for sound judgment and decision making. There is an almost constant demand for nurses who have expertise in highly specialized areas, so nurses must recognize the specialized skills and value the knowledge they require.

■ ■ ■ ■

RECOGNITION OF SPECIALIZATION

To minimize confusion, the CNA has provided an interpretation of the term *specialty:* "A specifically defined area of clinical and functional nursing with a narrowed, in-depth focus, necessary for the safe delivery of the full range of services required in that area of nursing" (1982, p. 25). Specialization has become an important phenomenon in nursing practice. Canadian nurses have sought certification from programs in the United States to demonstrate knowledge in their areas of practice. However, specialization in the United States developed rapidly, and many organizations set themselves up as certification bodies from the outset. The American Nurses Association (ANA) developed some certification programs but entered the scene somewhat later than the majority of organizations. Because of the number of organizations that initiated certification programs in the United States, the ANA and the National League for Nursing (NLN) sponsored a credentialing study that recommended a centre for coordinating all programs. However, no action was taken on this recommendation (Committee for the Study of Credentialing in Nursing, 1979).

Because of quality control problems, Canadians have not wanted to emulate the U.S. system. At the June 1980 Biennial Convention of the CNA, in Vancouver, the CNA Board passed a resolution to study the feasibility of developing certification examinations in major nursing specialties. Consideration of the issues involved led the CNA to develop a policy statement on credentialing in nursing and to make a commitment to facilitate the development of certification in nursing specialties (CNA, 1982). Guidelines for a certification mechanism were adopted, and a certification program was designed (CNA, 1986a). The process involved designation of a specialty for certification, development of a certification examination by the Canadian Nurses Association Testing Services (CNATS), and certification of individuals. The CNA differentiated those acquiring certification in this manner from the clinical nurse specialist, who is designated as a nurse with advanced preparation in a clinical area at the master's level (CNA, 1986b).

The response of the national association to the issues presented by specialization and certification has been positive and is likely to augur well for future developments. Although it is important for the provinces to consider these matters, this is an area for the national association to provide leadership, for membership in specialty groups tends to be small. It is unlikely that the cost of developing a quality program could be borne by the province, and reciprocity would be an issue if different programs were developed in each province. Because specialization and certification are not part of basic preparation for practice (regulated by provincial legislation pursuant to the jurisdiction of provinces as designated in the Constitution Act), development of programs at the national level appears to be the most appropriate and reasonable course of action.

The development of a CNA Advisory Council "to provide a forum for discussions between the Council and the CNA board of directors on health and nursing issues" (CNA Connection, 1989b, p. 10) has enabled special interest groups to address the CNA. The approach to the certification process taken by the CNA is broad: "The designation process applies to an area of nursing rather than to a group or an association, and the process may be initiated by any group of nurses that is able to provide evidence that a specific nursing area meets the required criteria" (CNA Connection, 1989b, p. 10). A discussion paper produced by the Canadian Association of University Schools of Nursing (CAUSN) (1989), *"Specialization in Nursing and Nursing Education,"* stimulated a rebuttal by the CNA, which interpreted the paper as criticism of the specialty designation and certification processes. The CNA expressed the view that CAUSN's view of specialization was "technologically-oriented and therefore, narrow, regarding skills and knowledge base," whereas its own view emphasized "nurses' knowledge of illness patterns and therapies [and] patterns of response in certain situations, including physical and psychosocial aspects" (CNA Connection, 1989b, p. 10).

In 1981, the CNA agreed to develop a certification examination for the Canadian Council of Occupational Health Nurses, which had received a grant to develop this program. They hired the CNATS to develop the examination. Consultation services relative to the development of the examination were offered "on the understanding they would join the CNA certification program when it became a reality" (CNA Connection, 1989a, p. 7). However, the disappointing announcement was made that "following discussion and correspondence between CNA and the Canadian Council of Occupational Health Nurses Inc., the process of integrating the occupational health nursing examination into the CNA certification program has been suspended" because the occupational health nurses "would like more time to consider integration criteria, and [have] suggested waiting until at least 1991 to begin the process" (CNA Connection, 1990, p. 14). At that point, the CNA decided that groups that had been scheduled to enter the certification program after the Canadian Council of Occupational Health Nurses would be accommodated first (CNA Connection, 1990). Thus, the first specialty groups to complete a certification program were neuroscience nursing and nephrology nursing. However, in March 1992, occupational health nursing was integrated into the CNA Certification Program, bringing the total number of specialty areas available for certification to three.

Meanwhile, demand for still other certification programs continued to grow, and the CNA recognized the need to expand the existing program. Based on recommendations of an ad hoc committee, the CNA Board of Directors reaffirmed its commitment to certification by adopting a plan for the accelerated expansion of the program to the year 2000. The expanded certification program will initially offer certification to any specialty area with 10,000 or more nurses employed in that area in Canada. L.A. Patry, Certification Coordinator for the CNA, believes that this approach will provide the CNA with sufficient financial support to continue expanding the program (personal communication, October 3, 1994).

Although the development of its certification program has taken time and has had its share of challenges, the CNA has successfully brought special interest groups into the mainstream of professional association activities by establishing the process, developing an advisory council of representatives from specialty associations, and creating a position on the CNA board of directors for a representative from this group. The profession has been strengthened by these initiatives, and it is likely that such efforts will continue as more specialty groups become part of the certification program.

REFERENCES

Canadian Association of University Schools of Nursing. (1989). Specialization in nursing and nursing education. Ottawa: Author.

Canadian Nurses Association. (1968). *The leaf and the lamp*. Ottawa: Author.

Canadian Nurses Association. (1982). Credentialing in nursing: Policy statement and background paper. Ottawa: Author.

Canadian Nurses Association. (1986a). CNA's certification program: An information booklet. Ottawa: Author.

Canadian Nurses Association. (1986b). Statement on the clinical nurse specialist. Ottawa: Author.

CNA Connection. (1989a). *The Canadian Nurse, 85*(1), 7.

CNA Connection. (1989b). *The Canadian Nurse, 85*(9), 10.

CNA Connection. (1990). *The Canadian Nurse, 86*(1), 14.

Committee for the Study of Credentialing in Nursing. (1979). Credentialing in nursing: A new approach, *American Journal of Nursing, 19*(4), 674-683.

Good, S.R., and Kerr, J.C. (Eds.). (1973). *Contemporary issues in Canadian law for nurses.* Toronto: Holt, Rinehart & Winston of Canada, Ltd.

Goode, W.J. (1960). Encroachment, charlatanism, and the emerging professions: Psychology, sociology and medicine. *American Sociological Review, 25,* 903.

International Council of Nurses. (1986). *Report on the regulation of nursing: A report on the present, a position for the future.* Geneva: Author.

Moloney, M.M. (1986). *Professionalization of nursing: Current issues and trends.* Philadelphia: J.B. Lippincott Company.

Prowse, A.J. (1983). *Nursing legislation in Canada: An overview for health services administrators.* Unpublished master's thesis, The University of Alberta, Edmonton, AB.

Sabin, H., Price, D., and Sellers, B. (1973). Nursing: What it is and what it is not. In S. Good and J. Kerr (Eds.), *Contemporary issues in Canadian law for nurses,* (pp. 63-82). Toronto: Holt, Rinehart & Winston of Canada, Ltd.

Wilensky, H.L. (1964). The professionalization of everyone. *American Journal of Sociology, 70*(2), 143-144.

CHAPTER TWENTY NINE

Developing Specialty Certificate Programs With Credit toward the Baccalaureate Degree in Nursing

JANET ROSS KERR

I n its seventh decade of growth and development in Canada, baccalaureate degree education in nursing centres on generalist rather than specialist preparation. Because a large amount of essential clinical knowledge must be taught in a basic program, theory and practice in specialty clinical areas cannot be included. Diploma programs in nursing must adequately cover basic material and associated clinical experience in a shorter time than the university degree programs in nursing. A problem for nursing administrators responsible for ensuring that specialty practice areas are staffed with suitably qualified staff is that few professional nurses with the necessary preparation to practise in these particular areas are available. Most staff nurses working in specialty clinical areas have had on-the-job training because there has been no integrated system of specialty courses or programs creditable to baccalaureate degree programs.

When nursing programs first appeared in Canadian universities, they offered preparation in specialized areas: first in public health, beginning in 1920, and later in nursing education and nursing administration. In the 1960s and 1970s, preparation for public health nursing was phased into basic and post-RN baccalaureate programs, and certificate courses in teaching and administration were discontinued to allow institution of baccalaureate programs. Many programs, however, allowed the student to select courses in these subjects within degree programs. Until recently, most Canadian universities have not offered certificate programs in clinical nursing areas of specialty. The most notable exceptions were the Certificate Program in Advanced Practical Obstetrics offered by the

University of Alberta from 1944 to 1984, when it was phased into the master's degree program as a midwifery option, and the two-year Certificate Program in Outpost Nursing offered by Dalhousie University beginning in 1967.

Hospitals operating schools of nursing have, in the past, offered postgraduate programs in a number of specialty clinical nursing fields, including operating room; emergency; orthopaedic; neurosurgical; psychiatric; rehabilitation; eye, ear, nose, and throat; neonatal intensive care; and critical care. The last two programs have been common since the early 1970s, after the widespread introduction of intensive care units in hospitals. Community college nursing programs, instituted in the 1950s, also offer continuing education programs in a more narrow range of clinical specialty areas, principally critical care, long-term care, mental health, and occupational health. In recent years, hospitals have reduced the number and range of programs offered, and many have withdrawn them almost entirely. These programs involve enormous costs, and when hospital budgets are closely monitored by provincial governments, it is difficult to justify the expenditures. It is likely that many of the postgraduate courses that were offered by hospitals were a form of intensive inservice education program designed both to prepare staff and to use the students as care providers on the apprenticeship model. Until recently, few of the postgraduate courses sponsored by hospitals sponsored credit toward baccalaureate degree programs. Community colleges, on the other hand, have added some specialty clinical courses, and a few universities have offered new certificate programs in clinical nursing specialties. Some of the community college courses have recently been approved for transfer credit to certain university degree programs, and several university courses have become creditable to degree programs. Since the 1960s, there has been an increase in the number of post-RN students entering university degree programs in nursing, which has increased the demand for clinical specialty courses and programs with degree credit.

Courses offered at the baccalaureate level in areas called *specialty areas* do not necessarily produce specialists. Any area could be considered a specialty area. Nurses develop areas of concentration or focus in health care. *Specialization* is a confusing term, for it means only certain designated clinical areas to some, knowledge and skills to others, and educational programs to still others. This chapter is based on the assumption that preparation of a specialist in clinical nursing involves study at the master's level, although there is also room for some education of a general nature in these areas at the baccalaureate level.

■■ ■■ ■■ ■■

PROFESSIONAL INTEREST IN SPECIALIZATION

The increase in the range and depth of knowledge in clinical fields has generated interest in specialization among members of professional nursing organizations. Since the 1970s, it has become necessary for every nurse to specialize in an area of practice after completing a program of basic nursing education. Concern has arisen about the competence of graduate nurses to function in the specialty areas without additional education. The safety question has prompted many tertiary-care institutions to provide intensive and substantive courses specific to areas of specialty in their orientation programs for new staff. The cost of these programs and the fact that hospitals are service, not educational, agencies have led nursing service administrators to cooperate with educational institutions to promote development of specialty programs.

Nurses have expressed doubt about whether an individual can function effectively when transferred from one hospital unit to another by nursing managers in the interest of maximum workload efficiency. The need for a complex array of skills and for good judgment based on knowledge in a particular specialty has led to questions about the wisdom of making short-term transfers of staff and of using the traditional float pool to cover shortages. Nursing unions have included these questions in contract negotiations and have been supported by members who are concerned about the professional issues involved. The opposite issue is the cost of not using these techniques in management, for the bottom line of the budget is maximum use of the health-care dollar. It is evident that special preparation in clinical specialty areas is a prerequisite for safe and competent practice (Woodrow and Bell, 1979) and that educational institutions have a major role in ensuring the provision of these programs.

The Canadian Nurses Association (CNA) has assumed a leadership role in developing initiatives for certification programs in various nursing specialties, spurred on by the situation in the United States, where many organizations are involved in credentialing and certification in nursing specialties and there is considerable variation in quality (Erickson, 1979; McCarty, 1979). With the lessons learned from the United States, the CNA's intent is that the process in Canada be rational and that quality be an important consideration for all specialty groups (Porter-O'Grady, 1985).

Most certification programs use examinations to determine how knowledge is acquired by the candidate. Some gain knowledge by practising in a specific area, attending workshops, and reading, whereas others enrol in short- or long-term courses in the specialty. There must be a means of acquiring the knowledge unique to an area to have safe and competent practice. It is probable that the most efficient way to learn is to enrol in programs that offer courses taught by experts and that include supervised clinical practice.

At the 1980 CNA Convention, in Vancouver, the CNA passed a resolution to "study the feasibility of developing certification examinations in various nursing specialties," (Canadian Nurses Association [CNA], 1986, p. 1). The CNA Board responded by launching a study of credentialing and developing certification examinations. The Policy Statement and Background Paper on Credentialing that resulted from this initiative is an important work that documents the processes and designations relevant to nursing education of all types in Canada (CNA, 1982). The statement was adopted by the CNA Board, which directed that an initiative be launched to establish guidelines for a credentialing mechanism. Three committees were established to study questions regarding specialization and certification, and a program was designed at the conclusion of the study. The CNA has emphasized that the program is not "carved in stone," that it will evolve over time, and that flexibility is needed to ensure that this can happen.

Recognizing that certification is a voluntary process that requires periodic updating, the CNA identified three purposes of a certification mechanism: "1) to provide an opportunity for practitioners to validate their expertise in a specialty; 2) to promote high standards of nursing practice in order to provide quality nursing care to the people of Canada; and 3) to identify, through a recognized credential, those nurses who have met the specialty standards" (CNA, 1986, p. 2). Three additional phases have been identified as part of the CNA certification process. Phase one is designation of a specialty for certification based on seven criteria that are applied to determine eligibility of a group: "[has] established standards, addresses recurrent phenomena in practice, role description for practitioners [is] available, [is] supported by literature, education and research, provides care for a defined population, has identified the number and distribution of nurses practising in the specialty, and has the human resources available to support the certification process" (L.A. Patry [personal communication, October 3, 1994]). Because of the costs involved, the CNA reserves the right to terminate a certification program. Phase two, development of a certification examination, involves a process similar to that used for development of registration examinations. Experts in the specialty determine the content of the examination, test plans and objectives are developed, and the examination is written, tested, and revised. The principle of cost recovery is applied in setting fees for the examination. Phase three involves certification of individuals. Several criteria are used to determine eligibility for the examinations: registration status, experiential background in the field of specialty, and a satisfactory performance record, as verified by a colleague and a supervisor or consultant in the specialty. Recertification criteria are similar. The CNA Committee on Certification is responsible for applying and implementing CNA certification policy. The CNA states that the nurse who successfully completes this process should be distinguished from the clinical nurse specialist who is prepared at the master's degree level in nursing (CNA, 1986).

▬ ▬ ▬ ▬

ORGANIZING CERTIFICATE COURSES AND PROGRAMS IN SPECIALITY CLINICAL AREAS FOR CREDIT TOWARD A BACCALAUREATE DEGREE

University nursing education administrators are often asked by registered nurses enroled in undergraduate degree programs in nursing to grant advanced degree credit for postgraduate clinical courses and certificate courses offered by other agencies. Most universities have been reluctant to award credit for work not completed under the auspices of a university, although some have recently recommended certain courses for credit. Because very few universities have offered certificate programs in nursing until recently, the issue of credit toward the bachelor's degree for these programs is relatively new. It seems that registered nurses attending universities to earn credentials related to their clinical areas of specialty want such programs to apply toward the baccalaureate degree.

Preparation for specialty practice continues to be a serious concern for nursing service administrators because of the increasing complexity of care, increasing acuteness of patients and wide use of specialty units. Recently, universities and hospitals have been collaborating to establish high-quality nursing certificate programs. These programs have been designed to enable nurses to gain university credit toward a degree and, at the same time, to meet the agencies' need for nurses who are prepared to assume complex responsibilities in specialty areas.

The Diploma Program in Outpost and Community Health Nursing offered by Dalhousie University, developed under a grant from Health and Welfare Canada in 1967, prepares nurses for practising primary health care in cross-cultural settings in the Canadian North. Although it initially provided no credit toward the baccalaureate degree, beginning in the fall of 1986, students earned 20 to 22 credit hours during a 15-month program (students spend two terms at the university, followed by a 28-week internship in northern Canada). These credits are applied to a 77-credit-hour BScN degree program. Studies in midwifery were emphasized until 1979, when the program was revised to respond to the changing needs of northern health care. The management of maternal and child health care continues to be emphasized along with experience in all aspects of primary health care. In 1988, a 9-month curriculum was developed for nurses holding baccalaureate degrees. The program has been funded by the federal Department of Supply and Services, and approximately 12 students per year are admitted (A. Vukic, personal communication, March 21, 1994).

Memorial University of Newfoundland also developed an outpost nursing program in 1978. The program was a two-year diploma program, consisting of six full semesters. A 1982 revision separated the outpost program into two distinct components: the Diploma in Nurse Midwifery and the Diploma in Community and Primary Care Nursing. These may be taken separately or together, as the Diploma in Outpost Nursing program. Partial program funding has come from the International Grenfell Association, and nursing stations of the Grenfell Regional Health Services are used for clinical experiences in the program. The midwifery component of the program is composed completely of nursing courses, whereas the community and primary care component includes courses in transcultural health care, health assessment, clinical management, community health, biology, sociology of the family, and developmental psychology. Since its initiation, the program has provided full credit toward the baccalaureate degree for work completed. Although this program continues to appear in the university calendar, the nurse midwifery component has not been offered since 1986 and the community and primary health care nursing component has not been offered since 1990 because of insufficient resources. (M.A. Lamb, personal communication, March 16, 1994).

The University of Alberta joined the University of Alberta Hospitals in 1982 to offer a certificate program in neonatal intensive care nursing. The program was designed as a part-time program so that nurses specializing in this area at several Edmonton hospitals could participate. The three courses in the program that incorporated theory and practice in the specialty were approved as University of Alberta courses and provided course credit toward the BScN degree. The cost of employing a faculty member to teach the program was borne jointly by the Faculty of Nursing and the University of Alberta Hospitals. The Faculty of Nursing soon realized that the program was popular with nurses working in this area; after completing the certificate program, many of them entered the post-RN baccalaureate program.

The success of the venture in neonatal nursing resulted in another joint effort, which involved the Faculty of Nursing at the University of Alberta and the

Misericordia Hospital School of Nursing, in emergency/intensive care nursing. This program, which began in September 1985, offered two courses on a full-time basis over 4 months. The two courses in this program were also established as Faculty of Nursing courses and were creditable toward the post-RN degree. In 1986, the University of Alberta Hospitals joined in the collaborative effort, making it a three-way arrangement. The Royal Alexandra and Grey Nuns Hospitals were to join later, and the name of the program was changed to Certificate Program in Critical Care Nursing. External funding to support the cost of the master's-prepared nurses engaged to teach the courses was sought and received. However, students were responsible for tuition, subsistence expenses, cost of books, and other incidental educational expenses. Funding cutbacks in 1994 prompted the Department of Advanced Education to withdraw funding for the program in Edmonton. A critical care program initiated at Foothills Hospital in Calgary several years earlier continued to receive funding. A similar arrangement to that at the University of Alberta and local hospitals was developed between the three Manitoba organizations: the University of Manitoba Faculty of Nursing, the Winnipeg Health Sciences Centre, and St. Boniface General Hospital for the certificate in adult intensive care program offered by those hospitals (Beaton, personal communication, March 29, 1994).

In 1986, the Faculty of Nursing responded positively to a request from nursing service administrators to develop a certificate program in nephrology nursing, based on part-time study and designed for students with a special interest in this area. Physicians supported this program, and a funded position for an instructor was made available (from the University of Alberta Hospitals) through their efforts. Subsequent problems led to the discontinuation of the program in 1990.

In Toronto, a collaborative certificate program in critical care nursing was developed in 1984 by Ryerson Polytechnical Institute and Toronto General Hospital. The program was initially financed by the Ministry of Health of Ontario as a research project and offered direct funding of full-time students. Over time, the program has expanded to include more students and is currently a collaborative venture, with seven hospitals providing clinical settings for practice. Although the Toronto Hospital (which now includes Toronto General and Toronto Western Hospitals) continues to be the key health-care agency, other hospitals involved include St. Michael's, Humber Memorial Hospital, Mt. Sinai Hospital, Wellesley, St. Joseph's Health Centre, and Women's College Hospital. Up to 300 students per year are prepared in the initial part of this program. The program consists of seven courses, three of which are taught during the first 7 weeks of full-time study and constitute the core program. Students become eligible for the certificate if they complete four other courses: two advanced nursing courses, one course in nursing theory or communication and teaching, and one liberal arts elective. The latter two courses in the certificate program provide credit toward the BScN degree. Currently, Ryerson provides funding for instruction, and the hospitals where the students are employed provide student funding. Reports of program outcomes indicate a high degree of satisfaction for the students and institutions. Although not all students complete the certificate, the opportunity is available for those who wish to take advantage of it.

The community colleges will probably continue to play a significant role in preparation for specialty practice in nursing. Many clinical specialty programs offered by these institutions across the country meet the needs of practitioners and agencies for nurses prepared in certain areas. Some universities are now giving partial credit for courses completed, but this is not universal. Some hospitals continue to offer postgraduate programs, but as previously noted, the number has declined since the mid-1960s. Tight budgets and a mandate to provide service rather than sophisticated educational programs will inhibit further expansion of the educational enterprise in hospitals. It is also unlikely that universities can meet all of the needs for specialty programs because of budget constraints and because of their efforts to expand programs at the baccalaureate and master's levels and to initiate or expand doctoral programs to support practice and research initiatives.

■ ■ ■ ■

ISSUES FOR THE FUTURE

That some university schools and faculties of nursing are considering involvement in certificate programs comprising courses that meet baccalaureate degree requirements may be a sign of their maturation. Nursing has entered the age of specialization, and given the increasing complexity of knowledge in health care and the performance expectations of nursing service administrators for registered nurses with expertise in clinical specialty nursing, there can be no retreat.

It is important, however, to note the changing philosophy of program models from the 1950s and 1960s to the present. In the past, specialty programs were offered primarily by hospitals and tended to be organized on an apprenticeship basis, with more emphasis on clinical practice, often unsupervised, than on theoretical knowledge in the field. Also, the instructional component tended to be provided by faculty members who had minimal preparation in nursing and would not qualify for faculty appointments in universities. Students in these programs were paid salaries because of the amount of service they provided, but these salaries were considerably lower than those paid to registered nurses. Often, no tuition charges were made. Students were not supernumerary to the unit, and they replaced higher-cost staff members. Thus the hospital gained financially and programs were self-sustaining. In many instances, programs were revenue-generating. The potential for exploitation of students by the hospital for financial reasons is evident here. Arguments to support the transfer of specialty programs to postsecondary institutions are the same as those raised to support the transfer of the basic nursing educational enterprise to the general educational system.

The new programs tend to be organized on a sound educational basis. Faculty are expected to have suitable academic qualifications for their positions, including considerable clinical expertise. The quality of faculty is important in universities, where the maintenance of standards must be demonstrated. Clinical experience is a significant part of the program and is carefully supervised. Programs will probably be financed in the usual manner, and students will not be expected to subsidize the cost of the program through service to the hospital. For this reason, the new certificate programs in clinical specialty areas are quite different from those that existed in earlier decades. Moreover, the increased complexity of nursing knowledge in all areas and the need for knowledgeable and competent practitioners in clinical specialities, with education beyond the basic level, makes education in specialty areas a professional necessity.

REFERENCES

Canadian Nurses Association. (1982). *Credentialing in nursing: Policy statement and background paper.* Ottawa: Author.

Canadian Nurses Association. (1986). *CNA's certification program: An information booklet.* Ottawa: Author.

Erickson, E.H. (1979). ANA's program of certification in nursing administration, *Journal of Nursing Administration, 9*(9), 32-33.

McCarty, P. (1979). Certification process: Complex but rewarding. *The American Nurse, 11,* 47.

Porter-O'Grady, T. (1985). Credentialing, privileging, and nursing bylaws: Assuring accountability. *Journal of Nursing Administration, 15*(12), 23-27.

Woodrow, M., and Bell, J.A. (1979). Clinical specialization: Conflict between reality and theory. *Journal of Nursing Administration, 1*(6), 73-78.

CHAPTER THIRTY

Distance Education in Nursing: Increasing Accessibility of Degree Programs

JANET ROSS KERR

T he entry to practice position, adopted and actively promoted by the Canadian Nurses Association (CNA) and the provincial professional associations, has many implications for the profession. Although the position addresses only graduates of nursing programs entering practice in the year 2000 and after, it implies that the profession is anticipating the baccalaureate entry standard for all at some time after the year 2000. Nurses qualified at the diploma level before the year 2000 will retire or otherwise cease to practise, and the baccalaureate standard will be implemented in its entirety.

Based on the direction the profession has taken, it is important that diploma-prepared nurses who wish to study for a baccalaureate degree be able to do so. Off-campus programs using distance education and outreach methods make it possible for university schools and faculties of nursing to extend their range and offer courses, even degree programs, over a larger geographic area than would otherwise be possible. These programs enhance and support the entry to practice position because they are accessible to those whose place of residence might preclude enrolment in a baccalaureate degree program in nursing located in a large urban centre. Canada's universities, a number of which are large and highly diversified "multiversities," are located primarily in these urban areas.

Increasingly, university faculties and schools of nursing have become very creative in designing BScN programs with greater accessibility. The size of the nation, some 5,000 miles from coast to coast, makes it the second largest nation on earth. Also, the variation in terrain, from rugged mountain ranges to bald prairie to impassable muskeg, with bitter winter weather conditions in many areas, presents a unique geographic and meteorologic picture. A relatively small population is scattered across this vast expanse of land, making transportation and communication challenging. Canadian history is replete with examples of people working together to overcome the obstacles of distance, geography, and climate to build a modern industrialized society. Much progress has been made in transportation since the last spike for the Canadian Pacific Railway was driven at Craigellachie in 1885, uniting East and West with a single transportation system for the first time. Today, there is a choice of transportation, and travel is faster and more efficient than ever before. After Sir Alexander Graham Bell invented the telephone, advances in technology were steady until, in the past two decades, a virtual explosion of developments took place. Sophisticated means of communication are available from one corner of the globe to another. Decreases in the price of new instruments and machines in the communications area have made them affordable. Electronic mail (e-mail) is revolutionizing global communications, and a nursing network recently established at the University of Toronto, *Nursenet,* is just one of many nursing groups using the Internet, a worldwide system of electronic communication. With more subscribers every day, this network unites nurses around the world and allows them to discuss and debate matters of professional interest.

It is interesting that the entry to practice goal has surfaced at a time of major technologic advance. Universities are being challenged to make the new technology accessible to everyone. The types of potential students at universities have also changed, and the character of the student population has shifted to include an increasing proportion of returning adults. The resolve of the nursing profession in Canada to achieve the entry to practice goal by the turn of the century heralds a new and important phase in the evolution of the profession. However, this development is predicated on a commitment to searching for the answers to nursing questions through research and a continuous redefinition of the nature and scope of nursing.

CHARACTERISTICS OF SUCCESSFUL OFF-CAMPUS PROGRAMS

Overcoming the barriers of distance in providing off-campus educational programming at the baccalaureate level may seem a formidable task. However, a positive approach, a commitment to achieving the entry to practice goal, and institutional support can facilitate program development. Many institutions have initiated programs by using outreach (in person) methods in off-campus locations exclusively. The inefficiency and cost, in human and monetary terms, of these methods prompt consideration of distance education methods, which include both interactive and noninteractive teaching methods.

STRUCTURE AND ORGANIZATION FOR LEARNING

Structure and organization for learning are key processes in establishing a successful off-campus program in nursing. When students are scattered across a wide geographic area, in locations remote from faculty members responsible for course instruction, these processes assume major importance, both at the course or program level and at the individual level. It is wise to define institutional intentions, in terms of courses and programs to be offered, at the outset. Students considering enrolment in a baccalaureate program in nursing need to know which courses will be offered in subsequent semesters, whether the entire program can be completed from a distance, and if not, what credit may be transferred for successfully completed courses. An outline of courses to be offered during the time period allotted for the program and any special requirements to be met should be available to students from the beginning to facilitate individual planning and commitment. Also, course content and expectations should be fully delineated in each course so that students are aware of requirements and make an informed commitment to the course.

It may be wise to give a faculty member responsibility for day-to-day planning, coordination, and administration of the off-campus program. This person can work with students and other faculty members to ensure that planning is appropriate and that there is ongoing communication of information about course and program activities. Academic advisement for off-campus students can also be provided by this individual, who becomes the students' link to the university faculty of nursing. The person who fulfils this role must have excellent communication skills, a commitment to the off-campus endeavour, and sensitivity to students' needs. If all requirements are met, the incumbent will serve as a stabilizing and unifying force, facilitating and enhancing the success of the program.

Designated opportunities for students to discuss questions with the professors teaching off-campus courses are important. Planning for this at a group or individual level can occur in a videoconference, teleconference, or by telephone. Financing of the particular program and location of the student may affect times and methods of communication between faculty member and student.

Variety in instruction is as important in distance programs as it is in traditional settings. Faculty members in traditional settings who think about and plan unique learning experiences frequently achieve success in terms of learning outcomes and student perceptions of the learning experience. Varied educational methods and experiences in off-campus courses are also important. They tend to help the learner view the subject in more depth and from a number of perspectives. In an off-campus mode, adjuncts to teaching, such as graphics, visual enhancements, outlines, and handouts, are essential for successful programs. Again, time and planning are necessary for optimum results.

■ ■ ■ ■

THE HUMAN ELEMENT

Important questions about off-campus programs address that elusive area known as "the human element," that is, an expectation by the student that the professor will demonstrate human qualities of thought, logic, and competence in the subject and, further, is interested in the student's learning needs, problems, and achievements. This may be an area in which concerns are expressed in both traditional and nontraditional programs and may be related to many factors, including class size and the workload of the particular faculty member. The quality of communication between student and faculty member is at issue, as well as the level of mutual understanding achieved. Ensuring that human feeling characterizes the learning encounter requires a slightly different approach in off-campus programs. In addition, student-to-student interactions and relationships constitute part of the human element in teaching-learning situations, for students learn from one another. Depending on the particular situation, the latter may be achieved in many different ways in off-campus programs.

■ ■ ■ ■

COLLABORATION

Cooperation and collaboration with other institutions has been a necessary and important defining characteristic of Canadian distance education programs in nursing. Because of the unique nature and extent of the arrangements required to provide off-campus courses and programs, it is unlikely that any one institution can "go it alone," without help from other organizations. There is usually a need to negotiate arrangements with agencies for space for computers and classes offered via teleconference or videoconference methods. These agencies include community colleges, continuing education centres, hospitals, educational consortia, and public libraries.

Other educational institutions may be an integral part of the program through the provision of courses, either on-site in community colleges or by other universities in distance format, using interactive or noninteractive methods. Athabasca University, situated in Athabasca, Alberta, is a postsecondary institution established with a mandate to develop distance learning programs. The majority of courses offered consist of learning packages of printed materials, although audio-cassettes, videocassettes, tutorials by telephone or in person in some regional settings, and teleconference sessions are used in some courses. Since the focus of this institution has been in the arts and science fields, Athabasca courses have provided the backbone of the liberal arts and science component of an off-campus baccalaureate program in nursing. Because the technology used in most of its courses is kept simple, it is possible to enrol in Athabasca courses from any location with postal service. This sector of educational activity has continued to grow and flourish in the 1990s. In 1994, Athabasca University had over 700 students from Alberta and 230 out-of-province students enrolled in post-RN baccalaureate courses, all receiving off-campus support from 250 tutors. In 1990 the university established a post-RN BScN degree program offering all required professional and arts and science courses through the distance learning system. The first students in this program convocated in 1993. A combination of the exponential growth in technology and the increasing affordability of sophisticated equipment has underscored the potential for providing educational programs at a distance in the future. It is likely that postsecondary institutions that have operated primarily in a traditional mode will move to develop the opportunity for students to study at a distance using sophisticated equipment such as videoconferencing. This may revolutionize higher education in the future and allow programs to be offered to students in locations that would have been thought inaccessible a short time ago.

▬ ▬ ▬ ▬

THE CLINICAL COMPONENT

The clinical component in nursing programs sets them apart from other university programs in traditional and nontraditional settings. A commitment to providing high-quality clinical instruction in regional and rural settings may seem to present insurmountable difficulties in developing off-campus programs in nursing. However, a variety of arrangements is possible for supervision of clinical learning experiences. These include using preceptors in some areas, using telephone, teleconference, or videoconference to communicate with faculty members on the main campus, hiring suitably qualified faculty members in off-campus locations, and sending faculty members to off-campus sites to supervise clinical learning. A program may be strengthened by securing clinical practice arrangements beyond the walls of large tertiary health-care institutions in urban areas; such arrangements are now being put into practice in traditional programs. Community general hospitals offer important clinical learning opportunities that can enhance programs. In addition, health units, home care programs, and other health-care agencies serving largely rural populations can offer a range and depth of experiences appropriate for baccalaureate courses in nursing. Many new ways of approaching arrangements for clinical practice in the context of baccalaureate-level programming will be formulated and explored in the future.

▬ ▬ ▬ ▬

TECHNOLOGY

The increasingly widespread availability and use of technology has begun to revolutionize higher education. For off-campus programs in nursing, technology can be very helpful, making possible interactive teacher-student communication and instructional enhancement of various kinds. The School of Nursing at the University of Victoria has been a pioneer in distance education in nursing. The use of learning packages in nursing courses for off-campus students in the post-RN baccalaureate program was innovative. These involve various modes of instruction, including printed materials, audiocassettes, and videocassettes. Through satellite transmission, televised nursing courses have been accessible to registered nurse students residing in the "footprint" region of western Canada. Questions telephoned in while the instructor is on the air allow for two-way interaction between students and the faculty member. The facilities of the "Knowledge Network," a public television broadcast station, and the Opening Learning Institute, which provides liberal arts courses via printed learning packages, both created by the British Columbia government, have been used by both of the university schools of nursing in that province for courses offered to students in off-campus locations.

In 1986, the University of Victoria announced that all courses in its degree program could be pursued on an off-campus basis, and they began to market their courses widely (Collins, 1987). By 1994 approximately 500 students completing one or more courses toward the baccalaureate program. The faculty act as tutors for both on- and off-campus students. Because of the demand for the off-campus courses, this program was restricted to B.C. residents. The majority of courses in the degree program are offered on an off-campus basis. A small number of courses have an on-campus requirement and are given in a condensed time frame to allow employed nurses to take them (Egan, 1994). For many nurses, the availability of these courses with emphasis on independent learning allowed study toward a degree not previously attainable. The University of British Columbia also implemented a distance model for its post-RN baccalaureate program. All courses are available in distance format, using print, video, and teleconferencing methods.

In Ontario, the University of Ottawa initiated a teleconferencing distance education program during the 1982 to 1983 academic year, with a satellite course in Cornwall, Ontario (DuGas, 1985; Styran, 1985). The teleconference sessions were part of the regular instructional program offered in the post-RN baccalaureate program in the evening. By the 1984 to 1985 academic year, students in four other centres—Brockville, Pembroke, Peterborough, and the Ottawa Civic Hospital—were permitted to enrol in the courses being offered in the evening program. During the 1983 to 1984 academic year, an electronic blackboard was purchased to enhance the instructional component (DuGas, 1985; DuGas & Casey, 1987; Styran, 1985). By 1994, eight additional teleconference sites—in Almonte, Belleville, Kingston, Montreal, Oshawa, Renfrew, Smith's Falls, and Toronto—were added, thus allowing over 100 students to be enrolled in off-campus courses and to complete the requirements for the baccalaureate program without having to attend classes on the main campus of the University of Ottawa.

St. Francis Xavier University in Antigonish, Nova Scotia is the only university in the Maritimes to offer the majority of nursing and arts and sciences courses using a distance model. Dalhousie University requires that all nursing courses in the post-RN baccalaureate program be taken on campus. However, Dalhousie has been a pioneer in developing a graduate program at the master's level in distance mode. All requirements for the Master of Nursing degree except one clinical nursing course can be completed off campus. The program is offered within the maritime region only.

In Alberta, the University of Calgary Faculty of Nursing decided to phase its existing post-RN baccalaureate program into one that would be offered only using distance methods. Implemented in the 1989 to 1990 academic year, this program continues to provide access to baccalaureate nursing education via distance delivery in the southern half of Alberta. The northern half has been served since 1984 by the University of Alberta Faculty of Nursing's distance delivery program and since 1989 by Athabasca University's new post-RN baccalaureate program.

■ ■ ■ ■

A MODEL OF DISTANCE EDUCATION AT ONE UNIVERSITY

The University of Alberta in Edmonton has since 1985 offered the entire post-RN degree program on an off-campus basis (Kerr, 1985; Kerr, 1987). At the time, it was the only university in Canada to offer an entire BScN degree program off campus. The University of Alberta first began to consider off-campus programming in 1978, with the submission of a proposal to the Alberta government for expansion of the post-RN baccalaureate program. The expansion was funded in 1979, and enrolment doubled. Half of the expansion enrolment was reserved for off-campus students.

At the beginning, outreach methods used to provide courses were primarily traditional classroom methods, and instructors went from the main campus to certain designated centres to offer courses on a weekly or biweekly basis. Teleconferencing was introduced in the fall of 1984. The program was initially conceived over 3 years, with 1 required year of full-time study on the main campus of the University of Alberta in Edmonton. This period was reduced to one term in 1982 to 1983 and was eliminated altogether for those centres beginning the program in 1985, when teleconferencing became the primary mode of instruction for courses. Residence requirements at the University of Alberta refer primarily to full-time study requirements on the campus; the campus is wherever University of Alberta faculty are providing courses. Residence requirements for undergraduate programs in the Faculty of Nursing were also eliminated in 1983 so that students could study on a part-time basis, provided that the post-RN program was completed within 5 years. The program was refined to the point that off-campus students could take the entire degree program on a part-time basis over 4 years. Currently, the University of Alberta's off-campus programming at the baccalaureate level has been directed to only one of the four original regions served by the program, in view of the role of Athabasca University in providing the post-RN degree program at a distance. However, beginning in 1992, the University of Alberta undertook to offer the Master of Nursing program to students living in central Alberta in Red Deer, using videoconferencing. The University, in cooperation with Red Deer College and Alberta Motor Transport, initiated a pilot project in which courses were offered in a variety of disciplines. Compressed-format videoconferencing equipment in Edmonton and Red Deer was used for teaching courses. Both the project itself and the students who entered the program were highly successful.

Teleconferencing was the original technology that revolutionized the off-campus program at the University of Alberta. Equipment was purchased, a Darome bridge was rented through the Alberta Hospital Association (AHA), and long-distance telephone charges were assumed by the faculty. In many instances, students used convenors and microphones owned by local hospitals, and hospital FX lines (flat rate for long-distance use) were made available for use in the evening program sessions. Use of the AHA bridge continued for 2 years but was discontinued because of expensive rental charges. Alternatives were explored, and the University of Alberta purchased a Confertech full-duplex bridge of its own in the spring of 1986. Six faculties of the University, committed to the need for this bridge, were able to raise sufficient funds to purchase it. Through the cooperative organization of educational agencies using teleconferencing in the province, the Alberta government made its government RITE-line system (provincial telephone exchange operated by the Alberta government) available to the institutions, for educational purposes, at no cost after 4:30 p.m. Thus the Faculty of Nursing could offer programming in centres throughout Alberta served by the RITE-line system without incurring long-distance telephone charges.

The Faculty of Nursing obtained a grant from the university to finance the purchase of three Telewriter II units for use in the off-campus program. The Telewriter system is a software package that allows production and storage of graphic materials for transmission during teleconference sessions. The associated modem allows two-way transmission of data over one telephone line. The system was implemented in September 1986, and an educational assistant with computer expertise was engaged in October to prepare graphics for faculty and to ensure that technical arrangements for teleconference sessions were managed. Since several courses are in progress at any one time, a competent person must assume responsibility for details. In 1987, three more systems were purchased for use in off-campus centres, and the Telewriter II software was upgraded to Telewriter III; the new software and additional equipment, such as graphics boards in the computers and use of a video camera, allow for transmission of video images to and from the off-campus sites.

A cooperative approach among faculties at the University and the efforts of the Distance Education Group have encouraged sharing of facilities and expertise. The intent of the group was to place videoconferencing systems in several locations in the province to which the University of Alberta delivers programs to facilitate instruction by all academic units. Cooperation with other universities and postsecondary institutions will also enhance the possibilities.

Other instructional methods involving technology used in regular and off-campus post-RN programs at the University of Alberta included computer-assisted learning and computer-managed learning. In 1981, a health assessment course was developed in this format and implemented in the program. The program was adapted from the PLATO (specialized computer language) format for use on an IBM computer, with provision for communication via modem and the TINA network (a provincial system for lowering long-distance telephone charges for computer use), and was used by instructors in the Faculty of Nursing. Thus it was necessary to hold only the laboratory sessions for practice in regional centres.

With the establishment of the collaborative degree program with Red Deer College in 1990, distance education programming was extended to include basic baccalaureate nursing students, whereas it had originally been used solely for post-RN baccalaureate students because they were the only ones studying at a distance. Distance delivery methods, an important part of this collaborative model, can be employed to capitalize on the expertise of faculty members in courses in both Edmonton and Red Deer.

■■■ ■■■ ■■■ ■■■

CONCLUSION

Higher education in this country is undergoing a technologic revolution that is rapidly changing the character of instruction in traditional settings and in centres outside main university campuses. Students will benefit from these changes and from the efforts of a growing number of institutions to make programming available to adult students in nontraditional settings. University libraries are rapidly placing their information on computers, and the ability to search the catalogue is available to anyone who owns a computer terminal and modem and is allowed access to the university computer system.

The technology for distance learning is not really foreign to most people. It is as available as the communication devices used in everyday living. The technology does not need to be highly sophisticated, although the use of two-way compressed-format videoconferencing using telephone lines will be rapidly incorporated into existing systems of distance delivery as the cost of the equipment drops dramatically. The telephone (both for voice and fax) will continue to be the mainstay of most current distance programs and will be an adjunct to even the most highly sophisticated ones. Its potential significance in distance education has not always been universally appreciated, but the success of programs, particularly those involving computers along with video enhancements as well as full videoconferencing capability, has consolidated its place in the system.

The effort to develop off-campus programs at the undergraduate-degree level in nursing, although challenging, has become an important one in Canada. It requires the effort and commitment of many people and the pooled resources of educational institutions and health-care agencies. There is a new appreciation of the vital role that technology has in extensive programs of study offered to students in remote locations. Achievement of the entry to practice goal of the profession will be facilitated by extending the campus and offering baccalaureate-degree programs in other than traditional university settings. The development of graduate programs in distance format will undoubtedly continue to be an important development in the future, as there is a large group of potential students whose access to programs in traditional format is limited by their geographic location. A larger cadre of nurses prepared to engage in advanced nursing practice in a variety of settings is urgently needed. Distance methods provide the means to take educational programs to those who both need and want to pursue them.

REFERENCES

Collins, F. (1987). Update on distance education at the University of Victoria. *The Canadian Nurse, 83*(2), 10-11.

DuGas, B.W. (1985). Baccalaureate entry for practice: A challenge that universities must meet. *The Canadian Nurse, 81*(5), 17-19.

DuGas, B.W., and Casey, A.M. (1987). Teleconferencing. *The Canadian Nurse, 83*(5), 22-25.

Hart, G., Crawford, T., and Hicks, B. (1985). RN to BN: Building on education and experience. *The Canadian Nurse, 81*(5), 22-23.

Kerr, J.C. (1985). Taking the campus to the student. *The Canadian Nurse, 81*(5), 30-31.

Kerr, J.C. (1987). History of off-campus programs and distance education at the University of Alberta. *AARN Newsletter, 43*(3), 19-20.

Styran, P. (1985). Winds of change. *The Canadian Nurse, 81*(5), 20-21.

CHAPTER THIRTY ONE

Primary Health Care: The Means for Reaching Nursing's Potential in Achieving Health for All

JANNETTA MacPHAIL

P rimary health care has been purported by the World Health Organization (WHO) as the means for promoting and maintaining the health of nations around the world. What is the meaning of the concept of primary health care? Why is it endorsed and proclaimed as the solution to many ills in existing health-care systems? Is it a feasible goal for Canada? What reforms will be required in Canada's health-care system to implement the concept? Does the profession of nursing support the concept? Are nursing students being educated to function effectively in a primary health-care system? These questions are addressed as the meaning and significance of primary health care are explored.

■ ■ ■ ■

HEALTH FOR ALL BY THE YEAR 2000

The goal of Health for All by the Year 2000 was established in 1978 at an international meeting held at Alma-Ata in Kazakh Republic of the Soviet Union, under the auspices of the World Health Organization (WHO) and the United Nations International Children's Emergency Fund (UNICEF) (WHO, 1978a). The meeting, attended by representatives of 127 nations and 72 international organizations, was to promote the concept of primary health care as the only viable means of attaining equitable distribution of health resources to enable people to attain "a level of health that will permit them to lead a socially and economically productive life" (WHO, 1978b, p. 429). The report of the conference challenges all countries and governments of the world to employ a primary health-care approach with emphasis on the development of their health services. The approach is "based on practical, scientifically sound, and socially acceptable methods and technology made universally accessible to individuals and families in the community through their full participation and at a cost that the community and country can afford" (WHO, 1978b). The International Council of Nurses (ICN) pledged its full support to making primary health care a reality in all countries of the world. Recognizing that most health care in the world is delivered by nursing personnel, ICN encouraged nurses in each country to participate in developing a primary health-care system that is relevant to the country's needs and uses nurses effectively in its implementation (WHO, 1978b, p. 429).

Commitment to the goal of Health for All by the Year 2000 led to another conference, held in Ottawa, Canada in November 1986, which was jointly organized by WHO, Health and Welfare Canada, and the Canadian Public Health Association (CPHA). It was attended by 212 participants from 38 countries who met to exchange experiences, share knowledge, and develop a plan of action to achieve the goal. Those attending the meeting were representative of a wide range of governmental, voluntary, and community organizations, as well as active practitioners and academics. The three main aims of the conference were to promote:

> . . . *visibility:* to encourage and enhance health promotion development by assessing past and current achievements;
> *sharing:* to put people in contact with each other, sharing examples of success and failure; and
> *consensus:* to develop through the active participation of conference members a conference statement on the future development of health promotion (Nutbeam and Lawrence, 1987, p. 1).

The conference was primarily a response to growing expectations for a new public health movement around the world. It was built around five major issues, which participants discussed in workshops conducted over a 1-week period. The issues were building healthy public policy, creating supportive environments, strengthening community action, personal skills, and reorienting health services (Nutbeam and Lawrence, 1987). One outcome of the conference was the publication of the *Ottawa Charter for Health Promotion,* which identifies three elements basic to health promotion: advocating health, enabling people to achieve their fullest health potential, and mediating differing interests for the pursuit of health (Nutbeam and Lawrence, 1987).

The Honourable Jake Epp, Minister of National Health and Welfare Canada, chose the occasion of the conference to launch the Canadian government strategy document, *Achieving Health for All: A Framework for Health Promotion.* He emphasized that the purpose in releasing the document was to promote dialogue among Canadians interested in health and to achieve better health for ourselves and contribute to better health for the people of the world. His goal was to move health promotion from the periphery of the health field to a central position (Nutbeam and Lawrence, 1987).

■ ─ ─ ─

THE CANADIAN APPROACH TO ACHIEVING HEALTH FOR ALL

The Canadian approach to achieving health for all is to focus on health promotion, which is perceived as the best strategy. Figure 31.1 identifies the overall aim, health challenges, health promotion mechanisms, and implementation strategies.

Self-care, a mechanism supported by nurses, is defined in Epp's document as *the decisions and actions individuals take in the interest of their own health.* This concept supports nursing's goal of helping people to become increasingly responsible for their own health. However, creating conditions and surroundings conducive to health, which is implied in creating healthy environments, goes beyond the individual and requires community action. One example of this philosophy is creating a smoke-free environment, which cannot be accomplished by an individual; there must be agreement by groups, such as health-care institutions and educational institutions. Today there is a definite trend to promote smoke-free environments because of the harmfulness of smoke to nonsmokers, who should not have to suffer from the poor health habits practised by smokers.

Achieving healthy environments will require developing the political will "to overcome likely conflicts between public health interests and commercial and other vested interests" (Nutbeam and Lawrence, 1987, p. 2). This offers a real challenge to governments in relation to creating a smoke-free environment. They must provide alternatives for farmers who have made a living for many years by growing tobacco and deal with animosity and resistance from tobacco companies who have made millions producing products that are harmful to the health of smokers and those exposed to secondhand smoke, including the unborn fetus, who is more likely to be premature if the mother smokes during pregnancy. Achieving the goal of health for all will require governments to take unpopular stands, which could jeopardize the party in power in an election. Those committed to promoting the public's health must remain firm and serve as role models for others in promoting healthy behaviours. This has implications for the positions taken by associations of health professionals and for the education of health professionals.

Reorienting health services to focus on health rather than illness presents another challenge to health professionals and governments. One of the major objectives is to effect change in the roles of health professionals, which may necessitate the development of new skills and expertise and require moving away from intervening to do what we consider best for patients to a mediating role for health professionals. The Ottawa Charter for Health Promotion (1986) states:

> The prerequisites and prospects for health cannot be ensured by the health sector alone. More importantly, health promotion demands coordinated action by all concerned: by governments, by health and other social and economic sectors, by non-governmental and voluntary organizations, by local authorities, by industry and by the media. People in all walks of life are involved as individuals, families and communities. Professional and social groups and health personnel have a major responsibility to mediate between differing interests in society for the pursuit of health (p. 1).

FIGURE 31.1   A framework for health promotion.

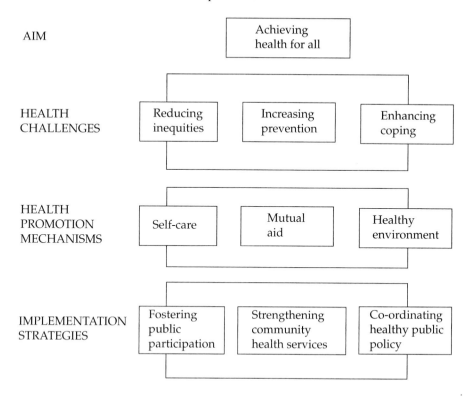

Modified from Ottawa Charter for Health Promotion. (1986). Ottawa: World Health Organization, Health and Welfare Canada, and the Canadian Public Health Organization.

At present, government funding of health services in Canada strongly favours cure and sickness care, with a minor proportion of the health-care dollar going to support health promotion and prevention of illness. Change in financial incentives will be needed to support health promotion activities. Similarly, changes will be needed in the initial and continuing education of health professionals to change their focus and priorities to primary health care and prepare them to help people achieve their fullest health potential and make decisions about matters that affect their health and well-being.

Maglacas, chief scientist for nursing with WHO, points out that although the aim of the Health for All movement has been interpreted by many as making health services available to everyone, the actual goal is to have all people in all countries achieve at least a level of health that allows them to work productively and participate actively in the social life of the community in which they live (CNA Connection, 1988). In 1987, almost 10 years after the WHO declaration at Alma-Ata, Maglacas (1988) assessed nursing's response to the Health for All challenge as "fragmented, sporadic, unplanned, and uncoordinated, and [as involving] few, if any, other disciplines or sectors" (p. 67). Primary health care, as envisioned by Maglacas and other nursing leaders, is perceived as the way to achieve the goal.

■■ ■■ ■■ ■■

PRIMARY HEALTH CARE

Primary health care has been confused with primary medical care and primary nursing, but it is distinctly different from both. In the United States and in some parts of Canada, the concept of primary health care is limited and tends to be equated with the nurse practitioner role. It is portrayed as a nurse, practising in an ambulatory setting or a remote site, who assesses the health and illness status of clients through "health history, physical examination, and diagnostic tests; develops and implements therapeutic plans; [and] engages in appropriate referrals, health counselling, and collaboration with other health care providers" (Ulin, 1982, p. 532). It is much like primary medical care, and seems to be so when comparing nurse practitioner and physician practice in ambulatory care, such as that reported by Diers, Hamman, and Molde (1986). Studies of nurse practitioner effectiveness, as compiled by Feldman, Ventura, and Crosby (1987) and as reviewed by Molde and Diers (1985), lend credence to this evaluation of the nurse practitioner role by Ulin.

Initial efforts to expand the role of the nurse in Canada in primary health care followed the pattern of two types of practice, as identified by Allen (1977). The first type of practice is the assistant to the physician, which involves performing tasks delegated by the physician and is seen most commonly in physicians' offices and family practice units. The second type is replacement of the physician, which signifies that the nurse performs the same tasks as the physician, although not those of the specialist, such as a surgeon. This type of practice is prevalent in remote areas in the north; in private practice, by nurses serving such populations as psychiatric patients; and in family practice units, where patients are allocated randomly to physicians and nurses depending on the availability of staff. Some nurses support the perspective of nurses replacing or substituting for physicians, as practised in the United States and carried out at McMaster University in the 1970s (Spitzer, Kergin, and Yoshida 1975).

In 1972 the Boudreau Committee, which was established to address a gap in health-care services in Canada, recommended that short-term practitioner programs be developed in selected Canadian universities to prepare nurse practitioners to practise in remote sites, such as the far north, where physicians did not wish to reside and practise (Report of the Committee on Nurse Practitioners, 1972). Such programs were established, and all but one have been phased out. The remaining program is at Dalhousie University, which has continued because it includes a nurse-midwifery component that meets a need in outlying areas in the Atlantic region. The intent was to incorporate primary health-care concepts and physical assessment and history-taking skills into basic baccalaureate programs so that this essential content would be an integral part of the preparation of all nurses graduating from baccalaureate degree programs. This has been achieved, but the baccalaureate programs do not include preparation for the "physician substitute" skills that were included in some of the Canadian nurse practitioner programs to prepare them to practise in remote areas, where consultation was provided by physicians by telephone. Some of the nurse practitioners have practised in urban areas, usually in central city, under-served areas, where the poor, the unemployed, and the indigent seek health-care services from clinics. With the rapid expansion of knowledge and the knowledge base and skills needed to make clinical decisions, it is recognized that short-term programs are not adequate to prepare nurses to practise in relatively independent, autonomous roles in which they actually substitute for physicians in remote areas.

The concept of primary health care envisaged by WHO is "essential health care made universally acceptable to individuals and families in the community by means acceptable to them, through their full participation and at a cost the community and country can afford" (Mahler, 1981, p. 5). It includes four major facets: health promotion; illness prevention; illness care; and rehabilitation at individual, family, and community levels (Canadian Nurses Association [CNA], September, 1988). Thus the concept is much broader than primary medical care and health promotion, although health promotion is the central focus, designed primarily to improve health potential and thereby maintain balance or stability. To achieve this goal "the focus in nursing must be moved to health and actions must move beyond the health sector and must involve the people themselves" (Maglacas, 1988, p. 67).

The key role for health professionals in this concept of primary health care is "empowering people to improve their lives and life styles, develop self-reliance and self-determination and take control of their health actions" (CNA Connection, 1988, p. 14). Fundamental changes in structure, roles, and relationships will be required to move from the present health-care system, which is increasingly expensive and emphasizes high technologies aimed at curing the few, to a very different and more widely available service built around health needs, with individuals, families, and communities taking increased responsibility for their own health. The focus would be on community health and social centres in the community rather than a system centred in acute-care hospitals, for which 95% of the health-care dollar is now expended (Weller, 1980),

■ ■ ■ ■

NURSING'S RESPONSE TO THE CHALLENGE

Are Canadian nurses and organized nursing in Canada prepared to support the changes needed to move to such a system of primary health care? In the past few years the CNA has given high priority to considering the possibility and accepting the challenge. In September 1988, the CNA published a major document, *Health for all Canadians: A Call for Health Care Reform*, which provides an analysis of inadequacies in the existing health-care system and a vision of the changes needed and strategies to effect them to move to a system based on the philosophy and principles of primary health care. The CNA supports individuals, families, and communities being active partners in their health care and recognizes the need for a major reorientation of health-care policies and health-care professionals to meet the challenges of the future.

In March 1989 the CNA Board of Directors approved a 5-year plan aimed at implementing this vision of primary health care in Canada. It includes steps to define and clarify the roles of nurses in primary health care, to establish stable and adequate funding to facilitate demonstration projects, to examine the implications for educational programs in nursing, and to establish a lobbying campaign to expedite the development of primary health care. "The major goals of the plan are to provide support for member associations to adopt and implement primary health care and to communicate the primary health care position at the national level" (*CNA CONNECTION*, 1989). In March 1989, the CNA published a *Position Statement on the Nurses' role in Primary Health Care*. Nurses are portrayed as having a key role that has four main aspects: "direct care provider; teacher and educator of health personnel and the public; supervisor and manager of primary health-care services; and researcher and evaluator of health care" (CNA, 1989).

Nursing already has a number of examples of their participation in primary health care on which to build. Nurses practising in remote parts of Canada integrate principles of primary health care, in varying degrees, in their daily practice (Chamberlain and Beckingham, 1987). In addition to the replacement model of practice seen in remote areas, Allen (1977) identified a complemental model. It differs from that of other health professionals, yet is complementary, so the client is provided with a more complete range of health-care services by experts. Allen developed such a practice in a "Health Workshop" staffed by faculty and students of the McGill University School of Nursing. The workshop, or health centre, was located in two middle-income, suburban communities, selected as representative of persons who consume large proportions of expensive medical services for life-style-related difficulties. They were also selected because existing models for improving health care were based largely on information from medically indigent populations and because families with young children tend to predominate in such suburban communities (Allen, 1981). The centre gave nurses the opportunity to help families "to examine their health habits and strategies for coping with life, practise new health behaviours, and search out healthy ways of living" (Warner, 1981, p. 34). The model was evaluated by Allen (1983), who reported that 83.2% of the persons brought health situations and 16.8% brought illness problems. "Approximately half the health contacts related to life-style and health behaviour, 20% to adaptation and management of illness, and 23% to changes in the family and interpersonal relationships combined" (p. 55). Although the model demonstrated that the health-care services provided were not available elsewhere and were needed, it did not continue because there was no mechanism for reimbursement of services through the existing health-care system. A need for change is indicated when a model that helped people become more self-reliant about their health and reduced the use of costly medical care services could not be supported and financed.

Increasing evidence suggests that alternative models for primary health care are cost-effective and enhance the quality of care. For example, home visits by public health nurses in Ottawa resulted in greater mobility and higher morale among the elderly and fewer admissions to hospital (Flett, Last, and Lynch, 1980).

In Manitoba, Ramsay, McKenzie, and Fish (1982) reported that patients who attended a clinic staffed by nurses achieved a greater decrease in blood pressure and greater weight loss than the patients attending a physician-staffed clinic. Similarly, persons in Newfoundland who received primary health care delivered by nurses had a decrease in admission to acute-care hospitals, whereas those receiving traditional, physician-based care had a 39% increase in the use of acute-care hospitals (Denton, Gafini, Spencer, and Stoddart, 1982). The length of hospital stay was shortened for patients who had members of the Victorian Order of Nurses (VON) involved in their discharge planning and follow-up care; and physical, social, and emotional outcomes were improved for these patients, in comparison to patients who did not have VON nurses' care (Chambers and West, 1978). In a comparative study of the health behaviours of mothers in three primary-care settings in Quebec—a hospital clinic, a private physician's office, and a community health centre—nurses' care made a difference in the health behaviours of the mothers and the health status of children under 5 years of age (Thibaudeau and Reidy, 1977). Other examples have been cited in the literature, but they have not had a systematic evaluation component to assess outcomes. Hence there is need for designing and testing more primary health-care models, in which nurses are the primary caregivers, and incorporating a sound evaluation component.

Approximately 40 government-funded community health centres have been developed in Ontario since 1973. It is estimated that there are also 160 in Quebec, 29 in the Atlantic provinces and 35 in the Prairie Provinces and British Columbia. They use a multidisciplinary approach, employing a variety of health professionals, such as community, home care and palliative care nurses, nurse practitioners, nutritionists, physicians, physiotherapists and chiropodists, and nonprofessional staff to meet identified needs. Ontario's centres are reported to have reduced costs; the persons using them have had 16.7% fewer hospital days than those using the services of physicians in private practice. There is reported to be low turnover and increased accountability and commitment among nursing staff. While these centres are not the primary health-care model envisioned under nurse leadership, they have facilitated community outreach and provided opportunity for collaborative research, which is critical for health-care programming and evaluation (Innes, 1987).

The Association of Registered Nurses of Newfoundland (ARNN), in collaboration with the Danish Nurses Organization, embarked on such a demonstration project, which continued until 1991. Primary health care is being practised by nurses in selected communities in Newfoundland, and outcomes are being evaluated in terms of measurable improvement in the health status of individuals and families and in health-directed life-styles. The communities were involved in all aspects of program planning, implementation, and evaluation, which is an important concept in primary health care. A major objective was to demonstrate that nurses can provide safe and effective primary health-care services in an affordable and cost-effective manner, and to develop a prototype of primary health care that could be tested in other communities in Newfoundland, in other provinces, and worldwide (AARN, 1987).

Because of concerns about the availability of primary health care to the citizens of Alberta, the cost of health-care, and the need for changes in the health-care system to fully utilize the potential of nurses, the Alberta Association of Registered Nurses (AARN) established a Task Force on Increased Direct Access to Nursing Services Provided by Registered Nurses in 1991. It included wide representation from consumers, government, other health-care providers, and nurses. "The AARN views increased direct access to registered nurses' services as a key component to successful, fundamental health care reform" (AARN, September 1993, p. 13). The challenge to the Task Force was to formulate strategies to increase direct access to nursing services in the community, and increase opportunities for remuneration of registered nurses through public funding. The outcome in 1993 was publication of a brochure and a booklet, both of which are entitled: *NURSES: KEY TO HEALTHY ALBERTANS*, to be used in educating the public, government, nurses, and other health-care professionals. They contain basic aspects of the AARN proposal including the services that could be provided; the benefits of direct access in terms of health promotion and cost savings; and a recommendation to the Alberta government to fund nursing services that can be accessed directly by reallocating present health-care funding from acute-care to a community-based system. Examples of cost savings included are: (l) a 1990 study that showed the cost of immunization by nurses in Alberta to be one-third the cost of immunization by physicians in Ontario (Sadoway, Plain, and Soskolne, 1990); (2) introduction of home care services for low birth weight infants that resulted in an average savings of $18,000 per infant with no reduction in quality of care; (3) provision of home care services through a community health center employing nurses and volunteers resulted in 15% of clients choosing to be discharged from nursing homes and a 25% reduction in hospitalization (Jamieson, 1990); and (4) A 1979 study that showed the cost of home care for dying patients to be 25% less than hospital care (Kassakian, Bailey, Rinker, Stewart, and Yates, 1979). Moreover, there was evidence of improvement of quality of life for the subjects involved in these studies. To implement the goal of increased direct access to services provided by registered nurses, four targets have been identified: nurses, the public, government, and the AARN regions. An organized campaign is underway to maintain and increase support for the initiative, to increase the services provided by nurses in the community, and to make those services more visible to the public through the media and presentations within communities.

■■ ■■ ■■ ■■

OPPORTUNITIES FOR NURSING LEADERSHIP IN PRIMARY HEALTH CARE

The development of other demonstration projects, with an evaluation component designed by experts, is of crucial importance to obtaining data to convince the policy makers and the public in all provinces that a community-focused, primary health-care system with nurses as leaders is the way for the future in Canada. The CNA Board of Directors has emphasized their strong commitment to the concept of primary health care and has established a plan to work toward that goal and lobby to influence and change health policy in Canada. Similar evidence of commitment to the cause is needed in the provinces and territories, where both health-care policy and educational policy are determined. There is increasing evidence of support, as reflected in the AARN proposal for change, to make more registered nurses a point of entry to the health-care system and reallocate health-care funds to provide much more support of primary health-care services. To facilitate changes in the health-care system and in nursing education, both must be changed to enable nurses to provide leadership and function effectively.

To achieve this goal, nurses must be prepared to accept shared responsibility with people for their own health, rather than use the traditional, authoritative approach as providers of care. Nurses must be willing to support communities in addressing matters concerning their health, life-styles, and well-being. They must develop new skills in enabling people to increase control over and improve their health; in empowering people for self-care, self-help, and environmental improvement; and in promoting healthy coping strategies to maintain health (Maglacas, 1988).

Nursing educators must examine curricula to ensure that they are teaching the concept of primary health care as previously interpreted. This is particularly important if the findings of a study of nursing education programs, as reported by Edwards and Craig (1987), are representative of all programs in Canada. The purposes of their study were to determine: (1) the primary health-care concepts in Canadian nursing curricula, (2) faculty's familiarity with primary health-care concepts, (3) the perceived importance of a primary health-care focus in various settings, and (4) the extent to which primary health-care concepts are taught by nursing educators. Their findings revealed that 31.4% of the respondents were aware of the Alma-Ata Declaration and 19.6% had read the ICN statement on primary health care. Approximately 88% were unaware of the Canadian government's position on primary health care. Responses indicated poor differentiation between the concepts of primary care, primary nursing, and primary health care. The inclusion of primary health-care knowledge and skills was minimal and significantly less than expected.

■ ■ ■ ■

THE DEVELOPMENT OF MIDWIFERY IN CANADA

A current issue related to primary health care is the status of midwifery in Canada. Until 1994 Canada was one of the eight WHO countries that did not recognize midwifery as a profession. This changed when Ontario became the first province to license midwives with regulations governing the practice of midwifery coming into effect January 1, 1994, ending a decade of struggle for recognition. The seven WHO countries that still do not recognize midwifery are "Venezuela, Panama, New Hebrides, El Salvador, Dominican Republic, Colombia, and Burundi" (McCourt, 1986, p. 285).

Over the past 4 decades, the public has had increasing influence on the delivery of maternal and infant care. Since the days of the introduction of natural childbirth by Dr. Grantly Dick Read in England, young parents have sought to have more control over the type of care for pregnancy and childbirth and have demanded more participation in decision making. Although some childbearing families in Canada and the United States have been allowed more control over the process of childbirth since the early 1950s, changes of this nature have been slow in developing. In fact some parents believe that medical technology has been allowed to advance at the expense of their rightful control over a normal physiologic process. As a result, some have opted for home birth attended by a practising midwife or occasionally a physician. The hazards of home birth are well known and midwives who provide such care are practising illegally. Young people are likely to continue to pursue this option if not given more voice in the type of care available.

Despite the lack of legal recognition of midwives in Canada until very recently in Ontario, some continued to practise in almost all provinces. In 1987 it was estimated that "approximately 50 midwives were practising in Ontario outside the official health care system" (Task Force on the Implementation of Midwifery in Ontario, 1987). The number practising in other provinces has not been documented, although the Canadian Confederation of Midwives Newsletters (1988 and 1989) include reports from provinces that indicate strong support from midwives across the country to have midwifery recognized legally as a separate profession. Some of these midwives are practising midwifery, whereas others are practising as nurses in obstetric units in hospitals, particularly in labour and delivery units. It is not known what proportion are lay midwives without formal training, nurse midwives, or nonnurse midwives who have earned their credentials to practise midwifery in other countries through approved educational programs. In countries such as Great Britain and the United States, only nurses are admissible to midwifery programs, whereas preparation as a nurse is not an admission requirement in many European countries, including Germany, Denmark, Switzerland, and the Netherlands. Nurses employed by the federal government in Canada in nursing stations/outposts provide comprehensive care to women living in remote areas during the prenatal and postpartal periods and may give emergency labour and birth care when it is not possible to fly a woman to a hospital. Although some of these nurses have had midwifery training in another country, which is considered invaluable, they are not recognized as midwives.

The viability of nurse-midwifery has been demonstrated in the hospital setting in three pilot projects: namely, the Grace Hospital Nurse-Midwifery Project in Vancouver (Weatherston, Carty, Rice, and Tier, 1985), The Chedoke-McMaster Hospitals Nurse-Midwifery Project in Hamilton (Task Force on the Implementation of Midwifery in Ontario, 1987), and The Misericordia Hospital Pilot Project in Edmonton (Marcos, 1983). In these projects the nurses function under the aegis of delegated medical functions, which means that ultimate responsibility resides with the physicians who are available for consultation and referral. The Grace Hospital Project was the first to use nurses, trained as midwives in other countries, in a primary health-care role. It was the result of a collaborative effort by a team of obstetricians and nursing instructors who organized a joint practice. A total of 61 families were cared for in the low-risk clinic, which was a small portion of the families who applied for the service. The approach to care supported the principles of health promotion and primary health care as stated in the Canada Charter. Self-responsibility for care was encouraged, and the care provided a great deal of support and teaching. The parents were active participants during labour and delivery, and the midwife was responsible for delivery of the baby. Midwives made postpartum physical assessments of mother and baby, provided emotional support when necessary and taught maternal self-care, care of the baby, and breastfeeding. They were on call to the mother for 6 weeks after the birth and checked the mother at 2 weeks and 6 weeks postpartum. Weatherston et al (1985) conclude:

> The way the health care system provides for the needs of childbearing women is a major women's health issue. The low-risk clinic provided a different approach to meet the health care needs of women in the perinatal period. Pregnancy and birth were viewed as normal processes and routine medical interventions were avoided. Women were involved in their own care; there was an emphasis on teaching and self-responsibility. The families involved were all extremely positive about the project and the approach taken to providing care. The midwifery approach provided safety as well as recognition of the broader significance of the event in the women's lives and those of their families (p. 37).

Although all of the pilot projects used nurse-midwives or nurses who had considerable experience and skill in maternity nursing, active support has developed across Canada for legalizing midwifery separately from nursing so that it will be an autonomous profession. Midwifery associations have been established to head this movement in all provinces except New Brunswick and Prince Edward Island. In addition, the Canadian Confederation of Midwives (CCM) serves as a mechanism for communication and coordination of efforts. The trend to organize and license midwifery separately from nursing has been opposed by the provincial nursing associations in Ontario, Alberta, British Columbia, and Saskatchewan, and the CNA, whose position is that registration as a nurse should be a prerequisite for admission to a midwifery program and that nurse-midwifery should be a nursing specialty. This position is adamantly opposed by the proponents of midwifery as a separate profession, some of whom have been quoted by the press as stating: "Nurses look after sick people, midwives look after well people. Nurses do things that are designed to cure, which presupposes a person is unwell. Midwives act more as supports, and as preventers of illness" and "A nurse is an adjunct to medicine and as in the medical model, is treating sick people. We don't want to practise medicine. We don't want to care for sick people. We are not nurses. The nurse-midwife is a creation of doctors, a physician extender" (Prokaska, 1985, p. C1). Such perceptions of nursing practice are antithetical to those purported by the CNA and the provincial nursing associations and certainly to the concept of primary health care described here. Both of the persons quoted were trained in another country (Elizabeth McDonald in Australia and Rena Pourteous in Scotland), and it is possible that their concepts of nursing differ from the roles of nurses, as practised in Canada and as envisioned for the future, applying concepts of primary health care.

The greatest progress in the current midwifery movement has occurred in Ontario, where the Minister of Health announced in 1986 "the government's intention to establish midwifery as a recognized part of the Ontario health care system and that midwifery would become a regulated health profession" (Task Force on the Implementation of Midwifery in Ontario, 1987, p. 7). A bill making midwifery 1 of 24 health professions was passed in 1993 and regulations governing the practice of midwifery came into effect January 1, 1994. A College of Midwifery was established through which midwives are to be licensed/registered, regulated and disciplined, as are other health professionals, including nursing through the College of Nursing within the Ontario Ministry of health. Thus midwifery was established as a self-regulating profession independent of nursing and medicine with the "scope of practice based on the international definition of a midwife" (Kaufman, 1991, p. 101.)

Preparation for midwifery in Ontario is through a multiple-entry educational program leading to a baccalaureate degree in midwifery as the entry to practice requirement. The curriculum was designed by a committee composed of midwives, nurses, physicians, educators, and consumers, that "would enable graduates to meet standards of safe midwifery practice within the unique political, sociocultural and geographical environment of Canada" (Relyea, 1992, p. 167). The concept of a multiple-entry program is to permit admission of persons from related backgrounds such as nursing, as well as direct entry (Kaufman, 1991). The first such baccalaureate degree program was established in September 1993, through a partnership involving three universities—McMaster University in Hamilton; Ryerson Polytechnical Institute in Toronto; and Laurentian University in Sudbury. The 4-year program to be offered within 3 calendar years is to include a balance of theory and practice in a variety of practice sites. Plans are to admit 26 students in 1993 and achieve a combined enrollment of 122 in all 3 years by 1996 (CNA News, 1993). In addition, "it is expected that 50-75 practising independent midwives will apply for a license after completing a 6 to 12 month program designed to ensure their competence (Vanwyck, 1992, p. 17). Kaufman (1991) states that the goal is to have midwifery a part of publicly provided services with midwives salaried, and to have midwifery care "accessible through a variety of existing facilities, such as hospitals, birth centres, office practices, community health centres, and women's health clinics, with the provision that the full scope of practice be available in each service" (p. 101). Undoubtedly, the legalization of midwifery practice will have an impact on nurses practising in hospitals and community settings. Vanwyck (1992) believes that "the opportunity to create a new collegial relationship with midwives can empower nurses who recognize and appreciate the benefits and challenges of the changing system" (p. 17).

On July 8, 1992, Alberta became the second province to pass legislation designating midwifery as a profession (Relyea, 1992). Efforts to reach this goal began in 1980 when "the Domiciliary Midwives Council of Alberta presented a brief to the Health Occupations Board for registration as a licensed body as their members were engaged in home delivery. There was strong consumer support for this move, but it was not granted because the domiciliary midwives were viewed as a sub-occupational group" (Alberta Association of Midwives [AAM], 1988, p. 1). The AAM was established in 1986 and includes nurses with midwifery training as well as empirically trained midwives who are practising in Alberta. Their position is the same as those taken in Ontario, and they have been opposed by the Alberta Association of Registered Nurses and the Alberta Medical Association, both of whom support nurse-midwifery but not direct entry into midwifery without prior education as a nurse. Field and Campbell (1986) emphasized that midwifery needs its own professional act to be accepted as part of the health-care system in Alberta. Both are nurse-midwives with advanced education in nursing, but regard it inappropriate to consider only nurse-midwifery and to consider midwifery as a specialty of nursing. They raise many issues that need to be discussed, such as how midwives will work with their colleagues in nursing, the most appropriate method for educating midwives, how midwives will be financed and insured, and whether they will increase or decrease the costs of the system. Field is in charge of the certificate program in nurse-midwifery implemented by the University of Alberta Faculty of Nursing in 1987, which may be taken only in conjunction with the Master of Nursing Program. The Faculty of Medicine has collaborated in the development of the certificate program, as they did in the operation of the Advanced Practical Obstetrics program offered by the Faculty of Nursing from 1944 to 1984. It was designed to better prepare nurses for practice in remote areas and for delivering babies in the absence of a physician. Since midwifery practice is now legalized in both Ontario and Alberta, the graduate students who complete this program will be well prepared for leadership roles in maternity nursing and for teaching in universities, and now will be able to continue to practise nurse-midwifery in those two provinces, which is essential to maintaining competence to teach and guide others in practice. From 1987 to 1995 there were eight graduates of this program (Relyea, 1992).

In their effort to have midwifery legalized in Alberta, the AAM had defined standards of midwifery practise and prepared a position paper on the scope of midwifery practice. In 1988 they presented a brief on the need for midwives in Alberta and documented ideas about role and functions, educational preparation, licensure, liability insurance, and costs to the Premier's Commission on Future Health Care for Albertans. The AAM has collaborated with the Alberta Task Force on Midwifery, which was established for publicity and lobbying purposes, in designing materials for educating the public and politicians about the need for and potential of legalized midwifery practice in Alberta. In 1989 the AAM was encouraged by the government department responsible for professional legislation, to target legislation in 1990 (Scriver, 1989). They succeeded in getting that legislation passed in July 1992. The next step was to establish a Regulatory Advisory Board to develop standards of practice, scope of practice and standards of education, using the Report of the Midwifery Services Review Committee prepared in the process of seeking legislation. This committee was charged with addressing principles, whereas the Regulatory Advisory Board has to address implementation (Field, 1992). "The regulatory review committee will have membership from the AAM [as the representatives of the group to be legislated]; consumers [representing those who will receive the services]; the AARN, the Alberta Hospital Association and the College of Obstetricians and Gynecologists [representing major stakeholders in the change]" (p. 10). The question of educational preparation for the practice of midwifery will have to be addressed. The

Midwifery Services Review Report recommended a baccalaureate degree in midwifery or other equivalent preparation, such as a baccalaureate degree in nursing plus appropriate education in midwifery (Field, 1992). "If a midwifery programme is established in Alberta it would need to be flexible, able to be delivered at a distance, open to challenge by experienced maternity nurses in appropriate areas, and cost effective" (Field, 1992, p. 10). Other issues to be addressed are hospital admitting privileges for midwives and the interface between them and maternity nurses, physicians, and other relevant groups. Collaboration and cooperation is critical to ensuring safe and functional midwifery service in any province (Field, 1992).

The Midwives Association of British Columbia (MABC) has been actively involved in efforts to have midwifery recognized as a separate and autonomous profession in that province. They also provided testimony for a coroner's inquest into the death of a baby, of which the outcome was "strong recommendations to the ministry of health, Grace Hospital, and (the MABC) to legalize autonomous midwifery into the health services of British Columbia and to establish a college of midwives to regulate education and practice" (Scriver, 1989, p. 6). This was not the first attempt to establish midwifery education in this province. In 1984 the British Columbia School of Midwifery was established without government funding and without any clinical practice sites in Canada since midwifery was not yet legalized. Clinical practice for students was obtained in countries, such as Jamaica, Holland, and Germany, that recognized direct-entry midwifery. "After graduating two classes, a total of twenty-two students from the three-year programme, the school ceased to admit students because of lack of economic and legal support" (Relyea, 1992, p. 166). The MABC reports that they have established good professional relationships with both the Registered Nurses Association of British Columbia (RNABC) and the Ministry of Health. They are able to discuss differences with RNABC, but that has not changed the position of RNABC that midwifery should be a nursing specialty and not a separate, autonomous profession that admits persons without nursing preparation to its educational programs. To date, no midwifery proposal has been produced, but an internal working paper is reported to have been drafted (K. Kaufman, personal communication, April 16, 1990).

It is evident that the leaders in midwifery in Canada are networking and helping and supporting each other in their attempts to have midwifery recognized as a separate, autonomous profession in Canada, and that they do not wish to be another nursing specialty or limit their ranks to nurses only, although they support and apply the principles of primary health care in their practice. With the goal of legalizing midwifery practice already achieved in Ontario and Alberta and a midwifery educational program established at the baccalaureate level in Ontario, it will be interesting to follow the progress of this new direction in Canada in these times of severe financial constraints in health care and education.

■ ■ ■ ■

CONCLUSION

The opportunities for nurses to practise primary health care as envisioned by the CNA, Maglacas, and other nursing leaders, are unlimited if they believe in the concept and accept the challenge to work with communities and help them assume responsibility for their own health and well-being. The vision of primary health care is relevant for midwifery practice and would respond well to the wishes of childbearing families to have more control over this important event in their lives. If ever there was a need for unity in nursing, this is the time, as we move forward into the 21st century, to advance the cause of primary health care. To attain nursing's goals and achieve Health for All by the year 2000, will require changes in the health-care system and reorientation of perceptions of nursing and the education needed to function effectively in the primary health-care system. As nurses, why not join forces with the public and work toward these goals?

REFERENCES

Alberta Association of Midwives. (1988, June 30). Brief on the need for midwives in Alberta to the Premier's commission of future health care for Albertans. Unpublished manuscript.

Alberta Association of Registered Nurses. (September 1993). *Nurses Key to Healthy Albertans: Position of AARN on increased direct access to services provided by registered nurses.* (2nd ed.) Edmonton: Author.

Alberta Association of Registered Nurses. (1993). *Nurses key to healthy Albertans: A proposal for change.* Brochure available from 11620 - 168 St., Edmonton, Alberta T5M 4A6.

Alberta Association of Registered Nurses. (1993). *Nurses key to healthy Albertans.* Booklet available from 11620 - 168 St., Edmonton, Alberta T5M 4A6.

Alberta Association of Registered Nurses. (1994 February). Update of AARN initiative on increased direct access to services provided by registered nurses. *AARN Newsletter, 50*(2), 12-13.

Allen, M. (1977). Comparative theories of the expanded role and implications for nursing practice. *Nursing Papers, 9*(2), 38-45.

Allen, M. (1981). The health dimension in nursing practice: Notes on nursing and primary health care. *Journal of Advanced Nursing, 6*(3), 63-64.

Allen, M. (1983). Primary care nursing: Research in action. In L. Hockey (Ed.), *Primary Care Nursing,* (pp. 32-77). Edinburgh: Churchill Livingstone.

Association of Registered Nurses of Newfoundland. (1987). *Primary health care: A nursing model: An overview.* St. John's, Newfoundland: The Association.

Canadian Nurses Association. (1988, September). *Health for all Canadians; A call for health care reform.* Ottawa: The Association.

Canadian Nurses Association. (1989, March). *Position statement on the nurse's role in primary health care.* Ottawa: The Association.

Chamberlain, M.C. and Beckingham, A.C. (1987). Primary health care in Canada: In praise of the nurse? *International Nursing Review, 34*(6), 158-160.

Cambers, L.W. and West, A.E. (1978). The St. John's randomized trial of the family practice nurse: Health outcomes of patients, *International Journal of Epidemiology, 7*(2), 153-161.

CNA Connection. (1988). Keynote speaker: Empowerment key role says Maglacas. *The Canadian Nurse, 84*(8), 14-15.

CNA Connection. (1989). CNA board endorses primary health care. *The Canadian Nurse, 85*(5), 8.

CNA News. (1993). Midwifery goes to college. *The Canadian Nurse, 89*(2), 8.

Denton, F., Gafini, D., Spencer, B., and Stoddart, G. (1982). *Potential savings from the adoption of nurse practitioner technology in the Canadian health care system,* Hamilton, Ontario: McMaster University.

Diers, D., Hamman, A., and Molde, S. (1986). Complexity of ambulatory care: Nurse practitioners and physician caseloads. *Nursing Research, 35*(5), 310-314.

Edwards, N.C. and Craig, H. (1987). *Does nursing education reflect the goals of primary health care?* Hamilton, Ontario: McMaster University.

Feldman, M.J., Ventura, M.R., and Crosby, F. (1987). Studies of nurse practitioner effectiveness. *Nursing Research, 36*(5), 303-308.

Field, P.A. and Campbell, I. (1986). An opinion: midwifery in Alberta. *AARN Newsletter, 42*(7), 17-18.

Field, P. A. (1992). Midwifery: A designated profession. What next? *AARN Newsletter, 48*(8), 10, 12.

Flett, J.E., Last, J.M., and Lynch, G.U. (1980). Evaluation of the public health nurse as primary health care provider for elderly people. In V. Marshall, (Ed.). *Aging in Canada: Social perspec-*

tives, (pp. 177-188). Don Mills, Ontario, Fitzhenry and Whiteside.

Innes, J. (1987). Health care reform: Sketching the future. *AARN Newsletter, 43*(8), 1, 5-6.

Jamieson, M.K. (1990). Block nursing: Practicing autonomous professional nursing in the community. *Nursing & Health Care, 11*, 250-253.

Kassakian, M.G., Bailey, L. R., Rinker, M., Stewart, C.A., & Yates, J.W. (1979). Cost and quality of dying: A comparison of home and hospital. *Nurse Practitioner, 4*(2), 18-23.

Kaufman, K. (1991 June). The introduction of midwifery in Ontario, Canada. *BIRTH, 18*(2), 100-103.

Maglacas, A.M. (1988). Health for all: Nursing's role. *Nursing Outlook, 36*(2), 66-71.

Mahler, H. (1981). The meaning of health for all by the year 2000. *World Health Forum, 2*(1), 5-22.

Marcos, F. (1983). Obstetricians and nursemidwifes: An "inquiry" into a team approach. Unpublished manuscript. Edmonton, Alberta, Misericordia Hospital.

McCourt, C. (1986). Legalization of midwifery and the issue of home births. *Canadian Medical Association Journal, 135*(4), 285-288.

Molde, S. and Diers, D. (1985). Nurse practitioner review: Selected literature review and research agenda. *Nursing Research, 34*(6), 362-367.

Nurse-Midwifery Program of Chedoke-McMaster Hospitals. (1986). Brief to the task force on the implementation of midwifery in Ontario. Unpublished manuscript.

Nutbeam, D. and Lawrence, J. (1987). *Positive health: An update on health promotion in action: A charter for action.* Cardiff: Institute for Health Promotion, College of Medicine, University of Wales.

Ottawa charter for health promotion. (1986). Ottawa: World Health Organization, Health and Welfare Canada, and the Canadian Public Health Association.

Prokaska, L. (1985, August 8). New approach to midwifery at Mac. *The Hamilton Spectator*, p. C1.

Ramsay, J., McKenzie, J.K., and Fish, D.G. (1982). Physicians and nurse practitioners: Do they provide equivalent care? *American Journal of Public Health, 72*(4), 55-57.

Relyea, M. J. (1992). The rebirth of midwifery in Canada: An historical perspective. *Midwifery, 8*, 159-169.

Report of the committee on nurse practitioners. (1972). Ottawa: Department of National Health and Welfare. The Committee.

Sadoway, D.T., Plain, R.H.M., and Saskolne, C.L. (1990). Infant and preschool immunization delivery in Alberta and Ontario: A partial cost-minimization analysis. *Canadian Journal of Public Health, 81*(2), 146-151.

Scriver, B. (ed.) (1988, Summer). *Canadian Confederation of Midwives Newsletter, 2*(1): Calgary, Alberta.

Scriver, B. (1989, Summer). *Canadian Confederation of Midwives Newsletter, 2*(2): (CCM Coordinator, Station G, 50 Couture, Sherbrooke, Quebec. J1H 5M4).

Spitzer, W., Kergin, D.J., and Yoshida, M.A. (1975). Nurse practitioners in primary care: The Southern Ontario randomized trial. In Leininger, M. (Ed.), *Health care dimensions.* Philadelphia: F.A. Davis Co.

Task Force on the Implementation of Midwifery in Ontario. (1987). *Report of the task force: Executive summary and summary of recommendations.* Toronto: Ontario Ministry of Health.

Thibaudeau, M.F. and Reidy, M.M. (1977). Nursing makes a difference: A comparative study of the health behaviours of mothers in three primary care agencies. *International Journal of Nursing Studies, 14*, 97-107.

Ulin, P.R. (1982). International nursing challenge. *Nursing Outlook, 30*(6), 531- 535.

Vanwyck, D.M. (1992). The "New" Profession. *The Canadian Nurse, 88*(2), 15-18.

Warner, M. (1981). The health workshop: A nursing model of primary health care in a rural community. *The Canadian Nurse, 77*(1), 34-36.

Weatherston, L., Carty, E., Rice, A., and Tier, D. (1985). Hospital-based midwifery: Meeting the needs of childbearing women. *The Canadian Nurse, 81*(1), 35-37.

Weller, G.R. (1980, Fall). The determinants of Canadian health policy. *Journal of Health Politics, Policy and Law, 5*, 408-409.

World Health Organization. (1978a). *Report of the international conference on primary health care:* Alma-Ata, USSR, Geneva, September 6-12, 1978.

World Health Organization. (1978b). The Alma-Ata Conference on Primary Health Care. *Who Chronicle, 32*(11), 409-430.

CHAPTER THIRTY TWO

The Growth of Graduate Education in Nursing in Canada

JANET ROSS KERR

T he first half century of university education in nursing in Canada might be termed *the era of the undergraduate basic degree program.* The development of graduate education has become an identifiable thrust in recent years with achievement of improved access to master's degree programs (Fig. 32.1). The start-up phase of bona fide doctoral programs in nursing is well underway with the establishment of five programs by the 1994-95 academic year. Increased research activity in nursing has occurred gradually as a result of a slowly increasing pool of nurses with preparation in research and the wider availability of funding for nursing research investigations. This development goes hand in hand with, and is a necessary condition for, establishment of graduate education in nursing. Most of the research in any field takes place in university settings, and teaching research methods is an important facet of graduate education. Approval of new programs by universities is unlikely without evidence of substantial research activity and the doctoral degree as a standard qualification for faculty appointment.

■ ■ ■ ■

THE ROOTS OF GRADUATE EDUCATION IN NURSING

Although the primary educational problems confronting the profession in the 1940s and 1950s centred around issues of quality in baccalaureate and diploma nursing education, the critical need for nursing leaders prepared at the master's and doctoral levels was recognized. In her study of the needs and resources for graduate nursing education in Canada, Hart observed (1962) that:

> . . . an increasing number of Canadian nurses recognized that graduate education was necessary to qualify for other specialized functions besides teaching. Canadian nurses had enrolled in programs leading to the master's degree to prepare for positions such as administration, supervision and consultation. Canadian nurses secured

407

FIGURE 32.1 Chronology of the growth and development of university degree programs in nursing in Canada.

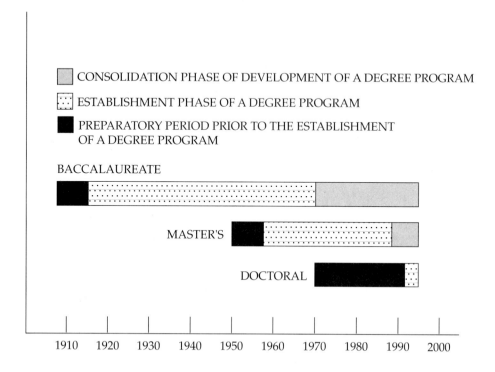

preparation for the specialized functions in nursing education as well as in nursing service in hospitals and health agencies. In spite of increasing demands for graduate education, by the time the study was undertaken there was still no provision for graduate study in nursing in Canada (p. 51).

Hart (1962) concluded that the need to leave the country to pursue graduate study meant that relatively few Canadian nurses were qualified for leadership positions. Good (1969) concurred with this assessment 10 years later. "Canadian nurses too have followed the pattern of study abroad for graduate education. The country of focus was, and still is, the United States of America" (pp. 3-4).

The Canadian Nurses Association (CNA) was in the forefront of developments and strongly supported the call for graduate programs in nursing. Its Committee on Nursing Affairs reported to the 31st Biennial Convention in 1962.

> We should promote immediately an assessment of present facilities, both university and clinical, in order to ascertain what is needed by way of the expansion of university nursing education. . . . On the principle that one can never go wrong with an investment in human beings, a crash program for the development of qualified faculty for Canadian schools of nursing should be undertaken by CNA. . . . CNA might also interest itself in giving some leadership to the development of graduate programs in nursing education, especially in terms of the pooling of university resources in particular specialties (Canadian Nurses Association, 1962, pp. 23-25).

The Committee on Nursing Education also recommended that:

Programs in nursing at the baccalaureate level should be expanded.

The director of the school of nursing should be a nurse with preparation at a master's level and should have the necessary qualifications to assume the responsibility for administration of the school.

All nurses responsible for teaching nursing students should have professional and academic preparation at least at the baccalaureate level and have demonstrated professional competence.

Programs should be developed at the master's and doctoral level to prepare nurses who will be qualified as nursing specialists and for administration, consultation, research and teaching (CNA, 1962, p. 46).

Thus the focus of the profession was broadened to include graduate education as a necessary adjunct in the quest for quality in basic professional education.

As was the case when baccalaureate programs were in their incipient stages, the first thrust was to be for the development of fellowship programs to prepare nurse faculty to take on the responsibilities associated with graduate education. Hart (1962) reported that in 1957

. . . a few unrestricted scholarships and fellowships were found to be available for graduate study in Canadian colleges and universities. Some scholarships were available specifically for nurses and other members of the health professions. . . . If programs for graduate study were available in Canada, it is likely that students in the nursing field would utilize such scholarship and fellowship aid (p. 47).

However, the Kellogg Foundation fellowship program, which spanned 2 decades, provided a much needed source of funds for graduate students who had to incur the expenses associated with taking up residence in a foreign country to find appropriate educational opportunities at the graduate level (Table 32.1). In 1962 the Canadian Nurses Foundation (CNF) was formed with the assistance of a grant of $136,639 from the Kellogg Foundation for the establishment of a fellowship program for study at the master's and doctoral levels and for research assistance for nurses. The CNF completed its first mandate admirably, with a total of 494 graduate fellowships awarded between 1962 and 1994: 339 for study at the master's level and 155 for doctoral work. The total amount given for fellowship awards over the 32-year period of the fund has been $1,595,460 (E. Mountain [personal communication, April 21, 1978]; B.A. Smith [personal communication, April 23, 1987]; B. Campbell [personal communication, March 4, 1994]). It should be noted that the CNF has been very active in fund raising and that provincial professional associations have been regular and substantial donors, and many individuals, institutions, and businesses have contributed funds. A summary of the number and amounts of awards for graduate study from 1962 to 1994 is presented in Table 32.2. Due to problems in maintaining the size of the fund in the first decade of its existence, the Research Committee of the CNF "formulated plans for developing nursing research in Canada but unfortunately, due to lack of funds, these could not be implemented" (Imai, 1971, p. 90). The CNF later initiated a program of research grants. The first such grant was one given to the Canadian Association of University Schools of Nursing

TABLE 32.1 Kellogg Foundation Grants to Canadian University Schools of Nursing and Selected Other Agencies, 1940 to 1978

Organization	Type of Grant	Date	Amount of Grant
Alberta			
University of Alberta, Edmonton	Fellowships in nursing	1949 to 1954	$ 10,862
British Columbia			
University of British Columbia, Vancouver	To aid in establishing nursing education curricula leading to registered nurse licensure, baccalaureate, master's and doctoral degrees	1974 to 1977	333,225
	Fellowships in nursing	1940 to 1953	18,032
Vancouver Metropolitan Health Department	Fellowships in nursing	1946	675
Manitoba			
University of Manitoba, Winnepeg	Fellowships in nursing	1941 to 1949	2,815
New Brunswick			
New Brunswick Association for Registered Nurses, Fredericton	Fellowships in nursing	1953	715
University of New Brunswick, Fredericton	To aid in establishing a degree program in basic nursing	1958 to 1965	198,857
	To help establish a program of continuing education in nursing	1958 to 1961	17,504
Ontario			
Canadian Nurses Association, Ottawa (for Province of Ontario)	Fellowships in nursing	1950	1,493
McMaster University, Hamilton	Fellowships in nursing	1948 to 1954	19,787
	To help establish a graduate education curriculum in nursing	1973 to 1978	290,935
Quebec			
McGill University	Development of a master's degree program for non-nurse graduates	1981	86,279

TABLE 32.2 Canadian Nurses Foundation Fellowship Awards, 1962 to 1987

Awards Given in	Number of Master's Awards	Number of Doctoral Awards	Total Amount Awarded
1962 to 1963	9	1	$ 11,700
1963 to 1964	12	—	31,000
1964 to1965	8	3	35,700
1965 to 1966	6	2	27,250
1966 to 1967	11	3	37,175
1967 to 1968	11	2	36,700
1968 to 1969	15	2	52,550
1969 to 1970	16	1	42,100
1970 to 1971	14	5	56,537
1971 to 1972	11	2	32,500
1972 to 1973	12	2	36,200
1973 to 1974	9	1	31,000
1974 to 1975	3	1	13,500
1975 to 1976	5	1	17,900
1976 to 1977	8	0	21,900
1977 to 1978	12	2	35,500
1978 to 1979	12	2	37,800
1979 to 1980	9	4	61,500
1980 to 1981	5	5	34,000
1981 to 1982	4	3	15,000
1982 to 1983	15	6	37,208
1983 to 1984	12	5	37,700
1984 to 1985	9	6	32,500
1985 to 1986	9	2	36,000
1986 to 1987	7	5	44,000
1987 to 1988	6	6	45,000
1988 to 1989	8	9	65,000
1989 to 1990	17	14	122,000
1990 to 1991	18	14	126,000
1991 to 1992	14	17	129,340
1992 to 1993	15	15	124,500
1993 to 1994	17	14	128,000
TOTAL	339	155	1,594,760

Personal communication with Eileen Mountain, Assistant to the Secretary-Treasurer, Canadian Nurses Foundation, April 21, 1978; Bette Anne Smith, Assistant to the Secretary-Treasurer, Canadian Nurses Foundation, April 23, May 15, 1987; and Bev Campbell, Executive Director, Canadian Nurses Foundation, March 4, 1994.

(CAUSN) for a research project on accreditation of university schools of nursing. With the establishment of the Ad Hoc Research Committee in 1983, the CNF Board of Directors initiated a program of research grants, which, although small, has been important in encouraging nurses to undertake research.

■■ ■■ ■■ ■■

ESTABLISHMENT OF MASTER'S DEGREE PROGRAMS

The efforts of the University of Western Ontario (UWO) to develop a 1-year diploma program in nursing service administration led to the establishment of a master's level program in that area, a program that became the first graduate program in nursing in Canada (Overduin, 1970). In 1957, when the President of the University, Dr. G.E. Hall, applied for Kellogg funding to implement the diploma program that had received the approval of the University Senate as early as 1956, he:

> ... requested $100,000 from the Foundation ... $50,000 of which was slated for the 'intensive development' of the new DNSA program—the Foundation indicated its willingness to support the school of nursing in its educational efforts in nursing administration. It supported the development of a master's program in Canada, to be supported by the Foundation over a five-year period just as it had done earlier in American universities (Overduin, 1970, p. 84).

A brief was prepared and submitted to the Kellogg Foundation.

> [It] showed that Western met all the requirements set by the Foundation, described in detail the programs and courses offered by the school of nursing, and a projected budget for a five-year period indicating the cost of five major areas which would be supported by the Foundation: the master's program, and project of case-writing in administration, two fellowships per year to be granted during each year of the grant— each fellow to receive $2,000 per year for each year of her two-year program, an annual seminar for senior nursing executives, and continuing education for faculty (Overduin, 1970, p. 84).

Although it is reported that $142,000 was awarded by the Foundation for the establishment of this program (Overduin, 1970; University of Western Ontario [UWO] School of Nursing, 1967 to 1968), Kellogg records indicate that $128,618 was in fact expended between 1959 and 1965 "to help establish a program of graduate education in nursing service administration" (W.K. Kellogg Foundation [cited in Kerr, 1978, p. 261]) (Table 32.1). Planning for the implementation of the new program began in March of 1959, and "on October 30, 1959, the Senate approved the first year of the program, and the entrance requirements" (Overduin, 1970, p. 85). Of note was the recognition that "the great need for research, especially research in appraising nursing care and service, was instrumental in the decision that a student would be required to produce a thesis" (Overduin, 1970, p. 85).

At McGill University, much progress had occurred since 1944, when the baccalaureate degree program was established. The transition to the integrated program occurred in 1957. However, planning for a master's level program began even earlier:

> Research in nursing at McGill had been urged in Miss Green's report of 1953. The following year students in the second year degree programme undertook small research projects under the direction of staff members. Miss Chittick began to press for the creation of a Master's programme in nursing at the School for Graduate Nurses (Tunis, 1966, p. 11).

After a resolution was passed at the 1958 CNA convention expressing the need for opportunities for graduate study in nursing in Canadian universities, "at McGill a two-year programme leading to a degree of M.Sc. (Applied) was drawn up for approval by the Faculty of Graduate Studies and Research" (Tunis, 1966, p. 112). Senate approval, in principle, was received in September 1959, and again the Kellogg Foundation provided financial support to make the program plans operational with a grant of $195,000 over 5 years (Tunis, 1966). This brought the total amount of Kellogg Foundation assistance to McGill for the development of curricula to $221,252 between 1946 and 1967 (Tables 32.1 and 32.3). Once again in the vanguard of developments in university nursing education in Canada, the W.K. Kellogg Foundation expressed its rationale for the assistance. "Graduate programs in Canadian universities are greatly needed. Better teachers of nursing produce better practitioners and, hence, improve patient care" (W.K. Kellogg Foundation, 1966, p. 56).

There was a considerable lapse of time after the early activity in the establishment of master's programs at UWO and McGill University sponsored by the Kellogg Foundation grants. However, demonstrations had begun and it was up to the institutions to obtain their own resources if they wished to initiate graduate programs in nursing. Given the historical reluctance of universities to approve the development of new and costly graduate programs requiring ongoing and increasing operating expenditures, it is not surprising, particularly in the absence of financial inducements, that 5 years passed before another program was established. The year 1966 witnessed the inception of the graduate program at l'université de Montréal, the first master's program in the French language in the world, and in 1968, a program was developed at the University of British Columbia (Good, 1971).

The W.K. Kellogg Foundation again offered support for development in master's programs with an award of $178,000 to the Faculty of Nursing at the University of Toronto "to establish a graduate program to prepare clinical nurse specialists" (W.K. Kellogg Foundation, 1971, p. 28). In her annual report to the President, Dean Helen Carpenter (1970) describes the nature of the program in its first year of operation.

> The Master's Degree programme embodies specialization, mastery in depth of a specific area of knowledge, independent and critical study, and research. The purposes of the course are to make available advanced preparation for leadership roles in selected areas of nursing, and to advance nursing knowledge and skills through analytical study and investigation. Opportunity is provided for the students to acquire knowledge from nursing and the related sciences to provide the rationale for the management of complex health problems. (p. 74)

Another indication of interest in innovative developments in nursing curricula in Canada is the Foundation support, granted in 1973 for a 5-year period, to the School of Nursing at McMaster University for an "interdisciplinary graduate program to prepare clinical nurse specialists in primary and ambulatory care" (W.K. Kellogg Foundation, 1975, p. 19). This program award was for $290,196. An excerpt from the Foundation's *Annual Report* (1974) discusses the nature of this unique program.

TABLE 32.3 Kellogg Foundation Support for Development of Master's Degree Programs in Nursing in Canada*

	Univ. of B.C.	Univ. of West. Ont.	McMaster Univ.	Univ. of Toronto	McGill Univ.	CNA	Total
1959		19,233					19,233
1960		24,453					24,453
1961		25,406			48,159		73,565
1962		24,427			22,812	13,920	61,159
1963		25,948			28,209	27,717	81,874
1964		17,985			26,672	27,837	72,494
1965					14,567	69,668	84,235
1966					21,425		21,425
1967					18,499		18,499
1968				34,852			34,852
1969				28,159			28,159
1970							0
1971				72,006			72,006
1972				28,968			28,968
1973			135,143				135,143
1974	76,838		79,798	8,738			165,374
1975	131,316			75,436			206,752
1976	84,337		46,984				131,321
1977	40,734		20,936		108,797		170,467
1978			8,074		111,673		119,747
1979					159,884		159,884
1980					186,586		186,586
1981					23,830		23,830
1982							0
TOTAL	333,225	137,452	290,935	248,159	771,113	139,142	1,920,026

*Since 1982 no grants have been made for Canadian health projects, as new guidelines have restricted grants outside the United States to Latin America and Southern Africa.

From Annual Reports of the WK Kellogg Foundation from 1959 to 1982.

Foundation funds are helping the Division of Health Sciences of McMaster University, Hamilton, Ontario, develop an interdisciplinary graduate program to prepare nurses for advanced clinical practice in primary and ambulatory care. Students may choose clinical practice in maternal child health, family practice, or rehabilitation. Every attempt is made to include a true interdisciplinary experience, with members of several health professions learning together about issues in the delivery and management of health care. Nursing students will work with a physician preceptor during their clinical experience. The physician preceptor will also work with medical residents and will relate to both groups toward effective interdisciplinary clinical practice (pp. 10-11).

Although the master's program at the University of Alberta, established in 1975, did not receive external funding, it derived substantial benefit from the development of the Master's in Health Services Administration program in 1968. This program was initiated under the auspices of the Western Canadian Council on Education of Health Personnel, with a Kellogg Foundation grant of $212,250 for a 5-year period (W.K. Kellogg Foundation, 1970). This program incorporated a stream for nursing administrators and paved the way for the 1975 development of the Master of Nursing program by providing for a joint appointment between the Division of Health Services Administration and the Faculty of Nursing and by developing a strong research thrust in the program. Both developments were assets to the Faculty of Nursing and facilitated the development of its master's program in 1975.

At the University of British Columbia (UBC), the initiation of the master's program took place initially without external funding. However, 5 years later, a large W.K. Kellogg Foundation grant was awarded to the School of Nursing "to aid in establishing nursing education curricula leading to registered nurse licensure, baccalaureate, master's and doctoral degrees" (W.K. Kellogg Foundation [Cited in Kerr, 1978, p. 259]) (Table 32.1). Although the basic elements of such a *ladder system* approach were developed before the termination of the grant in 1977, the doctoral part of the program was not established during the 5-year time frame. Noteworthy too, is the fact that UBC dropped the ladder concept before the end of the decade to concentrate on its basic and post-RN baccalaureate and master's programs. Another development in the availability of master's programs was the establishment of the first program in the Atlantic area at Dalhousie University in 1975.

Documentation of Kellogg Foundation support for the initiation of graduate programs on an annual basis between 1959 and 1982 provides a clear picture of financial resources expended by the Foundation in the first phase in the development of graduate education in nursing in Canada (Table 32.1). The resources, which were awarded to the CNA for the establishment of the CNF and are also included as CNF awards for graduate study, were a critical factor in the development of the faculty resources needed to offer graduate programs in Canada. Total support from 1959 to 1976 amounted to $1,920,026 with an average award of $2730 in any one year. Awards were made to five universities for this purpose. All awards, with the exception of the 1974 award to the UBC, were designed to assist with the establishment of new master's degree programs in nursing. In the case of UBC, support was designated for an articulated nursing program from baccalaureate through doctoral levels, although, as previously noted, this program did not materialize. Support was awarded for a 5-year period, after which the institution assumed full responsibility for all operating costs of continuing programs. Kellogg Foundation funding is no longer available for Canadian health projects, because "programming guidelines since 1982 have restricted grants outside the United States to Latin America and our beginning efforts in southern Africa" (Grace, personal communication, May 14, 1987).

▬ ▬ ▬ ▬

EXPANSION OF MASTER'S PROGRAMS IN NURSING

A great deal has occurred since the first master's programs were developed at the University of Western Ontario in 1959 and at McGill University in 1961

TABLE 32.4 Establishment of Master's Degree Programs in Nursing

Institution	Date program established
Faculty of Nursing, The University of Western Ontario	1959
School of Nursing, McGill University	1961
Faculté des sciences infirmières, l'université de Montreal	1965
School of Nursing, The University of British Columbia	1968
Faculty of Nursing, The University of Toronto	1970
Faculty of Nursing, The University of Alberta	1975
School of Nursing, Dalhousie University	1975
Faculty of Nursing, The University of Manitoba	1979
Faculty of Nursing, The University of Calgary	1981
School of Nursing, Memorial University of Newfoundland	1982
College of Nursing, The University of Saskatchewan	1986
École des sciences infirmières, l'université laval	1991
School of Nursing, The University of Ottawa	1993
School of Nursing, Queen's University	1994
School of Nursing, University of Windsor	1994
School of Nursing, McMaster University	1994

(see Table 32.4). The first programs offering study in clinical content areas were developed, beginning with the program at l'université de Montréal in 1966. The program at the University of British Columbia was begun in 1968. In the 1970s, three more new master's programs were established at the University of Toronto (1975), Dalhousie University (1975), and the University of Alberta (1975). As the impact of the slow growth and retrenchment of the early 1970s began to subside, three new master's degree programs in nursing appeared. These were located at the University of Manitoba (1979), University of Calgary (1981), and Memorial University of Newfoundland (1982). In 1986, another new master's program was initiated in the west, at the University of Saskatchewan. Further developments in the development of master's degree programs in nursing occurred in the first half of the decade of the 1990s, when programs were established at l'université laval (1991), the University of Ottawa (1993), the University of Windsor (1994), and at Queen's University (1994). Still other programs are in the planning stages, and it may be that there has been further pressure to develop greater access to master's degree programs in nursing from those who wish to enter doctoral programs in nursing.

The above statistics do not include interdisciplinary programs in which nursing may be one discipline of several that offer a master's degree program. Such programs have existed for some time and include the University of Alberta's Master of Health Services Administration program and McMaster University's interdisciplinary Master of Health Sciences program. More recently interdisciplinary programs have been developed at the University of Victoria in the Faculty of Human and Social Development of which the School of Nursing is one unit and at l'université de Sherbrooke where the School of Nursing operates as a unit of the Faculty of Medicine.

■■ ■■ ■■ ■■

ANALYSIS OF ENROLMENT TRENDS IN MASTER'S PROGRAMS

Considerable growth has occurred in master's programs since 1959 when the total enrolment at the UWO was two students (Overduin, 1970) or since the 1960-61 academic year when the combined enrolment at UWO and McGill University was 16. In the next 5 years, total enrolment grew by 56%. In the next 5-year interval, three more programs were established and there was an increase of 675 in total enrolment (see Table 32.5). During this time, programs that offered study in a clinical content area were developed, beginning with the program at l'université de Montréal in 1966. An analysis of early trends in the development of graduate education in nursing prompted one author to speculate on the reasons why Canadian nurses were still traveling to the United States for graduate study instead of enroling in the new Canadian programs.

1. Historical precedent
2. More and better qualified nurse faculty
3. Greater variety in programming

In the latter instance, US universities offer advanced study in five to eight clinical content areas, as well as in the functional specialties. At present, only one Canadian master's program offers study in a clinical area; all offer functional specialization (Good, 1969, p. 7).

Also interesting are enrolment trends since 1965. Erratic changes characterize the first 5-year period, probably due to the smaller aggregate numbers on which the calculations are based, and to the beginnings of retrenchment, as growth was replaced by shortfalls in enrolments nationally. The year 1969-70, when four programs were operational, was the only one of the decade in which there was a decrease in enrolment over the previous year. The next year saw a 35% increase, and a 26% increase occurred in 1971-72. In the period between 1970 and 1976, three more new master's programs were initiated, and total enrolment grew by 47%. For the academic years from 1971 through 1975, enrolment increases were lower, ranging from 3% to 8%, representing a slow but steady increase in student numbers and increased access to programs made possible by the addition of two programs after 1969-70. In 1975-76 there was a larger overall increase—

TABLE 32.5 Enrolment Changes in Master's Programs in Canadian Universities from 1965-66 to 1993-94

Year	Total Enrolment	Percentage Change in Enrolment From Year to Year
1965 to 1966	37	Base Year
1966 to 1967	51	+ 28
1967 to 1968	56	+ 9
1968 to 1969	79	+ 29
1969 to 1970	73	− 8
1970 to 1971	112	+ 35
1971 to 1972	151	+ 26
1972 to 1973	159	+ 5
1973 to 1974	172	+ 8
1974 to 1975	177	+ 3
1975 to 1976	203	+ 13
1976 to 1977	244	+ 17
1977 to 1978	278	+ 12
1978 to 1979	263	− 6
1979 to 1980	304	+ 13
1980 to 1981	345	+ 12
1981 to 1982	381	+ 9
1982 to 1983	381	0
1983 to 1984	526	+ 28
1984 to 1985	524	0
1985 to 1986	699	+ 25
1986 to 1987	632	− 9.6
1987 to 1988	729	+ 13.3
1988 to 1989	674	− 7.6
1989 to 1990	783	+ 13.9
1991 to 1992	847	+ 7.6
1992 to 1993	904	+ 6.3

Note: 1. Prior to 1991, data collected were from January to December.
       2. 1991 data were collected for the period ending July, 1991.
       3. 1992 data were collected for the period January to December 31, 1992.
       4. Totals include part-time and full-time students.

From annual statistical collection on university nursing students and faculty profiles collected by the Canadian Association for University Schools of Nursing and prepared by the Canadian Nurses Association, 1975-1994.

about 13%—in the total enrolment figures. The new programs accounted for the larger percentage increase. Exponential increases occurred over the next decade with the addition of new programs and increases in the size of existing ones. By 1993, total enrolment in master's programs had reached 904. Demand was apparent as more students applied for admission than could be accommodated in programs.

— — — —

ANALYSIS OF ENROLMENT TRENDS IN DOCTORAL PROGRAMS

With the establishment of the first fully funded doctoral program in nursing at the University of Alberta on January 1, 1991, followed shortly thereafter in September, 1991, by the implementation of a second funded program at the University of British Columbia, nursing students no longer had to study in other disciplines or be admitted as special case doctoral students in nursing. Programs at the University of Toronto and a joint program between McGill University and l'université de Montréal were initiated in the fall of 1993, and a fifth program commenced at McMaster University in September, 1994. As doctoral programs become established, enrolments will begin to climb. The first students were enrolled in doctoral programs in nursing between 1976 and 1988, and by 1992 enrolment across the country had reached 18 (see Table 32.6).

— — — —

DEVELOPING THE FACULTY RESOURCES FOR GRADUATE PROGRAMS

The element that constitutes the most essential resource in successfully operating a graduate program is its faculty. Securing faculty members with the requisite skills to offer such a program is the most critical and difficult task. This was recognized earlier by Kathleen Russell (cited in Carpenter [1970]) as she laid the foundations of the basic baccalaureate degree program at the University of Toronto.

> Among the criteria established for faculty positions were: the capacity for independent and creative thought and critical analysis, a broad concept of nursing, a university degree representing sound, general education in the humanities, and preparation for teaching. As nurses with these qualifications were difficult to find, fellowships were secured to assist those selected to undertake additional study and to broaden their understanding of nursing through travel and observation in other countries (p. 93).

Although skills such as creative thinking and critical analysis, complemented by a broad knowledge of nursing and research skills, can be learned in other than formal university settings, Stinson (1977) observed the following about the development of research skills: "One must consider the point that a great deal about research can be learned from participating in increasingly more complex projects" (p. 29). However, she also notes that "it is only in the rare instance that sound research preparation and high research productivity can occur in the absence of substantial amounts and kinds of formalized instruction" (Stinson, 1977, p. 29).

University nursing administrators have experienced difficulty in securing suitably qualified faculty for teaching in university programs. This was a major concern during the formative years in the establishment of baccalaureate programs, and there were times when schools were forced to operate with fewer staff than was desirable because of unfilled faculty positions. Supply and demand questions aside, there is still the leadership connection-that is, whether or not administrators of university schools were sufficiently perceptive and aggressive in recognizing the necessary skills and in encouraging their development in faculty members who showed promise.

TABLE 32.6   Enrolment Changes in Doctoral Programs in Canadian Universities from 1987 to 1993

Year	Total Enrolment	Percentage Change in Enrolment From Year to Year
1987 to 1988	2	Base Year
1988 to 1989	6	66.7
1989 to 1990	6	0
1990 to 1991	8	+ 25
1991 to 1992	8	0
1992 to 1993	18	+ 55.6

Note: 1. Prior to 1991, data collected were from January to December.
2. 1991 data were collected for the period ending July, 1991.
3. 1992 data were collected for the period January to December 31, 1992.
4. Totals include part-time and full-time students.

From annual statistical collection on university nursing students and faculty profiles collected by the Canadian Association for University Schools of Nursing and prepared by the Canadian Nurses Association, 1975-1994.

Fellowship programs for faculty development have been available since the 1920s. In the early years these were, for the most part, under the sponsorship of private foundations and were earmarked for faculty development. They were also often awarded directly to the institutions to offer to suitable candidates. However, in the late 1950s public funds became available from federal sources administered through the provinces. With the establishment of the CNF, fellowship funds for graduate study also became available from that source. Although they have been used to a great extent for faculty development, the new funds were not specifically earmarked for this purpose and have also been used for graduate preparation of nurses for practice, educational, and administrative settings.

The dearth of prepared faculty prompted Good (1969) to conclude that "the void in qualified nurse faculty in Canada has deterred development of Canadian graduate nurse education, and subsequent nursing research" (p. 8). The situation in 1960-61, shortly after master's programs were first initiated, was that among faculty teaching in university schools, 58% held baccalaureate degrees and 38% held master's degrees (Mussallem, 1965).

> . . . Although the academic qualifications of faculty in university schools of nursing are higher than those for hospital schools, it should be recognized that university instructors are teaching at the baccalaureate level and their preparation should be beyond that of their students (Mussalem, 1965, p. 84).

The situation changed slowly throughout the next decade as more master's programs became available, and by 1970-71, 1.43% of faculty in university programs held doctoral degrees, 44% held master's degrees, and 49% held baccalaureate degrees (CNA, 1971). In the 5-year period ending in 1975-76, there was evidence of additional progress, as 3.74% now held doctoral degrees, 31.28% held master's degrees, and 58.02% held the baccalaureate qualification (Statistics Canada, 1976). In 1980, Larsen and Stinson (1980) conducted a national survey to learn the number of nurses holding doctoral degrees. Of the 81 qualified at the doctoral level, 69% were employed in universities. A 1989 update of these statistics indicated that 257 held doctoral degrees; of these, 79% were employed in universities (Lamb and Stinson, 1990, p. 9).

PREPARING TO ESTABLISH DOCTORAL PROGRAMS IN NURSING

In 1975, at the Fourth National Nursing Research Conference held in Edmonton, Alberta, a group of participants interested in facilitating the establishment of doctoral programs in the country held an informal meeting to discuss how this might be accomplished. Other discussions were held at national nursing meetings, and in 1976, a resolution passed at the CNA Biennial Convention directing the Association to provide leadership in the quest to establish doctoral education in Canada. Through a joint initiative of the CNA, CNF, and CAUSN, a national seminar on doctoral education in nursing was convened in 1978. The W.K. Kellogg Foundation provided funding for the seminar, which brought together deans/directors of university schools of nursing and deans of graduate studies at those institutions to consider issues in planning for the establishment of doctoral education in Canada. The meeting produced a commitment to establishing one or more PhD programs in nursing (Zilm, Larose, and Stinson, 1979). This was the first public recognition of the need to develop one or more programs in this country. As had happened when access to baccalaureate and later master's programs was limited, Canadian nurses emigrated to the United States to take advantage of the educational programs there. Some never returned to Canada, as they were offered attractive positions in the United States.

Another initiative at the national level was the establishment of the Working Group on Nursing Research in 1982, by the Medical Research Council (MRC). This occurred as the result of efforts by the CNA to document the low level of nursing research funding provided by the national granting councils. Although the smallest funding body, the National Health Research and Development Program, provided limited funding, funds were not specifically designated for nursing; many other disciplines depended on it for the major share of their funding. Also, although both the MRC and the Social Sciences and Humanities Research Council stated that nursing was included among the disciplines that could be funded, nurses had difficulty getting either council to review nursing proposals. Consequently, few nursing proposals had been funded by either body. The Working Group was created to address these difficulties. Final recommendations in the Report of the Working Group in 1985 addressed the need to assist in creating opportunities for the establishment of PhD in Nursing programs. Also addressed was the need to designate nursing research for funding within the MRC (Medical Research Council of Canada, 1985). A special initiative to support nursing research was established in 1988 jointly by the MRC and the National

Health Research Development Program (NHRDP) but meagre results have emerged from this venture thus far. The broadening of the mandate of the MRC to include health research in 1994 was an initiative that the MRC has struggled with for many years. Nursing research was clearly included as eligible for funding under this broadened mandate.

■■ ■■ ■■ ■■

THE ESTABLISHMENT OF DOCTORAL PROGRAMS

After the Kellogg National Seminar in 1978, McGill University and l'université de Montréal prepared a joint submission for a cooperative, bilingual PhD program, but several factors prevented the approval of the program when it was proposed in 1980. The University of Toronto developed an arrangement with the Institute of Medicine whereby nurses could be admitted to the PhD program offered by that unit to pursue studies in nursing. This arrangement included some Faculty of Nursing input in the program and allowed nurses to take a program more closely related to their own discipline. In 1980, the Council of the Faculty of Nursing of the University of Alberta approved the development of a proposal for a PhD program. Consequently, a proposal was developed and approved by that Faculty Council by 1985 and was approved by the Board of Governors of the University in 1986. The program was funded by the Alberta government on January 1, 1991, which allowed the admission of students to the first fully funded PhD program in nursing in Canada (see Table 32.7). A second doctoral program in nursing was funded at the University of British Columbia in September, 1991, and two additional programs began in the fall of 1993 at the University of Toronto and a joint program at McGill University and l'université de Montréal. In the fall of 1994, a fifth program got underway at McMaster University. A number of special case students had been admitted to McGill University and the University of Alberta prior to the funding of bona fide PhD programs. The first graduate to receive a PhD in nursing from a Canadian university was a special case student, Francine Ducharme, from McGill who graduated in the fall of 1990. The School of Nursing at the University of Victoria has moved to develop a "PhD by Special Arrangement," an individualized PhD program of studies similar to the special case arrangements developed in other universities including McGill and Alberta prior to the establishment of their PhD in nursing programs (School of Nursing, University of Victoria, 1995). Although access to doctoral education in nursing is still very limited, enrolment is growing across all programs. It is likely that research in nursing will also continue to grow with the preparation of doctoral candidates with expertise in research.

■■ ■■ ■■ ■■

POSTDOCTORAL EDUCATION IN NURSING

Postdoctoral education in nursing is relatively new on the horizon, although this form of socialization to the academic world has been common in other disciplines for decades. The National Health Research and Development Program offers such fellowships to the various disciplines that receive research funding

TABLE 32.7 Doctoral Programs in Nursing in Canada: Historical Overview

Institution	Date program accepted first students	Preceded by a special case arrangement
Faculty of Nursing, University of Alberta	January 1, 1991	Yes
School of Nursing, Faculty of Applied Sciences, University of British Columbia	September 1, 1991	No
Faculty of Nursing, University of Toronto	September 1, 1993	No*
School of Nursing, Faculty of Medicine, McGill University/ Faculté des sciences infirmières, l'université de Montréal	September 1, 1993	Yes
School of Nursing, Faculty of Health Sciences, McMaster University	September 1, 1994	No
School of Nursing, Faculty of Human and Social Development, University of Victoria	N/A	Yes**

*The Faculty of Nursing at the University of Toronto had some involvement in a doctoral program established in the Institute of Medicine. Prior to the establishment of the PhD in nursing program, a number of nurses enrolled in and graduated from that program.

**The School of Nursing at the University of Victoria initiated the PhD by Special Arrangement in the 1994-95 academic year. The first student/s are expected to enrol in the 1995-96 academic year.

from it. The Social Sciences and Humanities Research Council also offers post-doctoral fellowships. The latter are limited to those who do not hold academic appointments at a Canadian university. This stipulation is somewhat of a detriment to university faculties and schools of nursing as nursing is developmentally at a different stage than most other academic disciplines in the university. There is a need for such fellowships among university nursing faculty members who are pursuing doctoral education in nursing in other institutions and who are on leave from their home university. The Alberta Foundation for Nursing Research established a new funding category for postdoctoral fellowships in 1990. However, fiscal problems being experienced by the organization make it likely that such fellowships will not be offered in the immediate future.

Postdoctoral educational opportunities in nursing are essential if graduates of the new PhD in nursing programs are to have an opportunity to develop research programs that they can continue as they take up academic appointments in nursing in universities in the future. Experience has shown that new PhD graduates require support from more experienced researchers and the time to plan their research and submit research proposals funding agencies. If they have the opportunity to work on a collegial basis with established researchers, they are much more likely to be successful when they take up their appointments in faculties and schools of nursing. Given the time and resources that have been invested in the brightest and the best, it would seem worthwhile to set up neophyte researchers for success!

REFERENCES

Canadian Nurses Association. (1962). *Folio of reports 1962*. Ottawa: Author.

Carpenter, H.M. (1970). The University of Toronto School of Nursing: An agent of change. In M.Q. Innes (Ed.), *Nursing education in a changing society*, (pp. 86-108). Toronto: University of Toronto Press.

Good, S.R. (1969). *Submission to the study of support of research in universities for the Science Secretariat of the Privy Council*. Ottawa: Canadian Nurses Association and Canadian Nurses Foundation.

Good, S.R. (1971). *Submission to the Association of Universities and Colleges of Canada*. Calgary: University of Calgary.

Hart, M.E. (1962). *Needs and resources for graduate education in nursing in Canada*. Unpublished doctoral dissertation. New York: Teacher's College, Columbia University.

Imai, H.R. (1971). Professional associations and research activities in nursing in Canada. In *National Conference on Research in Nursing Practice*. Ottawa: School of Nursing, The University of British Columbia.

Kerr, J.C.R. (1978). *Financing university nursing education in Canada: 1919-1976*. Ph.D. dissertation. Ann Arbor, MI: The University of Michigan.

Lamb, M. and Stinson, S.M. (1990). *Canadian nursing doctoral statistics: 1989 update*. Ottawa: Canadian Nurses Association.

Larsen, J. and Stinson, S.M. (1980). *Canadian nursing doctoral statistics*. Ottawa: Canadian Nurses Association.

Medical Research Council of Canada. (1985). *Report to the Medical Research Council of Canada by the Working Group on Nursing Research*. Ottawa: Author.

Mussallem, H.K. (1965). *Nursing education in Canada*. Ottawa: Queens University Printer.

Overduin, H. (1970). *People and ideas: Nursing at Western 1920-1970*. London, Ontario: The University of Western Ontario.

School of Nursing, University of Victoria. (1995). PhD by Special Arrangement: Brochure. pp. 1-5. Victoria, B.C.: Author.

Statistics Canada. (1976). *Nursing in Canada: Canadian nursing statistics, 1976*. Ottawa: Author.

Stinson, S.M. (1977). Central issues in Canadian nursing research. In B. LaSor and M.R. Elliott (Eds.), *Issues in Canadian nursing*, (pp. 3-42). Scarborough, Ontario: Prentice-Hall of Canada Ltd.

Tunis, B. (1966). *In caps and gowns*. Montreal: McGill University Press.

University of Western Ontario. (1967-68). *Calendar*. London, Ontario: Author.

W.K. Kellogg Foundation. (1966). *Annual Report*. Battle Creek, MI: Author.

W.K. Kellogg Foundation. (1970). *Annual Report*. Battle Creek, MI: Author.

W.K. Kellogg Foundation. (1971). *Annual Report*. Battle Creek, MI: Author.

W.K. Kellogg Foundation. (1974). *Annual Report*. Battle Creek, MI: Author.

W.K. Kellogg Foundation. (1975). *Annual Report*. Battle Creek, MI: Author.

Zilm, G., Larose, O., and Stinson, S. (1979). *Ph.D. (nursing)*. Ottawa: Canadian Nurses Association.

PART V

The View Beyond

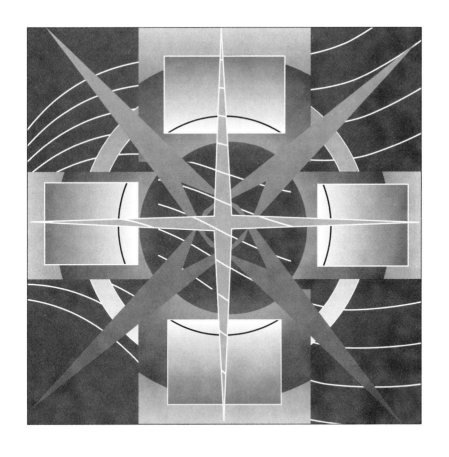

CHAPTER THIRTY THREE

International Nursing: Looking Beyond Our Borders

RICHARD SPLANE AND VERNA HUFFMAN SPLANE

T his chapter identifies issues relating to the complex and challenging field of international nursing. Although these issues are important to nurses everywhere, they are reviewed from a Canadian perspective. While the topic is approached developmentally, touching on international nursing's evolution and giving recognition to nurses who have played a role in its progress, most attention focuses on what now occupies the central stage—Health For All by the Year 2000, proclaimed by the United Nations. Through its unanimous adoption, all member nations, including Canada, have committed themselves to achieving that far-reaching objective.

The policy base for the Health For All goal was laid at the historic conference in Alma Ata, Union of Soviet Socialist Republic, in 1978. The conference, jointly sponsored by two of the United Nations' specialized agencies, the World Health Organization (WHO) and the United Nations Childrens' Emergency Fund (UNICEF), identified primary health care as the major strategy for achieving universal health and constituted the centrepiece of the Declaration of Alma Ata.

One of the 10 points that outline the scope and implications of the Declaration provides the core of its definition of primary health care as:

> . . . essential health care based on practical, scientifically sound and socially acceptable methods and technology made universally accessible to individuals and families in the community through their full participation and at a cost that the community and country can afford to maintain at every stage of their development in the spirit of self reliance and self determination (WHO, 1978, 3).

The definition also states that primary health care "forms an integral part both of the country's health system, of which it is the central function and main focus, and of the overall social and economic development of the community" (WHO, 1978, p. 3).

Advance notice of how the term *primary health care* is being defined throughout the chapter is one reason for this preface. A second reason is to provide an early indication of what will likely emerge as major international nursing issues of our time and of the foreseeable future. A third reason is to give visibility and emphasis to principles and strategies of the Alma Ata Declaration that should be part of the catechism of the well-informed nurse.

■■ ■■ ■■ ■■

STRUCTURES AND INSTITUTIONS: NONGOVERNMENTAL ORGANIZATIONS

Nongovernmental organizations (NGOs) include the International Council of Nurses (ICN) and other organizations, some of which involve nurses only and others in which nursing plays a role within a multidisciplinary or multipurpose structure. They include agencies functioning under religious auspices, universities, community colleges, research institutes, and ad hoc bodies that may convene a conference or address some problem that nurses from more than one country wish to explore.

The International Council of Nurses

Primary attention is focused on the ICN because of its central importance to world nursing. It is a remarkable organization in many respects. It was founded in 1899, less than 40 years after the first Nightingale nursing program was established, and to which the beginning of modern professional nursing is frequently ascribed. Although the ICN began with only three national associations, it had the distinction of being the first international professional organization in the health field. It attracted the attention of nurses everywhere who were struggling in their local settings with issues of nursing standards, training, status, recognition, and interdisciplinary relationships. In country after country, specialized nursing groups and local and provincial groups recognized the opportunity the ICN provided for them to become members of a world family of nurses. To accomplish this goal they needed to form national associations, and membership in the ICN constituted a strong force for the development of national nursing associations. This was true in Canada where, in 1908, 16 nursing groups from across the country formed the national organization, destined to become the Canadian Nurses Association (CNA), that sought and secured membership in ICN the next year. The CNA became the seventh member of ICN, which by 1993 had 111 national member associations and 1.25 million nurses.

It is individual nurses on whom the entire structure of nursing depends, a structure that extends, in Canada, from the local chapter through the provincial association and through the CNA to the ICN. Every nurse who is a member of a provincial or national organization should take pride in the vital part she or he plays in the endeavours of the global organization.

The ICN has served as the official voice of nursing throughout this century. As an independent professional body and through its consultative status with the World Health Organization, it represents the nursing profession in the international community. It has a twofold objective: the development and enhancement of strong national professional associations capable of providing the nursing component in national health-care systems, and the promotion of favourable conditions of life and work for its members. It maintains a continuous review of its standards and guidelines for nursing education, practice, research, and ethics.

The policies of the ICN are determined by a Council of National Representatives composed of the presidents of the national nursing associations. The Council meets every 2 years, and every 4 years convenes an international congress open to all nurses. At each Congress a board of directors, a president, and three vice presidents are elected.

The presidents of ICN, for much of ICN's history, were drawn from developed countries and that pattern was resumed in 1993 with the election of Margretta Styles of the United States. At the three previous quadrennial congresses those elected to the presidency were from developing countries: Eunice Muringo Kiereini from Kenya, in 1981; Nelly Garzón, from Colombia, in 1985; and Mo Im Kim, from Korea, in 1989. The emergence of strong leadership from developing countries gave evidence of the worldwide range of the organization and of its capacity to address environmental and socioeconomic problems of global dimensions that are critical to the Health For All objective.

Since 1981 the Secretariat of the ICN, located in Geneva, Switzerland, has been led by Constance Holleran, an American nurse with extensive experience in influencing governmental policy on nursing. She has developed close working relationships with WHO and other United Nations agencies, with NGOs having related socioeconomic concerns, and with international foundations.

Canadian nurses have played major roles in the ICN from its inception. Mary Agnes Snively, the first president of the CNA, served as Honourary Treasurer early in the century and Alice Girard, also a president of the CNA, was President from 1965 to 1969. There have been three Canadian vice presidents: Grace Fairley, 1949 to 1953; Verna Huffman Splane, 1973 to 1981; and Helen Glass, 1985 to 1989. Other Canadian nurses have served as members of the Board of Directors, the Council of National Representatives, and the Professional Services Committee, and have been presenters at quadrennial congresses and key figures involving ICN collaboration with other international bodies. Canada's participation was strongly in evidence at the 20th Congress in Madrid in 1993. Among the 160 Canadians who attended, many were involved in different aspects of the program from plenary presentations to poster sessions. Prominent roles were played by Helen Evans, retiring from the Board of Directors, and Alice Baumgart, newly elected to the Board, both former presidents of CNA. Of special importance was ICN's acceptance of the invitation extended by Eleanor Ross and Judith Oulton, the President-Elect and Executive Director, respectively, of the CNA, for the convening of the 21st Quadrennial Conference, in Vancouver in 1997.

This will be the second Congress held in Canada. The first, the 10th Congress, held in Montreal in 1969 and attended by more than 10,000 nurses, was notable for two associated events. One was a meeting in Ottawa of chief nursing officers in national ministries of health from some 30 countries—a meeting that recognized the important role senior nurses play in the formulation and implementation of national health policy. The second historic event was the inaugural meeting of the Commonwealth Nurses' Federation (CNF).

The Federation, facilitated by a grant from the Commonwealth Foundation, was established to strengthen nursing and midwifery throughout the Commonwealth by promoting and facilitating closer working relationships among the nursing associations of member countries (CNF, 1981). From 1971 to 1993 the extensive activities of the Federation were directed by its executive head, Margaret Brayton, a British nurse with wide international experience. Prior to her retirement she was a member of the steering committee of the Commonwealth Meeting of Chief Nursing Officers and Professional Associations held in Malta in 1992 (Commonwealth Secretariat, 1992). This conference, chaired by Dame Anne Poole, the recently retired Chief Nursing Officer for the United Kingdom, and hosted by the Government of Malta was sponsored by seven organizations, one of which was the CNA. The conference was a landmark event in bringing together governmental and nongovernmental nurses in a focused discussion of the pivotal role of nursing and midwifery in the provision of health care; it may also be seen as representative of the key role that nurses in Commonwealth countries have played in nursing worldwide. Two Canadian nurses who have played important roles in the Commonwealth Nurses Federation are Helen Musallem, one of its founding members, and Helen Taylor, president of CNF from 1980 to 1984 and a former president of CNA.

The Canadian Nurses Association

The roles that the CNA has played internationally extend beyond those linked wholly to ICN. The CNA has extensive networks of nurses throughout the world who look to it for professional help in strengthening their capacity to serve the nursing needs of their countries. From the mid 1960s to the mid 1980s, requests for assistance of this kind increased dramatically, prompting the Board of Directors in 1984 to establish an International Affairs Department charged with the review, coordination, and evaluation of international proposals and projects. The government of Canada, through its Canadian International Development Agency (CIDA), has encouraged and promoted this development through funding, consultation, and collaboration.

Through the International Affairs Department, Canadian nurses have been actively engaged in international health endeavours in many parts of the world, of which the following are illustrative: the promotion of primary health care in Upper Volta; consultation on educational programs respecting the health needs of the elderly in Thailand; assistance in the development of the West African College of Nurses; support of nursing education and curriculum development in the Peoples Republic of China; assistance to the nurses associations in Nepal and Colombia in the formulation of legislation for self-regulation; collaboration in research and leadership seminars and the production of nursing publications in Argentina; development of documentation centres for nursing and health resources in Chile; advice and participation in immunization programs in Benin and Uganda; consultation on clinical and management issues in countries in eastern Europe (CNA, 1993a).

Provincial Nurses Associations

A less publicized area of international work in nursing is that being undertaken by provincial nurses associations. An example is the Registered Nurses Association of British Columbia (RNABC), which is negotiating formal partnerships with nurses organizations in a number of countries where informal ties have previously existed. A notable example of this approach is the linkage that has been established between the Association of Registered Nurses of Newfoundland and the Danish Nurses Organization. This has involved a well-planned and substantially supported project to demonstrate primary health-care services managed and largely provided by nurses. This project, carried out in quite dissimilar communities, is attracting wide interest as a model that could be adopted throughout the world.

Educational Institutions

The interest in international nursing expressed by the university schools of nursing and other educational institutions in Canada has varied over the years. An international study published in 1993 (Splane and Splane, 1993) involving interviews with nurses who have held senior government posts in the past 100 years, has revealed the historically important role played by the nursing schools of the universities of McGill, Montreal, and Toronto. These institutions provided special programs and consultations for what might be called the "international circuit" of nursing administrators and educators in the prewar and early postwar periods. These included Eli Magnussen of Denmark, Venny Snellman of Finland, Majsa Andrell of Sweden, Yvonne Henstch of Switzerland, Fernanda Alves Diniz of Portugal, Kathleen Raven and Phyllis Friend of Britain, Tehmina Adranvala of India, Nita Barrow of Barbados, Antonia Fernandez of Venezuela, Leman Virol of Turkey, and Matsu Kameko of Japan.

In more recent years, the increased interest of Canadians in international affairs has been demonstrated in numerous connections formed between Canadian educational institutions and agencies with those in other countries. An interesting example was the role played by the Faculty of Nursing of McMaster University in its collaboration with the Aga Khan Foundation in the founding of the Aga Khan School of Nursing in Pakistan. This project, initiated in the 1970s by the late Dorothy Kergin, then Dean of Nursing at McMaster, has led to an unbroken relationship involving an exchange of faculty and students between the two institutions.

From the mid 1980s to the mid 1990s an upsurge in specialized international nursing conferences, too numerous to describe, has been held in centres across Canada, largely under the sponsorship of educational institutions. Notable among them was the International Nursing Research Conference held in 1986 in Edmonton. Sponsored jointly by the University of Alberta and the University of Calgary and superbly organized by a nursing committee under the leadership of Shirley Stinson, this conference attracted some 800 registrants from 38 countries. That event gave prominence to the extent and quality of existing nursing research, and to the measures needed for its support and expansion. Three other meetings of special note were: an International Colloquium on Primary Health Care, in Montreal, May 1992; the First International Nursing History Conference, in Saint John in 1992; and the International Conference on Community Nursing Research, in Edmonton in 1993. The first of these, sponsored and organized by the Faculté des sciences infirmières, Université de Montréal, attracted 125 abstracts from 23 countries with 85 oral presentations (Thibaudeau, personal communication, Feb. 3, 1992). The second was sponsored and organized jointly by the Canadian Association for the History of Nursing and the American Association for the History of Nursing, attracting more than 200 participants. The third, sponsored by the Board of Health of the City of Edmonton (a first in itself) was organized under the leadership of two internationally recognized public health nurses, Karen Mills and Shirley Stinson. It attracted more than 800 registrants from 35 countries.

Intercountry study of health care and nursing is assisted by travel grants and fellowships from such organizations as CIDA, the Canadian Public Health Association, the Association of Universities and Colleges of Canada, the International Development Research Centre, WHO, and the Commonwealth Foundation. Of special importance to student nurses is the International Health Exchange Program (IHEP) of the Canadian Society for International Health. The growing interest of nursing students in work or travel abroad and concern about international affairs has led to the formation of linkages with students in all health disciplines across the country and to requests for international health and nursing courses in their curricula. The number of nursing programs in Canada offering such courses is expected to expand throughout the 1990s.

Religious Auspices

International nursing under religious auspices has a long history. Nursing was brought to French Canada by religious orders of the Roman Catholic faith in the 17th century. One of these served under the lay direction of Jeanne Mance, the first European woman to arrive in Montreal. This importation of European nurses within religious sisterhoods was complemented over the years by an outflow of Canadian nurses to countries in many parts of the world. During the later years of the 19th century, Protestant denominations sent nurses with missionary callings to numerous countries in Latin America, Asia, and Africa. In the last decade, nurses from Roman Catholic Orders have been seconded to work with WHO and in senior governmental nursing positions in a number of countries (Pilkington, 1988). The work of the missionary in improving health services and in developing nursing training programs constitutes a fascinating story.

The work of religious bodies in the health field has been greatly enhanced by the work of the World Council of Churches, based in Geneva, and composed of 300 churches from 115 countries. Through its Christian Medical Commission, it plays an active role in upgrading and monitoring church-related health services around the world. It influences the policies of the individual denominations in their recruitment and deployment of nursing and other personnel; but the recruitment and utilization of health-care personnel in the missions remain the responsibility of the denominations. The Council's Medical Commission was headed for a number of years by Nita Barrow, an outstanding nurse and world leader in many fields who added significantly to the visibility of international nursing and reinforced the Council's commitment to primary health care involving interdisciplinary collaboration.

Other Nongovernmental Organizations

Much of the work in the field of international health previously carried out under religious auspices is now performed by numerous nongovernmental agencies that deal with disaster relief, refugees, and populations with differing forms of handicaps or vulnerability. The International Red Cross stands out in this regard; within it, for many years, the League of Red Cross Societies, of which the Canadian Red Cross is a member, has played direct and catalytic roles in nursing and nursing education. A Canadian NGO that is making an outstanding contribution to Health For All is the Canadian Public Health Association (CPHA, 1989a). Its role in international immunization and contagious disease control involves nursing in many countries and reflects the leadership of the nurses in its key positions, including Karen Mills, Margaret Hilson, and Anne Wieler. Variants of the nongovernmental organizations that focus on existing problems of health and deprivation are those oriented toward longer term social and macroeconomic development.

■ ■ ■ ■

GOVERNMENTAL INSTITUTIONS

The focus now shifts to the governmental sector, the importance of which cannot be overstated. Here the reference is to national governments (though some provincial governments in Canada have significant international programs); to regional government structures, notably the European Economic Community; and to world government, as represented by the United Nations and its specialized agencies. Among the latter are the Food and Agriculture Organization (FAO), the United Nations High Commission for Refugees (UNHCR), UNICEF, the International Labour Organization (ILO), and WHO, which is the organization of greatest relevance to nurses and nursing.

Agencies of the National Government: Health and Welfare Canada and the Canadian International Development Agency (CIDA)

National governments express their commitments to international health in many ways. In Canada, the Department of National Health and Welfare plays a number of international roles concerned with health protection and promotion and with Canada's obligations under resolutions of the United Nations, including working to advance the goal of Health For All by the year 2000 through primary health care and related strategies. Matters related to nursing, both nationally and internationally, are the concern of the Principal Nursing Officer, Josephine Flaherty, who, in her official role, advises the Minister on how nursing can be most effectively used at home and abroad.

CIDA, a crown corporation of the government, expresses Canada's commitment to helping the countries of the developing world to improve their social and economic conditions. More than 100 countries have received aid through CIDA's multilateral and bilateral programs, many of which have to do with Canada's support and sponsorship of resolutions adopted by the General Assembly of the United Nations. Frequently, CIDA's aid is in support of initiatives that are also being promoted by the specialized agencies, notably WHO. CIDA directly recruits and funds individuals, including nurses, to assist in developmental projects when developing countries request such professional and technical help.

Increasingly, however, CIDA has turned to Canada's NGOs, including professional associations, for the skills needed to meet the wide variety of requests from countries seeking help with their health and other social and economic needs. Among the NGOs who have enlisted nurses, usually young nurses, for overseas assignments are the Canadian University Service Overseas (CUSO) and the World University Service of Canada (WUCS). CIDA has also supported the CNA in many of the international projects referred to previously, most of which assist nurses in developing their associations and improving nursing's role in national health systems. CIDA has also collaborated with Canadian universities, including schools and faculties of nursing, as they have taken on projects to assist in education and training in developing countries. For Canadian nurses two scholarship programs are available from CIDA: the professional award providing opportunity for short-term study or work experience in a developing country, and the award for academic study or a practical work/study assignment that includes a fieldwork component in a developing country (CNA, 1993b).

In the early 1990s CIDA's emphasis shifted to include the former communist states in eastern Europe. Under CIDA and other auspices, Canadian nurses, some with ethnic roots in eastern Europe, have been assisting in the reconstruction of national health and nursing programs. A further shift in CIDA's aid policies in 1993 took the form of a move away from the least developed countries and toward more developed countries, exemplifying an entrepreneurial approach to economic development; the effects of this change may not be known until the mid or late 1990s.

Regional Government: The European Economic Community

Groupings of countries in some parts of the world are developing structures to deal with common interests on health and personnel issues that have crucial importance for international nursing. One regional governmental structure where this has emerged in a formal and highly significant way is the European Economic Community (EEC), which by 1995 consisted of 12 European countries. The EEC aims ultimately to integrate the countries' economies, coordinate social developments, and create a common labour market. To achieve the goal of labour mobility without endangering the public, the EEC has had to establish standards of qualification. For nurses, the EEC has passed legislation in the European Parliament to set out the minimum levels of education and training needed for a nurse to assume professional nursing positions in member states. The enactment of the legislation was preceded by difficult negotiations by nursing associations, and its implementation is monitored by a standing committee of nursing representatives from the member states. The EEC legislation has had a significant impact on the education of nurses in Europe, and its influence is likely to affect the debate on nursing standards in northern European countries, three of which

(Norway, Sweden, and Finland) are not yet members of the EEC. It will also provide guidelines for advances in nursing in the countries of eastern Europe that, in 1989, broke through the ideological and military barriers separating them from the West.

The EEC is the most advanced of the regional groupings of governments. As revealed in the 1993 book by Sheila Quinn and Susan Russell, *Nursing: The European Dimensions*, many complex problems continue to affect progress on nursing, and the existing measures have not yet significantly advanced the mobility of nurses throughout the community. The reference to the European experience is to suggest that nurses in Canada need to be aware of the stake they have in the future formation and policies of comparable regional structures in North America, the Western Hemisphere as a whole, or other possible regional groupings.

World Government: The World Health Organization

The organization within the structure of world government that plays the largest role in international nursing is WHO, founded by the United Nations soon after its creation at the end of World War II. Building on the work of its international and regional predecessors, WHO established a highly creditable record in promoting world health, with particularly impressive successes in the control and elimination of communicable diseases.

Nursing was given a high priority in the early years of WHO. In the first sessions of the World Health Assembly the shortage of health personnel was identified as a major problem, particularly in developing countries, and measures were taken to deal with it. Recognizing the central role of nursing in health services, WHO set up a nursing unit at headquarters in 1949, directed by a chief nursing officer, and thereafter established nursing officer positions in the six regional offices. Experienced and well qualified nurses were recruited from many nursing specializations and from many countries to provide consultation, conduct and promote studies and research, and perform direct nursing services in demonstration projects.

The work of the nursing components of WHO at its headquarters and in the regions transformed nursing throughout the world and contributed immeasurably to WHO's objectives, including that of extending unequivocal support to Health For All, largely through the primary health-care strategy.

Nursing in WHO, however, experienced a serious setback in the early 1970s when the nursing unit and the position of chief nursing officer were abolished and the nurses were transferred to the organization's functional units. There were also reductions in the complement of nurses in the regions. In succeeding years, extending into the 1980s, the role of nursing in advancing the Health For All goal was not adequately recognized or provided for. Those years were referred to in 1985 by Dr. Halfdan Mahler, the Director General from 1973 to 1988, as "the years of doubt". The doubt was in the minds of those controlling WHO's policies, including Dr. Mahler, and the doubt was about the capability of nurses to assume roles other than "resources to physicians" (WHO, 1985a, p. 1).

The Director General's comments were part of a dramatic reappraisal of nursing resulting from a review of the extent to which the health professions were making the changes needed for the implementation of the primary health-care strategy. Noting that "the nursing profession was infinitely more ready for change than other professional groups," he stated that "it was now time that nurses were brought in much more than hitherto . . . as leaders and managers in the primary health care/Health For All team" (WHO, 1985b, p. 1). Referring to nurses worldwide "as a powerhouse for change" (WHO, 1985b, p. 1), Dr. Mahler called for the optimal use of nurses in program planning and evaluation and in senior management, policy development, and decision making.

What was not acknowledged by Dr. Mahler was that WHO's action in abolishing the chief nursing officer position and the associated nursing unit in the early 1970s had not only reduced the effectiveness of WHO itself but constituted a damaging precedent for similar action in national ministries of health in many parts of the world. On the advice of WHO throughout the 1950s and 1960s, numerous chief nursing positions had been established within national ministries of health. Accordingly, WHO's seeming repudiation of that model strengthened the hands of those in national ministries of health who wished to take similar action to remove nurses from senior positions in policy development and management. The loss of chief nursing officer positions in many national ministries of health since 1970 may be attributable to many factors, not the least of which is the example set by WHO. It was ironic that the Director General's call in 1985 for the training of an adequate number of nurses "to assume a greater managerial role and to participate in developing policy with assurance and confidence" (WHO, 1985a, p. 2) was made after the key positions where such roles could be creatively managed in national ministries had been lost, possibly irretrievably, through actions by governments that were following WHO's own ill-advised action in the early 1970s.

The gradual rebuilding of the influence of nursing within WHO is associated with the one designated nursing position established at the Geneva headquarters after the abolition of the nursing unit. The position, ultimately designated as Chief Scientist for Nursing, was held for 14 years by Amelia Mangay Maglacas, a nurse from the Philippines with extensive experience in international nursing, teaching, administration, and research. The functions of the position were expanded over the years and, as its role as the focal point for nursing affairs in WHO was creatively used by Dr. Maglacas, its status and influence grew. The means used to strengthen global nursing included actions relating to the implementation of resolutions of WHO's General Assembly, the convening of expert committees on nursing, measures to promote improved education and training of nurses, the continued use of experienced nurses as consultants to member countries, the provision of WHO educational fellowships, and close collaboration with nursing leaders and associations, most notably with the ICN.

Specific initiatives taken with the support of Dr. Mahler included the convening of a high-level invitational meeting in Tokyo, Japan in April 1986 on Leadership in Nursing for Health For All. Of great long-term significance was the unveiling, also in 1986, of the plan to establish a worldwide chain of Collaborating Centres for International Nursing Development. The first centre was launched in 1986 at the College of Nursing, University of Illinois in Chicago.

Of the 22 centres widely distributed throughout the WHO regions in 1993, two were in Canada: one in the Faculty of Nursing of McMaster University in Hamilton, directed by Dr. Andrea Baumann, and the second at Mount Sinai Hospital in Toronto, directed by Dr. Judith Shamian.

In 1988 Dr. Mahler was succeeded as Director General by Dr. Hiroshi Nakajima of Japan, and in 1989 Amelia Mangay Maglacas was succeeded by a nursing leader with strong qualifications in research and teaching, Dr. Miriam Hirschfeld of Israel. Dr. Nakajima's message to the Nineteenth Congress of ICN, in Seoul in 1989, appeared to indicate that he appreciated the potential of nursing and the roles nurses have in meeting the contemporary range of health needs and issues.

By the early 1990s, however, it was evident that the WHO Secretariat was failing to execute resolutions respecting nursing and midwifery of the World Health Assembly, the legislative arm of WHO. This led to a number of strategic measures by nursing leaders to have a new resolution enacted by the World Health Assembly and to ensure its implementation by the Director General. The resulting resolution (WHA 45.5) established a Global Advisory Group on Nursing and Midwifery with a mandate to propose, promote, and monitor actions to be taken by WHO and member countries to strengthen nursing and midwifery in all WHO regions. After an indication of resistance within the Secretariat was deftly countered within the Assembly, the Director General promised his full support of the Advisory Group (WHO, 1992a).

The Advisory Group, which held its first meeting in December 1992 and met again in 1993, consists of 18 leaders in nursing and other health disciplines, with WHO's Chief Scientist for Nursing, Miriam Hirschfeld, as Secretary (WHO, 1992b). It has laid the groundwork for wide-ranging improvements in nursing and midwifery programs. Its work merits the interest and support of nursing associations and individual nurses in every country.

The contributions of Canadian nurses to WHO are noteworthy. This was especially true of the work of Lyle Creelman, the chief nurse from 1954 to 1968, a period of remarkable growth and achievement. Lily Turnbull, her successor from 1968 to 1975, was also Canadian, and Canadian nurses held the senior positions in all six WHO regional offices at various times. Examples are Margaret Cammaert, the Chief Nursing Officer in the Pan American Health Organization, the WHO regional office for the Americas, and Dorothy Hall, who served as Regional Nursing Officer both in southeast Asia and in Europe. Over the entire history of WHO, scores of Canadian nurses have held positions as consultants, project leaders on both long-term and short-term assignments, and on WHO committees. To the extent that well-prepared nurses are cognizant of and committed to the principles of the Alma Ata Declaration, they will continue to have opportunities to participate in the global endeavours of WHO.

■■ ■■ ■■ ■■

ISSUES WITH INTERNATIONAL DIMENSIONS

Nursing issues with international dimensions are evident now and are likely to be prevalent during the remainder of the century. Two categories of issues are identified: one has to do with the capacity and willingness of nurses to retain strong national and international organizations based on the firm commitment to general nursing that is needed if nurses and their professional organizations are to play effective roles nationally and internationally; the second has to do with the issues associated with the Health For All objective and the primary health-care strategy required for its achievement. Three or four subordinate but important issues fall within this second category.

General Nursing and the Integrity of the Profession

Nursing, through its professional associations provincially, nationally, and internationally, has demonstrated that it is strong and influential, both in reality and potential. Its present and future strength, however, depends on three associated conditions: (1) that nurses receive sound education in general nursing, (2) that they maintain an enduring commitment to the general nursing core of the profession, and (3) that the professional associations, created to represent the interests and reflect the concerns of general nursing, continue to honour that commitment.

The issue of the threat to the general nursing core comes essentially from two rather divergent sources. One is the tendency that derives from a misapplication of the managerial concepts of efficiency and effectiveness, which seeks to shorten the duration and restrict the content of basic general nursing programs. It comes from the expanding demand for personnel with skills in the increasingly technical procedures in modern hospitals and clinics, and results in pressure to channel nursing students prematurely into one or other of nursing's more technical or complex specializations.

This trend is affecting the reciprocal recognition of nurses between some European countries where the country of migration does not accept those certified in the country of graduation, where the latter has reduced the duration and the quality of its basic general nursing certificate. Those opposing this trend believe that if it is not arrested and reversed, it will destroy nursing and the nursing profession. The pressure to reduce basic general nursing education continues to be strong, however, and comes both from health-system managers and from governments seeking to reduce costs. They tend to ignore or reject the case for broad general nursing as having enduring value for the health-care system and as forming the foundation for the profession of nursing.

The other source of threat to general nursing comes from the special interest groups in nursing. These groups are to be welcomed for their commitment to attaining the highest levels of knowledge and performance in their specific areas of interest. What is *not* to be welcomed is their tendency to separate from the general nursing profession and to form autonomous, sometimes competitive, organizations. The CNA's approach to arrest that type of development, through providing a process for linkages within its structure, may prove to be a model for countries where there is still time to prevent nurses from abandoning their general nursing affiliation. The importance of such action can hardly be over-stressed. It is only through strong and united national organizations capable of supporting a strong international professional association, the ICN, that the nurses of the world can speak with one voice on the great issues that are linked to the goal of Health For All.

Nursing and Primary Health Care

Since 1979 nurses around the world have been exploring the meaning and implications of the Alma Ata Declaration. Presented here are some succinct comments on three aspects of the question: attitudinal, educational, and political.

Attitudinal Issues

The Alma Ata Declaration presents a sweeping and comprehensive challenge. It challenges people to think of their health and its preservation and restoration in ways that are radically different from the accustomed norms. It also challenges governments and especially health providers, who are called on to question and to change the prevailing values that underlie both the existing systems of health care and the even more basic social, cultural, and economic systems within which the health system is situated. That challenge requires profound attitudinal changes, individually and collectively. None of the health professions will change the attitudes of its members without stress and trauma. As noted earlier, the former Director General of WHO has described the nursing profession "as infinitely more ready for change than other professional groups" (WHO, 1985b). That is heartening. Time will test its validity.

Educational Issues

The most promising and fruitful modality for attitudinal change is education; in this case, the professional education of nurses. The implication of the Alma Ata Declaration is that the education of nurses become "international." The objective of Health For All calls for a world view of nursing. Few of the existing curricula in programs of nursing education show a recognition that international nursing constitutes an important field of study. That situation and a meaningful acceptance of the Alma Ata Declaration cannot coexist. It is not sufficient for international nursing to be an elective in a few postbasic nursing programs. The Health For All objective calls for international health and nursing to be part of nursing education, basic and postbasic, everywhere.

Political Issues

The achievement of Health For All requires political decisions at every level of government. The decisions to be made extend beyond the health-care system as it is usually defined. They extend to the range of policies that determine, in the words of the Alma Ata definition, a country's "overall social and economic development" (WHO, 1978, p. 16). Health For All cannot be achieved for people who are homeless, are without income for necessities, and are without other services and facilities needed for their inclusion in the normal life of the community. Few countries can claim to meet these preconditions for Health For All.

Nurses and other human service workers see the impact on the lives of people of social and economic policies that fail to provide the preconditions to good health. What they see and know entails a moral imperative to political action at the community, provincial, national, and international levels.

Action begins at the grassroots level in conveying the principles and providing the aid needed to enhance self-help and individual responsibility. It extends to reformulating the policies and changing the practices over the entire range of the social services. It focuses on governments, provincial and national, with jurisdictional responsibility for social services, income support, income redistribution, and the economy in general. Finally, it must reach those international bodies where macropolicies are made and macroresources are deployed: the World Bank, the International Monetary Fund, the United Nations, and all its specialized agencies (United Nations Development Programme, 1992, pp. 1-11).

This action carries nurses and nursing organizations beyond their accustomed fields of political concern and action, but nurses have met formidable political challenges in the past in many jurisdictions around the world. The Alma Ata Declaration calls for more sustained action, but action that is carefully planned and implemented in concert with other agencies and organizations working for peace, social development, and human well-being. It can be undertaken in the faith that what *must* be done *can* be done to advance Health For All in this century.

REFERENCES

Canadian Nurses Association. (1993a). Collaboration in action. *The Canadian Nurse, 89(2), 14-15.*

Canadian Nurses Association. (1993b). CIDA study programs. *The Canadian Nurse, 89(3), 10.*

Canadian Public Health Association. (1989). *A miracle in the making: Canada's international immunization program.* Ottawa: Author.

Commonwealth Nurses Federation. (1981). *Report of the executive secretary for the period 1979-1981. Annex D.* London: Author.

Commonwealth Secretariat. (1992). *Challenges and opportunities. Report of the Commonwealth Meeting of Chief Nursing Officers and Professional Associations, 7-10 September 1992, Quwra, Malta.* London: Author.

Pilkington, P. (1988). An interview for the study of chief nursing officer positions. Vancouver: Splane Associates.

Splane, R., and Splane, V.H. (1993). *Chief nursing officer positions in national ministries of health:* *Focal points for leadership.* San Francisco: University of California.

United Nations Development Programme. (1992). *Human Development Report 1992.* New York and Oxford: Oxford University Press.

World Health Organization. (1978). *Primary health care: report on the International Conference on Primary Health Care. Alma Ata, USSR. 6-12 September 1978.* Geneva: Author.

World Health Organization. (1985a). *Nurses lead the way.* WHO Features. June 1985a No. 97. Geneva: Author.

World Health Organization. (1992a). *Resolution WHA 45.5 Strengthening nursing and midwifery in support of strategies for health for all. Forty-fifth World Health Assembly 4-15 May 1992.* Geneva: Author.

World Health Organization. (1992b). *Report of the rapporteurs on the first meeting of the Global Advisory Group on Nursing and Midwifery, Geneva Headquarters 30 November - 2 December 1992.* Geneva: Author.

CHAPTER THIRTY FOUR

Looking Ahead

JANNETTA MacPHAIL
AND JANET ROSS KERR

Many issues of importance to the nursing profession have been discussed in this book. Traversing nursing practice, education, administration, and research, current issues in nursing have been presented from a Canadian perspective. The historical developments relevant to the issues discussed have been presented, and in four chapters the focus has been entirely upon the history of nursing in Canada. It is essential for every nurse to develop an awareness of matters of professional significance, for these affect everyday practice, and knowledge and understanding can significantly improve approaches to practice. The future depends on nurses entering practice today and tomorrow and the profession's ability to attract and retain a cadre of intellectually able and visionary risk takers to provide future leadership. It is the same professional practitioner who will have the ability to understand the concept of primary health care as the way to empower and enable Canadians to assume increasing responsibility for their own health, and to press for changes in the health-care system to incorporate a focus on primary health care.

The story of the nursing profession in Canada is ongoing. Three-and-a-half centuries of rich tradition have provided a wonderful and distinguished background from which to move forward. Nursing was an integral part of the early settlements along the shores of the St. Lawrence, and health-care facilities established and operated by nurses were available before the arrival of most settlers. As founder of the city of Montreal, Jeanne Mance, along with Paul de Chomédy, Sieur de Maisonneuve, and a small company, laid the foundations for the nursing service that would meet the needs of the struggling colony for many years. In later years the importance of establishing educational programs for nurses was recognized, as was the need to develop legislation to differentiate between qualified and unqualified practitioners. Succeeding years brought important advances in health-care knowledge and technology and new issues and problems.

The challenges to the profession have never been greater. Health-care restructuring is well underway in many provinces and changes in health-care financing have been made that will affect the nature of nursing and the way in which it is practised. Nurses need to be at the forefront of health-care reform and to be proactive in arguing the case for community-based access to health care in which physicians are no longer the sole gatekeepers to the system. The potential and abilities of nurses will never be fully and appropriately utilized as long as there is medical domination of the system, both in terms of the access to it and in terms of its operation.

Other challenges to the profession include developing and strengthening the new doctoral programs that have been established. There is a need for continued expansion of nursing research and funding to support it. Both public and private funding for research in nursing need to be clearly earmarked so that there are no barriers to access by well-qualified nursing researchers. The remarkable progress made since 1991 in moving toward the entry to practice goal through collaboration between university nursing programs and diploma programs needs to be continued and supported by all nurses to achieve the entry to practice goal by the year 2000. All these challenges are aimed at achieving Health for All by the year 2000. These are all major thrusts of the profession and represent challenges that require careful thought and concerted action by politically astute leaders, supported by the majority of the professional membership. The nursing profession has accomplished a great deal in its three and one-half centuries in Canada. There is no doubt that even greater accomplishments are yet to be seen.

Index

A

AACN; *see* American Association of
    Colleges of Nursing
AARN; *see* Alberta Association of
    Registered Nurses
Abbis Report, 303
Abdellah, Faye, 148
Abortion, 263
Accreditation, 351
    definition of, 359
    nursing education and, 299, 350-351
    of nursing education programs, 355-
      360
Acquired immunodeficiency syndrome
    (AIDS), 256
Active euthanasia, 257
Administration, nursing; *see* Nursing
    administration
Adranvala, Tehmina, 431
Advance directives, ethics and, 260-261
Advances in Nursing Science, 132, 152
AFNR; *see* Alberta Foundation for
    Nursing Research
Aga Kahn Foundation, 431
Aga Kahn School of Nursing, 431
Agencies of national government, inter-
    national nursing and, 433-434
Agency-faculty joint appointment, 342
AHFMR; *see* Alberta Heritage
    Foundation for Medical
    Research
AIDS; *see* Acquired immunodeficiency
    syndrome
Alberta
    establishment of nursing unions in,
      273

Alberta—cont'd
    nursing education in, 302
    University of, 27, 28, 42, 43, 120, 124,
      132, 148, 156, 257, 265, 284, 308,
      314, 324, 327, 328, 329, 342, 344,
      345, 360, 366, 374, 377-378, 386-
      388, 403, 410, 414-415, 416, 417,
      419, 422, 431
Alberta Association of Registered Nurses
    (AARN), 41, 58-59, 124, 130, 139,
    164, 197, 204, 213, 273, 322, 398,
    403
Alberta Foundation for Nursing Research
    (AFNR), 124, 139, 156-159, 423
Alberta Heritage Foundation for Medical
    Research (AHFMR), 138
Alberta Hospital Association (AHA), 185,
    280, 387, 403
Alberta Law Reform Institute and Health
    Law Institute, 261
Alberta Medical Association, 403
Alberta Task Force on Midwifery, 403
Alberta Task Force on Nursing Education,
    322
Allen, Moyra, 147, 301
Allen Memorial Institute (Montreal), 255
Allocation of health-care resources, ethics
    and, 263-264
Alma-Ata, Declaration of, 427, 428, 437,
    439, 440
American Academy of Nursing, 340
American Assembly of Men in Nursing,
    79-80
American Association
    of Colleges of Nursing (AACN), 337
    of Critical Care Nurses, 131

American Association—cont'd
for the History of Nursing, 432
American Journal of Nursing, 15, 365
American Medical Association (AMA),
297
American Nurses Association (ANA), 15,
27, 79, 106, 252-253, 269, 369
American Organization of Nurse
Executives, 197, 204
American Society of Superintendents of
Training Schools for Nurses of
the United States and Canada,
15, 364
Amherst Hospital (Nova Scotia), 277
ANA; *see* American Nurses Association
ANA Commission on Nursing Services,
288
Analgesia, patient-controlled, research-
based nursing practice and, 175-
176
Analysis, secondary, of data, 113-114
Andrell, Majsa, 431
Annual nursing research conferences,
organization of, 153-156
Annual Reviews of Nursing Research, 155
ANPEI; *see* Association of Nurses of
Prince Edward Island
ANPQ; *see* Association of Nurses of the
Province of Quebec
Approval, nursing education and, 350-351
ARCAUSN; *see* Canadian Association of
University Schools of Nursing
ARNN; *see* Association of Registered
Nurses of Newfoundland
Associated Alumnae of the United States
and Canada, 364
Association
of Nurses of Prince Edward Island
(ANPEI), 278, 286, 303-304, 331,
353
of Nurses of the Province of Quebec
(ANPQ), 275, 300
professional, 282-284, 287-288
of Registered Nurses of
Newfoundland (ARNN), 278,
304, 397, 431
of Universities and Colleges of
Canada, 432
Athabasca University, 384, 386, 387
Atlantic provinces, nursing education in,
303-304

Attitudinal issues, international nursing
and, 439
Augustinian nuns, 292
Autonomy, ethics and, 254
Auxiliary grants, nursing research and,
137-138

B
Baccalaureate degree, 321-333, 345, 377
developing specialty certificate pro-
grams with credit toward, 373-
380
entry to practice position and; *see*
Entry to practice position
Bégin, Monique, 222-223
Barrow, Nita, 431, 432
Baumann, Andrea, 437
Baumgart, Alice, 32, 38, 63, 429
BCIT; *see* British Columbia Institute of
Technology
Behaviour
innovation adoption, research-based
nursing practice and, 174-178
responsibilities for changing, ethics
and, 261-262
Bellevue Training School for Nurses (New
York), 293
Beneficence, ethics and, 254
Berwick, Donald, 189
Besel, Lorine, 48
Bill C43, 263
Bioethics Rounds, 264
Blue Cross Plans, 219
Bolton, Frances Payne, 79
Boothills Hospital, 378
Borrowed theory, nursing knowledge
and, 90-92
Boudreau Committee, 394
Bowden, Sister Helen, 293
Brandon, University of, 330
Brandon General Hospital, 330
Brayton, Margaret, 430
Brink, Pamela, 132
British Columbia
establishment of nursing unions in,
272-273
nursing education in, 302
University of, 28, 42, 43, 120, 135, 147,
156, 284, 297, 307, 308, 314, 318,
324, 327, 328, 329, 335, 342, 344,
386, 410, 413, 415, 416, 419, 422

British Columbia Children's Hospital, 123
British Columbia Health Care Research
        Foundation, 139
British Columbia Hospitals Association,
        306, 307
British Columbia Institute of Technology
        (BCIT), 302
British Columbia School of Midwifery,
        404
British Journal of Nursing, 15
British North America Act of 1867, 216,
        365
Brockville, 331
Brotherson, Sir John, 118
Brouet, Jehan de, 3
Brown, Esther Lucile, 292, 317

C

CAAT; *see* Colleges of applied arts and
        technology
Calgary, University of, 43, 124, 329, 342,
        386, 416, 431
Cambrian College, 330
Cammaert, Margaret, 437
Camosun College, 329
Campbell, Beverly, 124
Canada Council, 137
Canada Evidence Act, 247
Canada Health Act of 1984, 23, 49, 71, 209,
        221-223, 225
Canadian Army Medical Corps, 18
Canadian Association
    for the History of Nursing, 156, 432
    of University Schools of Nursing
        (CAUSN), 17, 35, 46, 123, 142,
        143, 148, 153-156, 337, 345, 352,
        355-356, 358, 359, 368, 370, 409-
        411, 421
Canadian Bar Association (CBA), 257
Canadian Cancer Society, 139
Canadian Centre for Nursing Research,
        46
Canadian Confederation of Midwives
        (CCM), 401
Canadian Confederation of Midwives
        Newsletters, 400
Canadian Council
    of Health Service Executives (CCHSE),
        48
    on Hospital Accreditation (CCHA), 35-
        36, 47, 183, 184

Canadian Council—cont'd
    of Hospitals and Facilities
        Accreditation Survey Standards,
        194
    of Occupational Health Nurses, 370-
        371, 371
    of Occupational Health Nurses
        (CCOHN), 39
Canadian Education Association (CEA),
        297
Canadian Heart Foundation, 139
Canadian Hemophilia Society, 35
Canadian Hospital Association (CHA),
        36, 257, 265
Canadian International Development
        Agency (CIDA), 430, 432, 433-
        434
Canadian Joint Committee on Nursing, 47
Canadian Journal of Nursing Research, 132,
        147
Canadian Long Term Association, 50
Canadian Medical Association (CMA), 34,
        220, 223, 257, 297
Canadian Medical Procurement and
        Assignment Board, 47
Canadian National Association of Trained
        Nurses (CNATN), 16, 31, 294
Canadian Nurse, The, 16, 44, 257, 309, 323,
        345, 365
Canadian Nurses Association (CNA), 16,
        27, 54, 123, 140-141, 156, 164, 184,
        209, 213, 222, 223, 243, 252, 257,
        269, 271-272, 283, 286, 294, 298,
        300, 315, 318, 322, 323, 324, 326,
        364, 365, 369-370, 375-376, 381,
        395, 396, 398, 408-409, 410, 421,
        428, 430
    certification and, 38-40
    health care reform and, 49-50
    image of nurses and nursing and, 33
    nursing administration and, 46-49
    nursing education and, 40-44
    nursing practice and, 33-36
    nursing research and, 44-46
    role of, in development of nursing in
        Canada, 31-53
    work-life affairs and, 36-38
Canadian Nurses Association Testing
        Services (CNATS), 370
Canadian Nurses Foundation (CNF), 17,
        41, 123-124, 138, 409, 411

Canadian Nurses Protective Fund
(CNPF), 38
Canadian Nurses Protective Society
(CNPS), 249
Canadian Nursing Research Group
(CNRG), 46, 156
Canadian Panel on Violence Against
Women, 35
Canadian Psychological Association,
50
Canadian Public Health Association
(CPHA), 34, 307, 391, 433
Canadian Red Cross Society, 20-21, 308,
316, 433
Canadian Society
for International Health, 432
of Superintendents of Training Schools
for Nurses, 365
Canadian University Nursing Students'
Association (CUNSA), 35
Canadian University Service Overseas
(CUSO), 434
Care
versus cure, 61
managed, case management and, 236-
237
quality of; see Quality assurance
Career Scientist grants, 123
Cariboo College, 329
Carnegie Foundation, 297
Carpenter, Helen M., 140, 413
Carter, Henry Bonham, 295
Cartier, Jacques, 3, 74
Case assignment, 228, 229
Case management
definition of, 237
and managed care, 236-237
Case Western Reserve University, 79, 337,
338, 341, 346
Catholic Hospital Conference of Ontario,
301
Cause-and-effect diagram, total quality
management and, 193
CAUSN; see Canadian Association of
University Schools of Nursing
Cavell, Edith, 56
CBA; see Canadian Bar Association
CCHA; see Canadian Council on Hospital
Accreditation
CCHSE; see Canadian Council of Health
Service Executives

CCM; see Canadian Confederation of
Midwives
CCOHN; see Canadian Council of
Occupational Health Nurses
CEA; see Canadian Education Association
CEGEP; see Colleges d'Enseignement
General et Professionnel
Center for Nursing Research in Canada,
138
Centralized Teaching Program, nursing
education and, 298-299
Centres Locaux de Services
Communautaires (CLSC), 276
Certificate Program in Critical Care
Nursing, 378
Certification, Canadian Nurses
Association and, 38-40
Certified nursing assistant, 315
CHA; see Canadian Hospital Association
Chamberlain, Joseph, 18
Charter of Rights and Freedoms, 248
Check sheet, total quality management
and, 193
Chedoke-McMaster Hospitals Nurse-
Midwifery Project, 400
Childbearing, 262-263, 399-400
Cholera, 13
Chomédy, Paul de, 7, 441
CIDA; see Canadian International
Development Agency
Civil law, 242
Clinical component of distance education
in nursing, 385
Clinical knowledge, 94
Clinical nurse specialist roles, research-
based nursing practice and, 173-
174
Clinical Nursing Research: An International
Journal, 132
Clinical nursing researcher (CNR), 168-169
CLSC; see Centres Locaux de Services
Communautaires
CMA; see Canadian Medical Association
CNA; see Canadian Nurses Association
CNATN; see Canadian National
Association of Trained Nurses
CNATS; see Canadian Nurses Association
Testing Services, 370
CNF; see Canadian Nurses Foundation;
Commonwealth Nurses'
Federation

CNO; *see* College of Nurses of Ontario
CNPF; *see* Canadian Nurses Protective Fund
CNPS; *see* Canadian Nurses Protective Society
CNR; *see* Clinical nursing researcher
CNRG; *see* Canadian Nursing Research Group
Code of ethics, 26, 243, 252-254, 283
Collaborating Centres for International Nursing Development, 436
Collaboration
  criticism of, 339
  in distance education in nursing, 384
  evaluation of outcomes of, 345-347
  interinstitutional linkages to promote, 337-345
  between nursing education and nursing practice for quality nursing care, education, and research, 334-349
  between service and education, deterrents to, 340-341
  strategies to promote, 343-345
Collaboration model, unification model and, 337-345
Collaborative research, 113
Collective bargaining in nursing; *see* Nursing unions
College(s)
  of applied arts and technology (CAAT), 301
  of New Caledonia, 329
  of Nurses of Ontario (CNO), 274, 301, 352
College St. Jean, 302
Colleges d'Enseignement General et Professionnel (CEGEP), 300, 331, 352, 368
Columbia University, 310
Committee on Nursing Education (Alberta), 354
Commonwealth Foundation, 430, 432
Commonwealth Meeting of Chief Nursing Officers and Professional Associations, 430
Commonwealth Nurses' Federation (CNF), 430
Communication
  interpersonal, political awareness in nursing and, 212

Communication—cont'd
  nursing research and, 169
Community colleges, 374
Computerization, nursing records and, 247-248
Conceptual knowledge, 94
Conceptual models, theories derived from, nursing knowledge and, 94
Conduct and Utilization of Research in Nursing (CURN), 176
Conference of Federal and Provincial Ministers of Health in Ottawa, 223
Confidentiality
  ethics and, 254
  legal aspects of, 248
Conflict, unionism and professionalism and, 285-287
Consent to nursing care, legal aspects of, 244
Consultation, nursing research and, 169
Consumers' Association of Canada, 50, 243
Content encompassing nursing knowledge, 87-90
Cooperation, unionism and professionalism and, 285-287
COPS; *see* Corps des Organismes Professionels de la Santé
Cornwall, 331
Corporate culture, transformation of, total quality management and, 190
Corps des Organismes Professionels de la Santé (COPS), 275-276
Cost-effectiveness of research-based nursing practice, 163-164, 165-166
Council
  on Medical Education, 297
  of National Representatives, 429
  of the Nightingale Fund, 295
  of Ontario University Programs in Nursing, 368
CPHA; *see* Canadian Public Health Association
Credentialing, 351, 363-372
  case for mandatory licensure and, 366-367
  mechanisms of, 364
  movement to secure legislation for registration and, 364-366

Credentialing—cont'd
  recognition of specialization and, 369-371
  registration and licensure and, 368
  specialization in nursing and, 368-369
Credibility of nursing knowledge, criteria for, 98-100
Creelman, Lyle, 437
Crimea, 75
Cross Cancer Institute, 265
CUNSA; see Canadian University Nursing Students' Association
Cure versus care, 61
CURN; see Conduct and Utilization of Research in Nursing
Currie, Sir Arthur, 311, 312
CUSO; see Canadian University Service Overseas
Customer focus, total quality management and, 190

D

D'Aiguillon, Duchess, 5
Dalhousie University, 42, 43, 308, 309, 316, 324, 331, 342, 344, 374, 377, 386, 394, 415, 416
Danish Nurses Organization, 397, 431
de Bullion, Mme., 7
de Champlain, Samuel, 3, 74
de Maisonneuve, Sieur, 7, 441
de Paul, Vincent, 6
de St. Bonaventure, Marie Forestier, 5
de St. Ignace, Marie Guenet, 5
Death, right to make choices in relation to, ethics and, 256-257
Declaration
  of Alma-Ata of 1978, 427, 428, 437, 439, 440
  of Universal Human Rights of 1948, 243
Degner, Lesley, 130
Degree programs
  collaboration between diploma programs and, 329-332
  increasing accessibility of, 381-389
Deming, Edward, 188
Demonstration model, nursing education and, 298
Depression, 309-312, 313-314
Descriptive theory, nursing knowledge and, 92-94

Diagnostic-related group-based (DRG) payment systems, 234-235
Dignity of patients, 253
Diniz, Fernanda Alves, 431
Diploma programs, 329-332, 368
  collaboration between degree programs and, 329-332
  emergence and growth of, 291-305
Distance education in nursing, 345, 381-389
  characteristics of successful off-campus programs in, 382
  clinical component of, 385
  collaboration in, 384
  human element in, 383-384
  model of, 386-388
  structure and organization for learning in, 382-383
  technology and, 385-386
Do not resuscitate (DNR) orders, ethics and, 257-260
Dock, Lavinia, 15
Doctoral programs; see Graduate education in Canada
Documentation, nursing, legal aspects of, 246-248
Dorothy J. Kergin Research Grant, 46, 124, 341, 431
Douglas, T.C., 220
Douglas College, 329
Ducharme, Francine, 422

E

Edmonton Group Hospitalization Plan, 219
Education, nursing; see Nursing education
Education roles, research-based nursing practice and, 172-173
Educational institutions, international nursing and, 431-432
Educational issues, international nursing and, 439
Edufacts, 40
Eduneuf, 40
EEC; see European Economic Community
Electronic mail (e-mail), 382
Embury, Sheila, 125
Empirical knowledge, 94
Empirics, nursing knowledge and, 95-96

Employee, involvement of, total quality
management and, 190
Employment
of nurses; *see* Nursing workforce
and Social Insurance Act of 1935, 220
Enablers, public's perception of nurses
and nursing and, 57
Entry to practice position, 40, 127
baccalaureate degree as, 321-333
collaboration between diploma and
degree programs and, 329-332
development and rationale of, 321-324
provincial developments in, 328
Environment, discipline of nursing and, 88
EP2000, 322, 323, 326-327
Epp, Jake, 391
Epp Report, 21
Erie Family Health Center, 70-71
Esthetics, nursing knowledge and, 96
Ethical issues and dilemmas in nursing
practice, 251-267
advance directives in, 260-261
allocation of health-care resources in,
263-264
basic human rights about health and
health care in, 255-256
codes of ethics in, 252-254
do not resuscitate orders in, 257-260
ethical dilemmas related to childbearing in, 262-263
principles and concepts of ethics in,
254-255
responsibilities for changing behaviour
in, 261-262
right to live as persons in, 261-262
right to make choices in relation to
death in, 256-257
strategies for addressing ethical dilemmas in practice in, 264-266
Ethics
code of, 243, 252-254
definition of, 251
nursing knowledge and, 96
principles and concepts of, 254-255
European Economic Community (EEC),
433, 434-435
Euthanasia, 256-257
Evans, Helen, 429
Experimental school of nursing, development of, at Toronto, 312-313

F
Fabiola, 74
Factor-isolating research questions, 121
Factor-relating research questions, 121
Faculty practice, 339-340
Faculty-agency joint appointment, 342
Fairley, Grace, 429
Fanshawe College, 330
FAO; *see* United Nations, Food and
Agriculture Organization
Fast, G.R., 302
Federal legislation for health-care financ-
ing, 220-221
Federal support for nursing research, 137-
138, 139-141
Federation
of Civil Employees (Manitoba), 274
of Nurses of Quebec, 276
Female Benevolent Society, 13
Feminism, nursing and, 67-73
relationship between, 68-70
research and, 71-72
women's health and, 70-71
Fenwick, Ethel Bedford, 15
Fernandez, Antonia, 431
Financing
of accreditation of nursing education
programs, 357-358
of health care; *see* Health care, organization and financing of
of nursing research, 135-145
federal support for, 137-138, 139-141
sources of funding for, 138-139
by university schools of nursing,
141-143
Fiscal Arrangements and Established
Programs Financing Act of 1977,
221
Fish-bone diagram, total quality management and, 193
Flaherty, Josephine, 433
Flexner, Abraham, 24
Flexner Report, 297
Flora Madeline Shaw Endowment Fund,
316
Florida, University of, 336-337
Flow chart, total quality management
and, 193
Focus, 131
FOCUS-PDCA, 192

Foothills Hospital, 329
Friend, Phyllis, 431
Friesen, Gordon, 234
Friesen Concept, 234
FSPIIQ; *see* la Fédération des Syndicats
    Professionels d'Infirmières du
    Québec
Functional assignment, 228, 229

G

Garzon, Nelly, 429
Girard, Alice, 429
Glass, Helen Preston, 222, 429
Global Advisory Group on Nursing and
    Midwifery, 437
Goldmark Report, 296
Gottleib, Laurie, 132
Government institutions
    international nursing and, 433-437
    regional, 434-435
    world, 435-437
Grace Hospital, 330
Grace Hospital Nurse-Midwifery Project,
    400
Graduate education in Canada, 79, 416,
    420, 421-424
    analysis of enrollment trends in
        Master's programs in, 417-418
    analysis of enrolment trends in doctor-
        al programs in, 419
    developing faculty resources for, 419-
        421
    establishment of doctoral programs in,
        422
    establishment of Master's degree pro-
        grams in, 412-415
    expansion of Master's programs in
        nursing in, 415-417
    growth of, 407-424
    postdoctoral education in nursing in,
        422-424
    preparing to establish doctoral pro-
        grams in, 421-422
Grand theories, nursing knowledge and,
    94
Grandparenting, baccalaureate degree
    and, 322
Grant MacEwan Community College,
    302, 328, 329, 360
Grey Nuns, 8-9, 13, 14-15, 26, 75

Grey Nuns Hospital, 378
Grier, Mother Hannah, 18

H

Hébert
    Louis, 4
    Marie Rollet, 4
Hall
    Dorothy, 437
    G.E., 412
Hall Commission, 299
Hamilton General Hospital, 318
Hampton, Isabel Robb, 15, 293, 350, 365
Harmer, Bertha, 310, 311, 312
Harper Hospital (Detroit, Michigan), 252
Harvard University, 189, 291
Hayes, Patricia, 132
Hôtel Dieu of Quebec, 6, 11, 12
HEAL; *see* Health Action Lobby
Healing Health Care, 189
Health
    for All by the Year 2000, 390-391, 393,
        427, 429, 433, 435, 436, 438, 439,
        440, 442
    basic human rights about, ethics and,
        255-256
    discipline of nursing and, 88
    and Welfare Canada, 35, 36, 45, 137,
        138, 377, 391, 433-434
    women's, feminist approach to, 70-71
Health Action Lobby (HEAL), 50
Health care
    basic human rights about, ethics and,
        255-256
    comparative view of, 216-217
    organization and financing of, 216-227
        Canada Health Act of 1984 and,
            221-223
        early health insurance plans and, 219
        federal legislation for, 220-221
        Medicare and, 218-219
        national health insurance and, 219-
            220
        philosophical basis of health-care
            financing legislation and, 224-
            225
        privatization of health care and,
            223-224
        restructuring health-care system
            and, 225-226

Health care—cont'd
  primary; *see* Primary health care
  privatization of, 223-224
Health Disciplines Act of 1977 (Ontario),
    284, 352, 368
Health insurance
  early plans of, 219
  national, 219-220
Health maintenance organization (HMO),
    237
Health-care agencies, nursing research in,
    143-144
Health-care consumer, legal rights of, 243-
    244
Health-care reform, Canadian Nurses
    Association and, 49-50
Health-care resources, allocation of, ethics
    and, 263-264
Henderson, Virginia, 70
Henstch, Yvonne, 431
Hilson, Margaret, 433
Hippocratic Oath, 252
Hirschfeld, Miriam, 437
Histogram, total quality management
    and, 193
HIV; *see* Human immunodeficiency virus
HMO; *see* Health maintenance organiza-
    tion
Holleran, Constance, 429
Holt, Mabel, 296
Hospital Council of Metro Toronto, 197
Hospital Disputes Arbitration Act of 1965,
    279-280
Hospital Employees Union, 273
Hospital Insurance and Diagnostic
    Services Act of 1957, 23, 220
Hospitali Res De La Miséricorde De Jésus,
    5-6
Hospitals
  Allen Memorial Institute (Montreal),
    255
  Amherst Hospital (Nova Scotia), 277
  Boothills Hospital, 378
  British Columbia Children's Hospital,
    123
  Grace Hospital, 330
  Grey Nuns Hospital, 378
  Hamilton General Hospital, 318
  Harper Hospital (Detroit, Michigan),
    252

Hospitals—cont'd
  Hôtel Dieu of Quebec, 6, 11, 12
  Hospital for Sick Children (Toronto),
    20
  Hospital for Sick Children Foundation
    (Toronto), 139
  Humber Memorial Hospital, 378
  Johns Hopkins Hospital (Baltimore,
    Maryland), 365
  Kingston General Hospital, 13
  Metropolitan Hospital, 297
  Misericordia Hospital (Edmonton),
    328, 360, 378, 400
  Montreal General Hospital, 264, 294,
    295
  Prince Edward Island Hospital, 296
  Royal Alexandra Hospital, 378
  Saint John General Hospital, 296
  St. Boniface General Hospital, 378
  St. Joseph's Health Centre (Toronto),
    378
  St. Michael's Hospital (Toronto), 378
  St. Thomas' Hospital (London,
    England), 292
  Toronto General Hospital, 237, 294,
    318, 365, 378
  Toronto Hospital, 378
  University College Hospital, 293
  University Hospitals of Cleveland, 337,
    338, 341, 346
  University of Alberta Hospitals
    (Edmonton), 28, 131, 265
  Vancouver General Hospital, 28, 42,
    296, 328
  Veterans Administration Medical
    Centre (Buffalo, New York), 185,
    233
  Victoria General Hospital, 331
  Victoria Public Hospital, 296
  Wellesley Hospital (Toronto), 378
  Winnipeg General Hospital, 18, 295-296
  Women's College Hospital, 378
Houston, Mary Renfrew, 130
Human element in distance education in
    nursing, 383-384
Human immunodeficiency virus (HIV),
    256
Humber College, 301
Humber Memorial Hospital, 378
Hunter, Trennie, 20

I

ICC; *see* Intraclass correlation coefficient
ICN; *see* International Council of Nurses
IHEP; *see* International Health Exchange
    Program
Illinois, University of, 436
ILO; *see* United Nations, International
    Labour Organization
Image: Journal of Nursing Scholarship, 132
Immigration, effects of, on nursing, 12-13
Implied consent, 244
Index of Canadian Studies, 147
Industrial Relations Act (New
    Brunswick), 277
Informed consent, 244
Innovation adoption behavior, research-
    based nursing practice and, 174-
    178
Integrity of nursing profession, interna-
    tional nursing and, 438
Interinstitutional linkages to promote col-
    laboration, 337-345
International Affairs Department, 430
International Colloquium on Primary
    Health Care, 431
International Community Health Nursing
    Research Conference, 345
International Conference on Community
    Health Nursing Research, 156
International Conference on Community
    Nursing Research, 432
International Council of Nurses (ICN), 16,
    27, 36, 243, 252, 283, 294, 366,
    391, 428-430, 438
International Development Research
    Centre, 432
International Grenfell Association, 377
International Health Exchange Program
    (IHEP), 432
International law, 242
International Monetary Fund, 440
International nursing, 427-440
    agencies of national government and,
        433-434
    attitudinal issues and, 439
    Canadian International Development
        Agency and, 433-434
    Canadian Nurses Association and, 430
    educational insitutions and, 431-432
    educational issues and, 439

International Nursing—cont'd
    European Economic Community and,
        434-435
    governmental institutions and, 433-437
    Health and Welfare Canada and, 433-
        434
    integrity of profession and, 438
    International Council of Nurses and,
        428-430
    issues with international dimensions
        and, 437-440
    nongovernmental organizations and,
        428-433
    political issues and, 439-440
    primary health care and, 439-440
    provincial nurses associations and, 431
    regional government and, 434-435
    religious auspices and, 432-433
    structures and institutions and, 428-
        433
    world government and, 435-437
    World Health Organization and, 435-
        437
International Nursing History
    Conference, 431-432
International Nursing Research
    Conference, 148, 156, 345, 431
International Red Cross, 433
Internet, 382
Interpersonal communication, political
    awareness in nursing and, 212
Intraclass correlation coefficient (ICC),
    185

J

JCAH; *see* Joint Committee on
    Accreditation of Hospitals
Johns, Ethel, 26, 307, 324
Johns Hopkins Hospital (Baltimore,
    Maryland), 365
Joint Committee on Accreditation of
    Hospitals (JCAH), 183
Joint-Faculties Bioethics Project, 265
Justice, ethics and, 254

K

Kameko, Matsu, 431
Kellogg, W.K., Foundation, 17, 41, 43, 298,
    315-316, 341, 357, 409, 410, 412,
    413, 414, 415, 421, 422
Kelsey Institute, 330

Kenney, Sister, 56
Kergin, Dorothy, 46, 124, 341, 431
Kidney Foundation of Canada, 139
Kiereini, Eunice Muringo, 429
Kim, Mo Im, 429
King
    Imogene M., 105
    W.L. MacKenzie, 219
Kingston Compassionate Society, 13
Kingston General Hospital, 13
Knowledge
    nursing; see Nursing knowledge
    scientific, 27-28
Knowledge Network, 385
Kwantlen College, 329

L

la Fédération des Syndicats Professionels
        d'Infirmières du Québec (FSPI-
        IQ), 275
Labour Relations Act (Manitoba), 269, 274
l'Alliance des Infirmières et Infirmiers du
        Québec, 275
Lalonde Report, 21
Langara College, 329
Laurentian University, 330
Laval, Université, 43, 154, 416
Law(s)
    British North America Act of 1867, 216
    Canada Evidence Act, 247
    Canada Health Act of 1984, 23, 49, 71,
        209, 223, 225
    confidentiality and, 248
    consent to nursing care and, 244
    Employment and Social Insurance Act
        of 1935, 220
    Fiscal Arrangements and Established
        Programs Financing Act of 1977,
        221
    Health Disciplines Act of 1977
        (Ontario), 284, 352, 368
    Hospital Disputes Arbitration Act of
        1965, 279-280
    Hospital Insurance and Diagnostic
        Services Act of 1957, 23, 220
    Industrial Relations Act (New
        Brunswick), 277
    Labour Relations Act (Manitoba), 269,
        274
    Medical Care Act of 1968, 209, 221
    negligence and, 245-246

Laws—cont'd
    nursing documentation and, 246-248
    Nursing Profession Act (Alberta), 29,
        284, 354, 368
    overview of, 241-242
    practising nurse and, 241-250
    Prince Edward Island Labour Act, 277-
        278
    Prince Edward Island Nurses' Act, 270,
        277-278
    Public Service Act (Newfoundland),
        278
    Public Service Labour Relations Act
        (New Brunswick), 277
    Quebec Labour Code, 275
    Quebec Nurses Act, 275
    Registered Nurses' Act, 273
    Registered Nurses' Act (Alberta), 213,
        366
    responsibilities of nurse under, 242-243
    rights of health-care consumer and,
        243-244
    telephone orders and, 245
    Trade Union Act (Saskatchewan), 274,
        277
    understanding legal aspects of nursing
        and, 249
    Universities' Act (Alberta), 351-352
Lawson, Elizabeth, 20
Le Fonds de recherche en sante du
        Quebec, 344
Leadership, nursing, opportunities for, in
        primary health care, 398-399
League of Red Cross Societies, 433
Learned Societies, 148
Legislation
    federal, for health care financing, 220-
        221
    mandatory, credentialing and, 366-367
    movement to secure, for registration,
        credentialing and, 364-366
Leininger, Madeleine, 105
Lethbridge Community College, 302
Licensed practical nurse, 315
Licensure, 368
Likert scale, public's perception of nurses
        and nursing and, 59
Lindeburgh, Marion, 312
l'Institut Marguerite d'Youville, 314
Livingston, Nora, 295

Loeb Center for Nursing and
 Rehabilitation, 70-71
Loyalist College, 331
LSD, 255
L'université de Sherbrooke, 417
Luther Christman Award, 80

M

MABC; see Midwives Association of
 British Columbia
Macdonald, Margaret, 18, 19
MacEachern, Malcolm T., 306
Machin, Maria, 294-295
Mack, Theophilus, 293
MacLaggan, Katherine, 303
MacLeod, Agnes J., 20
MacMurchy, Helen, 309
Maglacas, Amelia Mangay, 393, 394, 436,
 437
Magnussen, Eli, 431
Mahler, Halfdan, 435, 436, 437
Malaspina College, 329
Male nurses; see Men in nursing
Malpractice, 245-246
Managed care, case management and,
 236-237
Management
 nursing unions and, 278-279
 from top, total quality management
 and, 189
 total quality; see Total quality manage-
 ment
Management Analysis and Planning sys-
 tem (MAPS), 185, 186
Mance, Jeanne, 7-8, 209, 292, 432, 441
Mandatory legislation, credentialing and,
 366-367
Manitoba
 establishment of nursing unions in,
 274
 nursing education in, 302
 University of, 42, 43, 130, 316, 330, 378,
 410, 416
Manitoba Association of Registered
 Nurses (MARN), 130, 274, 302
Manitoba Health Research Board, 139
Manitoba Health Sciences Centre, 330
Manitoba Hospital Service Association,
 219
Manitoba Nurses' Union, 274

Manitoba Nursing Research Unit, 130
Manitoba Organization of Nurses
 Association (MONA), 274
MAPS; see Management Analysis and
 Planning System
MARN; see Manitoba Association of
 Registered Nurses, 274
Mass media and image of nurses and
 nursing, 55-57
Master's degree programs; see Graduate
 education in Canada
McDonald, Elizabeth, 401
McGill University, 27, 43, 44, 120, 132, 135,
 138, 147, 156, 284, 301, 308, 309-
 312, 310, 312, 314, 315, 316, 324,
 327, 342, 396, 410, 412, 413, 415-
 416, 417, 419, 422, 431
McMaster University, 27, 135, 148, 154,
 204, 284, 316, 318, 325, 327, 341-
 342, 394, 402, 410, 413, 414, 416,
 417, 419, 422, 431, 437
Measurement
 of outcomes, research-based nursing
 practice and, 164-165
 and process improvement, total quality management and, 191
Medical Care Act of 1968, 209, 221
Medical Research Council (MRC), 45, 123,
 127, 137, 141, 421
Medicare, 217, 218-219, 221
Medicine Hat College, 302
Medicus Systems Corporation, 235
Memorial University of Newfoundland,
 42, 43, 331-332, 345, 377, 416
Men in nursing, 55, 74-81
 barriers to, 77-78
 efforts to support, 78-80
 historical perspective of, 74-75
 proportion of, 75-77
 research on, 80
Metaparadigm, nursing knowledge and,
 87-90
Metropolitan Hospital, 297
Micro-range theories, nursing knowledge
 and, 94
Midwifery, 71, 226, 399-404
Midwifery Services Review Report, 404
Midwives Association of British
 Columbia (MABC), 404
Mills, Karen, 432, 433

Misericordia Hospital, 328, 360, 378, 400

Modular nursing, definition of, 235

MONA; *see* Manitoba Organization of Nurses Association

Monitoring standards in nursing education; *see* Nursing education standards

Montréal, University de, 27, 43, 44, 120, 135, 156, 284, 301, 315, 327, 342, 344, 413, 416, 417, 419, 422, 431, 432

Montreal, Grey Nuns of, 8-9, 14-15, 75, 326

Montreal General Hospital, 13, 264, 294, 295

Mount Royal College, 302, 329

Mount Sinai Hospital, 378, 437

Mount St. Vincent University, 316

MRC; *see* Medical Research Council

Multiple triangulation, 113

Musallem, Helen K., 299-300, 318, 430

N

Nakajima, Hiroshi, 437

NANDA; *see* North American Nursing Diagnosis Association

National Demonstration Project on Quality Improvement in Health Care (NDP), 189

National Federation of Nurses' Union (NFNU), 271-272

National Health Grants Program, 23, 220

National health insurance, 219-220

National Health Research and Development Program (NHRDP), 45, 123, 127, 137, 148, 421-422

National Health Service (United Kingdom), 78, 217

National League
for Nursing (NLN), 15, 355, 356-357, 369
for Nursing Education, 355

National Male Nurses Association, 79-80

National Nursing Research Conference, 147-156, 421

National Plan
for Entry to Practice, 326
for Nursing Administration, 48, 49

National professional nursing organizations, establishment of, 15-18

National Research Council (NRC), 137

Natural Sciences and Engineering Research Council (NSERC), 123, 127, 137

NBARN; *see* New Brunswick Association of Registered Nurses

NBNU; *see* New Brunswick Nurses Union

NCAST; *see* Nursing Child Assessment Satellite Training

NDP; *see* National Demonstration Project on Quality Improvement in Health Care

Negligence, legal aspects of, 245-246

New Brunswick
establishment of nursing unions in, 276-277
University of, 42, 345, 410

New Brunswick Association of Registered Nurses (NBARN), 276-277, 303, 331, 410

New Brunswick Civil Service Nurses' Provincial Collective Bargaining Council, 277

New Brunswick Nurses' Provincial Collective Bargaining Council, 277

New Brunswick Nurses Union (NBNU), 277

New England Medical Center Model, 237

New France, first nurses in, 4-9

New Mount Sinai Hospital, 301

Newfoundland
establishment of nursing unions in, 278
Memorial University of, 42, 43, 345, 377, 416

Newfoundland Hospital Association, 278

Newfoundland Ministry of Health, 197, 204

Newfoundland Nurses' Union, 278

NFNU; *see* National Federation of Nurses' Union

NGOs; *see* Nongovernmental organizations

Nightingale, Florence, 13-14, 26, 55-56, 67, 75, 85, 106, 163, 183, 252, 292, 294-295, 324, 350, 364

Nightingale model, nursing education and, 292-293

Nightingale School of Nursing, 301

NLN; *see* National League for Nursing, 355
No cardiopulmonary resuscitation orders, 257, 258
No code orders, 257-260
Nongovernmental organizations (NGOs), international nursing and, 428-433
Nonmaleficence, ethics and, 254
North American Code of Ethics, 27
North American Nursing Diagnosis Association (NANDA), 95
North Island College, 329
Northern Lights Community College, 329
Northwest College, 329
No-strike policy of Canadian Nurses Association, 286
Nova Scotia, establishment of nursing unions in, 277
Nova Scotia Nurses Union (NSNU), 277
NRC; *see* National Research Council
NRC; *see* Nursing research committee
NSERC; *see* Natural Sciences and Engineering Research Council
NSNU; *see* Nova Scotia Nurses Union
Nurse Educators Interest Group, 331
Nursenet, 382
Nurses
    employment of; *see* Nursing workforce
    image of, Canadian Nurses Association and, 33
    practising, and law, 241-250
    registered, 26, 197-200
    responsibilities of, under law, 242-243
NURSES: KEY TO HEALTHY ALBERTANS, 398
Nurses' Associated Alumnae of the United States and Canada, 15
Nursing
    in Canada, 1-81
        1600-1760, 3-10
        from 1760 to present, 11-22
        in seventeenth and eighteenth centuries, 9-10
    definition of, 106-107
    discipline of, 85, 88
    effects of immigration on, 12-13
    and feminism; *see* Feminism, nursing and
    foundations of, 107

Nursing—cont'd
    image of, Canadian Nurses Association and, 33
    international; *see* International nursing
    men in; *see* Men in nursing
    modes of inquiry in, 95-98
    modular, definition of, 235
    in New France, 4-9
    political awareness in; *see* Political awareness in nursing
    primary, 228-240
    professional image of; *see* Professional image of nursing
    professional practice of, 171-174
    public health, emergence of, 20-22
    response of, to primary health care, 395-398
    specialization in; *see* Specialization in nursing
    understanding legal aspects of, 249
Nursing administration
    Canadian Nurses Association and, 46-49
    research-based nursing practice and, 172
Nursing Approach, 64
Nursing assistant, certified, 315
Nursing care
    case management and managed care and, 236-237
    comparison of, 231-232
    consent to, legal aspects of, 244
    delivery of, 181-288
    future of, 237-238
    organization of, 228-240
    primary nursing and, 228-240
    quality, 334-349
    types of, 228-231
Nursing Child Assessment Satellite Training (NCAST), 176
Nursing documentation, legal aspects of, 246-248
Nursing education
    accreditation and, 299
    in Alberta, 302
    approval of programs in, 351-355
    in Atlantic Provinces, 303-304
    in British Columbia, 302
    Canadian Nurses Association and, 40-44

Nursing education—cont'd
  centralized teaching program and, 298-299
  collaboration between nursing education and nursing practice for, 334-349
  collaboration between nursing practice and, for quality nursing care, education, and research, 334-349
  collaboration between service and, deterrents to, 340-341
  demonstration school and, 298
  distance; *see* Distance education in nursing
  early preparation for nursing practice and, 292
  first Canadian, 293-296
  future of, 289-424
  graduate; *see* Graduate education in Canada
  historical influences on separation between service and, 334-337
  in Manitoba, 302
  movement to establish 2-year schools and, 300-304
  Nightingale model and, 292-293
  in Ontario, 301
  origins of, in Canada, 291-305
  professional, 28-29
  in Quebec, 300-301
  recognizing need for improvement in standards for, 296-300
  Royal Commission on Health Services and, 299-300
  in Saskatchewan, 300
  total quality management and, 190
  university; *see* University nursing education
Nursing Education Committee, 352
Nursing education programs, accreditation of, 355-357
Nursing education standards, 41, 47
  historical perspective of, 324-325
  monitoring, 350-362
  recognizing need for, 296-300
Nursing knowledge, 83-180
  classification of, 94-95
  content encompassing, 87-90
  criteria for credibility of, 98-100
  development of, 85-103

Nursing knowledge—cont'd
  future directions for, 100
  levels of, 92-94
  nursing theory and, 108
  and research utilization, 116
  sources of, 90-92
  substantive structure of, 87-100
  syntactical structure of, 95
  world view of, 86-87
Nursing leadership, opportunities for, in primary health care, 398-399
Nursing model, nursing knowledge and, 87-90, 91-92
Nursing organizations, national professional, establishment of, 15-18
Nursing outcome, 164
Nursing Papers, 132, 147
Nursing paradigm, theory-testing and theory-building and, 106-108
Nursing practice
  Canadian Nurses Association and, 33-36
  collaboration between nursing education and, for quality nursing care, education, and research, 334-349
  early preparation for, 292
  ethical issues and dilemmas in; *see* Ethical issues and dilemmas in nursing practice
  professional; *see* Professionalism
  research-based; *see* Research-based nursing practice
  scope of nursing research in, 146-161
Nursing Profession Act (Alberta), 29, 284, 354, 368
Nursing research, 62
  administrative roles and, 172
  Canadian Nurses Association and, 44-46
  choices of, 109
  classification of, 147
  clinical nurse specialist roles and, 173-174
  collaboration between nursing education and nursing practice for, 334-349
  definition of, 107
  demographic data and focus of, 149-151

Nursing research—cont'd
    design of, 109-110
    deterrents to conducting, 120-125
    deterrents to disseminating and apply-
        ing, 125-127
    development of, 146-147
    education roles and, 172-173
    feminism and, 71-72
    financing of; see Financing of nursing
        research
    future of, 178
    in health-care agencies, 143-144
    health-care system issues and, 163-171
    innovation adoption behavior and,
        174-178
    knowledge and, 116
    maximizing, 112-114
    men in nursing and, 80
    national conferences of, 147-156
    organization and funding of, 147-149,
        153-156
    partnerships and, 171
    patient-controlled analgesia and, 175-
        176
    professional practice of nursing and,
        171-174
    research-utilization framework and,
        176-177
    scope of, in nursing practice, 146-161
    strategies to promote, 127-132
    theory and, 108-109
    theory-generating, 110, 111
    theory-testing and theory-building
        and; see Theory-testing and theo-
        ry-building, nursing research
        and
    utilizing, in practice, 162-180
Nursing research committee (NRC), 168
Nursing research consultant, 130
Nursing Research, 126, 132, 152, 175, 177
Nursing science and knowledge, nursing
        theory and, 108
Nursing theory; see Theory-testing and
        theory-building, nursing
        research and
Nursing unions
    in Alberta, 273
    in British Columbia, 272-273
    emergence of, as social force in
        Canada, 268-281

Nursing unions—cont'd
    establishment and consolidation of,
        272-278
    impact of loss of right to strike and,
        279-280
    management and, 278-279
    in Manitoba, 274
    National Federation of Nurses' Unions
        and, 271-272
    in New Brunswick, 276-277
    in Newfoundland, 278
    in Nova Scotia, 277
    in Ontario, 274-275
    on Prince Edward Island, 277-278
    professional responsibility clauses and,
        279
    public impact of collective bargaining
        in nursing and, 280-281
    in Quebec, 275-276
    rise of, 269-271
    in Saskatchewan, 273-274
Nursing Unit Administration Program, 47
Nursing workforce, 196-207
    challenges facing, 202-204
    recommendations for change in, 204-
        206
    supply-demand imbalances and, 201-
        202
    trends in employment of nurses and,
        197-200
    trends in supply and, 200-201
Nutting, Mary Adelaide, 15, 293, 350

O
Off-campus programs; see Distance edu-
        cation in nursing
OIIQ; see Ordre des Infirmières et
        Infirmièrs du Québec
Okanagan College, 329
ONA; see Ontario Nurses Association
Ontario
    establishment of nursing unions in,
        274-275
    nursing education in, 301
Ontario Hospital Association, 275
Ontario Hospital Services Commission,
        301
Ontario Ministry of Health, 139, 204
Ontario Nurses Association (ONA), 32,
        197, 204, 271, 275

Opening Learning Institute, 385
"Operation Bootstrap," 17, 43, 45
ORCAUSN; *see* Canadian Association of
      University Schools of Nursing
Order(s)
    do not resuscitate, ethics and, 257-260
    no cardiopulmonary resuscitation, 257,
      258
    no code, 257-260
    of Nurses of the Province of Quebec
      (ONQ), 275, 285
    of Sisters of Charity of Montreal; *see*
      Grey Nuns
    telephone, legal aspects of, 245
Ordre des Infirmières et Infirmiers du
      Québec (OIIQ), 197, 204, 353
Orem, Dorothea, 105
Organization
    and financing of health care; *see* Health
      care, organization and financing
      of
    of nursing care, 228-240
Ottawa, University of, 43, 44, 314, 342,
      344, 416
Ottawa Charter for Health Promotion,
      391, 392, 393
Oulton, Judith, 429

P

Pan American Health Organization, 437
Paradigm
    definition of, 107
    nursing knowledge and, 87-90
Parent Commission, 300
Pareto chart, total quality management
      and, 193
Partial theories, nursing knowledge and,
      94
Partnerships, research-based nursing
      practice and, 171
Passive euthanasia, 257
Paternalism, ethics and, 254
Patient
    dignity of, 253
    legal rights of, 243-244
Patient-controlled analgesia (PCA),
      research-based nursing practice
      and, 175-176
Patry, L.A., 371
PCA; *see* Patient-controlled analgesia

PEI Labour Act; *see* Prince Edward Island
      Labour Act
PEI Nurses' Act; *see* Prince Edward Island
      Nurses' Act
PEI Nurses Union; *see* Prince Edward
      Island Nurses Union
Peltrie, Mme. de la, 5
Pennsylvania, University of, 337
Pennsylvania State Consultation Nursing
      Center, 70-71
Person, discipline of nursing and, 88
Personal knowledge, 96
Personhood, ethics and, 254
Phaneuf nursing audit, 185
Pharmaceutical Manufacturers
      Association of Canada Health
      Research Foundation, 46, 124
Pilot Project for Evaluation of Schools of
      Nursing, 318
PLATO, 388
Political awareness in nursing, 208-215
    creating, 211-212
    developing base of support for, 212
    enhanced, benefits of, 214
    importance of developing, 209-211
    international nursing and, 439-440
    interpersonal communication and, 212
    pursuit of goals and, 213-214
    understanding fundamentals of, 211-
      212
Poole, Dame Anne, 430
Pope, Georgina Fane, 18
Postdoctoral education; *see* Graduate edu-
      cation in Canada
Pourteous, Rena, 401
Practical nurse, licensed, 315
Practice, definition of, 366
Practising nurse and law, 241-250
Premier's Commission on Future Health
      Care for Albertans, 403
Prescriptive theory, nursing knowledge
      and, 92-94
Preventive systems, total quality manage-
      ment and, 190
Primary health care, 7-8, 42, 390-406
    Canadian approach to achieving, 392-
      394
    definition of, 394-395
    development of midwifery and, 399-
      404

Primary health care—cont'd
    Health for All by the Year 2000, 390-391
    international nursing and, 439-440
    nursing's response to challenge of, 395-398
    opportunities for nursing leadership in, 398-399
Primary nursing, 228-240
Prince Edward Island, establishment of nursing unions in, 277-278
Prince Edward Island Hospital, 296
Prince Edward Island (PEI) Labour Act, 277-278
Prince Edward Island (PEI) Nurses' Act, 270, 277-278
Prince Edward Island (PEI) Nurses Union, 272
Privatization of health care, 223-224
Process Chart Audit, 185, 186
Process focus, total quality management and, 190
Process improvement, measurement and, total quality management and, 191
Profession(s)
    characteristics of, 24
    development of, 24-26
    evolution of nursing as, 26-27
Professional associations and unions, 282-284, 287-288
Professional education for nursing, 28-29
Professional image of nursing, 54-66
    external and internal, 54-55
    mass media and, 55-57
    public's perception of, 57-60
    self-image of nursing and, 60-61
    strategies for changing, 61-65
Professional practice of nursing, 171-174
Professionalism, 23-30
    control of, 29
    emergence of scientific knowledge base and, 27-28
    facilitating, 29-30
    unionism and; see Unionism and professionalism
Provincial Advisory Council on Nursing Education, 352
Provincial Collective Bargaining Committee, 278

Provincial developments, entry to practice position and, 328
Provincial nurses associations, international nursing and, 431
Public health nursing, emergence of, 20-22
Public Hospital Act, 275
Public law, 242
Public Service Act (Newfoundland), 278
Public Service Labour Relations Act (New Brunswick), 277

Q

QRCAUSN; see Canadian Association of University Schools of Nursing
Qualitative/quantitative controversy, nursing theory and, 110-112
Quality assurance, 182-195
    future of, 193-195
    historical developments in, 183-186
    limitations of programs of, 186-187
Quality management, total; see Total quality management
Quality nursing care, collaboration between nursing education and nursing practice for, 334-349
Quality of care; see Quality assurance
QualPacs, 185
Quebec
    establishment of nursing unions in, 275-276
    nursing education in, 300-301
Quebec Federation of Labour, 275
Quebec Labour Code, 275
Quebec Ministry of Health, 139
Quebec Nurses Act, 275
Queen's University, 154, 316, 331, 416
Quinn, Sheila, 435
Quo Vadis School of Nursing, 301

R

Raven, Kathleen, 431
Rayside, Edith, 19
RCAMC; see Royal Canadian Army Medical Corps
Read, Grantly Dick, 399
Reasonable standards, 242-243
Recognition and reward, total quality management and, 191
Red Cross, 298, 308-309, 324
Red Deer College, 42, 302, 328, 360, 387, 388

Red River Community College, 302
Regina Grey Nuns Hospital School of
    Nursing, 300
Regional government, international nurs-
    ing and, 434-435
Registered nurse (RN), 26, 197-200
Registered Nurses' Act, 213, 273, 366
Registered Nurses Association
    of British Columbia (RNABC), 166,
        167, 269, 272, 302, 404, 431
    of Nova Scotia (RNANS), 277, 303
    of Ontario (RNAO), 32, 271, 301, 354
Registered Nurses Management Data, 197
Registered nursing assistant, 315
Registration
    and licensure, 368
    movement to secure legislation for,
        364-366
    of nurses, 368
Regulated Health Professions Act
    (RHPA), 366, 368
Reid
    Alma, 341
    Helen, 310
Reidy, Mary, 301
Release time, nursing research and, 169
Religious auspices, international nursing
    and, 432-433
Research
    collaborative, 113
    nursing; see Nursing research
Research fellowships, 137-138
Research grants, 137-138
Research Imperative, 45
Research in Nursing and Health, 132, 152
Research reports, critical evaluation of,
    114-116
Research-based nursing practice, 162-180
    benefits of, 163-164
    cost-effectiveness of, 163-164, 165-166
    examples of, 170-171
    infrastructures of, 167-170
    as investment, 166-167
    measuring outcomes of, 164-165
    purpose of, 163
    research-mindedness and, 118-134
    strategies to promote, 127-132
Research-mindedness
    deterrents to conducting research and,
        120-125

Research-mindedness—cont'd
    deterrents to disseminating and apply-
        ing research findings and, 125-
        127
    research-based nursing practice and,
        118-134
    strategies to promote research and
        research-based practice and, 127-
        132
Research-utilization frameworks,
    research-based nursing practice
    and, 176-177
Reward and recognition, total quality
    management and, 191
RHPA; see Regulated Health Professions
    Act
Right(s)
    about health and health care, ethics
        and, 255-256
    legal, of health-care consumer, 243-244
    to live as persons, ethics and, 261-262
    to make choices in relation to death,
        ethics and, 256-257
    to strike, loss of impact of, 279-280
Risk analysis, 213
Ritchie, Judith, 32
RITE-line system, 387
RN; see Registered nurse
RNABC; see Registered Nurses
    Association of British Columbia
RNANS; see Registered Nurses
    Association of Nova Scotia
RNAO; see Registered Nurses Association
    of Ontario
Robert Wood Johnson Foundation, 340
Rochester, University of, 337-338
Rockefeller Foundation, 296, 312, 313, 317,
    325
Rogers
    Lina, 20
    Martha E., 105
Role theory, 338
Ross, Eleanor, 429
Roy
    David, 264
    Sister Callista, 105
Royal Alexandra Hospital School of
    Nursing, 328, 360, 378
Royal Canadian Army Medical Corps
    (RCAMC), 19

Royal Commission
on Health Services, 47, 220, 225, 299-300
of Inquiry on Education, 300
on the Status of Women, 270
Run chart, total quality management and, 193
Rush University, 337-338
Rush-Medicus process audit, 185, 186
Russell
Edith Kathleen, 312, 313, 317, 318, 324-325, 335, 419
Susan, 435
Rutgers University, 337
Ryerson Polytechnical Institute, 301, 352, 378, 402

S

Saint John General Hospital, 296
Saint John School of Nursing, 303
Salvation Army Grace General Hospital, 332
Sandwich baccalaureate program, 335
Saskatchewan
establishment of nursing unions in, 273-274
nursing education in, 300
University of, 42, 314, 342, 416
Saskatchewan Health Research Board, 139
Saskatchewan Institute of Applied Arts and Technology (SIAST), 330
Saskatchewan Nursing Research Unit, 130
Saskatchewan Registered Nurses Association (SRNA), 130, 269, 273, 282, 298, 300, 330
Saskatchewan Relief Commission, 218
Saskatchewan Union of Nurses (SUN), 272, 274
Scatter diagram, total quality management and, 193
Scholarship programs, CIDA and, 434
Science, nursing, nursing theory and, 108
Scientific knowledge, emergence of, as base for nursing, 27-28
Secondary analysis of data, 113-114
Self-care, 392
Self-image of nursing, 60-61
Selkirk College, 302, 329
Service
collaboration between education and, deterrents to, 340-341

Service—cont'd
historical influences on separation between nursing education and, 334-337
nursing research and, 169
Service Employees International Union, 269, 282
Shamian, Judith, 437
Sharpe, Gladys, 19, 20, 318
Shaw, Flora Madeline, 310, 316
SIAST; see Saskatchewan Institute of Applied Arts and Technology
Situation-producing research questions, 121
Situation-relating research questions, 121
Smallpox, 5-6
Smellie, Elizabeth, 19
Smith, Dorothy, 336-337
Smoke-free environment, healthy environments and, 392
Snellman, Venny, 431
Snively, Mary Agnes, 16, 294, 365, 429
Social Sciences and Humanities Research Council (SSHRC), 123, 127, 137, 421, 422-423
South Carolina, University of, 337
Specialization in nursing, 369, 374
credentialing and, 368-369
professional interest in, 374-376
recognition of, credentialing and, 369-371
Specialty, 369, 374
Specialty certificate programs, development of, with credit toward Baccalaureate degree in nursing, 373-380
Splane, Verna Huffman, 429
SRNA; see Saskatchewan Registered Nurses Association
SSHRC; see Social Sciences and Humanities Research Council
St. Bernard, Anne Lecointre de, 5
St. Boniface General Hospital, 378
St. Catharine's Training School for Nurses, 293
St. Clare's Mercy Hospital, 332
St. Francis Xavier University, 314, 386
St. Joseph's Health Centre (Toronto), 378
St. Lawrence College-St. Laurent, 331
St. Michael's Hospital (Toronto), 378

St. Thomas' Hospital (London, England), 292

Staff Nurses' Association of Nova Scotia, 277

Standards of nursing education; *see* Nursing education standards

Statistics Canada, 358

Stewart
Isabel Maitland, 293, 310
Norma, 130

Stinson, Shirley, 431

Strike, right to, loss of impact of, nursing unions and, 279-280

Structure, definition of, 336

Styles, Margretta, 429

Substantive structure of discipline of nursing, 85

Suffragette movement, feminism and, 67

SUN; *see* Saskatchewan Union of Nurses

Supply-demand imbalances, nursing workforce and, 200-202

Surveys of nursing education, 318-319

Syntactical structure of discipline of nursing, 85

T

Taylor
Frederick W., 228-229
Helen, 430

Team nursing, 228, 229

Teamwork, total quality management and, 191

Technology, distance education in nursing and, 385-386

Telephone orders, legal aspects of, 245

Telewriter system, 388

Theory, definition of, 107

Theory-testing and theory-building, nursing research and, 92-94, 105-117
critically evaluating research reports and, 114-116
definition of nursing and, 106-107
development of, 108-109
foundations of nursing and, 107
knowledge and research utilization and, 116
maximizing research and, 112-114
methods issues and, 110-114
nursing paradigm and, 106-108
nursing science and knowledge and, 108
purposes and objectives of, 106

Theory-testing and theory-building, nursing research and,—cont'd
qualitative/quantitative controversy and, 110-112
research and theory and, 108-109
research choices and, 109
research design and theory development and, 109-110
theory-generating and theory-testing research and, 110, 111

TINA network, 388

Toronto, University of, 27, 43, 44, 120, 135, 140, 156, 204, 284, 308, 312, 313, 314, 315, 317, 318, 324, 327, 335, 342, 343, 344, 382, 413, 416, 419, 422, 431

Toronto General Hospital, 237, 294, 318, 365, 378

Toronto Hospital, 378

Total quality management (TQM)
key concepts of, 189-191
process of, 191-192
quality assurance and; *see* Quality assurance
tools of, 192-193
transition to, 187-189

Trade Union Act (Saskatchewan), 274, 277

Triangulation, 112-113

Turnbull, Lily, 437

Two-year schools, movement to establish, 300-304

U

UCC; *see* Universities Coordinating Council

UMNInc.; *see* United Management Nurses' Inc.

UNHCR; *see* United Nations, High Commission for Refugees

UNICEF; *see* United Nations, International Children's Emergency Fund

UNICEF; *see* United Nations International Children's Emergency Fund

Unification model
collaboration model and, 337-345
criticism of, 339

UNInc.; *see* United Nurses' Inc.

Unionism and professionalism, 282-288
characteristics of professional associations and unions and, 282-284

Unionism and professionalism—cont'd
 factors influencing cooperation and
  conflict and, 285-287
 relationships between professional
  associations and unions and,
  287-288
Unions
 nursing; see Nursing unions
 professional associations and, 282-284,
  287-288
Unique theory, nursing knowledge and,
 90-92
United Empire Loyalists, 12
United Management Nurses' Inc.
 (UMNInc.), 275
United Nations, 433, 434, 440
 Food and Agriculture Organization,
  433
 High Commission for Refugees,
  433
 International Children's Emergency
  Fund (UNICEF), 390, 427, 433
 International Labour Organization,
  433
United Nurses' Inc. (UNInc.), 275
United Nurses of Montreal (UNM), 275
Universities
 Athabasca University (Alberta), 384,
  386, 387
 Case Western Reserve University
  (Cleveland, Ohio), 79, 338, 341,
  346
 Dalhousie University (Halifax), 42, 43,
  308, 309, 316, 324, 331, 342, 344,
  374, 377, 386, 394, 415, 416
 Harvard University (Boston,
  Massachusetts), 189, 291
 l'université de Sherbrooke, 417
 McGill, 27, 43, 44, 120, 132, 135, 138,
  147, 156, 284, 301, 308, 310, 312,
  314, 315, 316, 324, 327, 342, 396,
  410, 412, 413, 415-416, 417, 419,
  422, 431
 McMaster University, 27, 135, 148, 154,
  204, 284, 316, 318, 325, 327, 341-
  342, 394, 402, 410, 413, 414, 416,
  417, 419, 422, 431, 437
 Memorial University of
  Newfoundland, 42, 43, 331-332,
  345, 377, 416

Universities—cont'd
 Mount St. Vincent University (Halifax),
  316
 Queen's, 154, 316, 331, 416
 Rush University (Chicago), 337-338
 Rutgers University, 337
 Ryerson Polytechnical Institute, 301,
  352, 378, 402
 St. Francis Xavier University
  (Antigonish), 314, 386
 Université Laval, 43, 154, 416
 University de Montréal, 27, 43, 44, 120,
  135, 156, 284, 301, 315, 327, 342,
  344, 413, 416, 417, 419, 422, 431,
  432
 University of Alberta (Edmonton), 27,
  28, 42, 43, 120, 124, 131, 132, 148,
  156, 257, 265, 284, 308, 314, 324,
  327, 328, 329, 342, 344, 345, 360,
  366, 374, 377-378, 386-388, 403,
  410, 414-415, 416, 417, 419, 422,
  431
 University of Brandon, 330
 University of British Columbia (UBC),
  28, 42, 43, 120, 135, 147, 156, 284,
  297, 307, 308, 314, 318, 324, 327,
  328, 329, 335, 342, 344, 386, 410,
  413, 415, 416, 419, 422
 University of Calgary, 43, 124, 329, 342,
  386, 416, 431
 University of Florida, 336-337
 University of Illinois (Chicago), 436
 University of Lethbridge, 130
 University of Manitoba, 42, 43, 130,
  316, 330, 378, 410, 416
 University of New Brunswick
  (Fredericton), 42, 345, 410
 University of Ottawa, 43, 44, 314, 342,
  344, 416
 University of Pennsylvania, 337
 University of Prince Edward Island, 154
 University of Rochester, 337-338
 University of Saskatchewan, 42, 314,
  342, 416
 University of South Carolina, 337
 University of Toronto, 27, 43, 44, 120,
  135, 140, 156, 204, 284, 308, 312-
  313, 314, 315, 316-318, 324, 327,
  335, 342, 343, 344, 382, 413, 416,
  419, 422, 431

Universities—cont'd
   University of Victoria, 42, 154, 329, 342, 385, 417
   University of Western Ontario (UWO), 314, 315, 324, 330, 344, 412, 413, 415-416
   University of Windsor, 154, 416
   Yale University, 79, 188, 291
Universities' Act (Alberta), 351-352
Universities Coordinating Council (UCC), 284, 351-352, 354, 368
University College Hospital, 293
University Hospitals of Cleveland, 337, 338, 341, 346
University nursing education
   crisis at McGill and, 309-312
   in Depression years, 313-314
   development of experimental school of nursing at Toronto and, 312-313
   emergence of, 306-308
   historical approach to evolution of, in Canada, 306-320
   impact of Red Cross funding on, 308-309
   inception of basic degree program at University of Toronto and, 316-318
   new initiatives and incentives in, between 1940 and 1955, 314-316
   surveys of, 318-319
University schools of nursing, research supported by, 141-143
UNM; see United Nurses of Montreal
Ursuline nuns, 5-6
UWO; see University of Western Ontario

V

Vancouver City College, 302
Vancouver General Hospital, 28, 42, 296, 307, 328
Veracity, ethics and, 254
Verstraetes, Ursula, 123
Veterans Administration Medical Centre (Buffalo, New York), 185, 233
Victoria, University of, 42, 154, 329, 342, 385, 417
Victoria General Hospital, 331
Victoria Public Hospital, 296
Victorian Order of Nurses (VON), 18, 19, 21, 316, 341, 397

Virol, Leman, 431
VON; see Victorian Order of Nurses

W

Wascana Institute, 330
Weir, George, 297
Weir Report of 1932, 41, 298, 299, 350
Wellesley Hospital (Toronto), 378
Western Canadian Council on Education of Health Personnel, 415
Western Interstate Commission for Higher Education in Nursing (WICHEN), 176
Western Journal of Nursing Research, 131, 132, 152
Western Memorial Regional Hospital, 332
Western Ontario, University of, 314, 315, 324, 330, 344, 412, 413, 415-416
WHO; see World Health Organization
WICHEN; see Western Interstate Commission for Higher Education in Nursing
Wieler, Anne, 433
Wilson, Jean, 16
Windsor, University of, 416
Winnipeg Civic Registered Nurses' Association, 274
Winnipeg General Hospital, 18, 295-296
Winnipeg Health Sciences Centre, 378
Wollstonecraft, Mary, 291
Women's College Hospital, 378
Wood, Marilynn, 132
Workforce, nursing; see Nursing workforce
Working Group on Nursing Research, 141, 142
Work-life affairs, Canadian Nurses Association and, 36-38
World Bank, 440
World Council of Churches, Christian Medical Commission of, 432
World government, international nursing and, 435-437
World Health Assembly, 435, 437
World Health Organization (WHO), 204, 390, 391, 393, 395, 399, 427, 429, 432, 433, 434, 435-437, 439
World University Service of Canada (WUCS), 434
World wars, nursing during, 18-20

WRCAUSN; *see* Canadian Association of
　　University Schools of Nursing
WUCS; *see* World University Service of
　　Canada

Y

Yale University, 79, 188, 291
Yarmouth Regional Hospital School of
　　Nursing, 331